Cardiovascular Medicine

Series Editor

James T. Willerson
MC 3-116
Texas Heart Institute
Houston, TX, USA

Cardiovascular Medicine will offer today's most up-to-date, user-friendly guidance on the evaluation, diagnosis, and medical and surgical treatment of heart and vascular disease and will be on the wish list for every trainee and practising cardiologist, cardiac surgeon, vascular surgeon, diabetologist, cardiac radiologist and any physician who manages cardiac patients. The book and online package is dedicated to providing comprehensive coverage of every aspect of cardiovascular medicine from cardiac signs and symptoms through peripheral vascular disease and the genetic basis for cardiovascular disease to preventive cardiology. The Editors – and over 150 world authorities – will offer their decades of scientific and clinical experience. A major selling point will be the consistent chapter organization, clear design, and engaging text that includes user-friendly features such as tables, lists and treatment boxes. The reader will have all the guidance to diagnose and manage a full range of conditions in a series of textbook resources, while also having access to additional video material. More than 1600 illustrations over the eight volumes – including a wealth of color Doppler, nuclear imaging, surgical and pathological images – clarify complex principles and help in the understanding of the subtleties of technique and their application, so that they can be implemented in your practice. The eight volumes of Cardiovascular Medicine, 4th Edition will be the premier resource of its kind, which will advance readers' knowledge and stimulate further study in cardiovascular medicine. Each volume is designed as firstly as a standalone reference in its subject, breaking the field of cardiology down into logical learning modules.

More information about this series at http://www.springer.com/series/10474

Blase A. Carabello
Editor

Valvular Heart Disease

Springer

Editor
Blase A. Carabello
Brody School of Medicine
East Carolina University
Greenville, NC
USA

ISSN 2363-5053   ISSN 2363-5061 (electronic)
Cardiovascular Medicine
ISBN 978-1-4471-2839-7   ISBN 978-1-4471-2840-3 (eBook)
https://doi.org/10.1007/978-1-4471-2840-3

This Springer imprint is published by the registered company Springer-Verlag London Ltd. part of Springer Nature
The registered company address is: The Campus, 4 Crinan Street, London, N1 9XW, United Kingdom

Preface

The field of valvular heart disease has exploded during the past decade, driven by new and exciting therapeutic options. Normally functioning heart valves permit a one-way blood flow through the heart. However, when valve malfunction occurs, it is of two types: valve stenosis, wherein narrowed valve orifices impede blood flow, and valve regurgitation, wherein valve incompetence permits backward flow. In general, the most effective solutions to these mechanical problems are also mechanical, consisting of valve repair or replacement. Until a decade ago, these mechanical solutions were performed surgically and, while quite effective, entailed all the risks of open-heart operations. The advent of transcatheter aortic valve replacement and transcatheter mitral valve repair brought innovative, simpler, and non-operative mechanical solutions to the patient, making therapy available to patients too high risk to benefit from surgery. These therapies also added cardiologists to the providers capable of providing them, initiating the heart team concept wherein a multidisciplinary group of providers worked in concert to decide on the therapy best suited to each individual patient. At the same time, these new therapies dramatically increased the complexity of the patients now able to be treated. It is in this new era of cardiology at which this text is aimed.

In this textbook, the experts in the field marry the old with the new, discussing the physical examination of the major valve lesions by which most valve diseases are discovered, emphasizing the imaging techniques (and their pitfalls) by which valve disease is assessed, and taking a balanced approach to the indications for therapy and the type of therapy indicated. It offers a broad exposure to issues connected to valve disease, including rheumatic fever, aortic root dilatation, infective endocarditis, and heart disease in pregnancy. The text is capped off by an interactive group of case scenarios, testing the reader's skill in addressing complex problems confronted in the real world, often for which there is only a "best" therapy but no definitive right or wrong answer. Thus, the reader will be exposed not only to guideline-directed therapy but also to therapeutic decisions that must be made but which are not specifically spelled out in the currently available guidelines.

Greenville, NC, USA Blase A. Carabello

Contents

Contributors

Corinne M. Aberle, MD Cardiothoracic Surgery, Texas Heart Institute—Baylor College of Medicine, Houston, TX, USA

Division of Cardiothoracic Surgery, Baylor College of Medicine, Baylor St. Luke's Medical Center, Houston, TX, USA

Cardiovascular Surgery, Texas Heart Institute at Baylor St. Luke's Medical Center, Houston, TX, USA

Haziam Alwair, MD Division of Cardiac Surgery, Department of Cardiovascular Sciences, East Carolina Heart Institute, Greenville, NC, USA

Sukhdeep Singh Basra, MD, MPH UT Center for Advanced Heart Failure, Interventional Cardiology, Section of Cardiology, University of Texas McGovern Medical School Houston, Houston, TX, USA

L. Maximilian Buja, MD Department of Pathology and Laboratory Medicine, McGovern Medical School, The University of Texas Health Science Center at Houston (UTHealth), Houston, TX, USA

Department of Cardiovascular Pathology Research, Texas Heart Institute, Houston, TX, USA

Blase A. Carabello, MD Cardiology Division, Brody School of Medicine, East Carolina University, Greenville, NC, USA

Department of Cardiovascular Sciences, Vidant Medical Center, Greenville, NC, USA

Y. S. Chandrashekhar, MD, DM Division of Cardiology, Department of Medicine, Veterans Affairs Medical Center, Minneapolis, MN, USA

Stephanie A. Coulter, MD Cardiovascular Education, Texas Heart Institute, Houston, TX, USA

Department of Cardiology, Baylor St. Lukes Medical Center, Houston, TX, USA

Jennifer R. Cozart, MD Division of Cardiothoracic Surgery, Baylor College of Medicine, Baylor St. Luke's Medical Center, Houston, TX, USA

Cardiovascular Surgery, Texas Heart Institute at Baylor St. Luke's Medical Center, Houston, TX, USA

Swaminadhan Gnanashanmugam, MS, MD Cardiothoracic Surgery, Texas Heart Institute—Baylor College of Medicine, Houston, TX, USA

Richard J. Hamill, MD Department of Medicine and Molecular Virology and Microbiology, Baylor College of Medicine, Houston, TX, USA

Infectious Diseases Section, Department of Medicine, Michael E. DeBakey VA Medical Center, Houston, TX, USA

Benjamin Jenny, MD Department of Cardiovascular Surgery, Texas Heart Institute, Houston, TX, USA

Hani Jneid, MD, FACC, FAHA, FSCAI Department of Medicine, Baylor College of Medicine, Interventional Cardiology, Houston, TX, USA

Interventional Cardiology, Michael E. DeBakey VA Medical Center, Houston, TX, USA

Biswajit Kar, MD UT Center for Advanced Heart Failure, Interventional Cardiology, Section of Cardiology, University of Texas McGovern Medical School Houston, Houston, TX, USA

Department of Medicine, Baylor College of Medicine, Interventional Cardiology, Houston, TX, USA

Interventional Cardiology, Michael E. DeBakey VA Medical Center, Houston, TX, USA

Ganesan Karthikeyan, MD, DM Department of Cardiology, All India Institute of Medical Sciences, New Delhi, India

Joseph Lamelas, MD Division of Cardiac Surgery, CHI St. Luke's Health—Baylor St. Luke's Medical Center, Houston, TX, USA

Department of Cardiovascular Surgery, Texas Heart Institute, Houston, TX, USA

Jeanney Lew, MD Department of Cardiovascular Surgery, Texas Heart Institute, Houston, TX, USA

Brian R. Lindman, MD, MSCI Vanderbilt Medical school, Nashville, USA

Michael J. Mack, MD Cardiovascular Service Line, Baylor Scott & White Health, Dallas, TX, USA

Department of Cardiovascular Surgery, The Heart Hospital, Baylor Plano, Plano, TX, USA

Spencer J. Melby, MD Cardiothoracic Surgery Division, Department of Surgery, Washington University School of Medicine, St. Louis, MO, USA

Marc R. Moon, MD Cardiovascular Disease, Cardiothoracic Surgery, Barnes-Jewish Hospital, St. Louis, MO, USA

Jagat Narula, MD, PhD, MACC Cardiology Department, Mount Sinai Saint Luke's Hospital, New York, NY, USA

Rajasekhar Nekkanti, MD Department of Cardiovascular Sciences, Vidant Medical Center, Greenville, NC, USA

Chrisita L. Powlett, MD Cardiovascular Surgery, Texas Heart Institute at Baylor St. Luke's Medical Center, Houston, TX, USA

Nishath Quader, MD Vanderbilt Medical school, Nashville, USA

Kumudha Ramasubbu, MD, FACC New York-Presbyterian Brooklyn Methodist Hospital, Brooklyn, NY, USA

Tina Shah, MD New York-Presbyterian Brooklyn Methodist Hospital, Brooklyn, NY, USA

Marc A. Sintek, MD Vanderbilt Medical school, Nashville, USA

James T. Willerson, MD Department of Cardiology, Texas Heart Institute, Houston, TX, USA

Valvular Heart Disease: Pathological Anatomy and Pathogenesis

1

L. Maximilian Buja

Introduction

Valvular heart disease comprises a spectrum of congenital abnormalities and acquired degenerative and inflammatory conditions [1–4]. Degenerative valve disease is now the most common general etiology of valvular heart disease in developed countries [5]. The leading entities of degenerative valve disease are calcific aortic stenosis and myxomatous degeneration of the mitral valve. Inflammatory and infections conditions, while of lower prevalence, remain clinically important.

Summary of Valvular and Endocardial Abnormalities

- Congenital Lesions
  - Degenerative Lesions
    - Calcific aortic valve disease
  - Prolapse of mitral valve
  - Carcinoid heart disease
  - Calcification of mitral annulus
  - Inflammatory Lesions—endocarditis
  - Noninfective
  - Rheumatic
  - Libman-Sacks (atypical verrucous) (SLE)
  - Nonbacterial thrombotic (NBTE, marantic)
  - Rheumatoid
  - Infective
  - Infective endocarditis
  - Cardiovascular syphilis
  - Jet lesions—mechanical stress

L. M. Buja (✉)
Department of Pathology and Laboratory Medicine, McGovern Medical School, The University of Texas Health Science Center at Houston (UTHealth), Houston, TX, USA

Department of Cardiovascular Pathology Research, Texas Heart Institute, Houston, TX, USA
e-mail: l.maximilian.buja@uth.tmc.edu

Cardiac Valve Structure and Function

The four cardiac valves of the mature heart have a similar architecture consisting of a dense collagenous layer adjacent to the outflow surface that provides strength, a central core of loose connective tissue containing glycosaminoglycans (GAGs), and a layer with elastin fibers below the inflow surface [6, 7]. The valves are lined by endothelium and contain valvular interstitial cells (VICs) as the major interstitial cell type. The architecture is well suited for the dynamic changes which the valves undergo with each cardiac cycle.

Congenital Valvular Heart Disease

The most common congenital malformation of heart valves is the bicuspid aortic valve [8–10]. Unless it is the site of associated dysplasia, this valve is not inherently stenotic, although it frequently becomes stenotic in later life. Stenosis is secondary to fibrosis and calcification of the cusps and usually not to fusion of the commissures, as is seen in rheumatic aortic stenosis [9]. Classically, the calcific deposits form nodules at the base of the cusps in the sinuses of Valsalva and extend to, but frequently do not involve, the free edge of the valve cusps (Fig. 1.1). In addition, there are foci of calcification and extensive fibrosis within the substance of the cusps. Commissural fusion is usually minimal, involves only one commissure, and is only rarely extensive [8, 10]. Another common reason for surgical excision of a bicuspid aortic valve is infective endocarditis. The extremely high incidence of infective endocarditis in patients with bicuspid aortic valves is well known. Therefore, each of these valves must be examined closely by the surgical pathologist for superimposed infective endocarditis, and if suspicious lesions are noted, sections must be taken for microbiologic culture before fixation.

The quadricuspid aortic valve is far less common than the bicuspid valve. The most frequent indication for surgical excision of these valves is aortic insufficiency. Most

B. A. Carabello (ed.), *Valvular Heart Disease*, Cardiovascular Medicine, https://doi.org/10.1007/978-1-4471-2840-3_1

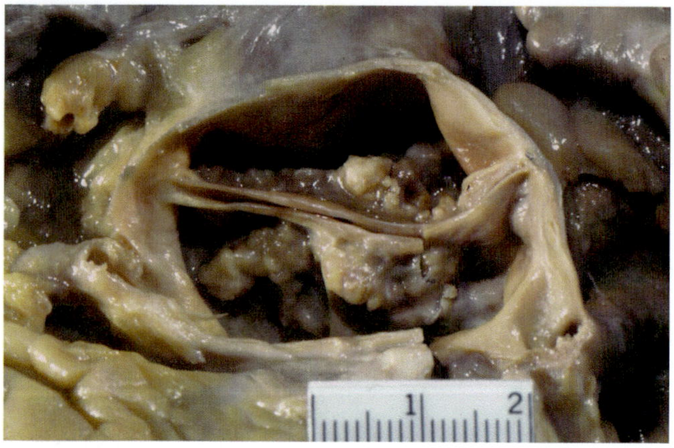

Fig. 1.1 This aortic valve was formed with two rather than the usual three cusps. This congenital bicuspid valve is subject to abnormal mechanical factors often leading to fibrosis, calcification, and stenosis in middle age. From McAllister HA Jr., Buja LM, Ferrans VJ. Valvular heart disease: anatomic abnormalities. In: Willerson JT, Cohn JN, Wellens HJJ, Holmes DR Jr., editors. *Cardiovascular Medicine*, third edition. London: Springer-Verlag, 2007. p. 369. Reprinted with permission from Springer

commonly, one of the cusps is rudimentary; however, the gross and microscopic appearance of the valves is usually otherwise normal [11]. Quadricuspid pulmonary valves rarely cause cardiac dysfunction unless there is associated dysplasia of the valve or a coexisting congenital cardiac defect. As in quadricuspid aortic valves, the fourth cusp is usually small and rudimentary, with the remaining cusps appearing morphologically normal [11].

Valve dysplasia may affect any of the cardiac valves, most frequently the aortic valve; however, 25% of patients have multiple valve involvement [12]. The dysplastic changes may be severe and extensive, so that the entire valve is distorted, or mild and focal, so that valve function is not impaired. A dysplastic stenotic pulmonary valve is frequently present in patients with Noonan's syndrome. The dysplastic semilunar valve may be unicuspid, bicuspid, or tricuspid; failure of development of the commissures also may occur, resulting in a dome-shaped valve. Stenosis is secondary to the marked thickening of the individual valve cusps. The spongiosa of the dysplastic valve is quite cellular and composed primarily of small spindle cells resembling fibroblasts, set in an acid mucopolysaccharides matrix and haphazardly arranged bundles of collagen [1]. This loose connective tissue encroaches on and often replaces the ventricularis and fibrosa of the valve cusps. The majority of involved cusps consist entirely of this loose connective tissue; however, remnants of the ventricularis and fibrosa, interrupted by accumulations of abnormal loose connective tissue, are often found at the base of the cusps. Inflammation and calcification are not features of the dysplastic valve. The abnormal valve tissue of the dysplastic or incompletely differentiated valve resembles the embryonic connective tissue of the cardiac valves in 8–12-week-old fetuses [10].

Calcific Aortic Valve Disease and Stenosis

The prevalence of valvular heart disease in the adult population of the USA is more than five million people [13, 14]. Aortic valve disease is now the third most common cause of cardiovascular disease. There are an estimated 95,000 surgical valve procedures performed each year in the USA. Aortic valve disease is responsible for more than 25,000 annual deaths. Untreated, calcific aortic stenosis has a fatal outcome within 2–5 years once the patient presents with angina, syncope, or heart failure due to the valve lesion.

Degeneration and calcification of a congenitally bicuspid aortic valve leads to clinical presentation of aortic stenosis in middle age whereas the disease process involving a tricuspid aortic valve progresses to clinical significance in older individuals (Figs. 1.1 and 1.2). The overall prevalence of degenerative aortic valve disease has risen as life expectancy has increased [6, 7, 13, 14].

The pathogenesis of calcific aortic stenosis involves a response of the valve to injury with common features to the pathogenesis of atherosclerosis (see schema below) [15–17]. Modulation of valvular interstitial cells (VICs) by transforming growth factor-ß is an important mechanism contributing to valve fibrosis. Subsequent expression of molecules that promote calcification occurs at a later stage. This basic information has led to therapeutic trials of interventions involving control of risk factors and use of statins, metal metalloproteinase inhibitors and angiotensin converting enzyme

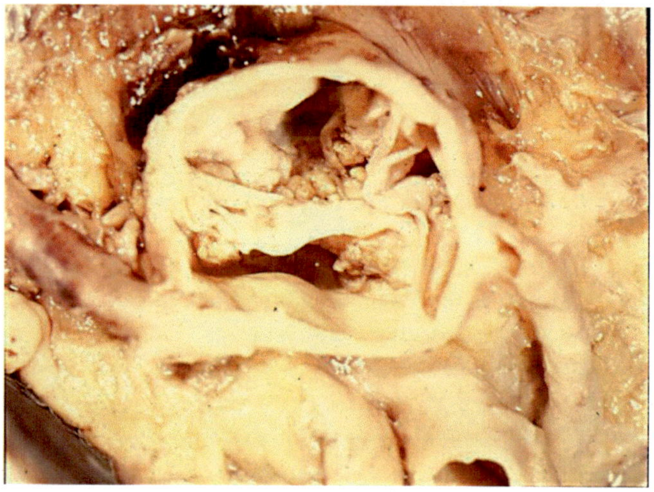

Fig. 1.2 This aortic valve with three cusps became stenotic in an individual in his seventies, and the condition is designated as senile calcific aortic stenosis. Stenosis is secondary to fibrosis and calcification of the midportion and hinge of the cusps and usually not to fusion of the commissures, as is seen in rheumatic aortic stenosis

inhibitors [13]. Most experience has been obtained with statin therapy for lipid control. Although the randomized trials did not confirm slowing of the progression of aortic stenosis, the largest trial did demonstrate improvement in primary end points of ischemic vascular disease [18].

Common Factors in the Pathogenesis of Calcific Aortic Stenosis and Atherosclerosis

Chronic Exposure to Altered Environment

Physical forces, hyperlipidemia, inflammation, reactive oxygen species, microorganisms

Activation and Modulation of Key Cell Types

Aortic valve—endothelium, valvular interstitial cells (VIC), macrophages

Arteries—endothelium, vascular smooth muscle cells (VSMC), macrophages

Response to Injury by VIC and VSMC

Proliferation, migration, matrix secretion, upregulation of matrix metalloproteinases (MMPs)

Tissue inhibitors of metalloproteinases (TIMPSs), apoptosis

Mediators and Modulators

Low-density lipoprotein (LDL), cytokines, chemokines, transforming growth factor β (TGF-β), fibroblast growth factor-2

Initial Lesion

Aortic valve—leaflet/cusp fibrosis

Arteries—intimal plaque with VSMC hyperplasia

Abnormal Repair

Aortic valve—leaflet/cusp thickening and stiffening due to progressive fibrosis

Arteries—Atherosclerotic plaques with central necrotic core and fibrous plaque

Calcification

Cbfa1, osteocalcin, osteopontin, bone morphogenic protein-2, other mediators

End Stage

Aortic valve—calcific aortic stenosis

Arteries—complicated atherosclerotic plaques

Floppy Valve (Myxomatous Degeneration) and Connective Tissue Dyscrasias

Mitral valve prolapse is a common disorder with a strong hereditary component which occurs in approximately 2% of the general population [19]. Mitral valve prolapse occurs in various genetic syndromes and as an idiopathic, nonsyndromic condition with an autosomal dominant inheritance pattern [20]. The pathological correlate is myxomatous valvular degeneration.

Although myxomatous degeneration has been described in tricuspid, aortic, and pulmonary values, the mitral value is most commonly involved, and the posterior leaflet is affected more often and more severely than is the anterior leaflet. Grossly, the most outstanding feature is marked increase in surface area of the affected leaflets (Fig. 1.3), which are voluminous, hooded, and white; however, they transilluminate with ease, especially before fixation. On sectioning, the myxomatous consistency of the center of the leaflet is often apparent on gross examination. Small foci of ulceration with occasional superimposed thrombi may be noted on the atrial surface of the affected mitral leaflet [1, 3, 4]. The chordae tendineae often are elongated and thin; however, some localized thickening may be present at their insertions into the valve leaflets (Fig. 1.4). Rupture of the chordae tendineae is common in myxomatous degeneration of the mitral valve: less frequently, myxomatous degeneration may result in aneurysmal dilatation and rupture of a mitral leaflet. Commissural fusion is not a feature of the floppy valve. Because these valves are predisposed to infective endocarditis, gross evidence of this complication must be sought by the surgical pathologist, so that appropriate sections can be obtained for culture before fixation of the valve.

Microscopically, the spongiosa contains stellate cells embedded in a matrix rich in proteoglycans (Fig. 1.5). Characteristically, there is focal to extensive replacement of the normal dense, homogeneous collagen of the fibrosa by this myxomatous tissue. This histologic pattern is in contrast to that seen in most valvular heart diseases, in which the spongiosa of the leaflets is partially or completely replaced

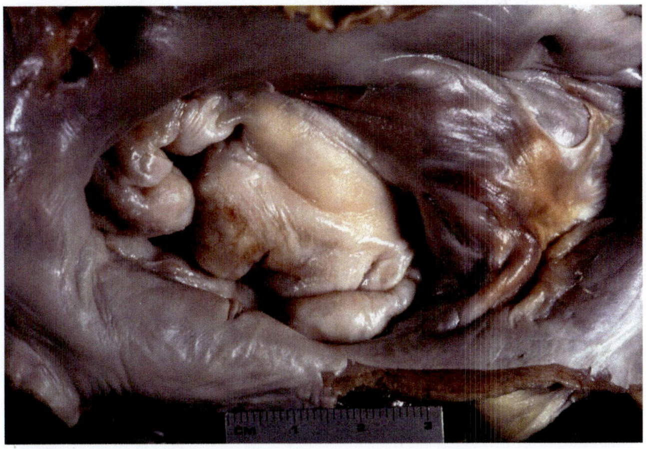

Fig. 1.3 Floppy mitral valve. The most outstanding feature is a marked increase in the surface area of the leaflets. They are voluminous, hooded, and white; however, they transluminate with ease. These are gross features of myxomatous degeneration. Commissural fusion is not a feature of the floppy valve. From McAllister HA Jr., Buja LM, Ferrans VJ. Valvular heart disease: anatomic abnormalities. In: Willerson JT, Cohn JN, Wellens HJJ, Holmes DR Jr., editors. *Cardiovascular Medicine*, third edition. London: Springer-Verlag, 2007. p. 369. Reprinted with permission from Springer

by dense fibrous tissue. The collagen in the chordae tendineae may show changes similar to those in the fibrosa. The atrialis of the leaflet generally contains a variable degree of fibroelastic proliferation, and superficial ulceration with microscopic fibrin deposition is not uncommon. Unless there is superimposed infective endocarditis, there is no evidence of inflammation or vascularization. Ultrastructurally, there is focal loss of the normal orderly cross-banding of collagen fibers. Microscopically, small areas of myxomatous degeneration may be found near the free edges of normal or diseased valves and should not be confused with the diffuse findings in floppy valves.

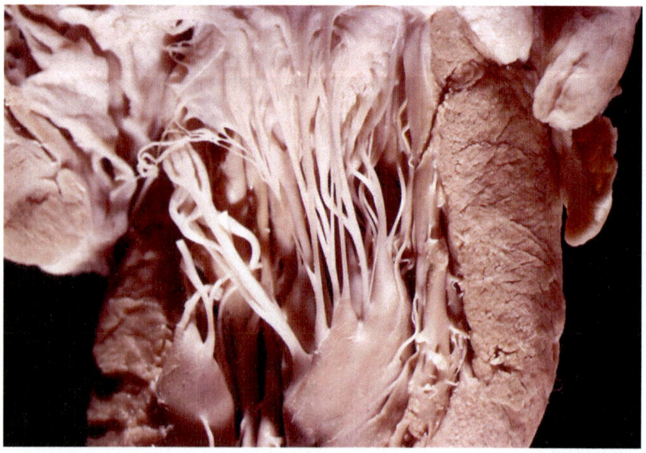

Fig. 1.4 Floppy mitral valve. The chordae tendineae are often elongated and thin; however, some localized thickening may be present at their insertion into the valve leaflets. From McAllister HA Jr., Buja LM, Ferrans VJ. Valvular heart disease: anatomic abnormalities. In: Willerson JT, Cohn JN, Wellens HJJ, Holmes DR Jr., editors. *Cardiovascular Medicine*, third edition. London: Springer-Verlag, 2007. p. 369. Reprinted with permission from Springer

Myxomatous degeneration of the cardiac valves, with resulting insufficiency, often occurs in connective tissue dyscrasias such as Marfan syndrome, osteogenesis imperfecta, cutis laxa, and relapsing polychondritis. This group of diseases may also be associated with cystic medial degeneration of the aorta. Adults with Marfan syndrome most commonly have myxomatous degeneration of the aortic valve; in children, however, the mitral valve is more commonly involved [21]. The affected mitral and aortic leaflets contain an accumulation of myxoid material mainly in the spongiosa. Recent studies have shown the importance of matrix metalloproteinases in the pathogenesis of these lesions in the Marfan syndrome [22]. The Ehlers-Danlos syndrome is a heterogeneous group of several genetically distinct disorders of connective tissue synthesis, which differ in major clinical features, inheritance patterns, and biochemical defects. Cardiovascular lesions have been described in types I–IV; however, myxomatous degeneration and prolapse of the mitral valve appear to be more common in type III, the benign hypermobile form [21]. The most common valvular lesion in osteogenesis imperfecta is aortic regurgitation; mitral regurgitation and combined aortic and mitral regurgitation are less common. The aortic regurgitation results from dilatation of the aortic root and deformity of the valvular leaflets, which become abnormally translucent, weak, and elongated. Aneurysms of

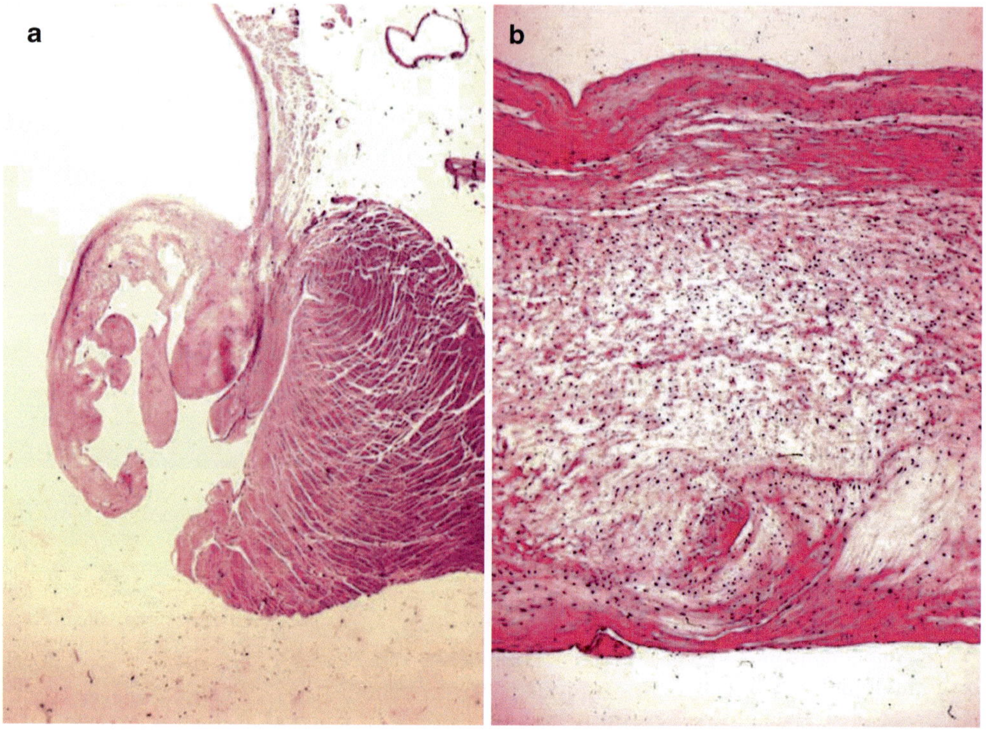

Fig. 1.5 Floppy mitral valve with histopathological features of myxomatous generation. (**a**) The whole mount section of left atrium, left ventricle, and mitral valve leaflet demonstrates a mitral valve leaflet which is thickened, elongated, and prolapsed into the left atrium [Hematoxylin and eosin, 1×]. (**b**) The thickened leaflet shows replacement of the normal fibrosa by loose myxoid connective tissue; the atrialis surface shows some secondary increase in dense collagen [Hematoxylin and eosin, 10×]

the sinuses of Valsalva also occur. The mitral annulus is dilated, the mitral leaflets are attenuated and redundant and tend to prolapse, and the chordae tendineae may rupture [21]. In cutis laxa, the most common cardiac lesions involve the aorta, pulmonary artery, and pulmonary veins; less commonly, there may be myxomatous degeneration of the aortic or mitral valves [2]. The aortic and mitral valves are the cardiac valves most commonly involved in relapsing polychondritis. Lesions may be microscopically identical to those in the other connective tissue dyscrasias [1].

The pathogenesis of myxomatous degeneration is thought to involve abnormal homeostasis of the valvular extracellular matrix related to complex genetic factors. The hypothesis has been advanced that genetic defects present at the time of valve morphogenesis, coupled with individual variation in genetic background, may lead to progressive alterations leading to clinical disease [23, 24].

Endocrine and Metabolic Valvular Diseases

In carcinoid heart disease, there is either focal or diffuse plaque-like thickening of valvular and mural endocardium and, occasionally, of the intima of the great veins, coronary sinus, pulmonary trunk, and main pulmonary arteries. The fibrous tissue is atypical and limited in the majority of instances to the right side of the heart. When the pulmonary valve is involved, deposition is almost exclusively on the arterial aspect of the valve cusps (Fig. 1.6). When the tricuspid valve is involved, however, the fibrous tissue is located predominantly on the ventricular aspect, often causing the leaflets to adhere to the adjacent ventricular wall [25]. Similar lesions may be observed in the mitral and aortic valves in patients with a patent foramen ovale or a functioning bronchial carcinoid tumor [26]. In some patients with predominant right-side carcinoid heart disease, the mitral and aortic valves also may be involved to a lesser degree. Microscopically, these lesions contain fibroblasts, myofibroblasts, and smooth muscle cells embedded in a distinctive stroma, which is rich in collagen and proteoglycans but lacking in elastic fibers. Blood vessels, often thick-walled, may be immediately adjacent to the valve leaflets. Lymphocyts and plasma cells are frequently located adjacent to these blood vessels.

Histologically, similar valvular and endocardial lesions have been described in patients taking methysergide [27] and ergot [28]; however, the mitral and aortic valves are most commonly involved in these cases. A decade ago, similar valvular lesions were described in patients taking fenfluramine and phentermine for appetite suppression [29].

The heart valves are involved in 50% of patients with cardiac amyloidosis. Valvular involvement is usually minimal, but discrete nodules measuring from 1 to 4 mm in diameter are occasionally present on the valves either in the cusps or in the annulus [21]. Rarely, valvular involvement is diffuse, resulting in thick, rigid cusps and stenotic or regurgitant orifices (Fig. 1.7). The four cardiac valves are affected with almost equal frequency.

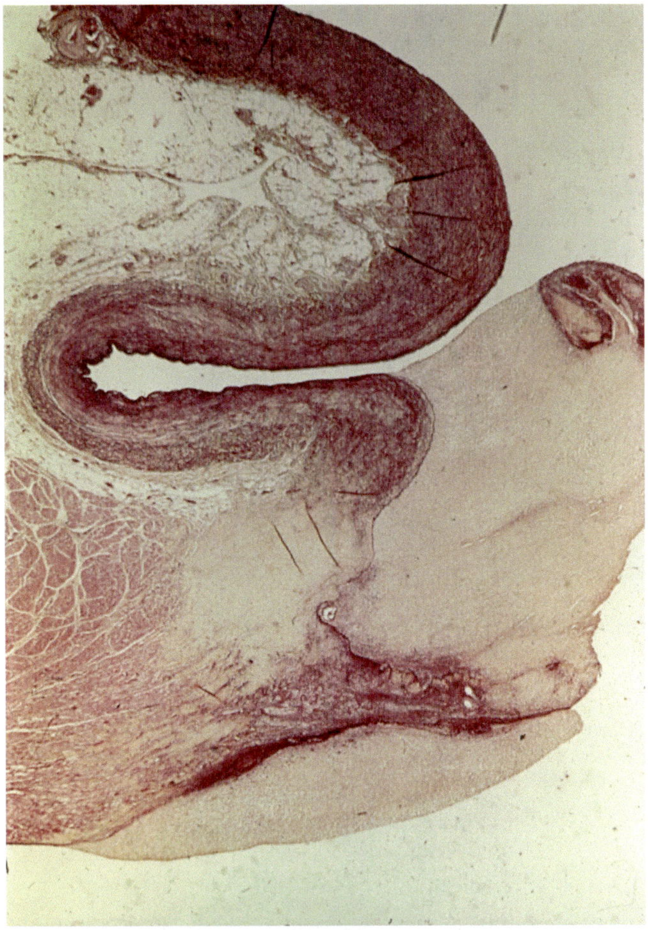

Fig. 1.6 Carcinoid heart disease, pulmonic valve. Heavy deposition of collagen, lacking in elastic fibers, occurs almost exclusively on the arterial aspect of the valve cusps, resulting in pulmonic stenosis [Movat pentachrome, 25×]. From McAllister HA Jr., Buja LM, Ferrans VJ. Valvular heart disease: anatomic abnormalities. In: Willerson JT, Cohn JN, Wellens HJJ, Holmes DR Jr., editors. *Cardiovascular Medicine*, third edition. London: Springer-Verlag, 2007. p. 369. Reprinted with permission from Springer

All heart valves and valvular annuli, especially the mitral and aortic valves, are sites of heavy pigment deposition in patients with ochronosis [21]. Although the pigment deposition is most prominent at the bases of the mitral and aortic valves and annulus fibrosus, the edges of the cusps may be roughened and fused for 1–2 mm at their bases; the cusps may be focally calcified. The ochronotic pigment appears blue-black on gross examination and yellow-tan in histologic sections. Infective endocarditis may occasionally be superimposed, especially when the valves are heavily calcified.

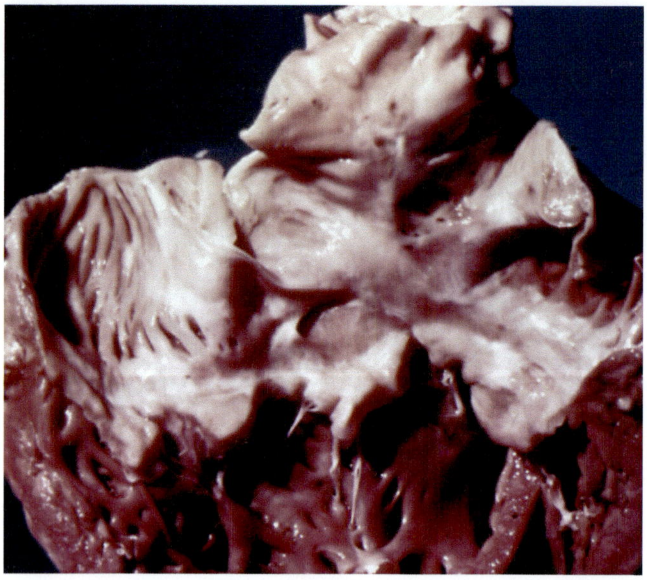

Fig. 1.7 Amyloid valve disease. Valvular involvement is usually minimal; however, diffuse involvement, as illustrated in this heart, can occur, resulting in thick, rigid cusps and stenotic or regurgitant orifices. From McAllister HA Jr., Buja LM, Ferrans VJ. Valvular heart disease: anatomic abnormalities. In: Willerson JT, Cohn JN, Wellens HJJ, Holmes DR Jr., editors. *Cardiovascular Medicine*, third edition. London: Springer-Verlag, 2007. p. 369. Reprinted with permission from Springer

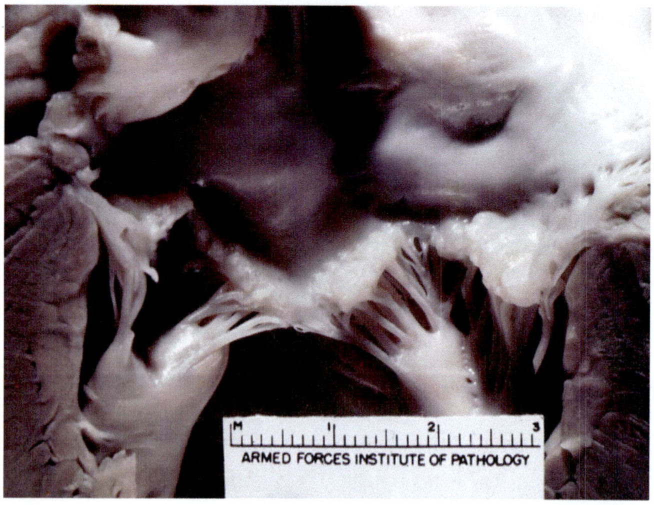

Fig. 1.8 Hurler's syndrome, mitral valve. The valvular thickening is most pronounced at the free margins, which have an irregular, nodular appearance. The commissures are not fused. The chordae tendineae are moderately shortened and thickened. From McAllister HA Jr., Buja LM, Ferrans VJ. Valvular heart disease: anatomic abnormalities. In: Willerson JT, Cohn JN, Wellens HJJ, Holmes DR Jr., editors. *Cardiovascular Medicine*, third edition. London: Springer-Verlag, 2007. p. 369. Reprinted with permission from Springer

The cardiac valves may be involved in any of the mucopolysaccharidoses, most frequently in Hurler's syndrome (mycopolysaccharidosis I) [21]. The valves are considerably thickened, particularly the mitral valve; right-sided cardiac valves are less severely affected than those in the left side of the heart (Fig. 1.8). The valvular thickening is most pronounced at the free margins, which have an irregular, nodular appearance. The commissures are not fused. The chordae tendineae of the atrioventricular valves are moderately shortened and thickened. Calcific deposits occur in the angle just beneath the basal attachment of the posterior mitral leaflet (mitral annular calcification), in the mitral leaflets, and in the aortic aspect of the aortic valve cusps. The valves contain large, oval or rounded connective tissue cells (Hurler cells) filled with numerous clear vacuoles, which are the sites of deposition of acid mucopolysaccharides [21]. This material is extremely soluble and difficult to preserve. In addition, small granular cells are present, which contain membrane-limited electron-dense material associated with fragments of collagen fibrils. The valve thickening is due to the presence of the cells and to an increase in the amount of fibrous connective tissue.

In Fabry's disease, the glycosphingolipid is deposited within the cardiac valves, occasionally resulting in valvular dysfunction [21]. The mitral and aortic valves are the two valves that most commonly present clinical problems. There may be thickening of the valves with interchordal hooding, or there may be attenuation of the chordae with thickening and ballooning of the mitral valve. Commissural fusion is not a feature of Fabry's disease.

Type II hyperlipoproteinemia (familial hypercholesterolemia) exists in homozygous and heterozygous forms, which differ in the severity and age of onset of clinical symptoms. Aortic valvular disease is frequent in homozygous patients but does not usually occur in heterozygous patients. The aortic valve may be markedly stenosed by fibrous tissue, deposits of foam cells, and cholesterol crystals in the cusps. Thickening of the mitral valve, which results in both stenosis and regurgitation, and thickening of the pulmonary valve and endocardium by foam cells also occur [21].

Patients with gout most commonly develop dysfunction due to hypertension secondary to renal damage; however, tophi occasionally may be present in the heart, most commonly in the mitral valve and the endocardium of the left ventricle and, less frequently, in the mitral annulus and aortic and tricuspid valve leaflets [21, 30]. To establish the diagnosis histologically, appreciable amounts of uric acid must be identified in the tophi to distinguish them from small amounts of uric acid that may be deposited on previously existing fibrocalcific lesions. Urate deposits are histochemically identifiable by fixation in absolute ethanol, followed by staining by the De Galantha method.

Collagen Vascular Diseases

Rheumatic Valvulitis

Acute rheumatic fever produces a pancarditis; however, valvular involvement is responsible for the most important long-term consequences. In the acute phase of rheumatic valvulitis, the most conspicuous lesions are minute, translucent nodules (verrucae) along the lines of closure of the valve cusps (Fig. 1.9). These are most frequently observed in the mitral and aortic valves, less often in the tricuspid, and rarely in the pulmonary valve. They vary in diameter from less than 1 to 3 mm and are located on the atrial surface of the atrioventricular valves and on the ventricular surface of the semilunar valves [25]. Occasionally, a few verrucae may be distributed elsewhere over the cusps. They are also characteristically present on the chordae tendineae, especially those of the mitral valve, and not infrequently, they extend over the posterior leaflet of the mitral valve onto the endocardium of the left atrium. The verrucae tend to conglomerate on the corpora arantii of the aortic valve and extend in a row along the semilunar cusps. Diffuse thickening of the valves, except the pulmonary, is a less conspicuous but frequent gross alteration.

Microscopically, the verrucae may have the appearance of either thrombi, formed by the deposition of platelets and fibrin on the surface of the valve, or extruded collagen that has undergone fibrinoid degeneration. The region immediately adjacent to the vegetation shows marked proliferation of fibroblasts, as well as edema and numerous lymphocytes [25]. The inflammatory process is observed most frequently in the auricularis layer of the atrioventricular valves and the ventricularis layer of the semilunar valves. A nonspecific inflammatory process, which may involve the entire valve and ring, consists of edema, increased numbers of capillaries, and a variety of inflammatory cells (mainly lymphocytes; occasionally polymorphonuclear leukocytes predominate). Plasma cells, fibroblasts, and other mononuclear cells are often present in variable numbers. Usually the valve also contains Anitschkow and Aschoff cells, which may be arranged in nodules or in rows and often surround foci of eosinophilic fragmented collagen, fibrinoid, or both. Aschoff cells may be multinucleated [31]. These lesions are typically accompanied by characteristic Aschoff nodules in the myocardium [25, 31, 32].

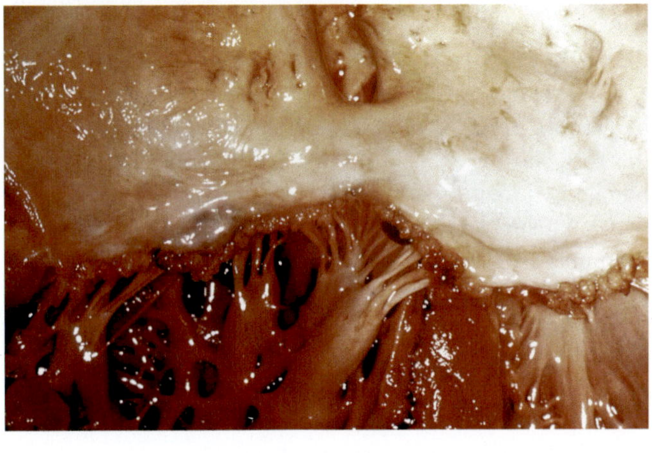

Fig. 1.9 Acute rheumatic valvulitis, mitral valve. Fibrinoid necrosis is represented by minute, translucent nodules (verrucae), 1–3 mm in diameter, along the lines of closure. From McAllister HA Jr., Buja LM, Ferrans VJ. Valvular heart disease: anatomic abnormalities. In: Willerson JT, Cohn JN, Wellens HJJ, Holmes DR Jr., editors. *Cardiovascular Medicine*, third edition. London: Springer-Verlag, 2007. p. 369. Reprinted with permission from Springer

Gross alterations of the cardiac valves become more pronounced as a result of recurrent rheumatic valvulitis. Thickening, irregularity of the surfaces, and gross vascularization are usually present. This thickening is usually most pronounced in the distal third of the valve leaflets [25]. The chordae tendineae become thicker and shorter, with especially prominent thickening at their insertions into the valve leaflets. Verrucae in various stages of activity and healing may be observed. In addition to being thickened, the aortic cusps may be considerably shortened, with their free margins rolled and inverted toward the sinus pocket. Fibrous adhesions are commonly present at the commissures, and verrucae in various stages of activity may extend across the commissures of aortic cusps. In recurrent valvulitis, there is a higher incidence of verrucae on the valves of the right side of the heart, and microscopic observation reveals considerable fibrosis, an apparent increase in elastic tissue, and inflammatory changes in various stages of activity [25, 32]. The fibrosis and inflammation involve the rings as well as the leaflets. This histologic pattern differs from that of acute valvulitis, in which the thickening of the valves is the result only of edema and inflammation. Also in contrast to the appearance of acute valvulitis are numerous arteries with thick muscular walls in the ring and proximal portion of the valve.

In chronic rheumatic valvulitis, the alterations described in recurrent valvulitis are most advanced. Usually, the diffuse thickening and fibrosis of the valves have resulted in loss of elasticity and in narrowing of the orifice (Fig. 1.10). Thickening, fusion, and shortening of the chordae tendineae of the mitral valve are usually pronounced (Fig. 1.11). In addition, focal deposits of calcium salts may be present. These deposits may be extensive and may project to the atrial and ventricular surfaces, causing further distortion. Ossification, complete with hematopoiesis, may occur, causing further distortion [32]. Verrucae are less frequent in chronic valvulitis than in recurrent valvulitis and are broad and flat. Active inflammation is less pronounced in chronic than in recurrent valvulitis and usually consists of scattered

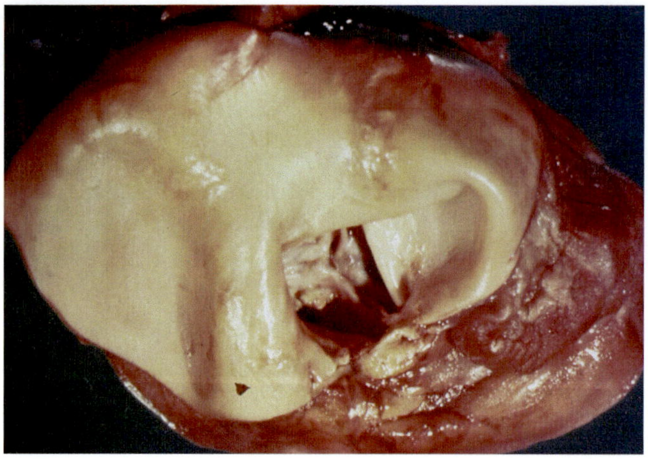

Fig. 1.10 Chronic rheumatic aortic stensosis. Diffuse thickening and fibrosis of the valve cusps with commissural fusion resulting in marked aortic stenosis. Also note the extensive poststenotic dilatation of the ascending aorta. From McAllister HA Jr., Buja LM, Ferrans VJ. Valvular heart disease: anatomic abnormalities. In: Willerson JT, Cohn JN, Wellens HJJ, Holmes DR Jr., editors. *Cardiovascular Medicine*, third edition. London: Springer-Verlag, 2007. p. 369. Reprinted with permission from Springer

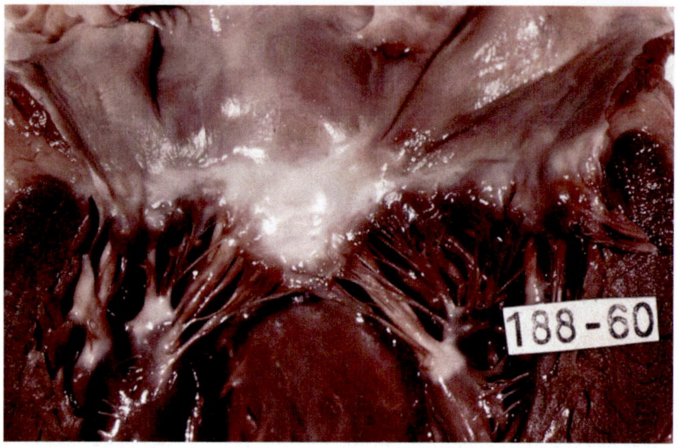

Fig. 1.12 Rheumatoid valve disease, mitral valve. Involvement may be focal or diffuse, as in this case, and is usually most prominent in the midportion of the base of the valve. The chordae tendineae are usually uninvolved, and commissural fusion is rare. From McAllister HA Jr., Buja LM, Ferrans VJ. Valvular heart disease: anatomic abnormalities. In: Willerson JT, Cohn JN, Wellens HJJ, Holmes DR Jr., editors. *Cardiovascular Medicine*, third edition. London: Springer-Verlag, 2007. p. 369. Reprinted with permission from Springer

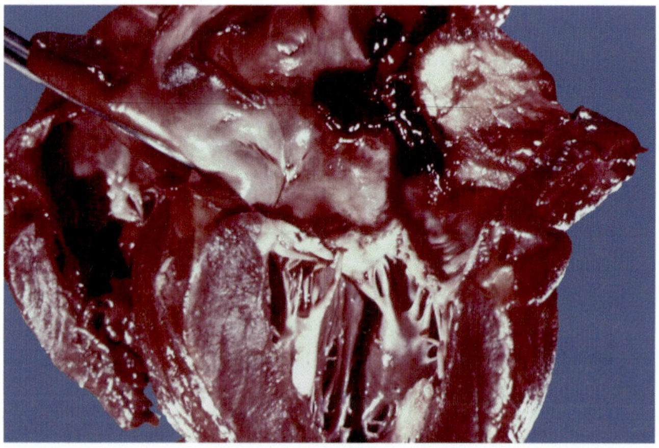

Fig. 1.11 Chronic rheumatic mitral stenosis. Note the thickening, fusion, and shortening of the chordae tendineae, as well as diffuse thickening and fibrosis of the valves, with commissural fusion. The left atrium is enlarged and contains a mural thrombus. From McAllister HA Jr., Buja LM, Ferrans VJ. Valvular heart disease: anatomic abnormalities. In: Willerson JT, Cohn JN, Wellens HJJ, Holmes DR Jr., editors. *Cardiovascular Medicine*, third edition. London: Springer-Verlag, 2007. p. 369. Reprinted with permission from Springer

foci of perivascular cuffing with lymphocytes. The grossly apparent thickening is due to an increase in fibrous and elastic tissue throughout the entire leaflet including the rings and the tips of the valves. The fibrous connective tissue is usually homogeneous and hyaline. These valves are vascularized by capillaries and thick-walled vessels, which are most numerous in the superficial layers. The verrucae no longer consist of material showing fibrinoid necrosis, but are organized and contain fibroblasts and collagen fibers. As chronicity progresses, the number of fibroblasts decreases, and the verrucae become dense, hyalinized scars.

Rheumatoid Valvulitis

Rheumatoid granulomas may occur in all of the cardiac valves but are most common in the mitral and aortic valves [33]. Involvement may be focal or diffuse and is usually most prominent in the midportion or base of the valve (Fig. 1.12). The chordae tendineae are usually uninvolved, but occasionally they may be fibrotic and shortened. Commissural fusion is rare. Rheumatoid nodules are most commonly located within the valve leaflets and are enclosed by fibrous tissue; rarely, a rheumatoid nodule may erode the surface of the valve, so that the necrotic center of the nodule communicates with a cardiac cavity (Fig. 1.13). In these unusual occurrences, there may be superimposed thrombus or infective endocarditis. Verrucae of fibrinoid necrosis, common in rheumatic valvulitis and systemic lupus erythematosus, are not a feature of pure rheumatoid valvulitis.

Lupus Erythematosus Valvulitis

Lupus erythematosus valvulitis (atypical verrucous endocarditis of Libman and Sacks) is recognized as a specific valvular abnormality occurring in systemic lupus erythematosus. Any valve may be involved, but the mitral and tricuspid valves are most often affected (Fig. 1.14). The verrucae

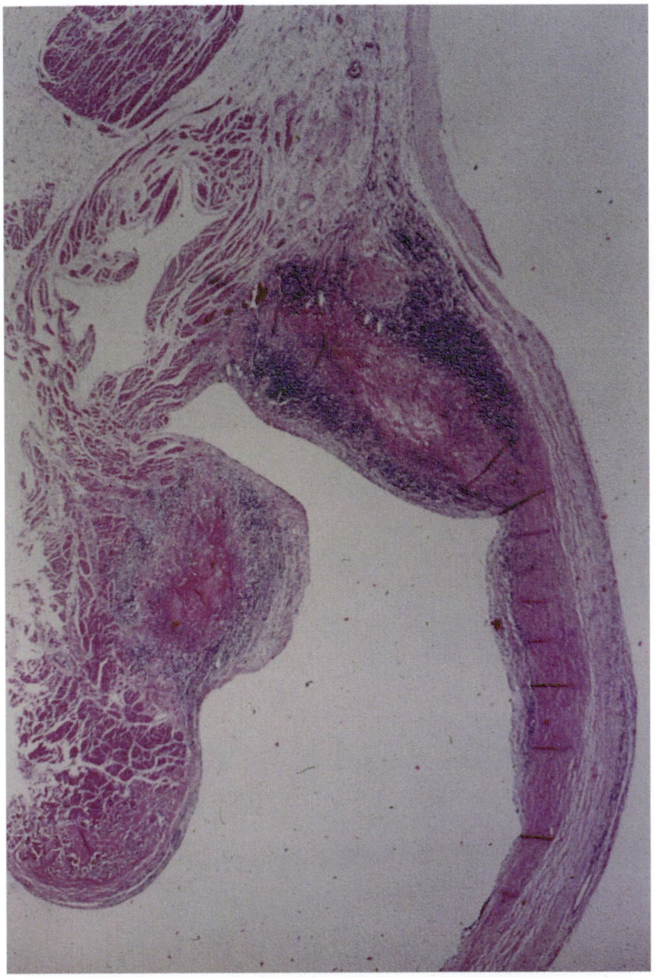

Fig. 1.13 Rheumatoid valve disease, mitral valve. Rheumatoid granulomas with extensive contiguous fibrosis involve the base and midportion of a mitral valve. Another rheumatoid granuloma is present in the adjacent subvalvular myocardium [Hematoxylin and eosin, 75×]. From McAllister HA Jr., Buja LM, Ferrans VJ. Valvular heart disease: anatomic abnormalities. In: Willerson JT, Cohn JN, Wellens HJJ, Holmes DR Jr., editors. *Cardiovascular Medicine*, third edition. London: Springer-Verlag, 2007. p. 369. Reprinted with permission from Springer

may be located on either side of a valve cusp but most frequently are present on the ventricular surface of the posterior mitral leaflet or in the valve ring; involvement of the anterior mitral leaflet is infrequent. The lesions have no special tendency to occur along the free edge of the valves and may be scattered on the chordae tendineae and atrial or ventricular mural endocardium. The lesions are small, usually ranging in size from 1 to 4 mm in diameter but, rarely, may reach a diameter of 8 to 10 mm. They are sterile, dry, granular pink vegetations that may be single or multiple in conglomerates [25]. Histologically, the verrucae consist of a finely granular, eosinophilic, fibrinoid material, which may contain hematoxylin bodies. In a general sense, these hematoxylin bodies are the tissue equivalent of the lupus erythematosus cell of the blood and bone marrow [25].

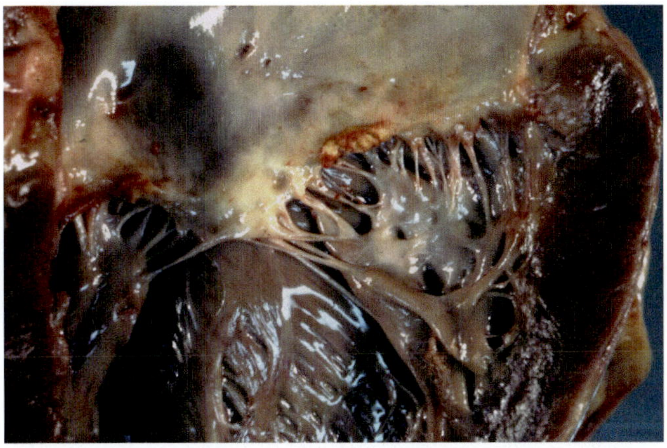

Fig. 1.14 Lupus erythematosus valvulitis (atypical verrucous endocarditis of Libman and Sacks), mitral valve. The lesions represent fibrinoid necrosis as sterile, dry, granular vegetations that may be single or multiple in conglomerates. They have no special tendency to occur along the free edge of the valves and may be scattered on the chordae tendineae and atrial or ventricular mural endocardium. From McAllister HA Jr., Buja LM, Ferrans VJ. Valvular heart disease: anatomic abnormalities. In: Willerson JT, Cohn JN, Wellens HJJ, Holmes DR Jr., editors. *Cardiovascular Medicine*, third edition. London: Springer-Verlag, 2007. p. 369. Reprinted with permission from Springer

The verrucous endocardial lesions result from degenerative and inflammatory processes of the endocardium and deeper layers of the valves. An intense valvulitis is present, which is characterized by fibrinoid necrosis of the valve substance and is often contiguous with the vegetations. Exudative and proliferative cellular reactions are present in the deeper layers of the valve. Healing of these lesions may produce foci of granulation tissue, which develop into focal fibrous thickening in the valves or in the mural endocardium. Rarely, bacterial endocarditis may be superimposed on the Libman-Sacks lesions [33].

Other Collagen Vascular and Related Diseases

Valvular lesions in scleroderma are distinctly rare; the most common lesion is nonbacterial thrombotic endocarditis. In patients with thrombotic thrombocytopenic purpura, nonbacterial thrombotic endocarditis frequently is present. In both diseases, the cardiac valves most commonly involved are the mitral and the aortic [33]. Valvulitis is most unusual in Wegener's granulomatosis. The mitral valve is most commonly involved by the inflammatory process, which may result in subsequent fibrosis with commissural fusion resembling rheumatic mitral stenosis [34]. Primary valvulitis is not a feature of dermatomyositis. Diseases that may result in valvulitis but are manifested most commonly by aortitis include syphilis, ankylosing spondylitis, psoriatic arthritis, Reiter's syndrome, and granulomatous aortitis.

Lesions Resembling Collagen Vascular Disease Valvulitis

Although not collagen vascular diseases, three entities that may result in fibrous thickening of the cardiac valves and thickening and fusion of chordae tendineae are Whipple's disease, endomyocardial fibrosis with eosinophilia, and radiation-induced disease. In Whipple's disease, the valve most commonly involved is the mitral, then the tricuspid and the aortic valves [35]. The gross deformity closely resembles that seen in chronic rheumatic heart disease, with diffuse thickening and fibrosis of the valve leaflets and chordae tendineae and rolling of the free edges of the leaflets (Fig. 1.15). Microscopically, the valve substance contains large macrophages filled with granules that are positive for the periodic acid-Schiff reaction; these granules are identical to those found in the epithelial cells of the small intestine in patients with this disease. Proliferating fibrous tissue and chronic inflammatory cells are commonly associated with the periodic acid-Schiff-positive macrophages. Scattered rod-shaped bodies, measuring 1.5–2.0 μm in length and 0.2–0.4 μm in diameter, are present intracellularly and extracellularly. These bodies, as well as membrane-bound masses of fibrillar material within the macrophages, are identical to those described in jejunal biopsies of patients with Whipple's disease [35] and are thought to represent bacteria (*Tropheryma whippelii*), which are known to be associated with this disease [36]. In endomyocardial fibrosis with eosinophilia, the valves most commonly involved are the mitral and the tricuspid, with a lesser incidence of aortic valve involvement.

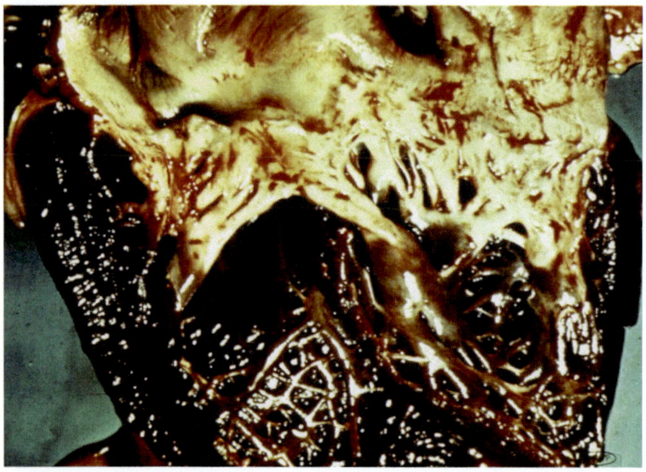

Fig. 1.15 Whipple's disease, mitral valve. The gross deformity closely resembles that seen in chronic rheumatic valve disease, with diffuse thickening and fibrosis of the valve leaflets and chordae tendineae and rolling of the free edges of the leaflets. From McAllister HA Jr., Buja LM, Ferrans VJ. Valvular heart disease: anatomic abnormalities. In: Willerson JT, Cohn JN, Wellens HJJ, Holmes DR Jr., editors. *Cardiovascular Medicine*, third edition. London: Springer-Verlag, 2007. p. 369. Reprinted with permission from Springer

There is fibrous thickening of endocardium, with superimposed fibrin thrombus beneath either the posterior mitral leaflet or the posterior or septal tricuspid leaflet. These leaflets become adherent to the underlying mural endocardium, which results in regurgitation [37]. The aortic valve cusps are occasionally thickened by vascularized fibrous tissue, which is superimposed on the ventricular aspects of the cusps. The commissures of the aortic valve may become fused by fibrous tissue with superimposed fibrin thrombus. Eosinophilic leukocytes in varying numbers are usually present at the periphery of the fibrous lesions.

Rarely, patients receiving mediastinal irradiation may develop lesions of the cardiac valves [8, 38]. The valves most commonly involved are the tricuspid and the mitral, followed by the aortic and the pulmonary. The fibrous valvular thickenings are focal, and the anterior tricuspid leaflet and the anterior mitral leaflet are usually more markedly involved than are the posterior leaflets. The chordae tendineae also may be focally thickened by fibrous tissue.

Infective Endocarditis

The relative frequency of involvement of the cardiac valves is similar for infective endocarditis and rheumatic heart disease; mitral, aortic, aortic and mitral, combined tricuspid, and pulmonary valves, in decreasing order of frequency. The tricuspid and pulmonary valves are not commonly involved, with the notable exception of intravenous drug abusers. In many cases of combined aortic and mitral involvement, the anterior leaflet of the mitral valve appears to be infected by regurgitation-induced deposition of organisms from the aortic vegetation. Lesions usually originate on the atrial surface of the atrioventricular valves and the ventricular surface of the semilunar valves and vary from tiny granular or flat vegetations to large polypoid masses. They may be single or multiple and may be firm or soft, but are usually friable. Grossly, they may appear yellow-white to red or brown [39]. The affected valve exhibits destruction and loss of tissue. Valvular ulceration, perforation, or formation of aneurysm of the valve may occur. Rupture of chordae tendineae is common. Infection may spread into the contiguous structures, resulting in annular or myocardial abscesses or aneurysms of the sinuses of Valsalva. Microscopically, the vegetations are composed of masses of necrotic tissue, fibrin, platelets, erythrocytes, leukocytes, and organisms. Classically, there is a superficial zone of fibrin, organisms, and leukocytes; and intermediate zone of amorphous necrotic material; and a basal zone of granulation tissue extending from the substance of the valve. Small foci of calcification are common.

Bicuspid aortic valves or valves with acquired deformities are most frequently involved in infective endocarditis; however, the disease may develop in previously normal valves, including the pulmonary and tricuspid valves, especially in patients over 60 years of age. Other risk factors are recent dental manipulation and diabetes mellitus [40]. In previously normal valves, the lesions tend to be larger, and tissue destruction is more extensive. Staphylococci and Gram-negative organisms are more likely to be the etiologic agents than in the case of infection of deformed valves, in which *Streptococcus viridans* is the most common organism encountered. Infected but previously normal valves often show marked necrosis and inflammation, which are less common findings in infected, previously scarred valves.

Although streptococci and staphylococci are the most common microorganisms responsible for infection, a wide variety of bacteria and fungi have been recovered from patients with infective endocarditis [40, 41]. *Candida* species in particular are recovered from addicts and patients with prosthetic heart valves. Gram-negative bacilli account for only a small percentage of infections, despite the relative frequency of Gram-negative bacteremia, and are more likely to be encountered in addicts or in patients with prosthetic heart valves. Rarely, infections are due to other organisms, such as meningococci, pneumococci, gonococci, *Brucella*, *Haemophilus*, *Cornebacterium*, mycobacteria, rickettsiae, and *Aspergillus* and other fungal species [41]. Fungal vegetations, in particular, tend to be large and friable, with a tendency to produce embolization. Because fungal endocarditis is frequently indolent clinically, it is important for the surgical pathologist to obtain appropriate special stains on any thromboembolus removed from a systemic artery. Any valve removed surgically that has gross lesions suggestive of infective endocarditis should have sections taken for microbiologic culture before fixation. Merely taking a swab of the surface of the valve for culture is not adequate. Indeed, even if the valve appears grossly normal, patients in whom the clinical history or physical findings suggest the possibility of infective endocarditis should have sections of the valve taken for culture.

Healing of vegetations may occur as a result of therapy or spontaneously, without antimicrobial therapy [39]. These healed vegetations often result in multiple, calcified, polypoid lesions on the surface of the valve. Contracture of scar tissue may further reduce the surface area of the valve. The healed vegetations in the heart valves or chordae tendineae are similar in gross appearance to those with active infection [39]. Occasionally, well-circumscribed defects with smooth edges remain in the heart valve after the healing of perforations that resulted from infective endocarditis. Usually, the etiology of these morphologic abnormalities cannot be identified, especially if there is no known antecedent infection. Histologic study rarely helps to resolve these issues because the alterations resulting from the healing of the inflammatory process tend to be similar in their end-state appearance [39].

Prosthetic Heart Valves

Types

Prosthetic heart valves in current use can be classified into two major groups: rigid-framed (mechanical) valves and tissue valves (bioprosthesis) [6, 7, 42–44]. Rigid-framed valves are of three types: (1) valves with a centrally placed occluder (ball or disc), which moves up and down in a metal cage and allows only lateral blood flow, (2) valves with a tilting disc, which permits semicentral flow, and (3) valves with two hinged, semicircular plates (St. Jude type), which allow central flow. The most prevalent caged ball valve, the Starr-Edwards valve ceased production in 2007 and the leading tilting disc valve, the Bjork-Shiley valve is also no longer manufactured. Thus bileaflet valves are the most common mechanical valves implanted today. Tissue valves include (1) fresh and variously treated homografts, (2) human dura mater or fascia lata valves, (3) bovine pericardial valves, and (4) porcine aortic valves. The metal and plastic mounting frames and the preimplantation chemical treatments vary from one type of tissue valve to another. Tissue valves without supporting frames (unstented porcine and human homograft valves) also are being used clinically. Knowledge of the frames and treatments is necessary to interpret morphologic findings in tissue valves. Radiographs may be useful in the identification and evaluation of explanted valves [42–44]. Essential for the evaluation of any prosthetic valve is knowledge of the length of time the valve was in place and the specific reason for its removal.

Complications

Certain complications are common to all types of prosthetic heart valves. Among these are thrombosis, embolization, infection, dehiscence of the valvular ring, paravalvular leak, disproportion, turbulent flow, and hemolysis. Complications limited to rigid-framed prostheses are related to wear and fracture of mechanical components, resulting in interference with proper motion of the occluder (and sometimes also in embolic phenomena), whereas complications peculiar to tissue valves are related to calcification or breakdown of the prosthetic tissue leaflets [6, 7, 45, 46]. Degenerative changes also develop in homograft human tissue valves [47, 48].

Complications Common to All Types of Prosthetic Valves

Thrombus formation in mechanical prostheses is most common at the base of the struts forming the cage. From this area, thrombi can spread and interfere with motion of the occluder, with seating of the occluder on the orifice, or with blood flow. These thrombi can undergo organization, become infected, or be sources of emboli. Ball valves with cloth-covered cage struts are less likely to form thrombi than are those with uncovered struts. Tissue valves are least likely to form large thrombi, although aggregates of platelets do develop on their surfaces. Thrombi can splint the cusps of bioprostheses and render them stenotic [49, 50]. Thrombi removed from prosthetic heart valves must be examined (by histology and by culture) for evidence of infection [32]. Dehiscence of a valvular ring must be regarded as due to infection until proved otherwise. Paravalvular leaks most frequently result from a prosthesis having been sutured to a ring that is heavily calcified or weakened (as occurs in patients with Marfan's syndrome or other connective tissue disorder). Anemia and renal hemosiderosis are typical findings in hemolysis produced by prosthetic heart valves.

Disproportion is caused by prosthetic heart valves that are too large for the chambers in which they are placed. This can result in interference with movement of the poppet, as in the case of large ball valves placed in a small ascending aorta (particularly in patients with combined mitral and aortic valve disease in whom the aortic root is usually not dilated) or in a small left ventricle (as in patients with combined mitral and aortic stenosis in whom the left ventricle is hypertrophied but not dilated). If a porcine bioprosthesis is improperly placed in the mitral orifice, one of its struts may obstruct the left ventricular outflow tract. In the case of the double valve replacement, the prosthetic mitral valve may be inadvertently placed in such a way as to interfere with proper seating of the poppet of the prosthetic aortic valve. Disproportion also may result from normal growth of the heart of a child in whom a small prosthetic valve was implanted at an early age.

Complications Limited to Rigid-Framed (Mechanical) Prosthetic Valves

Turbulent blood flow produced by caged-ball prostheses may lead to diffuse endocardial fibroelastotic thickening and to intimal proliferation in the ascending aorta, sometimes with extension of the thickening into the coronary arterial ostia. Degeneration (variance) of the silicone rubber poppet was common in the caged-ball prostheses implanted before 1967. This complication, which resulted from surface abrasion and lipid infiltration, has not been reported in the metallic hollow poppet. Wear of a caged disc, causing "grooving" and disc cocking, has been described in most caged-disc prostheses. Disc cocking remains a potential problem with all caged-disc valves, and it may be totally unrecognized as a cause of fatalities. Wear of the cloth covering on the struts and the orifice occurred in some of the older models of completely cloth-covered caged-ball prostheses, but strut cloth wear has not been reported in the newer Starr-Edwards model with metal tracts. Dislodgement of caged discs and poppets has been reported in association with wear of these components or with fracture of struts.

Complications Limited to Bioprosthetic (Tissue) Valves

The various types of bioprosthetic heart valves developed since the 1970s have the following characteristics in common: collagen is their major structural component; they are mounted (except for some of the homografts) on metal and plastic stents; the incidence of clinical episodes of thromboembolism is lower with these valves than with rigid-framed valves; and they have problems of long-term durability because they can become stenotic as a result of calcification or regurgitant due to alterations in collagen [6, 7, 51].

Porcine Aortic Valves

Porcine aortic valves treated with a low (<1%) concentration of glutaraldehyde (to crosslink tissue protein, to sterilize the tissue, and to eliminate problems of antigenicity) and mounted on flexible stents have become a widely used type of valvular bioprosthesis. During the first 5 years after implantation, these values usually have excellent function, although they can develop extensive anatomic changes. After the first 5 years, appreciable incidences of calcification and cuspal damage become evident. Calcific deposits develop more frequently and earlier in children and young adults than in older individuals and also are more frequent in patients with chronic renal disease [49, 50]. Cuspal perforations have no relation to patient age.

A bioprosthetic heart valve removed because of dysfunction should be first examined for evidence of infection, perforation, or calcification, and cultures should be taken as indicated by clinical or anatomic findings; then it should be radiographed and photographed before the cusps are detached from the frame for histologic sectioning. These valves are fragile and should be handled only by the mounting frame to avoid producing artifactual damage to the cusps. Connective tissue stains and stains for calcium are useful in evaluating these valves. Transmission electron microscopy provides the best method for studying the collagen, and scanning electron microscopy is the method of choice for examining the surfaces.

Histologically, porcine aortic valves are composed of the following three layers, which also are recognizable in the bioprosthesis even after having been in place for long periods of time: (1) the ventricularis, which faces the ventricular cavity when the valve is in its anatomic position and which contains collagen and abundant elastic fibers, (2) the spongiosa, which is the proteoglycan-rich middle layer, and (3) the fibrosa, which contains densely packed collagen but only small, scanty elastic fibers and which faces the aortic wall [6, 7]. Proteoglycans are lost from the spongiosa during commercial processing and soon after implantation of the bioprosthesis, leaving empty spaces that gradually are filled with deposits of plasma proteins. The surfaces of porcine valvular bioprostheses usually do not become endothelialized, although they may be covered by macrophages, multinucleated giant cells, platelet aggregates, and small fibrin deposits. Polymorphonuclear leukocytes are very scanty or absent unless infection is present. Macrophages show little tendency to invade the bioprosthetic tissue, and there is no evidence that immunologic rejection plays a role in its deterioration.

Calcific deposits usually develop in association with collagen in foci of loss of proteoglycans and with surface thrombi, especially in region near the commissures; they form yellow, plaque-like or raised lesions [52]. Calcific deposits also develop in the aortic wall just adjacent to the cusps and in cardiac muscle cells in a muscular shelf extending from the ventricular septum into the base of the right coronary cusp of the porcine aortic valve. This cusp is larger than the others, and its base is less translucent. Calcific deposits can also be associated with perforations, perhaps because collagen adjacent to those deposits undergoes severe mechanical stresses [52]. The collagen in bioprostheses undergoes a time-dependent process of degeneration, which may be related to material fatigue and many result in perforation of the cusps. Perforations in porcine valves occur most frequently near the basal attachment of the cusps. In pericardial valves, particularly those implanted in the mitral position, cuspal tears are likely to involve the free edge near the attachment to the post. It has been suggested that such tears begin at the attachment suture. Infection of porcine valvular bioprostheses differs from that of rigid-framed valves; it is likely to involve the cusps (rather than the sewing ring), is less likely to result in formation of a ring abscess, and usually extends into the collagen in the cusps [51]. The incidence of infection in the two types of valves appears to be similar.

Other Bioprosthetic Valves

Fresh, antibiotic-sterilized, freeze-dried, and chemically treated aortic valve homografts (allografts) have been used infrequently in the United States. However, cryopreserved aortic valve allografts have been used more extensively in recent years [47, 48]. In contrast to glutaraldehyde-treated bioprostheses, allografts tend to become covered with a fibrous sheath of host origin. These valves become completely acellular, and apoptosis has recently been shown to play an important role in the loss of the valvular cells [53]. Complications of allograft valves include calcification, cuspal rupture, and fibrous retraction of the edges of the cusps. Autologous fascia lata valves implanted without any chemical treatment have had a very poor record of durability and a high incidence of degeneration, thrombosis, calcification, and fibrous contraction of the cusps. Their use has been completely discontinued. Human dura mater valves preserved by glycerol treatment have been used extensively in Latin America. Bioprostheses made of glutaraldehyde-treated bovine pericardium have also been used as substitute cardiac valves and are becoming one of the most frequently implanted valves. Both dura mater and pericardium consist of dense collagenous sheets with sparse elastic fibers. Their layered structure is easily distinguishable histologically from that of porcine aortic valves. Complications of pericardial and dura mater valves are similar to those of porcine valves, consisting mainly of calcification and cuspal dehiscence [45].

Conduits

Conduits composed of various synthetic materials have been used to correct hypoplasia or atresia of the pulmonary artery. Valveless conduits were first used; subsequently, conduits containing mechanical (Björk-Shiley) valves were employed but were found to be prone to valvular thrombosis. More recently, extensive use has been made of pulmonic conduits with bioprosthetic (porcine or pericardial) valves; in addition, left ventricular apical-aortic conduits have had limited use for correction of tunnel aortic stenosis [45]. The most frequent complication of conduits is obstruction, which can result from one or more of the following causes: (1) muscular compression of the proximal end of the conduit during ventricular systole, (2) accumulation of thrombotic or fibrous material (fibrous peel) in the wall of the conduit, (3) compression of the conduit by the sternum, (4) calcific or thrombotic stenosis of the bioprosthesis, and (5) stenosis at the distal end (the most common cause of obstruction) because of the small size of the artery at the anastomotic site.

New Procedures

The contemporary management of patients with significant valvular heart disease is changing based on the advent of valve sparing surgical procedures and transcatheter valve replacement. Valve sparing repair of valves with prolapse and myxomatous degeneration is now performed extensively [54]. Repair of tricuspid or bicuspid aortic valves, coupled in some cases with aortic root re-implantation has yielded good results, whereas procedures on calcified bicuspid valves have been less successful [55]. Transcatheter aortic valve replacement is being used in selected patients as an alternative to surgical aortic valve replacement [56–58]. As noted in Chap. 10, transcatheter valves are approved for implantation for treatment of aortic stenosis. The Medtronic CoreValve is a self-expanding porcine valve while the Edwards Sapien valve is made of bovine pericardium. While the pathology of valve degeneration in these valves might be expected to be similar to surgically implanted bioprostheses, more data regarding this new therapy needs to be collected.

References

1. Vaideeswar P, Butany J. Valvular heart disease. In: Buja LM, Butany J, editors. Cardiovascular pathology. 4th ed. New York: Elsevier; 2016. p. 485.
2. Schoen FJ, Edwards WD. Valvular heart disease: general principles and stenosis. In: Silver MD, Gotlieb AI, Schoen FJ, editors. Cardiovascular pathology. 3rd ed. New York: Churchill Livingstone; 2001. p. 402.
3. Silver MD, Silver MM. Valvular heart disease: conditions causing regurgitation. In: Silver MD, Gotlieb AI, Schoen FJ, editors. Cardiovascular pathology. 3rd ed. New York: Churchill Livingstone; 2001. p. 443.
4. McAllister HA Jr, Buja LM, Ferrans VJ. Valvular heart disease: anatomic abnormalities. In: Willerson JT, Cohn JN, Wellens HJJ, Holmes Jr DR, editors. Cardiovascular medicine. 3rd ed. London: Springer; 2007. p. 369.
5. Soler-Soler J, Galve E. Worldwide perspective of valve disease. Heart. 2000;83:721–5.
6. Schoen FJ. Evolving concepts of cardiac valve dynamics: the continuum of development, functional structure, pathobiology, and tissue engineering. Circulation. 2008;118:1846–80.
7. Schoen FJ. Mechanisms of function and disease of natural and replacement heart valves. Annu Rev Pathol. 2012;7:161–83.
8. Roberts WC, Dangel JC, Bulkley BH. Nonrheumatic valvular cardiac disease: a clinicopathologic survey of 27 different conditions causing valvular dysfunction. Cardiovasc Clin. 1973;5:333–446.
9. Cheitlin MD, Fenoglio JJ, McAllister HA Jr, et al. Congenital aortic stenosis secondary to dysplasia of congenital bicuspid aortic valves without commissural fusion. Am J Cardiol. 1978;42:102–7.
10. Fenoglio JJ, McAllister HA Jr, DeCastro CM, et al. Congenital bicuspid aortic valve after age 20. Am J Cardiol. 1977;39:164–9.
11. Davia JE, Fenoglio JJ, DeCastro CM, et al. Quadricuspid semilunar valves. Chest. 1977;72:186–9.
12. Hyams VJ, Manion WC. Incomplete differentiation of the cardiac valves. A report of 197 cases. Am Heart J. 1968;76:173–82.
13. Goldbarg SH, Elmariah S, Miller MA, Fuster V. Insights into degenerative aortic valve disease. J Am Coll Cardiol. 2007;50:1205–13.
14. Rajamannan NM, Bonow RO, Rahimtoola SH. Calcific aortic stenosis: an update. Nat Clin Pract Cardiovasc Med. 2007;4:254–62.
15. Xu S, Liu AC, Gotlieb AI. Common pathogenic features of atherosclerosis and calcific aortic stenosis: role of transforming growth factor-beta. Cardiovasc Pathol. 2010;19:236–47.
16. Li C, Xu S, Gotlieb AI. The response to valve injury. A paradigm to understand the pathogenesis of heart valve disease. Cardiovasc Pathol. 2011;20:183–90.
17. Li C, Xu S, Gotlieb AI. The progression of calcific aortic valve disease through injury, cell dysfunction, and disruptive biologic and physical force feedback loops. Cardiovasc Pathol. 2013;22:1–8.
18. Rajamannan NM, Evans FJ, Aikawa E, et al. Calcific aortic valve disease: not simply a degenerative process: a review and agenda for research from the National Heart and Lung and Blood Institute Aortic Stenosis Working Group. Executive summary: calcific aortic valve disease-2011 update. Circulation. 2011;124:1783–91.
19. Hayek E, Gring CN, Griffin BP. Mitral valve prolapse. Lancet. 2005;365:507–18.
20. Levine RA, Slaugenhaupt SA. Molecular genetics of mitral valve prolapse. Curr Opin Cardiol. 2007;22:171–5.
21. Ferrans VJ. Metabolic and familial diseases. In: Silver MD, editor. Cardiovascular pathology. 2nd ed. New York: Churchill Livingstone; 1991. p. 1973.
22. Segura AM, Luna RE, Horiba K, et al. Immunohistochemistry of matrix metalloproteinases and their inhibitors in thoracic aortic aneurysms and aortic valves of patients with the Marfan's syndrome. Circulation. 1998;98(Suppl II):II331–7.
23. Guy TS, Hill AC. Mitral valve prolapse. Annu Rev Med. 2012;63:277–92.
24. deVlaming A, Sauls K, Hajdu Z, et al. Atrioventricular valve development: new perspectives on an old theme. Differentiation. 2012;84:103–16.
25. Baggenstoss AH, Titus JL. Rheumatic and collagen disorders of the heart. In: Gould SE, editor. Pathology of the heart and blood vessels. Springfield, IL: Charles C. Thomas; 1968. p. 701.
26. McAllister HA Jr. Endocrine disorders and the cardiovascular system. In: Silver MD, editor. Cardiovascular pathology. 2nd ed. New York: Churchill Livingstone; 1991. p. 1181.
27. Redfield MM. Ergot alkaloid heart disease. In: Hurst JW, editor. New types of cardiovascular diseases: topics in clinical cardiology. New York: Igaku-Shoin Medical; 1994. p. 63–76.
28. Redfield MM, Nicholson WJ, Edwards WD, Tajik AJ. Valve disease associated with ergot alkaloid use: echocardiographic and pathologic correlations. Ann Intern Med. 1992;117:50–2.
29. Connolly HM, Cresy JL, McGoon MD, et al. Valvular heart disease associated with fenfluramine-phentermine. N Engl J Med. 1997;337:581–8.
30. McAllister HA Jr. Pathology of the cardiovascular system in chronic renal failure. In: Lowenthal DT, Pennock RL, Likoff W, et al., editors. Management of cardiovascular disease in renal failure. Philadelphia, PA: FA Davis; 1981. p. 1.
31. Ferrans VJ, Butany JW. Ultrastructural pathology of the heart. In: Trump BF, Jones RT, editors. Diagnostic electron microscopy, vol. 4. New York: Churchill Livingstone; 1983. p. 319.
32. McAllister HA Jr, Ferrans VJ. The heart and blood vessels. In: Silverberg SJ, editor. Principles and practice of surgical pathology. New York: Churchill Livingstone; 1991. p. 787.
33. McAllister HA Jr. Collagen diseases and the cardiovascular system. In: Silver MD, editor. Cardiovascular pathology. 2nd ed. New York: Churchill Livingstone; 1991. p. 1151.
34. Fauci AS, Wolff SM. Wegener's granulomatosis and related diseases. Dis Mon. 1977;23(7):1–36.
35. McAllister HA Jr, Fenoglio JJ. Cardiac involvement in Whipple's disease. Circulation. 1975;52:152–6.
36. Eck M, Muller-Hermelink HK, Harmsen D, Kreipe H. Invasion and destruction of mucosal plasma cells by *Tropheryma whippelii*. Hum Pathol. 1997;28:1424–8.
37. Olsen EGJ, Spry CJF. The pathogenesis of Loffler's endomyocardial disease, and its relationship to endomyocardial fibrosis. Prog Cardiol. 1979;8:281.
38. McAllister HA Jr, Hall RJ. Iatrogenic heart disease. In: Cheng TO, editor. The international textbook of cardiology. New York: Pergamon; 1986. p. 871.
39. Titus JL. Infective endocarditis, active and healed. In: Edwards JE, Lev M, Abell MR, editors. The heart. Baltimore, MD: Williams & Wilkins; 1974. p. 176.

40. Castonguay MC, Burner KD, Edwards WD, Baddour LM, Maleszewski JJ. Surgical pathology of native valve endocarditis in 310 specimens from 287 patients (1985–2004). Cardiovasc Pathol. 2013;22:19–27.
41. Freedman LR. Endocarditis updated. Dis Mon. 1970;26(3):1–71.
42. Silver MD, Datta BN, Bowes FV. A key to identify heart valve prostheses. Arch Pathol. 1975;99:132–8.
43. Steiner RM, Flicker S. The radiology of prosthetic heart valves. In: Morse D, Steiner RM, Fernandez J, editors. Guide to prosthetic cardiac valves, vol. 53. New York: Springer; 1985.
44. Butany J, Ahluwalia MS, Munroe C, Fayet C, Ahn C, Blit P, Kepron C, Cusimano RJ, Leask RL. Mechanical heart valve prostheses: identification and evaluation. Cardiovasc Pathol. 2003;12:1–22.
45. Lefrak EA, Starr A. Cardiac valve prostheses. East Norwalk, CT: Appleton & Lange; 1979.
46. Zeien LB, Klatt EC. Cardiac valve prostheses at autopsy. Arch Pathol Lab Med. 1990;144:933–7.
47. Dagenais F, Cartier P, Voisine P, Desaulniers D, Perron J, Baillot R, Raymond G, Metras J, Doyle D, Mathieu P. Which biologic valve should we select for the 45- to 65-year-old age group requiring aortic valve replacement? J Thorac Cardiovasc Surg. 2005;129:1041–9.
48. Koolbergen DR, Hazekamp MG, de Heer E, Bruggemans EF, Huysmans HA, Dion RA, Bruijn JA. The pathology of fresh and cryopreserved homograft heart valves: an analysis of forty explanted homograft valves. J Thorac Cardiovasc Surg. 2002;124:689–97.
49. Platt MR, Mills LJ, Estrera AS, et al. Marked thrombosis and calcification of porcine heterograft valves. Circulation. 1980;62:862–9.
50. Croft CH, Buja LM, Floresca MZ, et al. Late thrombotic obstruction of aortic porcine bioprosthesis. Am J Cardiol. 1986;57:355–6.
51. Ferrans VJ, Tomita Y, Hilbert SL, et al. Evaluation of operatively excised prosthetic tissue valves. In: Waller BF, editor. Pathology of the heart and great vessels. New York: Churchill Livingstone; 1988. p. 311.
52. Hilbert SL, Ferrans VJ, McAllister HA Jr, Cooley DA. Ionescu-Shiley bovine pericardial bioprosthesis: histologic and ultrastructural studies. Am J Pathol. 1992;140:1195–204.
53. Hilbert SL, Luna RE, Zhang J, et al. Allograft heart valves: the role of apoptosis-mediated cell loss. J Thorac Cardiovasc Surg. 1999;117:454–62.
54. Yacoub MH, Cohn LH. Novel approaches to cardiac valve repair. From structure to function: part II. Circulation. 2004;109:1064–72.
55. Fattouch K, Murana G, Castrovinci S, Nasso G, Mossuto C, Corrado E, Ruvolo G, Speziale G. Outcomes of aortic valve repair according to valve morphology and surgical techniques. Interact Cardiovasc Thorac Sur. 2012;15:644–50.
56. Webb JG, Wood DA. Current status of transcatheter aortic valve replacement. J Am Coll Cardiol. 2012;60:483–92.
57. Himbert D, Pontnau F, Messika-Zeitoun D, et al. Feasibility and outcomes of transcatheter aortic valve implantation in high-risk patients with stenotic bicuspid aortic valves. Am J Cardiol. 2012;110:877–83.
58. Vahanian A, Himbert D, Brochet E, Depoix JP, Iung B, Nataf P. Transcatherter aortic valve implantation: our vision of the future. Arch Cardiovasc Dis. 2012;105:181–6.

Acute Rheumatic Fever

2

Y. S. Chandrashekhar, L. Maximilian Buja,
Ganesan Karthikeyan, and Jagat Narula

Rheumatic fever (RF) or acute RF (ARF) is a noninfectious consequence of pharyngitis caused by group A β-hemolytic streptococci (GABHS). Although it is rare in the developed world, RF remains a major problem worldwide [1–4]. However, RF continues to appear unexpectedly even in the First World, as evidenced by occasional outbreaks in the United States [5]. Furthermore, given the magnitude of international travel and immigration, clinicians everywhere are likely to encounter RF or its devastating cardiac sequelae. Acute RF most commonly presents as a combination of arthritis, carditis, chorea, erythema marginatum, and subcutaneous nodules, and valvular heart disease remains a major long-term consequence. It has thus been aptly said that "rheumatic fever licks the joints, but bites the heart."

Rheumatic Fever

Good quality data on the incidence of ARF from much of the developing world is lacking. Most studies from which incidence has been estimated are retrospective, and there are no studies from Africa, where incidence may be among the highest in the world. Acute RF is estimated to occur at annual rates varying between 1 and 194 per 100,000 population [4]. The highest rates are seen among the indigenous people living in the Northern Territory of Australia, and in countries in the South Pacific [4]. Data on the prevalence of rheumatic heart disease (RHD), which is the only permanent sequala of ARF, are more readily available. The most recent data from the Global Burden of Disease study suggest that there were over 34 million people with RHD in 2015 worldwide, with over 29 million of them living in developing countries [6]. Consequently, over 80% of the 319,000 annual deaths due to RHD occurred in developing countries. Two-thirds of deaths due to RHD occurred in three countries: India, China, and Pakistan [6].

In the United States, ARF was a major problem before the 1960s but has largely disappeared as a major cause of illness since then [1]. Improved socioeconomic status, less crowded housing conditions, the advent of antibiotics, and the widespread treatment of streptococcal throat infections have contributed to this decline. However, RF continues to appear all over the world, and several outbreaks have occurred in the United States, in portions of Utah and Ohio and at US Naval Training Centers [7]. Many of these outbreaks have involved middle-class suburbs, less crowded communities, and people with access to excellent health care—a situation entirely unlike the developing world, where socioeconomic issues are thought to be responsible for RF outbreaks. This emphasizes our limited understanding of RF.

Pathogenesis

A significant body of data implicates an autoimmune process in the development of RF. The salient features of the pathogenesis include (1) a human host who harbors "RF susceptibility factors," which are thought to increase the host's proclivity to developing ARF; (2) pharyngitis (but not other sites of streptococcal infection, interestingly); (3) the presence of an immune response against specific streptococcal antigens, the magnitude of which correlates with the occurrence of subsequent ARF;

Y. S. Chandrashekhar
Division of Cardiology, Department of Medicine,
Veterans Affairs Medical Center, Minneapolis, MN, USA

L. M. Buja
Department of Pathology and Laboratory Medicine,
McGovern Medical School, The University of Texas Health
Science Center at Houston (UTHealth), Houston, TX, USA

Department of Cardiovascular Pathology Research,
Texas Heart Institute, Houston, TX, USA

G. Karthikeyan
Department of Cardiology, All India Institute of Medical Sciences,
New Delhi, India

J. Narula (✉)
Cardiology Department, Mount Sinai Saint Luke's Hospital,
New York, NY, USA
e-mail: narula@mountsinai.org

B. A. Carabello (ed.), *Valvular Heart Disease*, Cardiovascular Medicine, https://doi.org/10.1007/978-1-4471-2840-3_2

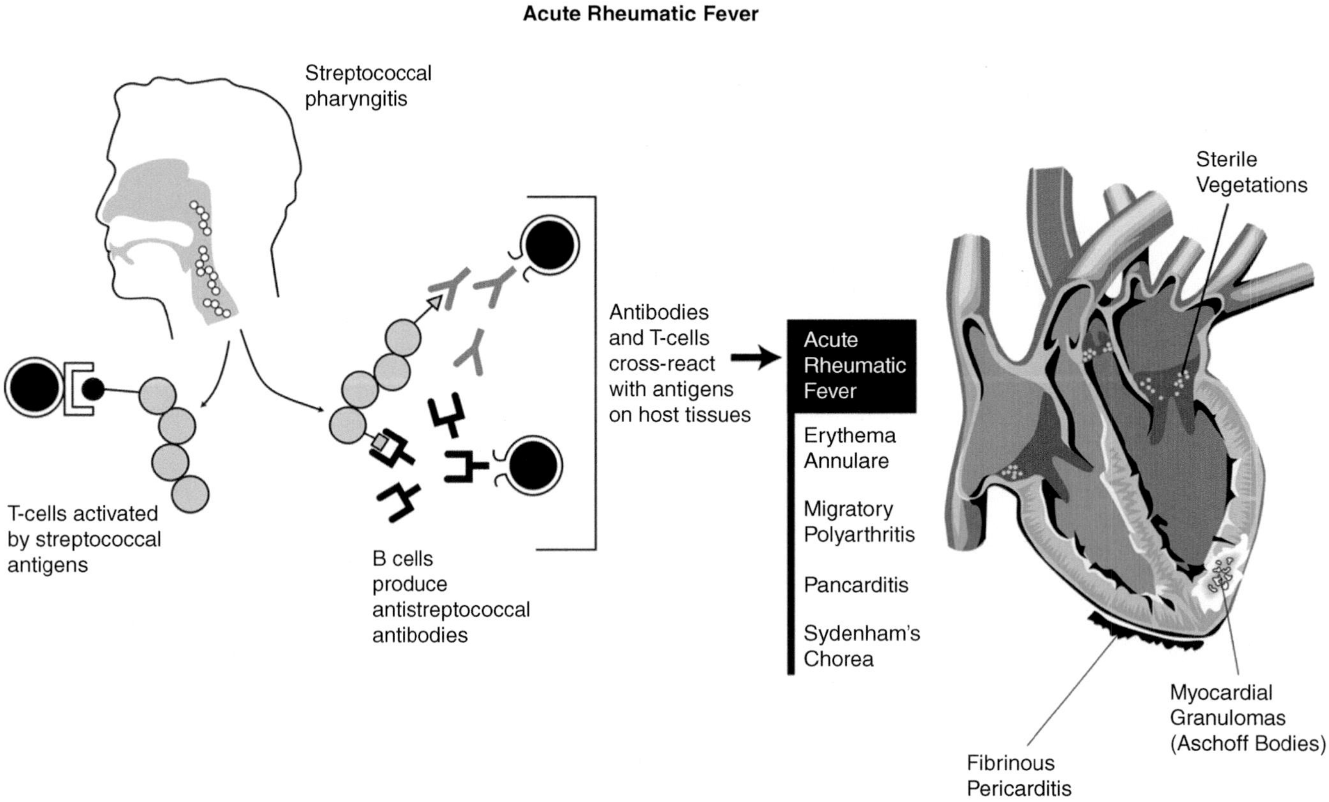

Fig. 2.1 Pathogenesis of acute rheumatic fever (ARF). In susceptible individuals, ARF develops as a delayed, noninfectious consequence of prior streptococcal pharyngitis. The initial event is a febrile illness due to an episode of pharyngitis produced by a group A β hemolytic streptococcus. During an asymptomatic interval, T lymphocytes become activated by streptococcal antigens and B lymphocytes produce anti-streptococcal antibodies. The activated T cells and anti-streptococcal antibodies cross-react with epitopes on the host tissues. The result is a febrile multisystem disorder known as ARF. The protean manifestations of ARF include erythema annulare, migratory polyarthritis, Sydenham's chorea, and pancarditis. The pancarditis manifests as fibrinous pericarditis, granulomatous myocardial lesions known as Aschoff bodies, and inflammation with sterile vegetations on the cardiac valves. ARF may be a limited illness, and many of the organ manifestations may be reversible, but it can have permanent sequelae, the most important of which is chronic rheumatic heart disease due to progressive damage and dysfunction of cardiac valves

and (4) an interval of 1–5 weeks between pharyngitis and the development of ARF (Fig. 2.1).

Only a few individuals with GABHS infection develop RF [8, 9], and the genetic makeup of the host may affect susceptibility to ARF. The putative susceptibility factor remains unclear so far, and indeed there may be many such factors. Identifying these factors is likely to help us target preventive measures. Belonging to certain racial groups (e.g., Samoans in Hawaii, Maori in New Zealand) and a history of previous episodes of RF increase one's susceptibility to streptococcal RF after pharyngitis. Another factor may be differences in the hosts' ability to mount a vigorous antibody response, which correlates with the occurrence of ARF. Familial or genetic susceptibility to RF has been proposed [4, 10, 11]. Several candidate gene studies [12], twin studies [13], and two genome-wide association studies [14, 15] provide further evidence for genetic susceptibility, and offer insights into the potential pathways through which genetic susceptibility may mediate the predisposition to develop ARF and RHD.

Among the various serotypes of GABHS, some appear more likely to initiate ARF (M-types 1, 3, 5, 6, 14, 18, 19, 24, 27, and 29), whereas others are not commonly associated with ARF (M2, 4, and 28). Furthermore, only throat and not skin infections mediate ARF. The exact mechanism by which GABHS initiates RF is unclear, and it is also not known why throat infections and not other streptococcal infections lead to RF [16]. In general, the RF-causing strains tend to be rich in M protein, provoke an intense M-type-specific immune response, and probably share epitopes with human tissue.

Mechanisms of Damage

Despite some claims of direct injury by streptococci, viruses, or toxins, most data suggest that RF occurs as a result of autoimmune injury. Antibodies (cross-reactive and polyspecific) that react to antigens shared between streptococci and human tissue (molecular mimicry) are thought to underlie this process (Fig. 2.1). Rheumatogenic streptococci contain multiple antigenic determinants that partially mimic normal human tissue antigen [9]. Thus, the hyaluronate capsule, the streptococcal membrane, and the M-proteins share similarity with valve glycoproteins, myocardial sarcolemma, and cardiac contractile proteins, respectively. After streptococcal pharyngitis, these antigens, which are recognized as foreign by the susceptible host, induce a hyperactive humoral and cellular immune response that damages native tissues bearing similar antigens. The type of damage is partly the result of which tissue shows what kinds of mimicry. For example, antibodies to the *N*-acetylglucosamine moiety of group A polysaccharide cross-react with the heart valve tissue [17], and this cross-reaction is thought to mediate valve damage; indeed, plasma levels of such antibodies are increased in patients with rheumatic heart valve disease [18].

Breakdown of tolerance is an important component of the pathogenesis of ARF. The M-protein epitopes not only can trigger heart cross-reactive antibodies and T-cell responses but also can act as superantigens [19]. This might explain the widespread immune response overriding the histocompatibility barrier. Both humoral and cellular immune responses are more vigorous in patients with ARF than in healthy individuals and might be related to the superantigenic property of streptococcal M protein. Significant T-cell infiltration is also observed in the valvular tissue, and T cells isolated from the valvular tissue of patients with RHD respond to streptococcal M5 protein and also cross-react with cardiac myosin [20, 21]. This homology with cardiac myosin can be expected to decrease tolerance and may enhance T-cell-mediated inflammatory damage [22]. The characteristic pathological findings (see below) suggest that the primary focus of ARF-induced damage is endothelium and subendothelial and perivascular connective tissue.

Both humoral and cell-mediated immune responses contribute to valve damage in ARF [4]. Binding of cross-reactive antibodies at the endothelial surface of the valve leads to upregulation of VCAM-1, which in turn induces adherence and infiltration by activated CD4 T cells and B lymphocytes [23]. Inflammatory cytokines released through a Th 1 immune response cause local tissue damage [24]. Binding to other antigens such as vimentin, laminin, and collagen cause further injury, which heals by neovascularization and fibrosis, resulting in the valve lesions typical of RHD [4].

The characteristic pathological findings (see below) suggest that the primary focus of ARF-induced damage is endothelium and subendothelial and perivascular connective tissue. Recently, a streptococcal M protein N-terminus domain has been shown to bind to the CB3 collagen type IV [25]. This binding may initiate an antibody response to the collagen and result in inflammation of the ground substance. Because these antibodies do not cross-react with M proteins, failure of the immune system and molecular mimicry may not be involved in their pathological effects. This alternative pathogenetic mechanism shares similarity with collagen involvement in both Goodpasture syndrome and Alport syndrome.

Pathology

The cardiac and non-cardiac tissues differ in how they react to ARF [26, 27]. The inflammatory process in the skin, joints, and brain tends to regress spontaneously without any significant residual effects. There is swelling with serous effusion in the joints. Inflammatory infiltration and edema are evident in the synovial membranes. Fibrinoid exudates frequently line the membranes. The blood vessels in the articular and periarticular areas are often inflamed and show infiltration by lymphocytes and polymorphonuclear leukocytes. On the other hand, the subcutaneous nodules have a center of fibrinoid necrosis with peripheral inflammatory reaction of lymphocytes and occasional polymorphonuclear leukocytes. Cardiac involvement in RF affects all three layers: pericardium, myocardium, and endocardium (resulting in pancarditis). The pericarditis is typically fibrinous (Fig. 2.2).

A fundamental pathological process in ARF is damage of the collagenous matrix of the cardiac and extracardiac tissue that elicits a granulomatous reaction called an Aschoff body. The process has early, intermediate, and late phases. The early and intermediate phases are characterized by fibrinoid necrosis. This is followed by a granulomatous reaction leading to the formation of the pathognomonic Aschoff body (Figs. 2.3 and 2.4) [28]. The Aschoff body consists of a central area of fibrinoid necrosis surrounded by cells of histiocytic-macrophage origin (Anitschkow cells), which show a typical owl's eye-shaped nucleus. These cells are usually found in the subendocardial or perivascular regions of the myocardium. There is surprisingly little histopathologic damage to the myo-

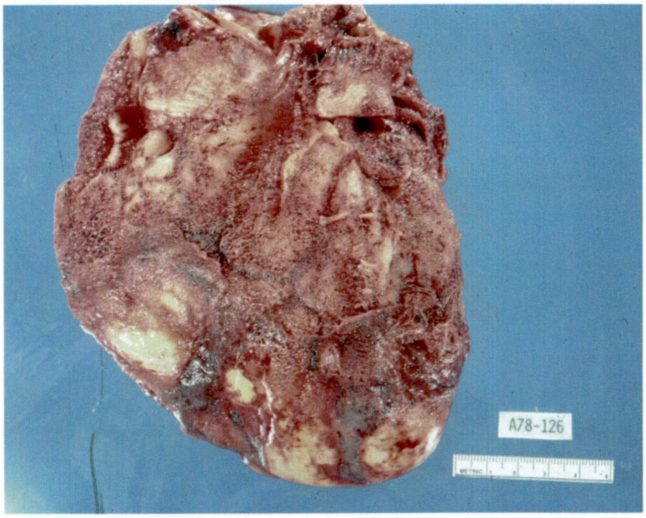

Fig. 2.2 Acute fibrinous pericarditis typical of ARF and other rheumatic diseases. The epicardial surface of the heart is covered with shaggy fibrinous exudates

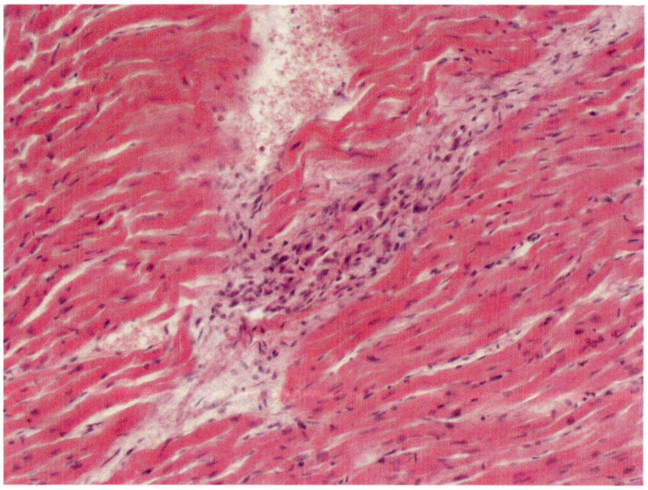

Fig. 2.3 Aschoff body in the myocardial interstitium consisting of a focus of granulomatous inflammation composed of T lymphocytes, occasional plasma cells, and plump activated macrophages called Anitschkow cells. The myocardial inflammation in ARF begins as foci of fibrinoid necrosis that evolve into foci of granulomatous inflammation. The cellular inflammation is confined to the interstitium, usually in a perivascular location. Myocardial necrosis is not seen even in patients with florid carditis and heart failure. The myocardial failure appears related to humorally mediated myocardial dysfunction leading to cardiac dilatation and mitral regurgitation due to dilatation of the mitral annulus. H&E stain; medium magnification

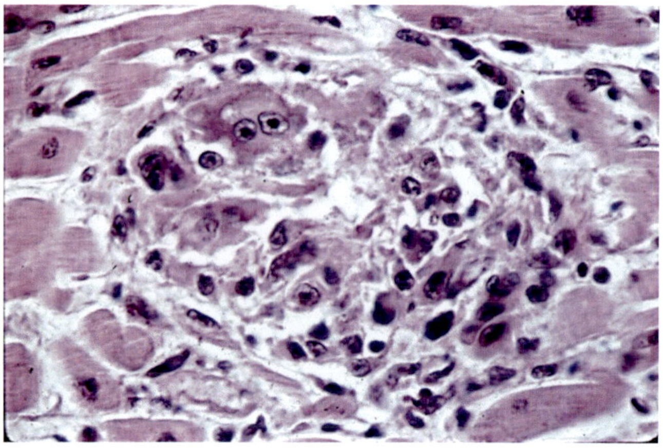

Fig. 2.4 Aschoff body with mononuclear Anitschkow cells and binucleate Aschoff cells. The nuclei of the Anitschkow and Aschoff cells are activated macrophages with central bars of chromatin, giving them an "owl-eye" appearance in cross-section. The Aschoff bodies are considered to be pathognomonic for the diagnosis of ARF. H&E stain; high magnification

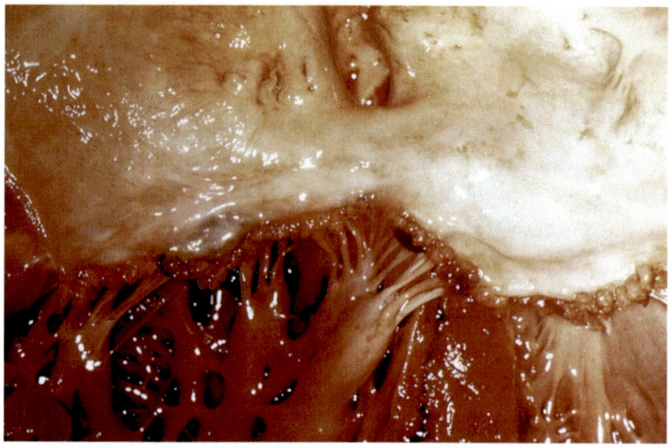

Fig. 2.5 Acute rheumatic valvulitis, mitral valve. Minute, translucent nodular vegetations called verrucae, 1–3 mm in diameter, are located along the lines of closure on the inflow (atrial) side of the leaflets. The nodules represent foci of fibrinoid necrosis and thrombosis devoid of micro-organisms. Systemic lupus erythematosus (SLE) also may exhibit a similar but distinctive type of sterile vegetative endocarditis. The Libman-Sacks endocarditis (LSE) caused by SLE has small or medium-sized vegetations on either or both sides of the valve leaflets. Both types of rheumatic vegetative endocarditis are distinct from the patterns of vegetative endocarditis seen in non-bacterial thrombotic endocarditis (NBTE) and infective endocarditis (IE). Reproduced with permission from: McAllister HA Jr., Buja LM, Ferrans VJ. Valvular heart disease: anatomic abnormalities. In: Willerson JT, Cohn JN, Wellens HJJ, Holmes DR, Jr., Editors. Cardiovascular Medicine, third edition. London: Springer Verlag, 2007, p. 372 (Fig. 14.6)

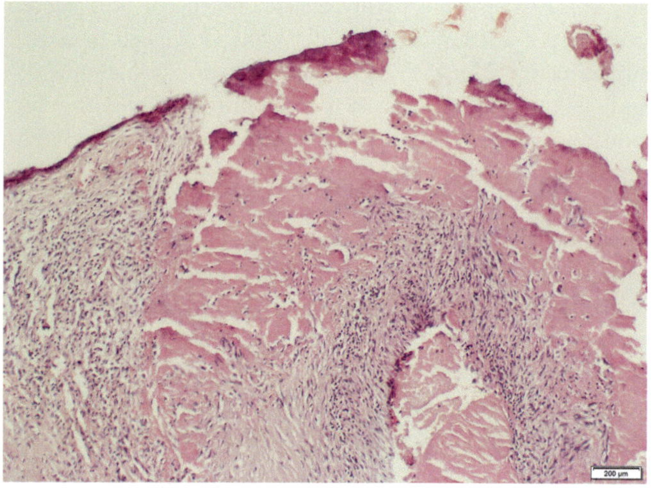

Fig. 2.6 Typical verrucae of ARF, composed of sterile fibrin-rich thrombus. There is surface necrosis and lymphohistiocytic inflammation in the underlying valve tissue. H&E stain; high magnification

cardium, even in patients with florid clinical carditis and heart failure [29, 30]. Myocyte necrosis is uncommon, and the cellular infiltrate is confined to the interstitium. This explains why even patients with frank rheumatic myocarditis do not have troponin leaks [31]. The conduction system shows little pathology, even in patients with clinical conduction defects. The valves are inflamed and thickened during the acute stage of the rheumatic activity. The surface of the valves develop small, sterile vegetations, or verrucae—particularly along the edges of the leaflets (Figs. 2.5 and 2.6)—that are not associated with thromboembolic sequelae. The inflammation is followed by a repair process involving ingrowth of blood vessels (neovascularization) and deposition of collagen (Fig. 2.7).

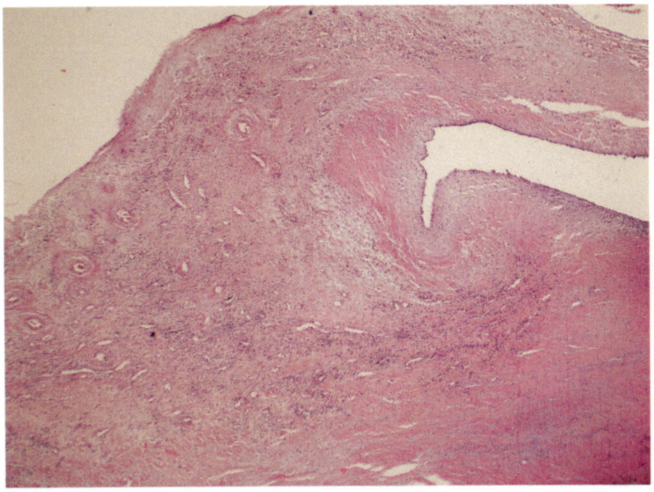

Fig. 2.7 Histology of mitral valve in healing phase of ARF. The autoimmune injury with necrosis, inflammation, and thrombosis triggers a repair process involving granulation tissue formation with the ingrowth of blood vessels and deposition of collagen. Thick-walled blood vessels that persist in the atrialis layer of the valve leaflets are recognized as neovascularization of the valve, as shown here. Contraction of the fibrous tissue leads to retraction of the leaflets. Organization of thrombus formed at the lateral margins of the leaflets leads to commissural fusion. H&E stain; medium magnification

A mild degree of inflammation leads to fusion of the cusps, whereas more severe inflammatory reaction extends to involve the chordae tendineae. This can result in early mitral or tricuspid regurgitation, caused by annular dilatation and leaflet prolapse. The scarring process typically occurs gradually, such that mitral and/or aortic regurgitation may not be initially manifest and then present months to years later clinically. Mitral and, rarely, aortic stenosis are late sequelae that result from scarring and inflammatory fusion of leaflet cusps (Fig. 2.8).

Clinical Features

Joint Symptoms

Arthritis is the earliest manifestation of RF and frequently brings the patient to clinical attention [32]. Arthritis occurs in at least two-thirds of patients and is more common in older patients. Although larger joints of the extremities are commonly involved, occasional involvement of smaller joints in the hands and feet may be seen; the hips, spine, and axial joints are rarely affected. The joints are swollen, hot, red, and tender.

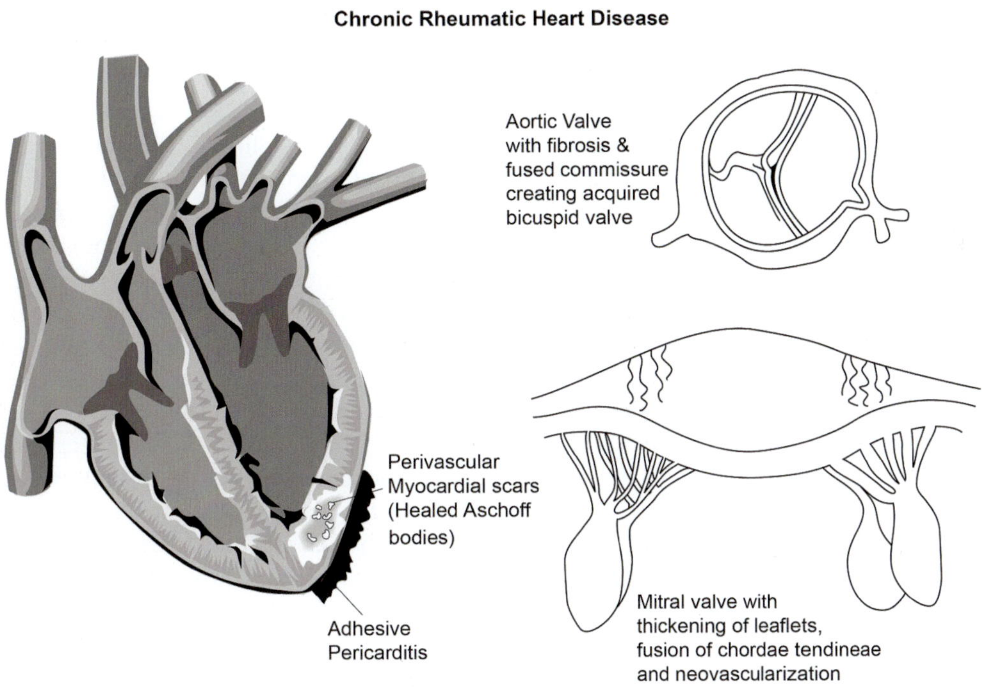

Fig. 2.8 Chronic rheumatic heart disease. The heart manifests sequelae after a single bout or recurrent episodes of ARF. The fibrinous pericarditis resolves with residual pericardial adhesions. Healing of the granulomatous Aschoff bodies results in areas of perivascular fibrosis. The repair of the acute injury to the valves results in variable combinations of fusion of chordae tendineae, fibrous thickening of leaflets or cusps, neovascularization, and commissural fusion. Over a period of months to years, progressive distortion of valvular architecture and function occurs as a result of chronic turbulence of flow across the valves and other mechanical factors rather than to ongoing autoimmune inflammatory insult. Secondary dystrophic calcification adds to the distortion of the valvular anatomy and can obliterate the characteristic feature of neovascularization. The end result is clinically significant stenosis, regurgitation of the mitral and/or aortic valves, or both, which is recognized clinically as chronic rheumatic heart disease. Chronic rheumatic heart disease shares similar pathologic features with the valve disease seen in systemic lupus erythematosus. The generic designation for the characteristic pathology is post-inflammatory valvulopathy

The joints are inflamed at different times and for various intervals, imparting a migratory character to joint pain. Aseptic monoarthritis may be frequent in endemic countries [33]. Arthritis usually resolves in 3–4 weeks, even without treatment, but it responds instantly to aspirin therapy and does not lead to permanent damage. Arthralgia without objective signs of inflammation is common in younger patients with carditis, particularly during rheumatic recurrences and in RHD patients in developing countries [34]. Some forms of polyarthritis after streptococcal pharyngitis may represent a reactive phenomenon. Post-streptococcal arthropathy is characterized by recurrent, severe, prolonged polyarthritis that is not very responsive to nonsteroidal anti-inflammatory agents. Although other manifestations of RF are not associated with arthropathy, some patients end up with residual heart disease [35]. Prophylaxis against reactive arthropathy remains similar to that for patients with RF, but few data are available to support definitive recommendations.

Cardiac Involvement

Carditis is the only manifestation of RF that results in permanent deformity [36]. Cardiac involvement in RF has been reported in nearly one-third of almost all cases in various studies and in up to one-half of cases in a prospective series [37]. Clinical carditis was seen in 72% of patients in a resurgence of RF in Salt Lake City [5], which is similar to the prevalence in the early twentieth century in the United States [38]. Subclinical carditis is being increasingly detected with modern imaging methods; valvular regurgitation can be documented in such cases with the use of echocardiography [39, 40] in 70–90% of all patients with ARF. Active rheumatic carditis can present in several ways, including subclinical cardiac involvement, acute or even fulminant congestive heart failure, and, occasionally, chronic heart failure. Younger patients often present with carditis, whereas older patients more commonly have joint involvement [32]. Although episodes of carditis occur less frequently in many older patients, they present more often with unexplained worsening of congestive heart failure. The clinical findings may be suggestive of pericarditis, myocarditis, and valvulitis. The guidelines for the diagnosis of rheumatic carditis are summarized in Table 2.1.

Table 2.1 Acute rheumatic carditis[a]

Criteria	First attacks	Recurrences
Valvulitis	New-onset apical systolic murmur or aortic regurgitation murmur Carey-Coombs murmur	Change in murmur New-onset murmur
Myocarditis	Unexplained cardiomegaly Unexplained congestive heart failure/gallop sounds	Worsening cardiomegaly Worsening congestive heart failure
Pericarditis	Pericardial rub Pericardial effusion	Pericardial rub Pericardial effusion
Miscellaneous	Conduction disturbances or unexplained tachycardia[b] Echocardiographic imaging findings[c] Nuclear imaging findings[c] Morphologic evidence at surgery Histologic evidence at biopsy or pathology examination	

[a]Supportive evidence is required for the diagnosis of acute rheumatic fever according to the Jones criteria. In patients with known rheumatic heart disease, acute rheumatic fever can be diagnosed with minor criteria *along with* evidence of antecedent streptococcal infection
[b]These would be considered soft criteria
[c]The validity of these methods is controversial

Endocarditis

Endocardial inflammation most commonly affects the mitral and aortic valves, and the clinical diagnosis of rheumatic endocarditis is based on identifying mitral or aortic regurgitation murmurs. Mitral valve disease is seen in approximately 70% of patients, mitral and aortic valve disease occurs in an additional 25%, and isolated aortic valve disease occurs in 5–8%. Clinical tricuspid or pulmonary valve involvement is rare in the first attack of RF.

The use of echocardiography has clarified the mechanism of valve regurgitation in RF [39]. Although mild-to-moderate mitral regurgitation is due to left ventricular dilatation with mild or no annular dilatation, more severe degrees of mitral regurgitation are associated with marked annular dilatation, chordal elongation, and anterior mitral leaflet prolapse [41]. Rarely, chordae rupture and result in flail leaflets and severe regurgitation. Because mitral regurgitation frequently resolves on follow-up [32, 42, 43], it is likely that a functional mechanism, rather than a permanent structural alteration in the valve or annulus, underlies the development of mitral regurgitation. Inflammatory changes in the aortic valves and the aortic ring result in aortic regurgitation; aortic valve prolapse contributes occasionally.

Myocarditis

Myocardial involvement is generally associated with new-onset cardiomegaly, an interval increase in cardiac size, or the development of congestive heart failure [30, 36, 44]. The left ventricular systolic function and myocardial contractility indices are normal in patients with rheumatic carditis, and histopathological examination reveals only minimal myocyte damage. Some evidence suggests that hemodynamically significant valvular lesions lead to the development of congestive heart failure [44].

Pericarditis

Clinical rheumatic pericarditis occurs in up to 15% of patients during the acute stage of RF, and the presence of an evanescent pericardial friction rub in such patients is evidence of rheumatic carditis. Detectable pericarditis usually indicates severe carditis [36].

Rheumatic pericarditis is almost always associated with findings of valvular involvement. A pericardial rub can sometimes mask the underlying valvular murmurs. However, other causes need to be considered if no valvulitis-related murmur is audible after the pericarditis resolves [36]. Rheumatic pericarditis is often associated with a mild-to-moderate serosanguineous effusion, and the development of pericardial tamponade is rare.

Sydenham Chorea

Sydenham chorea is a late manifestation of ARF that is characterized by a series of involuntary movements that commonly involve the face and extremities and are associated with emotional lability [32]. It commonly affects children between the ages of 7 and 14 years and occurs more frequently in girls; it is rarely seen in adults. The chorea is often associated with carditis and subcutaneous nodules, but it appears several weeks after an acute attack of ARF, when the acute manifestations have disappeared. The patients thus do not fulfill the Jones criteria at this time. The course of chorea is gradual as the patient appears increasingly nervous, becomes dysarthric, makes grimacing gestures, develops difficulty in writing, and shows characteristic purposeless movements of the arms and legs, which may be associated with muscular weakness. The chronic movements are exaggerated during effort or excitement but subside during sleep. The chorea is usually a self-limited condition and resolves without residual damage, but the associated carditis can leave behind valvular damage.

Skin Manifestations

Subcutaneous nodules and erythema marginatum are two important skin manifestations of RF. Subcutaneous nodules appear late in the course of RF. They are observed in up to 20% of patients, and their presence is usually associated with carditis. Subcutaneous nodules occur on bony prominences, vertebral spinous processes, or extensor tendons and are painless. They usually appear in crops, are variable in size, and disappear within 2–3 months.

Erythema marginatum can be an early or a late manifestation. It occurs in fewer than 15% of patients and appears on the trunk and proximal extremities as a serpiginous, macular, non-pruritic, and evanescent rash.

Clinical Diagnosis

There is no single diagnostic test or pathognomonic sign that allows an absolute diagnosis of RF; rather, the condition is recognized through a constellation of signs and symptoms in patients with recent GABHS pharyngitis. In 1944, Jones [45] described the clinical manifestations of RF and categorized each of them as major or minor. Since that time, the Jones criteria have been modified several times and by the WHO [3, 46] (Table 2.2). The most recent modifications suggested by the AHA were published in 2015 [47].

Various combinations of major and minor criteria are used for diagnosing ARF. The major manifestations include carditis, chorea, subcutaneous nodules, migratory arthritis involving large joints, and erythema marginatum. The minor manifestations include fever, prolonged joint pain, prolonged electrocardiographic PR interval, and laboratory indicators of inflammation, including an increased plasma concentration of acute-phase reactants. An elevated antistreptolysin O (ASO) titer or other evidence of previous streptococcal infection is considered a prerequisite.

Although the Jones criteria remain the cornerstone of diagnosing ARF, they are continually being updated to balance sensitivity/specificity, address different forms of presentation, accommodate a variable diagnostic armamentarium in different regions of the world, and reflect new information.

The most recent revision of the Jones criteria have recommended three major changes: First, echocardiographically detected, subclinical carditis should be considered a major criteria. Second, risk stratification of the population based on

Table 2.2 Jones criteria for diagnosis of acute fever[a]

Major criteria	Minor criteria
Carditis	Arthralgia
Polyarthritis	Fever
Chorea	Elevated erythrocyte sedimentation rate
Subcutaneous nodules	Positive C-reactive protein
Erythema marginatum	Leukocytosis
	Prolonged PR interval

[a]Two major criteria or one major plus two minor criteria are required for the diagnosis of rheumatic fever. Supportive evidence of recent streptococcal infection is also required for all diagnoses. Chorea, indolent carditis, and post-streptococcal arthritis may not fulfill Jones criteria at the time of diagnosis [74]

disease endemicity and ARF incidence (populations with a known incidence of ARF <2/100,000, or all-age RHD prevalence of <1/1000 are considered low-risk, all others being considered moderate or high risk). Third, different implications of joint manifestations based on baseline risk of the population (aseptic monoarthritis and polyarthralgia are considered major manifestations, and monoarthralgia a minor manifestation in moderate- or high-risk populations) [47]. However, it should be remembered that these guidelines are general expert opinion and have not been prospectively tested in randomized trials.

Although the Jones criteria provide an excellent set of guidelines for the diagnosis of RF, it is important to remember that similar manifestations may be present to varying degrees in other systemic illnesses. For example, streptococcal infection is relatively common, and an elevated ASO titer indicates only previous infection. Similarly, arthralgia is commonly associated with several viral syndromes, and carditis can result from Coxsackie B virus, Lyme disease, or Kawasaki infection. The early manifestations of other collagen diseases, such as systemic lupus erythematosus, may also lead to confusion in diagnosis when they are associated with inflammatory abnormalities of the heart valves, particularly the mitral valve. Rheumatoid arthritis can cause aortic regurgitation, and inflammatory reaction within the pericardium or conduction system may result in pericarditis or heart block. There may be an erythema multiforme type of rash and laboratory evidence of an elevated erythrocyte sedimentation rate (ESR), anemia, and marked leukocytosis. For these reasons, rheumatoid arthritis is easily confused with RF. In a patient who has streptococcal infection and carditis, particularly with evidence of migratory polyarthritis, the diagnosis of RF should be assumed until proved incorrect.

Laboratory Investigations

Evidence of previous streptococcal infection is a prerequisite for the diagnosis of RF. Because RF is a postinfectious immunologic complication, microbiologic evidence is limited, and the evidence for recent streptococcal infection is usually obtained with antistreptococcal antibody tests. The most commonly used antibody assays include ASO and anti-deoxyribonuclease B (anti-DNase B); other antibody tests, such as hyaluronidase, streptokinase, and nicotinamide adenine dinucleotidase, are occasionally used [48]. The antibody response to various streptococcal antigens develops within the first month and remains detectable for 3–6 months after the infection. Antistreptolysin O (ASO) titers are determined by an agglutination test or a hemolytic inhibition test, and in healthy adults, the titers are usually less than 85 Todd units/mL, whereas school-age children can have ASO titers of up to 170 U. Generally, an ASO level of more than 240 U in adults or more than 330 U in children is used for diagnosis, but an interval increase in ASO in two serial samples is more conclusive. Because ASO titers rise and fall more rapidly, the anti-DNase B test can be performed if ASO is nondiagnostic. The streptozyme test, a rapid slide agglutination test for antibodies against five streptococcal antigens, has been proposed as an additional screening method to improve the detection of streptococcal infection.

The electrocardiogram may be normal in patients with ARF. In patients who have cardiac involvement, ST-segment change may signal pericarditis, whereas repolarization abnormalities, including QT prolongation and T inversion, may indicate myocarditis. Such patients may also have sinus tachycardia, ventricular extrasystoles, supraventricular tachycardia, and atrioventricular block. First-degree atrioventricular block is commonly seen in patients with RF but is equally common in patients with and without carditis. The chest radiograph has been traditionally used to evaluate cardiomegaly and is an inexpensive way to study the evolution of the patient under treatment.

Echocardiography has become the tool of choice in diagnosis and monitoring cardiac structure and function. Current echocardiographic techniques were not available during many of the major RF epidemics, so its utility remains unclear. An echocardiogram will quickly determine whether a clinically undetectable murmur is truly absent and will protect patients with clinical carditis from being grouped with non-carditic patients, who have a more benign prognosis and require a shorter secondary prophylaxis regimen. Echocardiography detects valve regurgitation more often than clinical examination alone [49]; this advantage is greater in cases with aortic valve involvement. More importantly, echocardiographic data also suggest that in a significant number of patients, echo-detectable valve regurgitation persists despite adequate prophylaxis, suggesting that echo-detectable cardiac involvement might represent clinically important cardiac damage [40].

The clinical situation is different in the developing world [50], where the incidence of recurrent RF and the prevalence of RHD are high and access to medical care is limited. First attacks are rarely witnessed, and patients present with recurrences and usually with established heart disease. Physical examination is the most commonly used method to detect cases with and without cardiac involvement. Moreover, there is some evidence, albeit controversial, that echocardiography has no incremental diagnostic benefit for patients with advanced disease who live in endemic areas; this is probably due to a cumulative effect of multiple clinical and subclinical recurrences [39]. In addition, a study found that most echo-detectable carditis was also clinically detected within a short period of follow-up [51]. Recurrences are common, and medical records are sparse; thus, one cannot be sure if trivial regurgitation represents new carditis or residua of previous episodes in patients with streptococcal pharyngitis or congenitally present mitral or tricuspid regurgitation, especially in females, in whom these findings are common even among those who are otherwise healthy. Echocardiographic facilities are not widely available, and the cost and additional workload imposed by the universal use of echocardiography in RF episodes are likely to be enormous. Therefore, detecting subclinical carditis in this population may not only be costly but also probably will not change the management strategy very much; none of the RF therapies available to date modify the natural history of carditis, and the initial period of prophylaxis is no different in patients without and with mild carditis [50]. In this population, carditis mandates lifelong prophylaxis, as does valvular disease. It is interesting to note that adding echocardiography to the initial workup did not seem to make prophylaxis more rigorous in the developed world; only a small proportion of patients were taking prophylactic medications on long-term follow-up [51]. Finally, the natural history of echo-detectable carditis is just being evaluated, and there may be merit in exercising caution [52] about making echocardiography the cornerstone of diagnosing carditis. Until there is a convincing body of data that demonstrates both the need to detect subclinical carditis and the possibility of actually modifying its natural history, echo-detectable carditis may divert scarce and valuable prophylaxis resources from more proven entities that need these urgently. Therefore, for patients in developing countries, echocardiography should be used only selectively in cases of RF [50]. Of course, the value of echocardiography for detecting and managing established RHD in any population is unquestioned.

Computed tomography and magnetic resonance imaging may also be useful in diagnosing myocarditis, but their usefulness in RF patients remains unclear [53]. Endomyocardial biopsies have been performed in persons with acute rheumatic carditis. Aschoff nodules, which are pathognomonic features of rheumatic carditis, are observed in 40% of patients, thereby offering a test with limited sensitivity [29]. However, because biopsy results are mostly normal in patients with chronic RHD or non-carditic manifestations of RF, the specificity of the test is very high. In addition, various radionuclide imaging approaches have been evaluated in rheumatic carditis, with variable success [54]; these approaches include imaging with indium 111 (111In)-labeled antimyosin antibodies, radiolabeled leukocytes, and gallium 67 (67Ga) scintigraphy. The utility of these techniques remains unproven, and they should be considered experimental at this time.

Natural History

A major problem with understanding the natural history of RF is that most data are old and have not been reevaluated in the current diagnostic and therapeutic milieu. It appears that the natural history of RF has changed significantly with the advent of prophylaxis, better recognition of antecedent streptococcal infections, and evolution in streptococcal virulence. Rheumatic fever appears to behave differently in developing countries than in the developed world. Presumably because of conducive socioeconomic factors, patients in developing countries have multiple recurrences and a particularly aggressive course [55]. However, it is heartening that even in this situation, regular prophylaxis favorably modifies this bleak natural history.

First attacks of RF in children characteristically occur between the ages of 5 and 15 years. Rheumatic fever rarely occurs in children younger than 2 years, and first attacks after the age of 40 years are also uncommon. Individuals who have RF are susceptible to recurrences of the disease, but this susceptibility again diminishes with time. Rheumatic fever can recur with various manifestations at intervals of weeks, months, or years, with apparent inactivity between these episodes. Congestive heart failure (CHF) is a seriously adverse prognostic indicator; cardiomegaly and CHF that do not improve with treatment are associated with the worst prognosis.

In patients without major valvular damage, preventing recurrent attacks substantially improves prognosis with regard to overall survival and freedom from heart disease. If there is valvular involvement, the scarring process may lead to long-term impairment of valve function that progresses over 10–30 years, with various combinations of stenosis and regurgitation. Perhaps the most insidious valvular lesion is mitral stenosis, which may develop very late—as long as 20 years after the onset of the acute infection—often with no symptoms until the onset of atrial fibrillation and heart failure. The onset of arrhythmias can be the beginning of rapid deterioration or thrombotic complications. Patients with valve dysfunction remain at risk for subacute bacterial endocarditis and should receive prophylactic antibiotics before procedures, as indicated by consensus guidelines.

Treatment

The primary objective in treating patients with acute RF is eliminating the offending streptococci with appropriate antibiotic therapy; penicillin remains the agent of choice (Table 2.3). The list of other options is long, but it is important to remember that some of the more commonly used ones may not be as effective as others in preventing recurrent ARF [56]. The second objective of treating acute RF is to eliminate the inflammatory state, particularly that involving vital organs such as the heart. Salicylates, predominantly aspirin, have been used for many years as anti-inflammatory agents in RF patients. They are very effective, and the diagnosis of RF is suspect if high-dose salicylates do not significantly resolve joint pain and inflammation within 48 h. Relatively high doses are needed: up to 8–10 g/day (100 mg/kg/day) for

Table 2.3 Secondary prevention of rheumatic fever

Agent	Dose	Mode	Schedule
Benzathine penicillin G[a]	1.2 million U	Intramuscular	Every 4 weeks[b]
Penicillin V[c]	250 mg 2×/day	Oral	Daily
Sulfadiazine[d]			Daily
For patients <27 kg (60 lbs)	500 mg		
For patients ≥27 kg (60 lbs)	1000 mg		
Erythromycin[e]	250 mg 2×/day	Oral	Daily

[a]Administer drug at room temperature and with procaine penicillin to reduce pain
[b]Consider three times weekly in high-risk situations, including in Third World countries
[c]May interfere with oral contraception
[d]Avoid use in pregnancy. More effective than oral penicillin
[e]For patients with penicillin and sulfa allergy

a period of 3–4 weeks. A gradual taper is recommended to avoid rebound worsening. Salicylates do not alter the natural history of the disease.

Corticosteroids are used in patients with severe carditis and heart failure. Steroids rapidly suppress the toxic state, relieve inflammation, help prevent the appearance of new murmurs, help murmurs disappear faster, allow faster resolution of pericardial effusions, and may be lifesaving in patients with critical illness [57]. Similar to other therapies for RF patients, they do not alter the disease's long-term natural history [57, 58]. However, most of the published studies are old, have serious methodologic problems, and did not study current immunosuppressive therapies. A short course of steroids is commonly used in patients with severe carditis [4]. Prednisone is given at 1–2 mg/kg/day for 3 weeks, with a tapering schedule once the acute symptoms resolve.

There are no definitive end points for discontinuing anti-inflammatory therapy in RF. General indicators include the absence of clinical symptoms and signs of rheumatic activity, in addition to normalization of acute-phase reactants, usually ESR and C-reactive protein. Too-rapid reduction can be accompanied by a symptomatic rebound. The steroid taper is occasionally covered with salicylates to prevent a relapse. If heart failure continues to persist despite steroid therapy, surgical repair of mechanical lesions should be considered instead of prolonged trials with high-dose steroids.

It was long believed that surgery should not be undertaken when the patient is an acute inflammatory state, because early studies showed higher surgical mortality rates in patients with acute RF. However, this is changing. Essop and associates [44] reported no deaths among patients with active carditis who underwent mitral valve or mitral and aortic valve replacement, and surgery was associated with rapid and substantial improvement, including a reduction in left ventricular dimensions. A subsequent series with a much longer follow-up period showed that surgery during acute rheumatic carditis may be associated with a somewhat less favorable outcome after mitral valve repair, and that during the acute episode, surgical treatment should be reserved for patients who are refractory to medical therapy [59]. In this series, there was a relatively high incidence of valve failure (27%), and acute carditis was the strongest predictor of reoperation. Cardiac surgery has been used with greater success in patients with chronic RHD. It appears that many of these patients have repairable valves [60, 61], although valve repair carries some risk of reoperation.

The third important objective in treating RF is to prevent recurrences of rheumatic activity [62]. This is achieved by long-term antibiotic prophylaxis to prevent streptococcal pharyngitis (Table 2.4). A secondary prophylaxis program should begin during the acute episode of RF and should be focused on preventing streptococcal pharyngitis. Though the practice of secondary antibiotic prophylaxis for preventing recurrences or progression of valve disease is based on low-quality evidence [63], it is supported by strong biologic plausibility. Rheumatic fever is a recurrent disease, and patients who had carditis in previous attacks have a higher recurrence rate per streptococcal infection than those without previous carditis [64–66]. The risk of recurrence per streptococcal infection may be as high as 40–60% in young patients with established RHD, and every recurrence further damages the heart. Rheumatic fever recurrences can be prevented by chemoprophylaxis of streptococcal infections, which may result in an eventual reduction in the prevalence of residual heart disease [43, 51, 62–66], reduced need for operations, and a possible subsequent reduction in RHD-related mortality. The duration of prophylaxis depends on the likelihood of acquiring streptococcal infection, the anticipated risk of RF recurrence with each streptococcal throat infection, and whether carditis develops during the index RF episodes. The risk of RF recurrence is likely to be higher in patients with carditis or residual heart disease, multiple previous attacks, and younger age, whereas the risk decreases with the interval after the last attack. Streptococcal infections are more common in schoolchildren, their parents, teachers, and health personnel in contact with children, and persons living in closed quarters or in crowded housing. Recommendations for the choice of antibiotics and duration of prophylaxis are listed in Tables 2.3 and 2.4 [3, 62]. The need for prophylaxis should be reassessed periodically. In all situations, the decision to discontinue prophylaxis should be made after discussing the potential risks and benefits with the patient. While it is obvious that this regimen has the potential to significantly reduce morbidity associated with ARF, rates of adherence to these guidelines has remained dismal [67]. This poses serious challenges to the ARF/RHD control effort.

Table 2.4 Duration of secondary rheumatic fever prophylaxis[a]

	Risk of streptococcal infection[b]		
Risk factor(s)	High	Not high	Not high
RHD	Lifelong	Age <40 years	Age ≥40 years[c]
History of carditis and no RHD[d]	Until age 40 years[c]	Until age 40 years[c]	None[c]
RF and no carditis	Until age 21 years[c] or 10 years from last attack[e]	Until age 21 years[c] or 10 years from last attack[e]	None[c]
		Until age 21 years[c] or 5 years from last attack[e]	None[c]

RF rheumatic fever, *RHD* residual rheumatic heart disease (of any severity)
Patients from developing countries who have large RF burden should be considered at high risk for recurrent infection
[a]Each case is judged individually after considering the clinical situation and the patient's wishes
[b]Modify prophylaxis in epidemic situations, especially if virulent streptococci reemerge
[c]Should be at least 10 years since last attack and should not have history of multiple attacks
[d]Use echocardiography if possible to prove or disprove RHD
[e]Whichever is longer in duration

Reviews of additional forms of therapy are beyond the scope of this chapter, but several such reviews are available for the interested reader [4, 68–74].

References

1. World Health Organization. Rheumatic fever and rheumatic heart disease. Report of a WHO study group. Technical report series no. 764. 1988.
2. World Health Organization. Joint WHO/ISFC meeting on rheumatic fever/rheumatic heart disease control, with emphasis on primary prevention. WHO document WHO/CVD 94.1. Geneva, 7–9, 1994.
3. World Health Organization. Rheumatic fever and rheumatic heart disease. Report of a WHO expert consultation. WHO technical report series no. 923. 2004.
4. Karthikeyan G, Guilherme L. Acute rheumatic fever. Lancet. 2018;392:161–74.
5. Veasy LG, Wiedmeier SE, Orsmond GS, et al. Resurgence of acute rheumatic fever in the intermountain area of the United States. N Engl J Med. 1987;316:421–7.
6. Watkins DA, Johnson CO, Colquhoun SM, Karthikeyan G, et al. Global, regional, and national burden of rheumatic heart disease, 1990–2015. N Engl J Med. 2017;377:713–22.
7. Kaplan EL, Hill HR. Return of rheumatic fever: consequences, implications, and needs. J Pediatr. 1987;111:244–6.
8. Hafez M, el-Battoty MF, Hawas S, et al. Evidence of inherited susceptibility of increased streptococcal adherence to pharyngeal cells of children with rheumatic fever. Br J Rheumatol. 1989;28:304–9.
9. Stollerman GH. Rheumatogenic streptococci and autoimmunity. Clin Immunol Immunopathol. 1991;61:131–42.
10. Ayoub EM. The search for host determinants of susceptibility to rheumatic fever: the missing link. T. Duckett Jones Memorial Lecture. Circulation. 1984;69:197–201.
11. Rajapakse CN, Halim K, Al-Orainey I, Al-Nozha M, Al-Aska AK. A genetic marker for rheumatic heart disease. Br Heart J. 1987;58:659–62.
12. Guilherme L, Köhler KF, Kalil J. Rheumatic heart disease: genes, inflammation and autoimmunity. Rheumatol Curr Res. 2012;S4:001.
13. Engel ME, Stander R, Vogel J, Adeyemo AA, Mayosi BM. Genetic susceptibility to acute rheumatic fever: a systematic review and meta-analysis of twin studies. PLoS One. 2011;6(9):e25326.
14. Gray LA, D'Antoine HA, Tong SYC, McKinnon M, et al. Genome-wide analysis of genetic risk factors for rheumatic heart disease in aboriginal Australians provides support for pathogenic molecular mimicry. J Infect Dis. 2017;216(11):1460–70.
15. Parks T, Mirabel MM, Kado J, Auckland K, et al. Association between a common immunoglobulin heavy chain allele and rheumatic heart disease risk in Oceania. Nat Commun. 2017;8:14946.
16. McDonald M, Currie BJ, Carapetis JR. Acute rheumatic fever: a chink in the chain that links the heart to the throat? Lancet Infect Dis. 2004;4:240–5.
17. Goldstein I, Halpern B, Robert L. Immunological relationship between streptococcus a polysaccharide and the structural glycoproteins of heart valve. Nature. 1967;213:44.
18. Dudding BA, Ayoub EM. Persistence of streptococcal group A antibody in patients with rheumatic valvular disease. J Exp Med. 1968;128:1081–98.
19. Tomai M, Kotb M, Majumdar G, Beachey EH. Superantigenicity of streptococcal M protein. J Exp Med. 1990;172:359–62.
20. Guilherme L, Cunha-Neto E, Coelho V, et al. Human heart-infiltrating T-cell clones from rheumatic heart disease patients recognize both streptococcal and cardiac proteins. Circulation. 1995;92:415–20.
21. Fae KC, da Silva DD, Oshiro SE, Tanaka AC, et al. Mimicry in recognition of cardiac myosin peptides by heart-intralesional T cell clones from rheumatic heart disease. J Immunol. 2006;176:5662–70.
22. Cunningham MW, Antone SM, Smart M, Liu R, Kosanke S. Molecular analysis of human cardiac myosin-cross-reactive B- and T-cell epitopes of the group A streptococcal M5 protein. Infect Immun. 1997;65:3913–23.
23. Roberts S, Kosanke S, Dunn ST, Jankelow D, Duran CMG, Cunningham MW. Pathogenic mechanisms in rheumatic carditis: focus on valvular endothelium. J Infect Dis. 2001;183(3):507–11.
24. Guilherme L, Cury P, Demarchi LM, Coelho V, et al. Rheumatic heart disease: proinflammatory cytokines play a role in the progression and maintenance of valvular lesions. Am J Pathol. 2004;165(5):1583–91.
25. Tandon R, Sharma M, Chandrashekhar Y, Kotb M, Yacoub MH, Narula J. Revisiting the pathogenesis of rheumatic fever and carditis. Nat Rev Cardiol. 2013;10:171–7.
26. McAllister HA Jr, Buja LM, Ferrans VJ. Valvular heart disease: anatomic abnormalities. In: Willerson JT, Cohn JN, Wellens HJJ, Holmes DR, editors. Cardiovascular medicine. 3rd ed. London: Springer; 2007. p. 369–79.
27. Vaideeswar P, Butany J. Valvular heart disease. In: Buja LM, Butany J, editors. Cardiovascular pathology. 4th ed. London: Elsevier/Academic Press; 2016. p. 485–528.
28. Virmani R, Roberts WC. Aschoff bodies in operatively excised atrial appendages and in papillary muscles. Frequency and clinical significance. Circulation. 1977;55:559–63.
29. Narula J, Chopra P, Talwar KK, et al. Does endomyocardial biopsy aid in the diagnosis of active rheumatic carditis? Circulation. 1993;88:2198–205.
30. Veasy LG. Myocardial dysfunction in active rheumatic carditis. J Am Coll Cardiol. 1994;24:581–2.
31. Williams RV, Minich LL, Shaddy RE, Veasy LG, Tani LY. Evidence for lack of myocardial injury in children with acute rheumatic carditis. Cardiol Young. 2002;12:519–23.

32. Massell BF, Narula J. Rheumatic fever and carditis. In: Braunwald E, editor. The atlas of heart diseases. Philadelphia, PA: Current Medicine; 1994. p. 10.11–20.
33. Cann MP, Sive AA, Norton RE, McBride WJ, Ketheesan N. Clinical presentation of rheumatic fever in an endemic area. Arch Dis Child. 2010;95(6):455–7. https://doi.org/10.1136/adc.2008.157107.
34. Padmavati S, Gupta V. Reappraisal of the Jones criteria: the Indian experience. N Z Med J. 1988;101:391–2.
35. Deighton C. Beta haemolytic streptococci and reactive arthritis in adults. Ann Rheum Dis. 1993;52:475–82.
36. Kothari SS, Chandrashekhar Y, Tandon RK. Rheumatic carditis. In: Narula J, Tandon R, Reddy KS, Virmani R, editors. Rheumatic fever. Washington, DC: AFIP Press; 1998.
37. Raju BS, Turi ZG. Rheumatic fever. In: Bonow RO, Mann DL, Zipes DP, Libby P, editors. Braunwald's heart disease: a textbook of cardiovascular medicine. 9th ed. Philadelphia, PA: Saunders/Elsevier; 2012. p. 1868–75.
38. Bland EF, Duckett Jones T. Rheumatic fever and rheumatic heart disease; a twenty year report on 1000 patients followed since childhood. Circulation. 1951;4:836–43.
39. Vasan RS, Shrivastava S, Vijayakumar M, Narang R, Lister BC, Narula J. Echocardiographic evaluation of patients with acute rheumatic fever and rheumatic carditis. Circulation. 1996;94:73–82.
40. Tubridy-Clark M, Carapetis JR. Subclinical carditis in rheumatic fever: a systematic review. Int J Cardiol. 2007;119:54–8.
41. Marcus RH, Sareli P, Pocock WA, et al. Functional anatomy of severe mitral regurgitation in active rheumatic carditis. Am J Cardiol. 1989;63:577–84.
42. Massell BF, Fyler DC, Roy SB. The clinical picture of rheumatic fever: diagnosis, immediate prognosis, course, and therapeutic implications. Am J Cardiol. 1958;1:436–49.
43. Tompkins DG, Boxerbaum B, Liebman J. Long-term prognosis of rheumatic fever patients receiving regular intramuscular benzathine penicillin. Circulation. 1972;45:543–51.
44. Essop MR, Wisenbaugh T, Sareli P. Evidence against a myocardial factor as the cause of left ventricular dilation in active rheumatic carditis. J Am Coll Cardiol. 1993;22:826–9.
45. Jones T. The diagnosis of rheumatic fever. JAMA. 1944;126:481–4.
46. Ferrieri P, Jones Criteria Working Group. Proceedings of the Jones Criteria workshop. Circulation. 2002;106:2521–3.
47. Gewitz MH, Baltimore RS, Tani LY, Sable CA, et al. Revision of the Jones Criteria for the diagnosis of acute rheumatic fever in the era of Doppler echocardiography: a scientific statement from the American Heart Association. Circulation. 2015;131(20):1806–18.
48. Burdash NM, Teti G, Hund P. Streptococcal antibody tests in rheumatic fever. Ann Clin Lab Sci. 1986;16:163–70.
49. Figueroa FE, Fernandez MS, Valdes P, et al. Prospective comparison of clinical and echocardiographic diagnosis of rheumatic carditis: long term follow up of patients with subclinical disease. Heart. 2001;85:407–10.
50. Narula J, Chandrasekhar Y, Rahimtoola S. Diagnosis of active rheumatic carditis. The echoes of change. Circulation. 1999;100:1576–81.
51. Abernethy M, Bass N, Sharpe N, et al. Doppler echocardiography and the early diagnosis of carditis in acute rheumatic fever. Aust NZ J Med. 1994;24:530–5.
52. Dajani AS, Allen HD, Taubert KA. Echocardiography for diagnosis and management of rheumatic fever-reply. JAMA. 1993;269:2084.
53. Gagliardi MG, Bevilacqua M, Di Renzi P, Picardo S, Passariello R, Marcelletti C. Usefulness of magnetic resonance imaging for diagnosis of acute myocarditis in infants and children, and comparison with endomyocardial biopsy. Am J Cardiol. 1991;68:1089–91.
54. Bhatnagar A, Calegaro JUM, Narula J. Radionuclide imaging in rheumatic fever. In: Narula J, Virmani R, Reddy KS, Tandon R, editors. Rheumatic fever. Washington, DC: American Registry of Pathology; 1999. p. 329–38.
55. Roy SB, Bhatia ML, Lazaro EJ, Ramalingaswami V. Juvenile mitral stenosis in India. Lancet. 1963;2:1193–5.
56. Congeni B, Rizzo C, Congeni J, Sreenivasan VV. Outbreak of acute rheumatic fever in northeast Ohio. J Pediatr. 1987;111:176–9.
57. Albert DA, Harel L, Karrison T. The treatment of rheumatic carditis: a review and meta-analysis. Medicine (Baltimore). 1995;74:1–12.
58. Skoularigis J, Sinovich V, Joubert G, Sareli P. Evaluation of the long-term results of mitral valve repair in 254 young patients with rheumatic mitral regurgitation. Circulation. 1994;90:II167–74.
59. Cilliers A, Adler AJ, Saloojee H. Anti-inflammatory treatment for carditis in acute rheumatic fever. Cochrane Database Syst Rev. 2015;(5):CD003176.
60. Choudhary SK, Talwar S, Dubey B, Chopra A, Saxena A, Kumar AS. Mitral valve repair in a predominantly rheumatic population. Long-term results. Tex Heart Inst J. 2001;28:8–15.
61. Grinda JM, Latremouille C, Berrebi AJ, et al. Aortic cusp extension valvuloplasty for rheumatic aortic valve disease: midterm results. Ann Thorac Surg. 2002;74:438–43.
62. Chandrashekhar Y. Secondary prevention: theory, practice and analysis of available trials. In: Narula J, Tandon R, Reddy KS, Virmani R, editors. Rheumatic fever. Washington, DC: AFIP Press; 1999. p. 399–442.
63. Manyemba J, Mayosi BM. Penicillin for secondary prevention of rheumatic fever. Cochrane Database Syst Rev. 2002;(3):CD002227.
64. Majeed HA, Batnager S, Yousof AM, Khuffash F, Yusuf AR. Acute rheumatic fever and the evolution of rheumatic heart disease: a prospective 12 year follow-up report. J Clin Epidemiol. 1992;45:871–5.
65. Sanyal SK, Berry AM, Duggal S, Hooja V, Ghosh S. Sequelae of the initial attack of acute rheumatic fever in children from north India. A prospective 5-year follow-up study. Circulation. 1982;65:375–9.
66. United Kingdom and United States Joint Report on Rheumatic Heart Disease. The natural history of rheumatic fever and rheumatic heart disease. Ten-year report of a cooperative clinical trial of ACTH, cortisone, and aspirin. Circulation. 1965;32:457–76.
67. Robertson KA, Volmink JA, Mayosi BM. Lack of adherence to the national guidelines on the prevention of rheumatic fever. S Afr Med J. 2005;95:52–6.
68. Bessen DE, Fischetti VA. Vaccines against Streptococcus pyogenes infections. In: Levine MM, Woodrow GC, Kaper JB, Cobon GS, editors. New generation vaccines. New York: Marcel Dekker; 1977. p. 83–802.
69. Dale JB, Chiang EC. Intranasal immunization with recombinant group A streptococcal M protein fragment fused to the B subunit of Escherichia coli labile toxin protects mice against systemic challenge infections. J Infect Dis. 1995;171:1038–41.
70. Dale JB, Simmons M, Chiang EC, Chiang EY. Recombinant, octavalent group A streptococcal M protein vaccine. Vaccine. 1996;14:944–8.
71. Ji Y, Carlson B, Kondagunta A, Cleary PP. Intranasal immunization with C5a peptidase prevents nasopharyngeal colonization of mice by the group A Streptococcus. Infect Immun. 1997;65:2080–7.
72. Kapur V, Maffei JT, Greer RS, Li LL, Adams GJ, Musser JM. Vaccination with streptococcal extracellular cysteine protease (interleukin-1 beta convertase) protects mice against challenge with heterologous group A streptococci. Microb Pathog. 1994;16:443–50.
73. Lancefield RC. Persistence of type-specific antibodies in man following infection with group A streptococci. J Exp Med. 1959;110:271–92.
74. Stollerman GH. Changing streptococci and prospects for the global eradication of rheumatic fever. Perspect Biol Med. 1997;40:165–89.

Infective Endocarditis

3

Tina Shah, Richard J. Hamill, and Kumudha Ramasubbu

Introduction

Endocarditis is the inflammation of the cardiac endocardium and may affect the cardiac valves, mural endocardium, or surface of catheters or devices implanted in the heart. The inflammation may be secondary to an infection or a noninfectious process. This chapter will focus on infective endocarditis.

Epidemiology

About 10,000–15,000 new cases of infective endocarditis (IE) are diagnosed each year in the United States. Studies have reported an incidence of anywhere from 0.6 to 11.6 cases per 100,000 person-years [1–3]. The differences in this rate are likely due to variability in the definition of endocarditis and regional differences in rheumatic heart disease and intravenous drug use. The incidence has been reported to be higher in men than women with a male to female ratio >2:1 [4]. The majority of cases occur in patients above the age of 60 with the median age at diagnosis increasing over the years [5]. The epidemiologic landscape of endocarditis is changing with less cases occurring as a result of rheumatologic heart disease and more cases noted in degenerative valvular disease, prosthetic valves, implanted devices, and catheters. This is attributed to the decreasing incidence of rheumatic heart disease and aging population and thus the rising prevalence degenerative valve disease [6].

T. Shah · K. Ramasubbu (✉)
New York-Presbyterian Brooklyn Methodist Hospital, Brooklyn, NY, USA
e-mail: kur9002@nyp.org

R. J. Hamill
Department of Medicine and Molecular Virology and Microbiology, Baylor College of Medicine, Houston, TX, USA

Infectious Diseases Section, Department of Medicine, Michael E. DeBakey VA Medical Center, Houston, TX, USA

About ¾ of the patients presenting with IE have prior structural heart disease including valvular disease, congenital heart disease, prosthetic heart valve replacement, and history of previous endocarditis. Other risk factors include intravenous drug use (IVDU), poor dentition/dental infection, presence of an intravascular catheter/device, impaired immune response/HIV, and invasive procedures. PVE accounts for 10–20% of cases of IE with a valve in the mitral position being more susceptible to infection. Healthcare associated IE (which includes nosocomially acquired cases and cases related to intravascular catheters and devices) comprises approximately 23–27% of all IE cases [7]. Prior endocarditis is a risk factor for subsequent endocarditis and recurrent endocarditis occurs in ~4.5% of cases. Incidence of IVDU-associated IE differs based on geographical location studied and the incidence of IVDU in the specific location. In Philadelphia, for example, the incidence of IVDU-associated IE was ~5.3 cases per 100,000 person-years, almost half of all IE cases [8].

Despite improvements in diagnosis and treatment, mortality in patients with IE remains high. In-hospital mortality in patients diagnosed with IE ranges from 18 to 23% and 6 month mortality has been reported to be 22–27%. Risk factors for poor outcome, apart from IE complications (discussed later), include female gender, diabetes mellitus, low serum albumin, and poor surgical candidacy [4, 9–11]. Prognosis varies considerably with patients with right-sided IE or uncomplicated left-sided native IE demonstrating the best prognosis (mortality <10%) and patients with *Staphylococcus aureus* prosthetic valve endocarditis exhibiting the highest mortality rate (~40%) [12, 13]. Death in IE is usually a result of heart failure, stroke, multi-organ failure, and sepsis.

The incidence of IE has not changed much over the past few decades despite improvements in diagnostic tests and treatment strategies. This apparent paradox is explained by a progressive evolution in risk factors [14]. Besides the classic predisposing conditions such as rheumatic heart disease, new risk factors like intravenous drug use, sclerotic valve

B. A. Carabello (ed.), *Valvular Heart Disease*, Cardiovascular Medicine, https://doi.org/10.1007/978-1-4471-2840-3_3

disease in elderly patients, use of prosthetic valves and other intracardiac devices, and nosocomial disease (often associated with more virulent pathogens) have emerged. Resistant organisms and poorly cultivable pathogens also present challenges.

Pathogenesis

Both host and organism factors play a role in the evolution of endocarditis. Typically, damaged valve endothelium is more susceptible to bacterial adherence and infection. Valve damage can occur through persistent turbulent blood flow, trauma through catheters or device leads, repeated injection of particulate matter as in the setting of intravenous drug use (IVDU), age-related valvular degeneration, and chronic inflammation/valvulitis (such as in rheumatologic conditions). The damaged valve surface is coated by sterile platelet and fibrin thrombus. Transient bacteremia can then result in the infection of this coating. Vegetations usually form on the low pressure aspect of valves, i.e., the atrial surface of the mitral valve and ventricular surface of the aortic valve. In the setting of a ventricular septal defect, the low-pressure side is the right ventricle, and the thrombus is usually found on the right side of the defect (Figs. 3.1 and 3.2). A further host factor that may predispose to endocarditis is a compromised immune system as seen, for example, in HIV infection.

Organism-related factors include virulence and adherence properties, and obviously procedures predisposing to bacteremia such as invasive dental procedures, colonoscopy, and insertion of indwelling hemodialysis catheters play an important role.

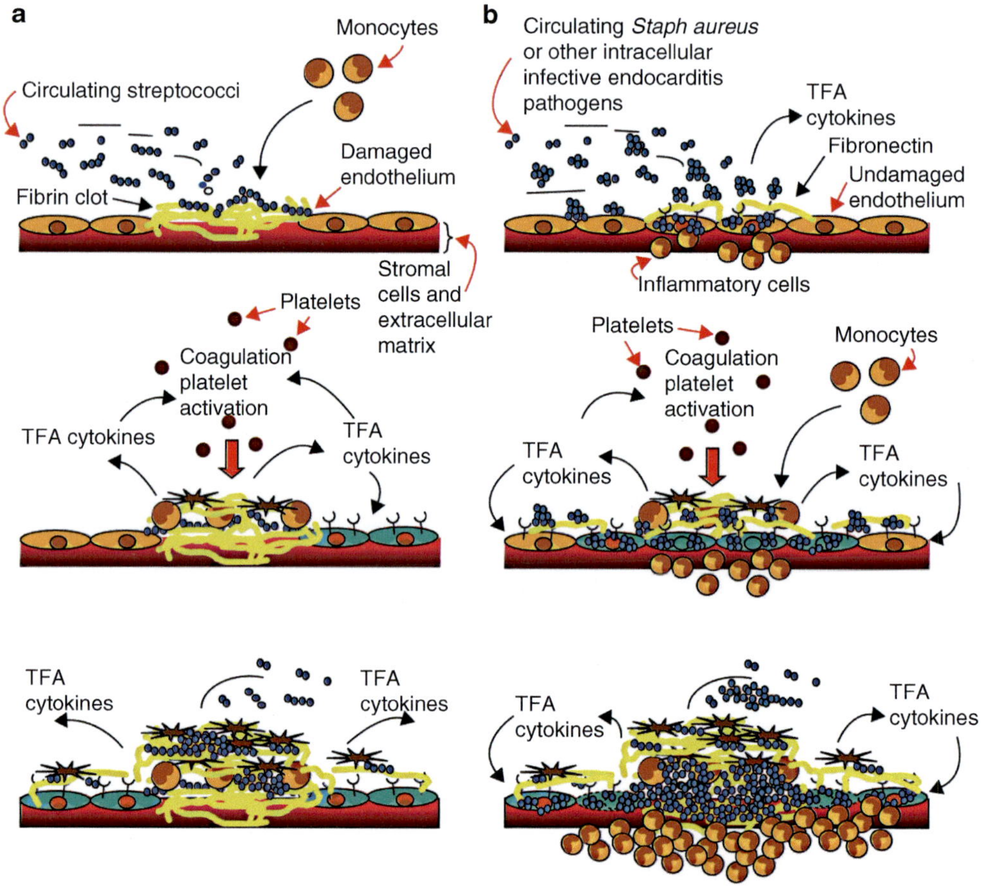

Fig. 3.1 Early steps in bacterial valve colonization. (**a**) *Colonization of damaged epithelium*: exposed stromal cells and extracellular matrix proteins trigger deposition of fibrin-platelet clots to which *Streptococci* bind (upper panel); fibrin-adherent *Streptococci* attract monocytes and induce them to produce tissue-factor activity (TFA) and cytokines (middle panel); these mediators activate coagulation cascade, attract and activate blood platelets, and induce cytokine, integrin, and TFA production from neighboring endothelial cells (lower panel), encouraging vegetation growth. (**b**) *Colonization of inflamed valve tissues*: in response to local inflammation, endothelial cells express integrins that bind plasma fibronectin, which microorganisms adhere to via wall-attached fibronectin-binding proteins, resulting in endothelial internalization of bacteria (upper panel); in response to invasion, endothelial cells produce TFA and cytokines, triggering blood clotting and extension of inflammation, and promoting formation of the vegetation (middle panel); internalized bacteria eventually lyse endothelial cells (green cells) by secreting membrane-active proteins—e.g., hemolysins (lower panel). From Philippe Moreillon, Yok-Ai Que. Infective endocarditis. The Lancet. 2004;363(9403):139–49. Reproduced with permission from Elsevier Limited

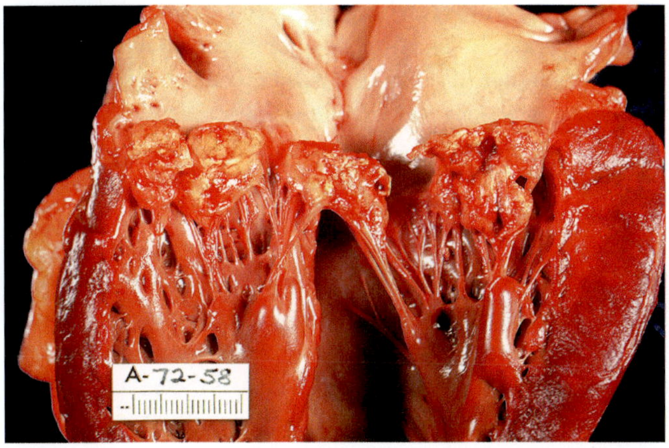

Fig. 3.2 Vegetations on the mitral valve (arrows) in a patient with infective endocarditis [Image courtesy of Dr. Edwin P. Ewing Jr. and the Centers for Disease Control and Prevention (CDC)]

Classification

Traditionally, endocarditis was classified into acute, subacute, and chronic depending on clinical course. Acute native valve endocarditis usually displays a rapidly progressive course with high mortality rates typically caused by virulent organisms such at *Staphylococcus aureus* or group B Streptococci. The course in subacute/chronic endocarditis is more indolent and associated with more nonspecific symptoms, typically associated with less virulent organisms. Other classifications differentiate between native and prosthetic valve endocarditis, endocarditis associated with intravenous drug use and right- and left-sided endocarditis. Classification is now mainly based on defining the clinical setting, organism, location, and mode of acquisition as these factors are more important in guiding choice of treatment strategy and outcome.

Microbiology of Infective Endocarditis

Table 3.1 shows the modern microbiology data from a large international collaborative study of infective endocarditis [7] and is consistent with changes seen in causative organisms in recent years. Whereas, in the past, infective endocarditis due to the viridans streptococci affecting individuals with rheumatic heart disease was most common, a shift in the microbiology has occurred as a result of the declining prevalence of rheumatic heart disease. *Staphylococcus aureus* is now the most prevalent causative agent in most large surveys. The increase in *S. aureus* is fueled by an increase in nosocomial infections. Infective endocarditis due to *S. aureus* frequently occurs in individuals without underlying structural heart disease, although infections involving indwelling cardiac devices are very common. The organism typically causes an acute syndrome and is associated with metastatic abscesses in many different organs. Mortality is high, particularly in cases due to methicillin-resistant staphylococci [13].

Table 3.1 Microbiologic etiology in 2781 patients with definite infective endocarditis

	Number (%) of patients			
	Native valve IE		Intracardiac device IE	
Microbial etiology	Drug abusers (*n* = 237)	Not drug abusers (*n* = 1644)	PVIE (*n* = 463)	Other devices[a] (*n* = 172)
Staphylococcus aureus	160 (68)	457 (28)	129 (23)	60 (35)
Coagulase-negative staphylococci	7 (3)	148 (9)	95 (17)	45 (26)
Viridans group streptococci	24 (10)	345 (21)	70 (12)	14 (8)
Streptococcus gallolyticus[b]	3 (1)	119 (7)	29 (5)	5 (3)
Other streptococci[c]	5 (2)	118 (7)	26 (5)	7 (4)
Enterococcus species	11 (5)	179 (11)	70 (12)	10 (6)
HACEK group[d]	0 (0)	30 (2)	13 (2)	1 (0.5)
Other[e]	6 (3)	62 (4)	38 (7)	10 (6)
Fungi/yeast	3 (1)	16 (1)	23 (4)	2 (1)
Polymicrobial	6 (3)	16 (1)	5 (0.8)	0 (0)
Negative cultures	12 (5)	154 (9)	65 (12)	18 (11)

Modified from Murdoch et al. [7] with permission from American Medical Association

[a]Includes pacemakers and implantable cardioverter defibrillators

[b]Formerly *Streptococcus bovis*

[c]Includes *Streptococcus pneumoniae*, groupable streptococci *A, B, C, and G*

[d]*Haemophilus* spp., *Aggregatibacter* (formerly *Actinobacillus*) *actinomycetemcomitans*, *Cardiobacterium hominis*, *Eikenella corrodens*, and *Kingella* spp.

[e]Includes *Enterbacteriaceae*, *Pseudomonas* spp., *Acinetobacter* spp., *Stenotrophomonas* spp., *Burkholderia* spp., *Neisseria* spp., Anaerobes, *Salmonella* spp., *Brucella* spp., and others

Coagulase-negative staphylococci (CNS) are an infrequent cause of native valve endocarditis. The infection is healthcare associated in one-half of patients, with a large proportion of patients having an indwelling pacemaker or implantable defibrillator. Compared with patients who have *S. aureus* native valve endocarditis, patients with CNS IE have a much more indolent course and are less likely to have vascular or immunologic evidence of infective endocarditis on physical examination. Heart failure is a frequent complication (>40%) and mortality rates are substantial (25%) [15]. Coagulase-negative staphylococci are a common cause of prosthetic valve endocarditis, with nearly one-half of cases occurring between 60 and 365 days following valve replacement [16]. One-half of patients develop intracardiac abscesses; mortality is approximately 24%.

Viridans streptococci (*S. mitis*, *S. sanguis*, *S. mitior*, *S. mutans*) are less frequent causes of infective endocarditis with the decreasing prevalence of rheumatic heart disease. These organisms cause a subacute syndrome resulting in symptoms that can last weeks to months. Valvular complications are less common than in IE cases caused by *S. aureus*. Organisms previously referred to as "nutritionally-deficient streptococci" include *Abiotrophia defectiva* and *Granulicatella adiacens*. Identification of these bacteria is more difficult because of their slow growth and the requirement for addition of pyridoxal hydrochloride to culture media. These organisms have been associated with large vegetations, embolic phenomena, and valvular destruction [17].

Organisms, formerly known as *Streptococcus bovis*, have undergone taxonomic reclassification, although this reclassification has not been enthusiastically embraced. *S. gallolyticus* is the newly recognized name for *S. bovis* biotype I. These organisms, usually categorized as group D streptococci, can occasionally be erroneously identified as viridans streptococci by the laboratory. *S. gallolyticus* causes disease most commonly in elderly individuals, usually with some underlying chronic illnesses. Up to 60% of patients with infective endocarditis due to *S. gallolyticus* will ultimately be found to have a concomitant adenoma or carcinoma of the bowel upon thorough investigation. Therefore, any patient with infective endocarditis due to this organism warrants an evaluation for gastrointestinal disorders [18].

Infective endocarditis due to *Streptococcus pneumoniae* is uncommon, accounting for only 1.4% of cases of endocarditis in one large Spanish cohort [19]. It is accompanied by a substantial mortality rate, in excess of 35%, because the diagnosis of endocarditis is often missed, overshadowed by other manifestations of pneumococcal disease, such as pneumonia and meningitis. Left heart failure is common due to aortic or mitral valvular involvement.

Enterococcal species are now the third most common cause of infective endocarditis with *Enterococcus faecalis* accounting for 90% of these cases and with *E. faecium* being less frequently implicated. These organisms tend to affect the elderly and debilitated, frequently patients with underlying cardiac disorders or valvular prostheses. Twenty-five percent of cases are healthcare associated, 30% of which affect prosthetic valves. Recently, trends in North America indicate an increasing number of cases caused by antimicrobial-resistant *E. faecium* strains. The mortality rate for enterococcal endocarditis has not changed according to recent surveys, ranging between 11 and 18% [20].

HACEK is an acronym assigned to a group of fastidious, gram-negative bacteria that colonize the oropharynx and are responsible for about 1.4% of cases of infective endocarditis. Organisms in this group include *Haemophilus parainfluenzae*, *Aggregatibacter* (formerly *Actinobacillus*) *actinomycetemcomitans*, *A. aphrophilus*, *A. paraphrophilus*, *A. snegnis*, *Cardiobacterium hominis*, *C. valvarum*, *Eikenella corrodens*, *Kingella kingii*, and *K. denitrificans*. HACEK organisms tend to cause disease in younger individuals, and produce a subacute syndrome characterized by a higher prevalence of immunologic and vascular phenomena, including emboli. Patients infected with HACEK organisms suffer from heart failure less frequently than IE caused by other agents. Despite the higher incidence of embolic manifestations, the overall prognosis of endocarditis due to the HACEK group of organisms tends to be excellent with a lower mortality (4%), and good outcomes with either medical or surgical therapies [21].

Non-HACEK gram-negative bacilli are unusual causes of infective endocarditis, and include various members of the *Enterobacteriaceae* and *Pseudomonas* spp., most frequently. The portal of entry is also changing. While previously, parenteral drug abusers were more commonly afflicted, recent data indicate that the disease is often nosocomially acquired, and involvement of implanted endovascular devices is frequent. Forty percent of cases occur on native valves, and 60% on prosthetic valves and devices. These patients are more likely to have undergone previous invasive gastrointestinal or genitourinary procedures before diagnosis of IE, with symptoms frequently being present for longer than a month [22, 23].

Fungal causes of endocarditis account for 2–4% of all cases [24]. Several different host risk factors predispose to infection by fungi, including parenteral drug abuse, individuals with indwelling vascular catheters and prosthetic devices, and patients with a compromised immune system. Clinical manifestations of fungal endocarditis are nonspecific, although vascular embolic manifestations are not uncommon. *Candida* spp. are the most frequently implicated fungi, with *C. albicans* and non-*albicans Candida* accounting for equal numbers; however, recent data suggests an increase in the frequency of non-*albicans Candida* spp. which has significant implications for antifungal therapy. *Aspergillus* IE most commonly occurs as a prosthetic valve infection, and can be difficult to diagnosis because of the infrequency of positive blood cultures; diagnosis is occasionally made from examination of embolectomy specimens.

Despite improved blood culture systems, the increased utilization of molecular biological techniques and serological methodologies, 5–10% of cases of endocarditis are still unidentified. Culture negative cases can result from previous antibiotic therapy, endocarditis due to fastidious organisms, and true blood culture negative cases that result from organisms that cannot be grown using conventional techniques. The latter group includes such organisms as *Coxiella burnetti*, *Bartonella* sp., and *Tropheryma whipplei*, the causative agent of Whipple's disease [25].

Diagnosis

Key to the outcome of IE is the rapid identification of patients with highly probable or definite IE and subsequent institution of treatment (antibiotics with and without surgery). Diagnosis is made based on a combination of clinical, microbiologic, and echocardiographic features. Although certain guidelines such as the Duke criteria can assist in diagnosing IE, a comprehensive individual evaluation is critical.

Clinical Features

The clinical manifestations of IE can range from subtle and nonspecific symptoms to fulminant symptoms. The rate of progression depends on the extent of preexisting cardiac disease, virulence of the organism, and age and immunity of the patient. The diagnosis of endocarditis is straightforward in patients who present with the four cardinal Oslerian manifestations of IE: the presence of persistent bacteremia or fungemia, the presence of active valvulitis, the occurrence of large-vessel embolic events, and the presence of immunologic vascular phenomena. In many patients, however, especially patients with right-sided endocarditis, the peripheral stigmata are absent.

Symptoms

Fever is almost universal and is present in 80–90% of the patients. However, fever is less frequent in the elderly and immunocompromised patients, and hence a high index of suspicion and low threshold for investigation to exclude IE are essential in these groups. Patients can present with symptoms of heart failure, neurologic symptoms and demonstrate symptoms from embolic phenomena. Other nonspecific symptoms that are observed include fatigue, weight loss, malaise, chills, night sweats, arthralgias, and myalgias, especially back pain.

Physical Findings

Virtually all organ systems can be affected by IE. Thus, a comprehensive physical exam is critical in recognizing signs that may suggest IE. Cardiovascular exam may demonstrate new or changing murmurs indicative of valve damage, which are more prevalent in acute endocarditis and are frequently harbingers of heart failure. However, murmurs may be absent with right-sided endocarditis or intracardiac device infection. The murmur of acute and fulminant aortic regurgitation or mitral regurgitation may also be particularly difficult to hear. Signs of congestive heart failure may be present, and depending on the acuity of the disease process, patients' symptoms can range from mild heart failure symptoms to acute decompensated heart failure with hemodynamic compromise.

Neurologic findings are most commonly caused by embolic complications of endocarditis. They include embolic strokes, intracranial hemorrhage secondary to rupture of mycotic aneurysms and less frequently meningitis, brain abscess or encephalopathy.

Various mucocutaneous manifestations of endocarditis are often observed. Petechiae are present in 20–40% of patients presenting with IE and can be found on the conjunctiva, buccal or palatal mucosa and extremities. Splinter hemorrhages are red, linear, flame-shaped streaks seen in the proximal nail bed of fingers or toes. Whereas both petechiae and splinter hemorrhages are nonspecific, Osler's nodes, Janeway lesions, and Roth spots are more specific for IE. Osler's nodes are small, tender, violaceous, subcutaneous nodules usually seen in the pulp of the digits. Roth spots are retinal hemorrhages with a pale center. Osler's nodes and Roth spots are a result of immune complex deposition. Janeway lesions are non-tender, erythematous skin lesions that often appear in crops on the palms or soles and are a result of septic emboli to the skin with formation of microabscesses.

Other organ manifestations include abdominal symptoms due to bowel ischemia secondary to emboli to mesenteric arteries. Splenomegaly can be encountered and is the result of splenic infarcts and/or activation of the immune system. Flank tenderness can be present due to renal infarction as a result of emboli and a splenic friction rub may be present in cases of embolic splenic infarction.

The diagnosis of IE is based upon clinical suspicion derived from signs and symptoms and, most importantly, the demonstration of associated bacteremia. Over the years, there has been a drive to develop strategies to aid in the diagnosis of IE [26]. In 1994 the Duke criteria incorporated echocardiographic data into the diagnostic mix [27]. These criteria have been validated subsequently by many other studies, including the most recent modifications [28]. A diagnosis of IE is based on the presence of either major or minor clinical criteria. It uses both clinical and pathologic criteria to classify cases as definite IE (Tables 3.2 and 3.3). Major criteria in the Duke strategy included IE documented by data obtained at the time of open heart surgery or autopsy

Table 3.2 Diagnosis of infective endocarditis based on Duke criteria

Definitive IE *Pathological criteria* • Microorganisms demonstrated by culture or histological examination of a vegetation, a vegetation that has embolized, or an intracardiac abscess specimen or • Pathological lesions; vegetation or intracardiac abscess confirmed by histological examination showing active endocarditis *Clinical criteria (using definitions listed in Table 3.3)* • Two major criteria or • One major criterion and three minor criteria or • Five minor criteria
Possible IE • One major criterion and one minor criterion or • Three minor criteria
Rejected IE • Firm alternative diagnosis explaining evidence of IE or • Resolution of IE syndrome with antibiotic therapy for ≤4 days or • No pathological evidence of IE at surgery or autopsy, with antibiotic therapy for ≤4 days

From Li et al. [28] with permission from Oxford University Press

Table 3.3 Definition of terms used in the modified Duke criteria for the diagnosis of IE

Major criteria *Positive blood cultures* • Typical microorganisms consistent with IE from two separate blood cultures: *Viridans streptococci*, *Streptococcus bovis*, *HACEK group*, *Staphylococcus aureus* or community acquired *enterococci* in the absence of a primary focus or • Microorganisms consistent with IE from persistently positive blood cultures defined: at least two positive cultures of blood samples drawn >12 h apart; or all of three or a majority of four or more separate cultures (with first and last sample drawn at least 1 h apart); or • Single positive blood culture for *Coxiella burnetii* or anti-phase 1 IgG antibody titer >1:800 *Evidence of endocardial involvement* • Echocardiogram positive for IE defined as follows: – Oscillating intracardiac mass on valve or supporting structures, in the path of regurgitant jets, or on implanted material in the absence of an alternative anatomic explanation or – Abscess or – New partial dehiscence of prosthetic valve • New valvular regurgitation (worsening or changing or preexisting murmur not sufficient)
Minor criteria • Predisposition, predisposing heart condition, or intravenous drug use • Fever, temperature ≥38 °C • Vascular phenomena, major arterial emboli, septic pulmonary infarcts, mycotic aneurysm, intracranial hemorrhage, conjunctival hemorrhages, and Janeway's lesions • Immunologic phenomena: glomerulonephritis, Osler's nodes, Roth's spots, and rheumatoid factor • Microbiological evidence: positive blood culture but does not meet a major criterion as noted above or serological evidence of active infection with organism consistent with IE

From Li et al. [28] with permission from Oxford University Press

(pathological criteria) or by well-defined microbiological criteria plus echocardiographic data (clinical criteria).

Definite diagnosis of IE requires pathologic evidence (histologic and/or bacteriologic examination of vegetations, intracardiac abscess or emboli demonstrating typical pathology or cultured microorganisms) or clinical evidence that includes two major criteria or one major criterion and three minor criteria or five minor criteria.

Possible cases of IE do not meet the criteria for definite IE but satisfy one major criterion and one minor criterion or three minor criteria.

A rejected diagnosis of IE is present when there is no pathological evidence of IE at autopsy or surgery, rapid resolution of the clinical syndrome with either no treatment or short-term antibiotic therapy or when a firm alternative diagnosis has been found. The usefulness of the Duke criteria is limited in early stages of IE, in the setting of negative blood cultures and in the presence of prosthetic valves and device leads [29].

Microbiologic Diagnosis

Blood cultures remain the cornerstones for the diagnosis of IE and therefore should be obtained prior to initiation of antibiotic therapy. Three separate sets of blood cultures, each from a separate venipuncture site, obtained over 24 h, are recommended to evaluate patients with suspected endocarditis. Each set should include a bottle containing an aerobic and anaerobic medium, and at least 10 mL of blood should be placed in each bottle. Blood cultures may be collected at any time; they do not need to be obtained at the time of fever or chills since patients with IE typically have continuous bacteremia. With this strategy, a microbiological diagnosis can be made in ~90% of patients. However, blood cultures can be negative in up to 30% of cases, often due to prior exposure to antibiotics or infection with intracellular bacteria, fungi, or fastidious organisms [30, 31]. A microbiologic diagnosis in these situations may require special media, longer culture time (due to slower growth of certain organisms), and serologic tests. Serologic tests can be used to make diagnosis of endocarditis caused by *Brucella* species, *Legionella* species, *Bartonella* species, *Coxiella brunetti*, or *Chlamydia* species. Special techniques such as polymerase chain reaction (PCR) allow rapid and reliable detection of fastidious and non-culturable microorganisms. Moreover, if patients go to surgery, organisms can be identified in the valve tissue by culturing, immunohistochemical staining, or PCR.

Other abnormal laboratory tests that can be encountered include anemia, which is found in 70–90% of patients but may be absent in acute endocarditis. Erythrocyte sedimentation rate (ESR) and C-reactive protein (CRP) are elevated in most patients with IE. A CRP level that is elevated at baseline and normalizes with therapy is associated with good outcomes [32]. Similarly, the outcome of surgery in patients with increasing preoperative CRP levels has been demonstrated to be poor [33]. Hematuria and proteinuria may be present in patients with renal dysfunction due to immune-mediated glomerulonephritis or septic emboli causing renal infarction.

Imaging

Echocardiography

Echocardiography is central to the diagnosis and management of IE. Not only does echocardiography provide evidence of IE, it also provides important data regarding the hemodynamic consequences of the infection and helps predict short- and long-term prognosis. Furthermore, it helps in identifying patients at high risk for complications, diagnoses those complications, and identifies patients who benefit from surgery.

Echocardiography should be performed as soon as possible after the diagnosis of IE is suspected. Transthoracic echocardiography (TTE) is usually performed first in all cases, because it is a noninvasive technique that provides rapid, useful information for both the diagnosis and the assessment of IE severity. However, image resolution is limited by TTE and lesions <3 mm in size may not be detected. Transesophageal echocardiography (TEE) is performed in the majority of patients with suspected IE, because of its better image quality and sensitivity, particularly for the diagnosis of complications. TEE is indicated in patients with a negative TTE but high clinical suspicion for IE, poor TTE quality and suspected IE of prosthetic valves or device leads. Some centers perform TEE even if TTE shows evidence of IE to better evaluate the vegetation and valve structure and identify complications. The only situation in which TTE may be considered sufficient is the case of good-quality negative TTE associated with a low level of clinical suspicion. Negative echocardiography (TTE and TEE) and high suspicion for IE should prompt repeat studies. Many findings identified by TEE can also be detected on transthoracic views. Thus, concurrent TTE images can serve as a baseline and follow-up for a noninvasive comparison of vegetation size, valvular insufficiency, or change in abscess cavities during the course of the patient's treatment and in case of clinical deterioration. TTE can be superior to TEE in certain settings. Anterior cardiac structures such as the tricuspid valve and the right ventricular outflow tract may occasionally be better visualized with TTE. Moreover, TTE is superior to TEE in acquiring hemodynamic information such as calculating left ventricular function, quantifying severity of regurgitant lesions, and assessing filling pressures and pulmonary artery pressures. Thus, information acquired by TTE and TEE is complementary.

Several echocardiographic findings suggest the diagnosis of IE but the vegetation is the hallmark lesion. Typically, a vegetation presents as an oscillating mass attached to a valvular structure, with a motion independent to that of the valve (Fig. 3.3). Vegetations typically occur on the low pressure side of a high velocity jet. Hence, they are most often visualized on the atrial side of the mitral and tricuspid valves

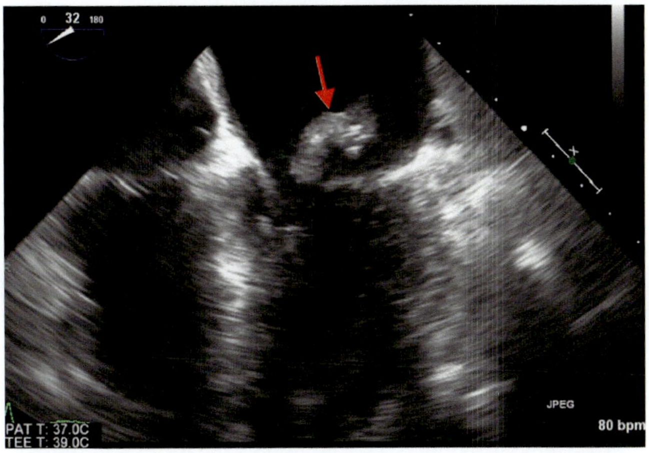

Fig. 3.3 Transesophageal echocardiogram demonstrating a large vegetation (arrow) on the mitral valve in a patient with infective endocarditis. From Shah T: Endocarditis. In Levine G (ed.): Color Atlas of Cardiovascular Disease. 2015, Jaypee Brothers Medical Publishers, Philadelphia, with permission

and ventricular aspects of the aortic and pulmonic valves. Although cardiac valves are the most common sites of infection, vegetations may also occur in other intracardiac locations, such as atrial or ventricular surfaces (where a high velocity jet of blood has damaged the endothelial integrity) or on intracardiac devices.

Echocardiography can detect structural damage and dysfunction of the valves. Valve leaflet perforation is the result of destruction of valve tissue by the infection and is generally associated with a virulent microorganism or when the infection continues undetected for a substantial amount of time. The endocarditis process can cause significant valvular regurgitation without perforation of the leaflets. Vegetations on the valve leaflets can obstruct coaptation and cause regurgitation. Less frequently, obstruction of the valve orifice by a vegetation can cause valvular stenosis. Moreover, significant regurgitation can be caused by chordal rupture and flail leaflet. Infection of a prosthetic valve typically affects the valve ring leading to valve dehiscence. Dehiscence occurs through infectious destruction of the sutures and ring leading to partial detachment of the ring from the surrounding tissue. This can result in a rocking motion of the prosthetic valve and perivalvular regurgitation.

Echocardiography is critical for the diagnosis and management of complications of endocarditis and in strategizing the timing of surgery. Heart failure, perivalvular extension of infection, and embolic events represent the three most frequent and severe complications of IE and the three main indications for early surgery [34]. Valve destruction causing acute regurgitation is the most characteristic mechanism leading to HF in native valve IE. Echocardiography provides (1) a detailed assessment of the mechanism (valve perforation, cusp fenestration, torn leaflet, flail leaflet due to ruptured infected chordae, or interference of the vegetation mass with leaflet closure) and (2) a reliable quantification and evaluation of the hemodynamic impact of the regurgitation.

Echocardiography plays a key role in the assessment of perivalvular extension of infection. Transesophageal echocardiography is the technique of choice for the diagnosis of perivalvular extension and its resulting complications. The infectious process can extend into the adjacent structures resulting in the formation of abscesses, pseudoaneurysms and fistulae. A fistulous connection is formed if the infectious process extends through the myocardium and ruptures into a cavity.

TTE and particularly TEE should be performed in the setting of any embolic event. By assessing the size, mobility, and location of vegetations, echocardiography is useful in predicting embolic risk and therefore plays a key role in identifying a subgroup of patients who might benefit from early surgery to avoid embolism. The size and mobility of vegetations are powerful echocardiographic predictors of new embolic events. Vegetations greater than 10 mm are at higher risk of embolism and risk is even higher in patients with very large (>15 mm) and highly mobile vegetations [35]. Embolism occurs more frequently in patients with vegetations located on the mitral valve (in particular on the anterior mitral leaflet) and when increasing or decreasing size of the vegetation is observed under antibiotic therapy.

When surgery is undertaken, intraoperative TEE evaluation includes assessment of the infected, dysfunctional valve, other valves, and contiguous structures. TEE also aids in confirming the adequacy of valve repair or replacement and documents the successful closure of fistulous tracts. Perivalvular leaks should be recognized and documented to avoid later confusion about whether the leaks are new and possibly the result of recurrent infection [36].

Repeat echocardiographic imaging is indicated if the initial exams did not show evidence of endocarditis but clinical suspicion remains high, in the setting of a new complication and as a follow-up in patients on medical therapy. The type and timing of repeat echocardiographic examinations depend on the clinical presentation and the initial echocardiographic findings.

Multi-Slice Computer Tomography

Although echocardiography is the "gold standard" method used to assess the anatomy of the cardiac valves and perivalvular apparatus, its effectiveness may be limited by the patient's anatomy and by artifacts due to valvular calcifications or prosthetic material [37]. Also echocardiography requires a highly trained operator and results are to a certain degree operator dependent. Multi-slice computer tomography (MSCT) offers another modality for imaging valvular and perivalvular damage, providing high-resolution anatomic information and affording multiplanar reformations. CT scanning offers the possibility to rapidly image the heart and other organs and thus to identify cardiac lesions and extracardiac complications, such as embolic events, infectious aneurysms, hemorrhages, and septic metastases, which can modify the therapeutic strategy. It also provides an anatomical assessment of the coronary bed, which is important in the preoperative evaluation. In a small study of 37 consecutive patients with clinically suspected IE, Feuchtner et al. found good results in detecting valvular and perivalvular damage using MSCT. Although small leaflet perforations were missed, CT provided more accurate anatomical information regarding presence of abscess/pseudoaneurysm than TEE [38]. Fagman et al. recently investigated the role of MSCT in the diagnosis of aortic prosthetic valve IE. The authors showed that MSCT had comparable diagnostic performance to TEE. Moreover, intraoperative findings demonstrated that MSCT detected three additional pseudoaneurysms not found by TEE [39].

MRI may be indicated in some instances in the evaluation of infective endocarditis. Although it is less accurate than TTE and TEE in identifying valvular vegetations, it can be used primarily for the evaluation of complications such as paravalvular and myocardial abscesses and infectious pseudoaneurysms. Moreover, MRI is useful in the identification of embolic complications to the brain and spinal cord and identification of mycotic aneurysms of the aorta and its branches.

Molecular imaging with 18-fluorodeoxyglucose (FDG)-PET and localizing low dose CT for attenuation correction (PET/CT) has shown promise in the diagnosis of IE in prosthetic valves and intracardiac devices. This imaging modality enables measurement of metabolic activity within an organ obtained from the emission of positrons after disintegration of the injected radioactive product (Fig. 3.4). In prosthetic valve endocarditis, TTE and TEE may occasionally fail to recognize vegetations and periannular extension due to acoustic shadowing by components of the prosthetic heart valve. In these difficult cases, the use of FDG-PET/CT can help in identifying intracardiac areas of increased metabolic activity suggesting infection [40].

Gallium-67, indium-111, or technetium-99m-hexamethylpropyleneamine oxime labelled leukocyte scintigraphy is another option for imaging of infection, with or without incorporation of CT images. Compared to PET/CT, this method is more specific for infection, however is more time-consuming. The sensitivity and the specificity of ^{99m}technetium radiolabelled leukocyte scintigraphy in patients with a suspicion of prosthetic valve IE and an inconclusive echocardiogram have been reported as 57% and 78%, respectively [41]. Because of a better specificity in detection of infection, this modality might be better than PET/CT in differentiating early prosthetic valve IE from postoperative inflammation.

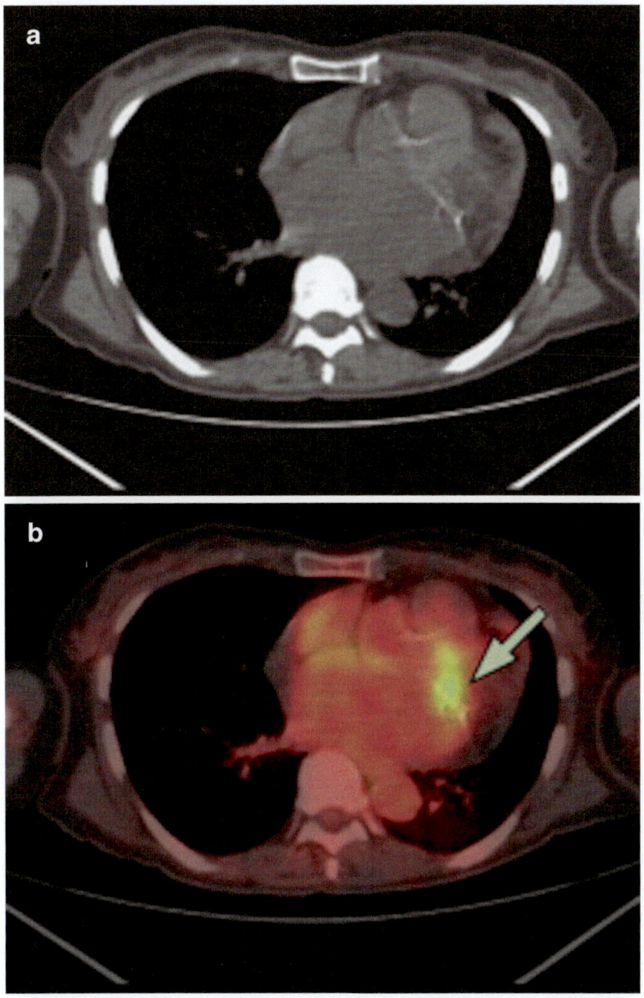

Fig. 3.4 PET-CT of a 64-year-old woman with a mass on thickened mitral valve but no pathogen identified by blood cultures or serology. *FDG* fluorodeoxyglucose. (**a**) Transaxial CT scan. (**b**) Transaxial PET-CT fused image showing an increase FDG uptake in the area of the mitral valve (green arrow). The endocarditis diagnosis was confirmed by pathological examination after surgery (recurrent emboli) showing vegetation but no pathogen could be identified. From Thuny F, Grisoli D, Collart F, Habib G, Raoult D. Management of infective endocarditis: challenges and perspectives. Lancet. 2012;379(9819):965–75. Reproduced with permission from Elsevier Limited

IE Complications

Despite advances in diagnosis and management, IE still remains a disease with high morbidity and mortality usually resultant from complications which can alter the outcome and influence management. Complications can be intracardiac or extracardiac (Table 3.4). While cardiac complications are related to local spread of infection, extracardiac complications result from vegetations embolizing to various organs, immune-mediated damage, and complications related to treatment of IE. Heart failure, perivalvular extension, and embolic events represent the three most frequent and severe complications of IE [34].

Table 3.4 Complications of IE

Complications of infective endocarditis
Structural
• Leaflet perforation
• Ruptured chordae/flail leaflet
• Perivalvular extension
• Abscess
• Aneurysm
• Fistula
• Valve dehiscence
• Pericardial effusion
Hemodynamic—heart failure
• Acute valvular or perivalvular regurgitation
• Valve obstruction
• Intracardiac shunt
• Myocarditis
• Myocardial infarction
Extracardiac manifestations
• Renal
• Infarct (embolic)
• Immune-mediated glomerulonephritis
• Neurologic
• Stroke
• Embolic
• Mycotic aneurysms
• Meningitis
• Encephalitis
• Pulmonary embolism (right-sided or device-related IE)
• Emboli to other abdominal organs
• Spleen
• Liver
• Mesenteric vessels
• Spine
• Coronary emboli
Treatment related
• Drug toxicity
• Secondary bacteremia due to intravenous lines
• Thrombosis of vascular lines

Cardiac Complications

Local, intracardiac extension of the infection can lead to tissue destruction of the valve apparatus and surrounding cardiac tissue resulting in cardiac complications. Cardiac complications include heart failure, perivalvular abscess formation, fistula formation, and pericarditis.

Heart failure is usually caused by destruction of the valve apparatus (valve leaflets, chordae) leading to significant valvular regurgitation (Figs. 3.5 and 3.6). Improper coaptation of the leaflets due to the vegetation can also lead to significant valvular regurgitation. In rare cases, a large vegetation can obstruct the valve orifice leading to valvular stenosis and heart failure or vegetation fragments can embolize into the coronary arteries resulting in myocardial infarction and subsequent heart failure. Heart failure is the most common cause of death and the most common indication for surgery in patients with IE [42].

Extension of the infectious process outside the valve leaflets into surrounding structures such as the annulus,

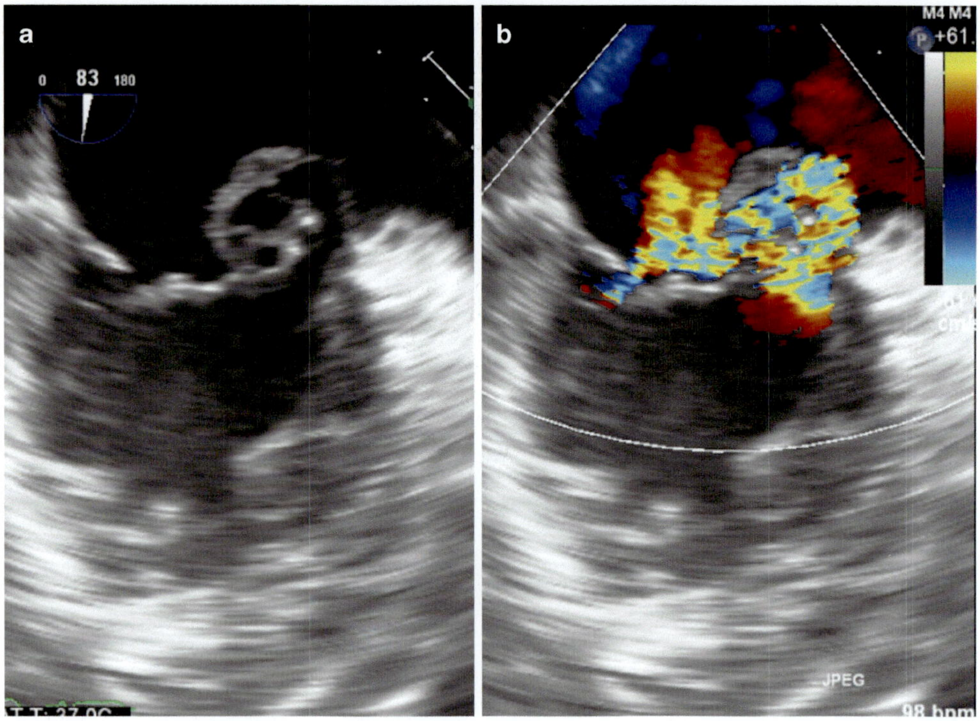

Fig. 3.5 TEE (**a**) Large vegetation (arrow) on the posterior mitral valve leaflet complicated by formation of aneurysm. (**b**) Color Doppler imaging demonstrates mitral regurgitation at the leaflet coaptation and regurgitation through the posterior leaflet consistent with leaflet perforation

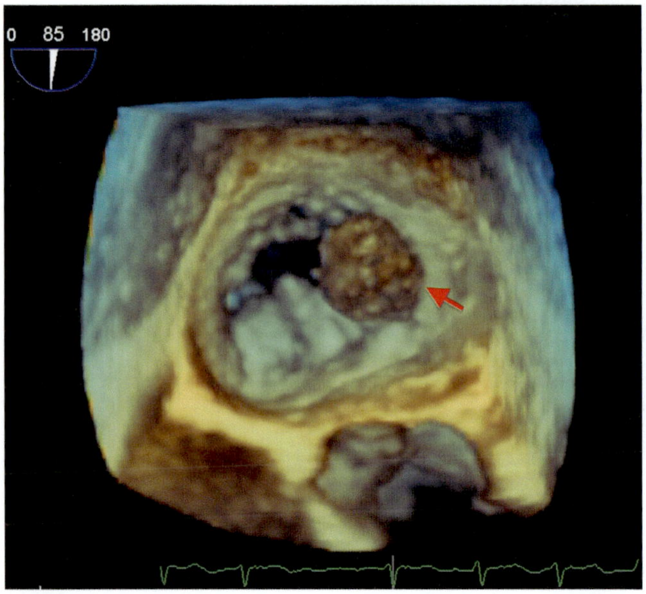

Fig. 3.6 3D TEE images of en face view of the mitral valve demonstrating large vegetation on the posterior leaflet

the myocardium, the conduction system, or the intervalvular fibrosa can lead to abscess formation. Perivalvular infection appears to be more frequent in aortic valve IE than in mitral valve IE [43] (Fig. 3.7). Rarely, these abscesses can rupture and lead to myocardial perforation and suppurative pericarditis. Further contiguous spreading of the infection especially in the region of the intervalvular fibrosa can lead to pseudoaneurysm and fistula formation. Extension of a perivalvular abscess into the adjacent conduction system tissue can lead to conduction disturbances. The latter is more frequently seen in aortic valve endocarditis. In rare cases, extensive perivalvular abscess formation can lead to compression of coronary ostia and myocardial ischemia [44].

The presence of a perivalvular abscess should be suspected in the setting of persistent bacteremia despite appropriate antibiotic therapy or new onset conduction abnormalities. Thus, the PR interval and intensity of the first heart sound should be monitored daily. Although TEE remains the diagnostic tool of choice for detecting perivalvular complications, MSCT has been shown to give useful complementary information for the assessment of the perivalvular extent of abscess and aneurysms [37]. Perivalvular complications are one of the most serious complications of IE and are associated with a higher rate of embolic complications and death, and thus surgery is indicated in these patients.

Lastly, pericarditis (purulent or non-purulent) can also develop in the setting of IE [45]. Purulent pericarditis is usually caused by spread of the infectious process into the pericardial space, but can also be caused by blood borne spread of the infection to the pericardium. Non-purulent pericarditis may occur as a result of systemic inflammation or immunological phenomena in the setting of IE [46]. The signs and symptoms of pericarditis are similar to those found in patients with pericarditis due to other etiologies.

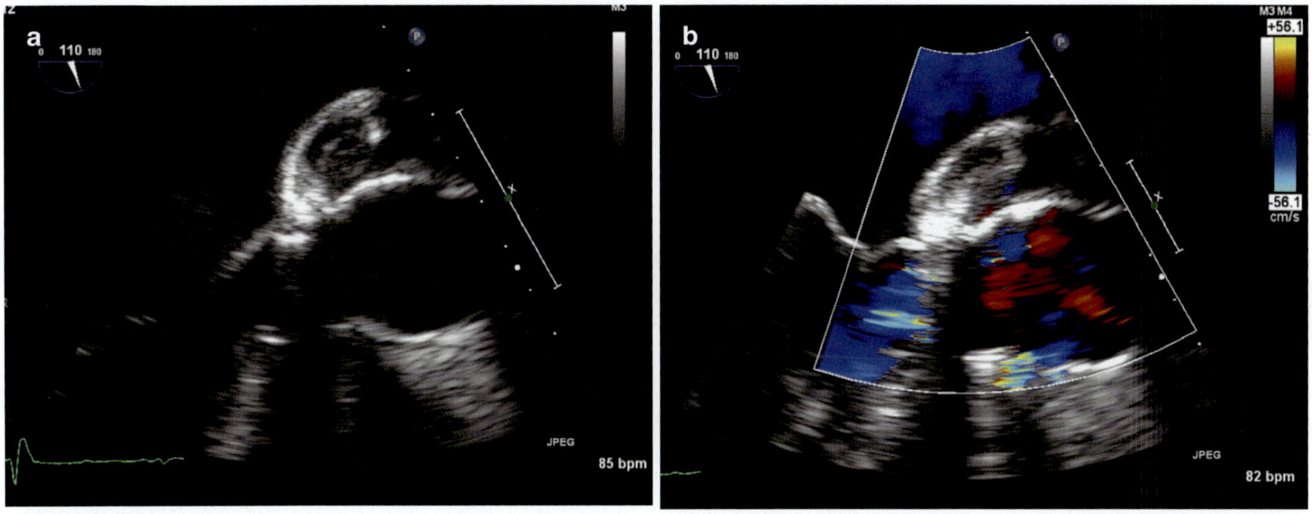

Fig. 3.7 TEE (**a**) short-axis and (**b**) long-axis images showing aortic root abscess formation (arrows) in a patient with aortic valve endocarditis. (*TEE* Transesophageal echocardiogram). From Shah T: Endocarditis. In Levine G (ed.): Color Atlas of Cardiovascular Disease. 2015, Jaypee Brothers Medical Publishers, Philadelphia, PA, with permission

Extracardiac Complications

Peripheral embolic events are caused by fragments of the vegetation embolizing into the peripheral vascular bed. It is the second most common complication of IE occurring in 20–50% of patients [34]. Risk factors predicting embolization are the presence of left-sided IE, mitral valve IE (rather than aortic valve IE), larger vegetation size (>10 mm), high mobility of the vegetation, IE due to *S. aureus* or fungi, history of prior embolization, age, diabetes and atrial fibrillation [10, 47–50]. Left-sided IE can result in systemic embolization whereas right-sided IE can lead to pulmonic embolization. Embolic events may be clinically silent in about 20% of IE patients. Brain and spleen are the most common sites for embolization in left-sided endocarditis. Stroke is the most commonly observed major clinical consequence of embolization affecting 60–80% of patients, and the risk of stroke appears much greater for mitral than for aortic valve endocarditis [51–53]. Clinical cerebrovascular events are noted in about 35% of patients and 50% of events remain clinically silent. In patients with IE undergoing systematic MRI examination any kind of cerebral abnormality was found in 80% of patients [54]. Other cerebral complications of IE include intracerebral hemorrhage, mycotic aneurysm, meningitis, and abscess formation. Mycotic aneurysms develop through septic embolization into the arterial lumen or into the vasa vasorum and subsequent infection of the vessel wall [55]. Apart from the brain and spleen, emboli may involve any vital organ, including the liver, kidney, spinal cord, abdominal mesenteric vessels and skin resulting in infarcts with or without abscess formation in these organs. Renal emboli can cause hematuria and flank pain. Splenic infarction may lead to abscess development and cause prolonged fevers or left shoulder pain from diaphragmatic irritation. Coronary emboli can result in myocardial infarction. Pulmonary emboli can be seen in intravenous drug users with right-sided endocarditis or in patients with intracardiac devices such as pacemakers or defibrillators.

Immune-mediated sequelae of IE include the development of glomerulonephritis and Osler nodes as a result of immune-complex deposition in the glomeruli and skin, respectively. Although control of the infection is important for resolution of renal dysfunction, antibiotic treatment-associated complications include aminoglycoside-induced nephro- and ototoxicity, interstitial nephritis, drug fever, allergic reactions to antibiotics, intravenous catheter-associated complications (thrombophlebitis, thrombosis, cellulitis), and *Clostridium difficile* infection.

Antimicrobial Therapy

If there is clinical suspicion for IE, empiric antimicrobial therapy can be started once blood cultures are drawn depending on the severity of the clinical course. In patients demonstrating an indolent course, microbiologic diagnosis can be awaited before starting antibiotics. In patients with a more fulminant course, antibiotics should be started immediately after blood cultures are drawn. Empiric antibiotic therapy should cover staphylococci (methicillin susceptible and resistant), streptococci, and enterococci and thus vancomycin is the recommended antibiotic. If there is clinical suspicion for gram-negative bacteremia, a fourth generation cephalosporin such as cefepime can be added to the vancomycin. After the antimicrobial diagnosis has been made, antibiotics are tailored to the susceptibility of the organism. It is critical that the type and dose of antibiotics are bactericidal. Thus, the minimum inhibitory concentration (MIC) of antibiotics against the organism should be determined in every patient. Table 3.5 outlines the antibiotic treatment combinations for various organisms.

After antibiotic therapy has been initiated, two sets of blood cultures should be obtained every 24–48 h until blood cultures are negative. In general, patients should be treated

Table 3.5 Antibiotic treatment for infective endocarditis

Organism	Drug and dose	Duration (weeks)	Comments
Streptococci			
Highly penicillin-susceptible viridans streptococci and *Streptococcus gallolyticus* affecting native valves	Aqueous penicillin G 2–3 mU IV Q4H *or* Ceftriaxone 2 g/day IV *or* Vancomycin 15 mg/kg IV Q12H	4	Vancomycin is recommended only for patients not able to tolerate penicillin or ampicillin
Native valve endocarditis due to strains of viridans streptococci or *S. gallolyticus* that are relatively resistant to penicillin	Aqueous penicillin G 2–3 mU IV Q4H *or* Ceftriaxone 2 g/day IV *plus* Gentamicin 3 mg/kg IV Q24H in 1 dose	4 2	
Prosthetic valve endocarditis due to penicillin-susceptible viridans streptococci and *S. gallolyticus*	Aqueous penicillin G 2–3 mU IV Q4H *or* Ceftriaxone 2 g/day IV *or* Vancomycin 15 mg/kg IV Q12H *with or without* Gentamicin 3 mg/kg IV Q24H in 1 dose	6 2	
Prosthetic valve endocarditis due to strains relatively or fully resistant to penicillin	Aqueous penicillin G 2–3 mU IV Q4H *or* Ceftriaxone 2 g/day IV *or* Vancomycin 15 mg/kg IV Q12H *plus* Gentamicin 3 mg/kg IV Q24H in 1 dose	6	
Enterococci			
	Ampicillin 2 g IV Q4H *or* Aqueous penicillin G 3–4 mU IV Q4H *or* Vancomycin 15 mg/kg IV Q12H *plus* Gentamicin 1 mg/kg IV Q8H	4–6	Vancomycin is recommended only for patients not able to tolerate penicillin or ampicillin Streptomycin 7.5 mg/kg IV Q12H can be substituted for gentamicin if no high level resistance
Staphylococci			
Methicillin-susceptible, affecting native valves	Nafcillin or oxacillin 2 g IV Q4H *or* Cefazolin 2 g IV Q8H *or* Vancomycin 15 mg/kg IV Q12H	4–6	Use vancomycin *only* in patients who cannot tolerate a β-lactam agent
Methicillin-resistant strains, affecting native valves	Vancomycin 15 mg/kg IV Q12H *or* Daptomycin 6 mg/kg IV Q24H	6	Daptomycin should only be used for strains with elevated vancomycin MICs
Methicillin-susceptible strains, affecting prosthetic valves	Nafcillin or oxacillin 2 g IV Q4H *plus* Rifampin 300 mg IV/PO Q8H *plus* Gentamicin 1 mg/kg IV Q8H	≥ 6	
Methicillin-resistant strains, affecting prosthetic valves	Vancomycin 15 mg/kg IV Q12H *or* Daptomycin 6 mg/kg IV Q24H *plus* Rifampin 300 mg IV/PO Q8H *plus* Gentamicin 1 mg/kg IV Q8H	≥ 6	Daptomycin should only be used for strains with elevated vancomycin MICs

Table 3.5 (continued)

Organism	Drug and dose	Duration (weeks)	Comments
HACEK organisms, affecting either native or prosthetic valves			
	Ceftriaxone 2 g/day IV *or* Ampicillin/sulbactam 3 mg IV Q6H *or* Ciprofloxacin 400 mg IV Q12H	4	
Non-HACEK gram-negative bacilli	Refer to guidelines in Ref. [36]		
Fungi/yeasts	Refer to guidelines in Ref. [36]		

[a]See Ref. [36] for full recommendations and details

with intravenous antibiotics for 6 weeks starting from the first day of negative blood cultures. Shorter regimens may be sufficient in certain patients with right-sided endocarditis or IE with highly susceptible organisms in the absence of complications. After valve surgery, the duration of antibiotic therapy is determined by the operative tissue culture results. If the culture results are negative, the duration should be calculated from the first day of negative blood cultures. If the cultures are positive, a complete course of antibiotic treatment is indicated starting from the day of surgery. Irrespectively, intravenous antibiotics should be administered for at least 2 weeks following surgery.

Surgical Therapy

In past publications, rates of surgery for IE vary considerably; however, there has been a trend towards an increase in surgery in the treatment of IE. A systematic review of 15 analyses demonstrated a 7% per decade increase in patients undergoing valve surgery for IE from 1969 to 2000 [1]. A clear mortality benefit with surgical treatment has not been demonstrated due to a paucity of prospective randomized trials. That said, delay in surgery once heart failure has intervened contributes to increased mortality.

In patients presenting with IE, the questions that have to be posed when considering surgical therapy include:

1. Whether to operate (indications)
2. When to operate (timing)
3. Choice of surgical procedure
4. Strategy of adjunctive antibiotic treatment

Indications for Surgery

Due to the complexities and uncertainties regarding the indication and timing of surgery in these patients, who often have other comorbidities, it is recommended that patients with IE are managed by a Heart Valve team involving cardiology, cardiothoracic surgery, and infectious disease specialists [56]. Cardiothoracic surgical consultation should be obtained promptly after the diagnosis of IE to assist with assessment of need for surgery and its optimal timing.

Each patient must be evaluated individually and all factors associated with increased risk of complications and death identified at the time of diagnosis so as to rapidly initiate antibiotic treatment and identify patients who require early surgery, realizing that the patient's comorbidities have to be taken into account and the risks versus benefits of surgery weighed. In patients with complicated endocarditis, antibiotic therapy combined with valve replacement results in higher survival rates and fewer relapses compared to antibiotics alone. Although surgical therapy during the active phase of the disease is associated with significant risk, it can be justified in patients with high-risk features in whom the possibility of cure with antibiotic treatment only is unlikely and in whom severe complications of IE have or are likely to occur. Early surgery during the active phase of the infection is reportedly performed in 40–60% of patients [57]. The benefit of early surgery has been difficult to demonstrate in observational studies due to various confounding factors. However, a clear trend towards improved outcomes with early surgery has been noted [58–61].

Despite the paucity of evidence-based data, the recommended indications for surgical treatment in native IE are significant valve dysfunction causing heart failure, paravalvular extension of infection, recurrent embolization, persistent bacteremia despite appropriate antibiotic treatment and pathogens which are less responsive to antimicrobial therapy (such as fungi and resistant organisms). However, not infrequently, the risk benefit assessment in patients with IE may not be very clear. Predictors of increased mortality include left ventricular systolic dysfunction, heart failure, shock, renal insufficiency, prosthetic valve IE, and high Euroscore [59, 62, 63]. Further factors that have been associated with worse outcome are large/enlarging vegetation, pulmonary hypertension, and objective measures of heart failure including elevated intracardiac filling pressures, depressed left ventricular function, and elevated BNP and troponin levels [10, 61, 64–66]. Several studies have attempted to develop a prognostic classification system for patients with native IE. In a retrospective analysis of 259 patients with complicated left-sided native valve IE, five baseline parameters were shown to be independently associated with increased 6-month mortality: abnormal mental status, moderate to severe congestive heart failure, bacterial etiology other than viridans streptococci, and medical therapy without valve surgery [66]. In another study of 192 patients with IE, the authors explored time-dependent risk stratification by identifying independent predictors of 6-month mortality on days 1, 8, and 15 [67]. The presence of thrombocytopenia, heart failure, and severe comorbidity (using Charlson comorbidity scale) was associated with increased 6-month mortality at all three time points, and several other predictors were identified at individual time points. Patients identified at low risk had a 6-month mortality of 2.4% whereas high risk was associated with a 6-month mortality of 78.2%. Although valve surgery for IE was associated with reduced 6-month mortality, the benefit of surgery cannot be deduced from this data as this was a retrospective analysis. In a further study of 263 patients with left-sided IE, parameters obtained within 72 h of admission were evaluated for their predictive power with respect to in-hospital mortality or urgent surgery [68]. Independent risk factors for this outcome were infection with *Staphylococcus aureus*, heart failure, and periannular complications. In a further analysis of The Society of Thoracic Surgeons Adult Cardiac Surgery Database, 13,617 surgeries performed for IE were examined [65]. The overall operative mortality rate was lower than reported in other studies at 8.2%, and even in patients with the highest score, operative mortality did not exceed 30%. Several factors were identified to independently predict operative mortality with the preoperative hemodynamic condition of the patient being the strongest predictor. Interestingly, preoperative cerebrovascular disease was not a significant predictor of mortality or morbidity. Even in patients with recent preoperative stroke, the rate of postoperative stroke was low at 4.3% considering a median time interval between admission and surgery of 7 days. Of note, the presence of active IE (as opposed to treated IE) was associated with an increased operative risk. In the individual patient, this increased operative risk must be counterbalanced against the risk of postponing the surgery and the patient suffering from complications such as embolic events, heart failure, and death. Although these risk prediction models aid in identifying patients with IE at high risk for mortality and morbidity, they do not necessarily help in deciding which patients should go to surgery and the ideal timing of surgery. These decisions are made individually, taking into account the overall risk due to IE, individual operative risk, and risk of complications with medical treatment only.

Heart failure is the most common cause for mortality in patients with IE and has been demonstrated to be the clearest and strongest indication for early surgery in all types of IE. In patients with IE and moderate to severe heart failure, mortality approaches 75% with medical treatment alone whereas surgical mortality in these patients is less than 25% [69, 70]. In patients who are hemodynamically stable and without heart failure, indications for surgery are less clear. In such cases, surgery after eradication of infection may be performed for adverse hemodynamic effects of valvular regurgitation that result from valve damage. In a retrospective, observational cohort study of 513 cases of complicated, left-sided endocarditis, investigators found that valve surgery was independently associated with reduced 6-month mortality (HR, 0.40; 95% CI, 0.18–0.91; $P = 0.03$) in propensity-matched subgroups [60]. Stratifying the data by congestive heart failure among propensity-matched patients undergoing surgery showed that among patients with none to mild congestive heart failure, valve surgery was not associated with reduced mortality compared with medical therapy (HR, 1.04; 95% CI, 0.43–2.48; $P = 0.93$). However, among propensity-matched patients with moderate to severe congestive heart failure, valve surgery was associated with a significant reduction in mortality compared with medical therapy (HR, 0.22; 95% CI, 0.08–0.53; $P = 0.01$).

Embolism occurs in 20–40% of patients with IE and is associated with an increased morbidity and mortality. In a smaller randomized trial of 76 patients, early surgery (within 48 h) in patients with vegetation size >10 mm resulted in a significant decrease in the composite endpoint of in-hospital mortality and embolic events (3% versus 23%) mainly driven by a decrease in embolic events. A randomized controlled trial of surgical intervention in patients with severe left-sided valve dysfunction and vegetations >10 mm in length (even in the absence of clinically apparent embolic events or HF) showed that early surgery performed within 48 h after diagnosis reduced the composite primary endpoint of death from any cause or embolic events by effectively reducing the risk of systemic embolism [71]. Moreover, these improvements in clinical outcomes were achieved without an increase in operative mortality or recurrence of infective endocarditis. Thus, early surgery is reasonable in patients who are at high risk for embolic events. Several factors are associated with increased risk of embolism, including the size and mobility of vegetations, the location of the vegetation on the mitral valve (specifically anterior mitral leaflet), the increasing or decreasing size of the vegetation under antibiotic therapy, particular microorganisms (*Staphylococci*, *Streptococcus bovis*, *Candida* spp.) and previous embolism. As noted above, size and mobility of the vegetations are the most potent independent predictors of a new embolic event. The risk of embolism is highest during the first days after initiation of antibiotic treatment and decreases significantly after 2 weeks of therapy. An analysis from the International Collaboration on Endocarditis–Prospective Cohort Study (ICE-PCS) study group showed that the crude incidence of stroke in patients receiving appropriate antimicrobial therapy was 4.82/1000 patient days in the first week of therapy and fell to 1.71/1000 patient days in the second week. This rate continued to decline with further therapy. Stroke rates fell similarly regardless of the valve or organism involved.

After a cerebral embolic event, the decision to proceed with surgery must take into account the risk of further embolism and the risk of neurologic deterioration caused by cardiopulmonary bypass in patients who have already experienced a cerebrovascular complication. A history of embolic stroke or transient ischemic attack is not in itself a contraindication to surgery. In general, postoperative neurologic deterioration has been reported to be low (0–6%) [72] and this is also true after a silent cerebral embolism or a transient ischemic attack [73]. After an ischemic stroke, surgery can be performed if the patient does not have severe neurologic damage and cerebral hemorrhage has been ruled out by cerebral imaging [58]. A recent study from The International Collaboration on Endocarditis–Prospective Cohort Study (ICE-PCS) showed that there is no apparent survival benefit in delaying surgery (>7 days) when indicated in IE patients after ischemic stroke [74].

Paravalvular extension of infection is usually an indication for surgery as medical therapy alone is rarely curative [75]. Although surgical mortality in patients with paravalvular extension is high (19–43%), prognosis with medical therapy only is dismal [43, 76–78]. In one case series of 20 patients, medical management was associated with a mortality rate of 40% at 6 months. Thus, surgical treatment is indicated in patients with paravalvular extension unless surgical risk is prohibitive.

In patients with IE due to documented infection of pacemaker and defibrillator systems, complete removal of the systems, including all leads and the generator is indicated as part of the early management (Class I, LOE B) [56]. Even without evidence of device or lead infection, it is reasonable to completely remove the pacemaker or defibrillator systems in patients with valvular IE caused by *S. aureus* or fungi or in patients undergoing valvular surgery for endocarditis (Class IIa) [56]. Surgery is also recommended for patients with prosthetic valve endocarditis and relapsing infection (defined as recurrence of bacteremia after a complete course of appropriate antibiotics and subsequently negative blood cultures) without other identifiable source for portal of infection (Class I, LOE C) [56].

Recently released ACC/AHA guidelines recommend early surgery for the conditions listed in Table 3.6.

Table 3.6 Indications for surgery in IE

Indications for surgery in endocarditis	
Indicated in patients with IE who present with valve dysfunction resulting in symptoms of heart failure	Class I, LOE B
Indicated in patients with left-sided IE caused by *S. aureus*, fungal, or other highly resistant organisms	Class I, LOE B
Indicated in patients with IE complicated by heart block, annular or aortic abscess, or destructive penetrating lesions	Class I, LOE B
Indicated in patients with evidence of persistent infection as manifested by persistent bacteremia or fevers lasting longer than 5–7 days after onset of appropriate antimicrobial therapy	Class I, LOE B
Reasonable in patients with IE who present with recurrent emboli and persistent vegetations despite appropriate antibiotic therapy	Class IIa, LOE B
May be considered in patients with native valve endocarditis who exhibit mobile vegetations greater than 10 mm in length (with or without clinical evidence of embolic phenomenon)	Class IIb, LOE B

1. Early surgery is indicated in patients with IE who present with valve dysfunction resulting in symptoms of heart failure (Class I, LOE B).
2. Early surgery is indicated in patients with left-sided IE caused by *S. aureus*, fungal, or other highly resistant organisms (Class I, LOE B).
3. Early surgery is indicated in patients with IE complicated by heart block, annular or aortic abscess, or destructive penetrating lesions (Class I, LOE B).
4. Early surgery is indicated in patients with evidence of persistent infection as manifested by persistent bacteremia or fevers lasting longer than 5–7 days after onset of appropriate antimicrobial therapy (Class I, LOE B).
5. Early surgery is reasonable in patients with IE who present with recurrent emboli and persistent vegetations despite appropriate antibiotic therapy (Class IIa, LOE B).
6. Early surgery may be considered in patients with native valve endocarditis who exhibit mobile vegetations greater than 10 mm in length (with or without clinical evidence of embolic phenomenon) (Class IIb, LOE B).
7. Surgery is recommended for patients with prosthetic valve endocarditis and relapsing infection (defined as recurrence of bacteremia after a complete course of appropriate antibiotics and subsequently negative blood cultures) without other identifiable source for portal of infection (Class I, LOE C).

Timing of Surgery

When deciding about the timing of surgery the risk of operating during active infection resulting in potential infection of the prosthesis must be weighed against increasing complications if surgery is postponed. In a small, randomized trial in patients with native left-sided endocarditis, large vegetation (>10 mm) and severe valvular regurgitation or stenosis, 37 patients underwent early surgery (within 48 h) and 39 patients underwent surgery either during initial hospitalization or during follow-up. The early surgery group demonstrated a lower rate of the primary endpoint (in-hospital mortality and embolic event) at 6 weeks than the conventionally managed group (3% versus 23% respectively). In another study, 138 patients underwent valve replacement in the setting of active infection. In these patients, early mortality was 11.5% (mainly due to heart failure and multi-organ failure) and early recurrent endocarditis occurred in 2% of patients. The optimal timing of surgery continues to remain unclear due to the lack of randomized controlled data, which will likely be difficult to obtain due to the heterogeneity in the patients presenting. From current data, early surgery for the appropriate indications appears to be feasible with low risk of prosthetic valve reinfection and evidence towards improved outcomes [71]. The indications for early surgery will hopefully be more clearly defined as more data emerges.

Choice of Surgical Procedure

Surgery for IE usually includes debridement of all affected areas, copious irrigation, reconstruction of any defects with autologous or bovine pericardium and either valve repair or replacement with a prosthetic valve [79]. Thorough removal of infectious tissue is more important for the outcome than choice of valve procedure [80]. The mode of surgery (replacement versus repair) or type of prosthesis used (mechanical versus biological) has no influence on operative mortality, although repair techniques, when applicable, offer long-term advantages, including a reduced risk of late complications (notably, recurrent IE) and obviation of the need for lifelong anticoagulation [42, 81]. Valve repair may be possible when a leaflet perforation occurs in the absence of extensive leaflet destruction or annular involvement.

Prosthetic Valve Endocarditis (PVE)

PVE occurs in about 1–6% of patients with prosthetic valves and can be separated into early and late forms [82]. Early PVE occurs within 60 days of valve implantation and typical organisms include coagulase-negative staphylococci, gram-negative bacilli, and *Candida* species. Late PVE occurs >60 days after valve implantation and associated organisms are similar to those encountered in native valve IE (staphylococci, alpha-hemolytic streptococci, and enterococci). With respect to fulminance, early PVE tends to be more acute and aggressive whereas late PVE usually is more indolent and

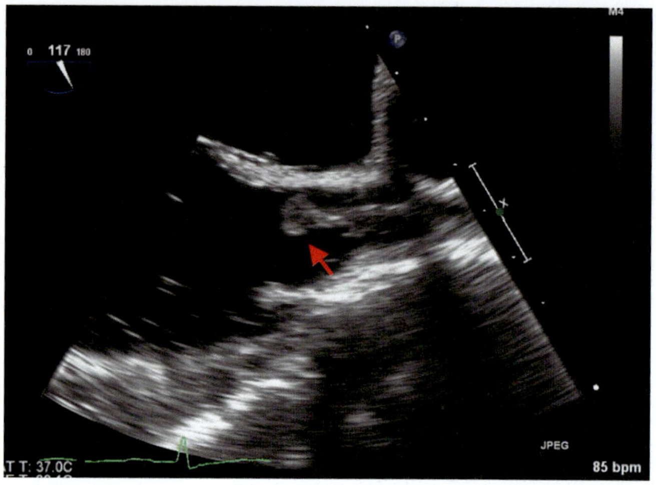

Fig. 3.8 Vegetation on an ICD lead (arrow) (*ICD* intracardiac defibrillator)

subacute similar to native valve IE. IE affects bioprosthetic and mechanical valves in equal frequency. Mitral valve prostheses are more prone to infection than aortic valve prosthesis. Complications such as abscess/fistula formation, valve dehiscence, and heart block are more frequently seen with aortic valve PVE. In-hospital mortality is higher than in native valve IE with a reported rate of 20–40% [82].

Device-Related Endocarditis

Device-related endocarditis usually involves implantable pacemakers and defibrillators and usually occurs within a few months of implantation (Fig. 3.8). The infection can involve the generator pocket, the intravascular portions of the leads, the intracardiac portions of the leads, or a combination of the components. The majority of device infections are caused by staphylococci, both coagulase-negative and coagulase-positive.

Right-Sided Endocarditis

Right-sided endocarditis is seen in patients with intracardiac devices and catheters (see below) and more frequently in patients with intravenous drug use (IVDU). Right-sided endocarditis accounts for 10% of all IE in population-based surveys and a higher proportion of IE in injection drug users [83, 84]. Diagnosis of endocarditis in IVDU can be difficult and requires a high index of suspicion. A murmur may be absent in those with tricuspid disease, owing to the relatively small pressure gradient across the valve (Fig. 3.9). Pulmonary manifestations like pneumonia and septic pulmonary emboli are prominent in patients with tricuspid infection. Peripheral manifestations, such as splinter or conjunctival hemorrhages,

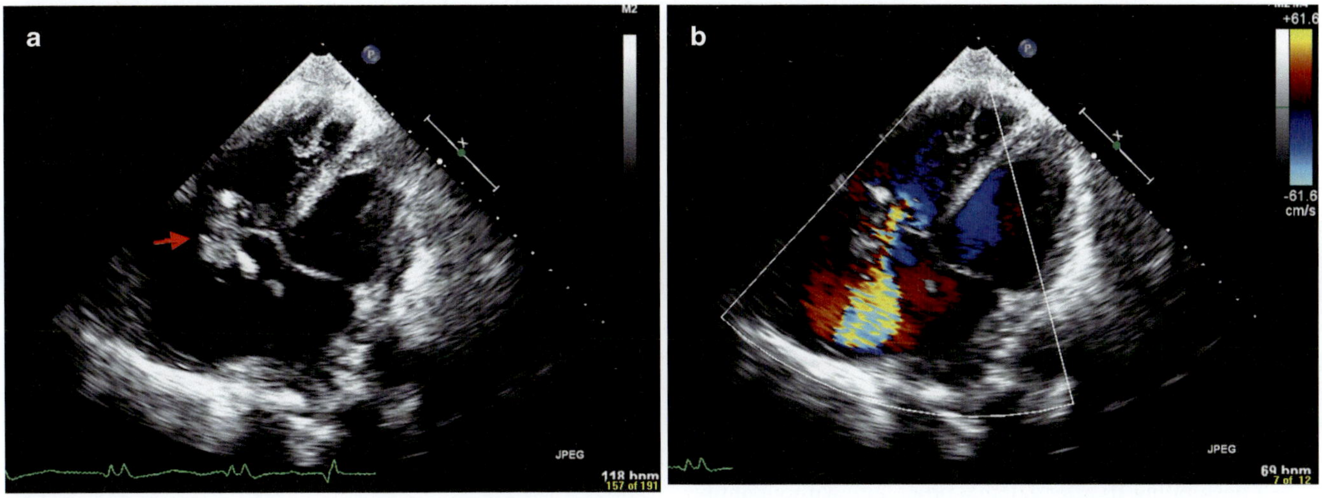

Fig. 3.9 TTE of large tricuspid valve vegetation. (**a**) Apical view. (**b**) Apical view with Color Doppler showing Tricuspid regurgitation

are observed less frequently. Among injection drug users (IDUs), *S. aureus* is the most common cause of right-sided IE, whereas left-sided IE can be caused by viridans streptococci or *S. aureus*. The successful management of a complicated case requires the close cooperation of a cardiologist, an infectious disease physician and addiction physicians in managing drug withdrawal and maintaining the patient in hospital [84]. Prognosis is relatively good with a quoted in-hospital mortality rate of <10%. Most patients can be treated medically, with surgery being necessary in only a small minority of cases [85]. Sepsis (which is uncontrolled despite adequate antibiotic treatment), intractable right heart failure (despite appropriate medical treatment), and paravalvular abscess or fungal endocarditis are the most important indications for surgical intervention [84].

Anticoagulation

The beneficial versus deleterious effect of anticoagulation in patients with IE is determined by a multitude of clinical, bacteriologic, radiological, and echocardiographic variables. Factors that may influence decision-making include native versus prosthetic valve endocarditis, size of the vegetation and its location on the mitral or aortic valve, virulence of the infective organism, size of the cerebral infarct(s), and presence of hemorrhagic transformation or mycotic aneurysms.

In patients with NVE, routine use of anticoagulation is not recommended unless a separate indication exists. There is no conclusive evidence that prophylactic anticoagulation reduces the incidence of emboli in patients with NVE who have no other indication for anticoagulation.

Alternatively, for patients already receiving anticoagulation with VKA or aspirin for other evidence-based indications at the time of diagnosis with IE, there is little information on the risks and benefits of continued anticoagulation therapy. Continuing anticoagulant therapy in the face of IE potentially increases the risk of hemorrhagic transformation of an embolic stroke or accentuation of bleeding from septic arteritis or mycotic aneurysms. Moreover, there is a theoretical risk of dislodging the vegetation and increasing the risk of embolic events with anticoagulation. The evidence and propensity of expert consensus suggest that anticoagulation be discontinued at the time of initial presentation with IE secondary to the combined risk of bleeding from potentially urgent invasive procedures and the risk of developing hemorrhagic stroke.

Decisions about continued anticoagulation and antiplatelet therapy should ultimately be directed by the patient's consulting cardiologist and cardiothoracic surgeon in consultation with a neurology specialist if neurological findings are present. Although there is no strong evidence base for screening neurological imaging studies, the data are strong that subclinical neurological abnormalities are common. Thus, in patients with valvular or nonvalvular indications for continued use of VKAs, strong consideration should be given to cerebral magnetic resonance imaging to evaluate for subclinical cerebrovascular complications to help guide anticoagulation management.

The 2014 ACC/AHA valve guidelines recommend the following [56]:

1. Temporary discontinuation of VKA anticoagulation might be considered in patients receiving VKA anticoagulation at the time of IE diagnosis (Class IIb, LOE B).
2. It is reasonable to temporarily discontinue anticoagulation in patients with IE who develop central nervous system symptoms compatible with embolism or stroke regardless of the other indications for anticoagulation (Class IIa, LOE B).

Prophylaxis for Endocarditis

Experimental studies have demonstrated that bacterial endocarditis can be induced when bacteria with a known ability to cause endocarditis are injected into laboratory animals following traumatization of the heart valves with vascular catheters. It has also been shown that if antibiotics with activity against streptococci are given prior to up to 30 min after injection of bacteria, endocarditis can be prevented in these experiments. Previously adopted recommendations for IE prophylaxis were mainly based on the results of these animal studies. However, there is no strong evidence supporting the use of antibiotic prophylaxis in patients with preexisting cardiac conditions. In fact, a French study demonstrated that the risk of developing IE after a dental procedure without antibiotic prophylaxis in patients with predisposing cardiac conditions was 1 in 11,000 in patients with prosthetic valves and 1 in 54,000 in patients with native valves. In patients who received prophylaxis, the risk of IE was 1 in 150,000 [86]. Thus, a large number of patients would need to be treated to prevent a very small number of IE cases. In the last decade the AHA and ESC dramatically revised the guidelines to restrict the use of antibiotic prophylaxis to a select group of patients. Several observations led to the revision of the guideline. Studies have shown that high-grade bacteremia is not necessary to induce endocarditis, but everyday exposure to low-grade endocarditis (caused by everyday-life actions like chewing or tooth brushing) represents a much greater cumulative risk in humans [87]. Also, the benefit of antibiotics needs to be balanced with the risk of their use like hypersensitivity, adverse effects, and antibiotic resistance due to widespread use. Thus, because of the lack of published evidence on the use of prophylactic antibiotics to prevent IE, antibiotic prophylaxis is now indicated for only a subset of patients who are at high risk for developing IE and at highest risk for an adverse outcome if IE occurs [88] (Table 3.7).

Antibiotic prophylaxis with dental procedures is reasonable only for patients with cardiac conditions associated with the highest risk of adverse outcomes from endocarditis in the setting of procedures likely to result in bacteremia with a microorganism that has the potential ability to cause endocarditis, including:

- Prosthetic cardiac valve or prosthetic material used in valve repair
- Previous endocarditis
- Congenital heart disease (CHD) only in the following categories:
  - Unrepaired cyanotic CHD, including those with palliative shunts and conduits
  - Completely repaired congenital heart defect with prosthetic material or device, whether placed by surgery or catheter intervention, during the first 6 months after the procedure
  - Repaired CHD with residual defects at the site or adjacent to the site of a prosthetic patch or prosthetic device (which inhibit endothelialization)
- Cardiac transplantation recipients with cardiac valvular disease

Table 3.7 Antibiotic prophylaxis regimens for IE

Situation	Agent	Regimen—single dose 30–60 min before procedure	
		Adults	Children
Oral	Amoxicillin	2 g	50 mg/kg
Unable to take oral medication	Ampicillin *or*	2 g IM or IV	50 mg/kg IM or IV
	Cefazolin *or* ceftriaxone	1 g IM or IV	50 mg/kg IM or IV
Allergic to penicillins or ampicillin—oral regimen	Cephalexin *or*	2 g	50 mg/kg
	Clindamycin *or*	600 mg	20 mg/kg
	Azithromycin *or* clarithromycin	500 mg	15 mg/kg
Allergic to penicillins or ampicillin and unable to take oral medication	Cefazolin *or* Ceftriaxone *or*	1 g IM or IV	50 mg/kg IM or IV
	clindamycin	600 mg IM or IV	20 mg/kg IM or IV

In patients in whom IE prophylaxis is reasonable, prophylaxis is only indicated before dental procedures that involve manipulation of gingival tissue or the periapical region of teeth or cause perforation of the oral mucosa [88]. Prophylaxis against IE is not recommended in patients with VHD who are at risk of IE for non-dental procedures (e.g., TEE, esophagogastroduodenoscopy, colonoscopy, or cystoscopy) in the absence of active infection.

Multiple epidemiological studies show no increase in the rate of IE since adoption of the AHA and European Society of Cardiology guidelines recommend more restrictive use of IE prophylaxis. The NICE (National Institute for Health and Clinical Excellence, United Kingdom) guidelines do not recommend antibiotic prophylaxis, regardless of the dental, genitourinary, or gastrointestinal procedure regardless of the cardiac condition [89]. Subsequent epidemiological studies performed in the wake of the NICE guideline revisions have demonstrated no increase in clinical cases or deaths from IE [90]. Table 3.7 lists the choice of recommended antibiotics when IE prophylaxis is indicated.

References

1. Tleyjeh IM, Abdel-Latif A, Rahbi H, Scott CG, Bailey KR, Steckelberg JM, et al. A systematic review of population-based studies of infective endocarditis. Chest. 2007;132(3):1025–35.
2. Griffin MR, Wilson WR, Edwards WD, O'Fallon WM, Kurland LT. Infective endocarditis. Olmsted County, Minnesota, 1950 through 1981. JAMA. 1985;254(9):1199–202.
3. Correa de Sa DD, Tleyjeh IM, Anavekar NS, Schultz JC, Thomas JM, Lahr BD, et al. Epidemiological trends of infective endocardi-

tis: a population-based study in Olmsted County, Minnesota. Mayo Clin Proc. 2010;85(5):422–6.
4. Hill EE, Herijgers P, Claus P, Vanderschueren S, Herregods MC, Peetermans WE. Infective endocarditis: changing epidemiology and predictors of 6-month mortality: a prospective cohort study. Eur Heart J. 2007;28(2):196–203.
5. Durante-Mangoni E, Bradley S, Selton-Suty C, Tripodi MF, Barsic B, Bouza E, et al. Current features of infective endocarditis in elderly patients: results of the International Collaboration on Endocarditis Prospective Cohort Study. Arch Intern Med. 2008;168(19):2095–103.
6. van der Meer JT, Thompson J, Valkenburg HA, Michel MF. Epidemiology of bacterial endocarditis in the Netherlands. II. Antecedent procedures and use of prophylaxis. Arch Intern Med. 1992;152(9):1869–73.
7. Murdoch DR, Corey GR, Hoen B, Miró JM, Fowler VG, Bayer AS, et al. Clinical presentation, etiology, and outcome of infective endocarditis in the 21st century: the International Collaboration on Endocarditis-Prospective Cohort Study. Arch Intern Med. 2009;169(5):463–73.
8. Wilson LE, Thomas DL, Astemborski J, Freedman TL, Vlahov D. Prospective study of infective endocarditis among injection drug users. J Infect Dis. 2002;185(12):1761–6.
9. Chu VH, Cabell CH, Benjamin DK, Kuniholm EF, Fowler VG, Engemann J, et al. Early predictors of in-hospital death in infective endocarditis. Circulation. 2004;109(14):1745–9.
10. Thuny F, Di Salvo G, Disalvo G, Belliard O, Avierinos JF, Pergola V, et al. Risk of embolism and death in infective endocarditis: prognostic value of echocardiography: a prospective multicenter study. Circulation. 2005;112(1):69–75.
11. Wallace SM, Walton BI, Kharbanda RK, Hardy R, Wilson AP, Swanton RH. Mortality from infective endocarditis: clinical predictors of outcome. Heart. 2002;88(1):53–60.
12. Sy RW, Kritharides L. Health care exposure and age in infective endocarditis: results of a contemporary population-based profile of 1536 patients in Australia. Eur Heart J. 2010;31(15):1890–7.
13. Selton-Suty C, Célard M, Le Moing V, Doco-Lecompte T, Chirouze C, Iung B, et al. Preeminence of Staphylococcus aureus in infective endocarditis: a 1-year population-based survey. Clin Infect Dis. 2012;54(9):1230–9.
14. Moreillon P, Que YA. Infective endocarditis. Lancet. 2004;363(9403):139–49.
15. Chu VH, Woods CW, Miro JM, Hoen B, Cabell CH, Pappas PA, et al. Emergence of coagulase-negative staphylococci as a cause of native valve endocarditis. Clin Infect Dis. 2008;46(2):232–42.
16. Chu VH, Miro JM, Hoen B, Cabell CH, Pappas PA, Jones P, et al. Coagulase-negative staphylococcal prosthetic valve endocarditis—a contemporary update based on the International Collaboration on Endocarditis: Prospective Cohort Study. Heart. 2009;95(7):570–6.
17. Lin CH, Hsu RB. Infective endocarditis caused by nutritionally variant streptococci. Am J Med Sci. 2007;334(4):235–9.
18. Fernández-Ruiz M, Villar-Silva J, Llenas-García J, Caurcel-Díaz L, Vila-Santos J, Sanz-Sanz F, et al. Streptococcus bovis bacteraemia revisited: clinical and microbiological correlates in a contemporary series of 59 patients. J Infect. 2010;61(4):307–13.
19. Martínez E, Miró JM, Almirante B, Aguado JM, Fernandez-Viladrich P, Fernandez-Guerrero ML, et al. Effect of penicillin resistance of Streptococcus pneumoniae on the presentation, prognosis, and treatment of pneumococcal endocarditis in adults. Clin Infect Dis. 2002;35(2):130–9.
20. Chirouze C, Athan E, Alla F, Chu VH, Ralph Corey G, Selton-Suty C, et al. Enterococcal endocarditis in the beginning of the 21st century: analysis from the International Collaboration on Endocarditis-Prospective Cohort Study. Clin Microbiol Infect. 2013;19(12):1140–7.
21. Chambers ST, Murdoch D, Morris A, Holland D, Pappas P, Almela M, et al. HACEK infective endocarditis: characteristics and outcomes from a large, multi-national cohort. PLoS One. 2013;8(5):e63181.
22. Morpeth S, Murdoch D, Cabell CH, Karchmer AW, Pappas P, Levine D, et al. Non-HACEK gram-negative bacillus endocarditis. Ann Intern Med. 2007;147(12):829–35.
23. Raza SS, Sultan OW, Sohail MR. Gram-negative bacterial endocarditis in adults: state-of-the-heart. Expert Rev Anti-Infect Ther. 2010;8(8):879–85.
24. Gould FK, Denning DW, Elliott TS, Foweraker J, Perry JD, Prendergast BD, et al. Guidelines for the diagnosis and antibiotic treatment of endocarditis in adults: a report of the Working Party of the British Society for Antimicrobial Chemotherapy. J Antimicrob Chemother. 2012;67(2):269–89.
25. Tattevin P, Watt G, Revest M, Arvieux C, Fournier PE. Update on blood culture-negative endocarditis. Med Mal Infect. 2015;45(1–2):1–8.
26. Pelletier LL, Petersdorf RG. Infective endocarditis: a review of 125 cases from the University of Washington Hospitals, 1963–72. Medicine (Baltimore). 1977;56(4):287–313.
27. Durack DT, Lukes AS, Bright DK. New criteria for diagnosis of infective endocarditis: utilization of specific echocardiographic findings. Duke Endocarditis Service. Am J Med. 1994;96(3):200–9.
28. Li JS, Sexton DJ, Mick N, Nettles R, Fowler VG, Ryan T, et al. Proposed modifications to the Duke criteria for the diagnosis of infective endocarditis. Clin Infect Dis. 2000;30(4):633–8.
29. Thuny F, Grisoli D, Cautela J, Riberi A, Raoult D, Habib G. Infective endocarditis: prevention, diagnosis, and management. Can J Cardiol. 2014;30(9):1046–57.
30. Raoult D, Casalta JP, Richet H, Khan M, Bernit E, Rovery C, et al. Contribution of systematic serological testing in diagnosis of infective endocarditis. J Clin Microbiol. 2005;43(10):5238–42.
31. Fournier PE, Thuny F, Richet H, Lepidi H, Casalta JP, Arzouni JP, et al. Comprehensive diagnostic strategy for blood culture-negative endocarditis: a prospective study of 819 new cases. Clin Infect Dis. 2010;51(2):131–40.
32. Heiro M, Helenius H, Sundell J, Koskinen P, Engblom E, Nikoskelainen J, et al. Utility of serum C-reactive protein in assessing the outcome of infective endocarditis. Eur Heart J. 2005;26(18):1873–81.
33. Okada Y, Hosono M, Sasaki Y, Hirai H, Suehiro S. Preoperative increasing C-reactive protein affects the outcome for active infective endocarditis. Ann Thorac Cardiovasc Surg. 2014;20(1):48–54.
34. Habib G, Badano L, Tribouilloy C, Vilacosta I, Zamorano JL, Galderisi M, et al. Recommendations for the practice of echocardiography in infective endocarditis. Eur Heart J Cardiovasc Imaging. 2010;11(2):202–19.
35. Thuny F, Disalvo G, Belliard O, Avierinos J-F, Pergola V, Rosenberg V, et al. Risk of embolism and death in infective endocarditis: prognostic value of echocardiography: a prospective multicenter study. Circulation. 2005;112(1):69–75.
36. Baddour LM, Wilson WR, Bayer AS, Fowler VG, Bolger AF, Levison ME, et al. Infective endocarditis: diagnosis, antimicrobial therapy, and management of complications: a statement for healthcare professionals from the Committee on Rheumatic Fever, Endocarditis, and Kawasaki Disease, Council on Cardiovascular Disease in the Young, and the Councils on Clinical Cardiology, Stroke, and Cardiovascular Surgery and Anesthesia, American Heart Association: endorsed by the Infectious Diseases Society of America. Circulation. 2005;111(23):e394–434.
37. Grob A, Thuny F, Villacampa C, Flavian A, Gaubert JY, Raoult D, et al. Cardiac multidetector computed tomography in infective endocarditis: a pictorial essay. Insights Imaging. 2014;5(5):559–70.
38. Feuchtner GM, Stolzmann P, Dichtl W, Schertler T, Bonatti J, Scheffel H, et al. Multislice computed tomography in infective endocarditis: comparison with transesophageal echocardiography and intraoperative findings. J Am Coll Cardiol. 2009;53(5):436–44.

39. Fagman E, Perrotta S, Bech-Hanssen O, Flinck A, Lamm C, Olaison L, et al. ECG-gated computed tomography: a new role for patients with suspected aortic prosthetic valve endocarditis. Eur Radiol. 2012;22(11):2407–14.
40. Tanis W, Scholtens A, Habets J, van den Brink RBA, van Herwerden LA, Chamuleau SAJ, et al. CT angiography and 18F-FDG-PET fusion imaging for prosthetic heart valve endocarditis. JACC Cardiovasc Imaging. 2013;6(9):1008–13.
41. Hyafil F, Rouzet F, Lepage L, Benali K, Raffoul R, Duval X, et al. Role of radiolabelled leucocyte scintigraphy in patients with a suspicion of prosthetic valve endocarditis and inconclusive echocardiography. Eur Heart J Cardiovasc Imaging. 2013;14(6):586–94.
42. Prendergast BD, Tornos P. Surgery for infective endocarditis: who and when? Circulation. 2010;121(9):1141–52.
43. Arnett EN, Roberts WC. Valve ring abscess in active infective endocarditis. Frequency, location, and clues to clinical diagnosis from the study of 95 necropsy patients. Circulation. 1976;54(1):140–5.
44. Attias D, Messika-Zeitoun D, Wolf M, Lepage L, Vahanian A. Acute coronary syndrome in aortic infective endocarditis. Eur J Echocardiogr. 2008;9(6):727–8.
45. Rose RL, Higgins LS, Helgason AH. Bacterial endocarditis, pericarditis and cardiac tamponade. Am J Cardiol. 1967;19(3):447–51.
46. Ribeiro P, Shapiro L, Nihoyannopoulos P, Gonzalez A, Oakley CM. Pericarditis in infective endocarditis. Eur Heart J. 1985;6(11):975–8.
47. Di Salvo G, Habib G, Pergola V, Avierinos JF, Philip E, Casalta JP, et al. Echocardiography predicts embolic events in infective endocarditis. J Am Coll Cardiol. 2001;37(4):1069–76.
48. Bayer AS, Bolger AF, Taubert KA, Wilson W, Steckelberg J, Karchmer AW, et al. Diagnosis and management of infective endocarditis and its complications. Circulation. 1998;98(25):2936–48.
49. Rohmann S, Erbel R, Görge G, Makowski T, Mohr-Kahaly S, Nixdorff U, et al. Clinical relevance of vegetation localization by transoesophageal echocardiography in infective endocarditis. Eur Heart J. 1992;13(4):446–52.
50. Hubert S, Thuny F, Resseguier N, Giorgi R, Tribouilloy C, Le Dolley Y, et al. Prediction of symptomatic embolism in infective endocarditis: construction and validation of a risk calculator in a multicenter cohort. J Am Coll Cardiol. 2013;62(15):1384–92.
51. Jones HR, Siekert RG. Neurological manifestations of infective endocarditis. Review of clinical and therapeutic challenges. Brain. 1989;112(Pt 5):1295–315.
52. Cabell CH, Pond KK, Peterson GE, Durack DT, Corey GR, Anderson DJ, et al. The risk of stroke and death in patients with aortic and mitral valve endocarditis. Am Heart J. 2001;142(1):75–80.
53. Anderson DJ, Goldstein LB, Wilkinson WE, Corey GR, Cabell CH, Sanders LL, et al. Stroke location, characterization, severity, and outcome in mitral vs aortic valve endocarditis. Neurology. 2003;61(10):1341–6.
54. Duval X, Iung B, Klein I, Brochet E, Thabut G, Arnoult F, et al. Effect of early cerebral magnetic resonance imaging on clinical decisions in infective endocarditis: a prospective study. Ann Intern Med. 2010;152(8):497–504, W175.
55. Corr P, Wright M, Handler LC. Endocarditis-related cerebral aneurysms: radiologic changes with treatment. AJNR Am J Neuroradiol. 1995;16(4):745–8.
56. Nishimura RA, Otto CM, Bonow RO, Carabello BA, Erwin Iii JP, Guyton RA, et al. 2014 AHA/ACC guideline for the management of patients with valvular heart disease: a report of the American College of Cardiology/American Heart Association Task Force on Practice Guidelines. J Am Coll Cardiol. 2014;63(22):e57–e185.
57. Thuny F, Grisoli D, Collart F, Habib G, Raoult D. Management of infective endocarditis: challenges and perspectives. Lancet. 2012;379(9819):965–75.
58. Habib G, Hoen B, Tornos P, Thuny F, Prendergast B, Vilacosta I, et al. Guidelines on the prevention, diagnosis, and treatment of infective endocarditis (new version 2009): the Task Force on the Prevention, Diagnosis, and Treatment of Infective Endocarditis of the European Society of Cardiology (ESC). Endorsed by the European Society of Clinical Microbiology and Infectious Diseases (ESCMID) and the International Society of Chemotherapy (ISC) for Infection and Cancer. Eur Heart J. 2009;30(19):2369–413.
59. Thuny F, Habib G. When should we operate on patients with acute infective endocarditis? Heart. 2010;96(11):892–7.
60. Vikram HR, Buenconsejo J, Hasbun R, Quagliarello VJ. Impact of valve surgery on 6-month mortality in adults with complicated, left-sided native valve endocarditis: a propensity analysis. JAMA. 2003;290(24):3207–14.
61. Lalani T, Cabell CH, Benjamin DK, Lasca O, Naber C, Fowler VG, et al. Analysis of the impact of early surgery on in-hospital mortality of native valve endocarditis: use of propensity score and instrumental variable methods to adjust for treatment-selection bias. Circulation. 2010;121(8):1005–13.
62. Alexiou C, Langley SM, Stafford H, Lowes JA, Livesey SA, Monro JL. Surgery for active culture-positive endocarditis: determinants of early and late outcome. Ann Thorac Surg. 2000;69(5):1448–54.
63. Jault F, Gandjbakhch I, Rama A, Nectoux M, Bors V, Vaissier E, et al. Active native valve endocarditis: determinants of operative death and late mortality. Ann Thorac Surg. 1997;63(6):1737–41.
64. Shiue AB, Stancoven AB, Purcell JB, Pinkston K, Wang A, Khera A, et al. Relation of level of B-type natriuretic peptide with outcomes in patients with infective endocarditis. Am J Cardiol. 2010;106(7):1011–5.
65. Gaca JG, Sheng S, Daneshmand MA, O'Brien S, Rankin JS, Brennan JM, et al. Outcomes for endocarditis surgery in North America: a simplified risk scoring system. J Thorac Cardiovasc Surg. 2011;141(1):98–106.e1–2.
66. Hasbun R, Vikram HR, Barakat LA, Buenconsejo J, Quagliarello VJ. Complicated left-sided native valve endocarditis in adults: risk classification for mortality. JAMA. 2003;289(15):1933.
67. Sy RW, Chawantanpipat C, Richmond DR, Kritharides L. Development and validation of a time-dependent risk model for predicting mortality in infective endocarditis. Eur Heart J. 2011;32(16):2016–26.
68. López J, Fernández-Hidalgo N, Revilla A, Vilacosta I, Tornos P, Almirante B, et al. Internal and external validation of a model to predict adverse outcomes in patients with left-sided infective endocarditis. Heart. 2011;97(14):1138–42.
69. al Jubair K, al Fagih MR, Ashmeg A, Belhaj M, Sawyer W. Cardiac operations during active endocarditis. J Thorac Cardiovasc Surg. 1992;104(2):487–90.
70. Larbalestier RI, Kinchla NM, Aranki SF, Couper GS, Collins JJ, Cohn LH. Acute bacterial endocarditis. Optimizing surgical results. Circulation. 1992;86(5 Suppl):II68–74.
71. Kang DH, Kim YJ, Kim SH, Sun BJ, Kim DH, Yun SC, et al. Early surgery versus conventional treatment for infective endocarditis. N Engl J Med. 2012;366(26):2466–73.
72. García-Cabrera E, Fernández-Hidalgo N, Almirante B, Ivanova-Georgieva R, Noureddine M, Plata A, et al. Neurological complications of infective endocarditis: risk factors, outcome, and impact of cardiac surgery: a multicenter observational study. Circulation. 2013;127(23):2272–84.
73. Thuny F, Avierinos JF, Tribouilloy C, Giorgi R, Casalta JP, Milandre L, et al. Impact of cerebrovascular complications on mortality and neurologic outcome during infective endocarditis: a prospective multicentre study. Eur Heart J. 2007;28(9):1155–61.
74. Barsic B, Dickerman S, Krajinovic V, Pappas P, Altclas J, Carosi G, et al. Influence of the timing of cardiac surgery on the outcome of patients with infective endocarditis and stroke. Clin Infect Dis. 2013;56(2):209–17.
75. Moon MR, Stinson EB, Miller DC. Surgical treatment of endocarditis. Prog Cardiovasc Dis. 1997;40(3):239–64.

76. Daniel WG, Mügge A, Martin RP, Lindert O, Hausmann D, Nonnast-Daniel B, et al. Improvement in the diagnosis of abscesses associated with endocarditis by transesophageal echocardiography. N Engl J Med. 1991;324(12):795–800.
77. Omari B, Shapiro S, Ginzton L, Robertson JM, Ward J, Nelson RJ, et al. Predictive risk factors for periannular extension of native valve endocarditis. Clinical and echocardiographic analyses. Chest. 1989;96(6):1273–9.
78. Choussat R, Thomas D, Isnard R, Michel PL, Iung B, Hanania G, et al. Perivalvular abscesses associated with endocarditis; clinical features and prognostic factors of overall survival in a series of 233 cases. Perivalvular Abscesses French Multicentre Study. Eur Heart J. 1999;20(3):232–41.
79. Pang PY, Sin YK, Lim CH, Tan TE, Lim SL, Chao VT, et al. Surgical management of infective endocarditis: an analysis of early and late outcomes. Eur J Cardiothorac Surg. 2015;47:826–32.
80. David TE, Gavra G, Feindel CM, Regesta T, Armstrong S, Maganti MD. Surgical treatment of active infective endocarditis: a continued challenge. J Thorac Cardiovasc Surg. 2007;133(1):144–9.
81. Feringa HHH, Shaw LJ, Poldermans D, Hoeks S, van der Wall EE, Dion RAE, et al. Mitral valve repair and replacement in endocarditis: a systematic review of literature. Ann Thorac Surg. 2007;83(2):564–70.
82. Vongpatanasin W, Hillis LD, Lange RA. Prosthetic heart valves. N Engl J Med. 1996;335(6):407–16.
83. Hoen B, Alla F, Selton-Suty C, Béguinot I, Bouvet A, Briançon S, et al. Changing profile of infective endocarditis: results of a 1-year survey in France. JAMA. 2002;288(1):75–81.
84. Moss R, Munt B. Injection drug use and right sided endocarditis. Heart. 2003;89(5):577–81.
85. Hecht SR, Berger M. Right-sided endocarditis in intravenous drug users. Prognostic features in 102 episodes. Ann Intern Med. 1992;117(7):560–6.
86. Duval X, Alla F, Hoen B, Danielou F, Larrieu S, Delahaye F, et al. Estimated risk of endocarditis in adults with predisposing cardiac conditions undergoing dental procedures with or without antibiotic prophylaxis. Clin Infect Dis. 2006;42(12):e102–7.
87. Veloso TR, Amiguet M, Rousson V, Giddey M, Vouillamoz J, Moreillon P, et al. Induction of experimental endocarditis by continuous low-grade bacteremia mimicking spontaneous bacteremia in humans. Infect Immun. 2011;79(5):2006–11.
88. Wilson W, Taubert KA, Gewitz M, Lockhart PB, Baddour LM, Levison M, et al. Prevention of infective endocarditis: guidelines from the American Heart Association: a guideline from the American Heart Association Rheumatic Fever, Endocarditis, and Kawasaki Disease Committee, Council on Cardiovascular Disease in the Young, and the Council on Clinical Cardiology, Council on Cardiovascular Surgery and Anesthesia, and the Quality of Care and Outcomes Research Interdisciplinary Working Group. Circulation. 2007;116(15):1736–54.
89. Richey R, Wray D, Stokes T, Guideline Development Group. Prophylaxis against infective endocarditis: summary of NICE guidance. BMJ. 2008;336(7647):770–1.
90. Thornhill MH, Dayer MJ, Forde JM, Corey GR, Chu VH, Couper DJ, et al. Impact of the NICE guideline recommending cessation of antibiotic prophylaxis for prevention of infective endocarditis: before and after study. BMJ. 2011;342:d2392.

Inflammation Injury and Selected Disease Processes Causing Aortic Root and Aortic Valvular Inflammation

4

James T. Willerson and L. Maximilian Buja

Marfan Syndrome

Marfan syndrome (MFS) is an autosomal dominant disease characterized by cardiovascular, ocular, and skeletal problems. The disorder has an estimated prevalence of 1 in 3000–5000 individuals. Although MFS is inherited as an autosomal dominant disorder, in approximately one-third of cases, the individual with MFS has unaffected parents. In these cases, the syndrome is believed to be caused by sporadic, new mutations in the affected individual.

Cardiovascular Manifestations

The most common cardiovascular complication in patients with MFS is progressive aortic root enlargement that initiates at the sinuses of Valsalva [1]. Ascending aortic aneurysms can lead to acute, type A aortic dissection; aortic rupture; or aortic regurgitation, which can result in premature death. Management of aortic disease in these patients consists of regular imaging to detect and assess the progression of aortic dilation, β-adrenergic receptor antagonist therapy (in the largest dose tolerable by the patient), and prophylactic aortic repair when the dilation becomes ≥5.0 cm or causes severe AR. Before surgical repair of the aorta became an option, the majority of patients with MFS died prematurely of aortic rupture, resulting in an average life expectancy of 45 years [2]. Improvements in the medical and surgical management of the aortic disease in these individuals have substantially increased their average life expectancy to 70 years [3, 4].

J. T. Willerson (✉)
Department of Cardiology, Texas Heart Institute, Houston, TX, USA
e-mail: jwillerson@texasheart.org

L. M. Buja
Department of Pathology and Laboratory Medicine, McGovern Medical School, The University of Texas Health Science Center at Houston (UTHealth), Houston, TX, USA

Department of Cardiovascular Pathology Research, Texas Heart Institute, Houston, TX, USA

Aortic root dilatation typically begins at the sinuses of Valsalva and progresses to involve the proximal ascending aorta. The rate of enlargement of the proximal aorta varies widely among individuals, and the progressive enlargement is usually asymptomatic. Therefore, the proximal aorta should be evaluated annually or more often, depending on the severity of the dilatation. Transthoracic echocardiography provides precise measurements of aortic root size for comparison over time. Magnetic resonance imaging and transesophageal echocardiography are also useful. Use of aortography is usually limited to studies performed before surgery to define the anatomy (Fig. 4.1).

Aortic valve insufficiency often occurs as the aorta dilates. The risk of the proximal aorta rupturing increases as the size of the aortic root increases. Consideration of prophylactic aortic root replacement is recommended when the diameter reaches 5.0 cm [6, 7]. Once an aneurysm is larger than 6 cm, there is a fourfold increase in the cumulative risk of aortic rupture or dissection [6]. In some cases, surgery may be performed when the aortic diameter is less than 5.0 cm, such as when the aortic diameter increases rapidly (>1 cm/year), when the patient has a family history of premature aortic dissection (dissection occurring when the diameter is <5 cm), and when the patient has moderate-to-severe aortic regurgitation.

Composite valve graft replacement is achieved by mobilizing buttons of aortic tissue around the coronary arteries for anastomosis to the aortic graft. These patients are maintained on beta blockers, and bacterial prophylaxis is recommended. The most common causes of late death after composite valve graft repair are undergoing dental work or invasive diagnostic or surgical procedures and dissection or rupture of the residual distal aorta. Approximately 10% of the patients who undergo composite valve graft repair subsequently require distal aortic surgery.

Other surgical procedures have been developed that preserve the patient's native aortic valve; these are called "valve-sparing" aortic root replacement procedures [8, 9]. The Yacoub procedure is referred to as the "remodeling" technique

B. A. Carabello (ed.), *Valvular Heart Disease*, Cardiovascular Medicine, https://doi.org/10.1007/978-1-4471-2840-3_4

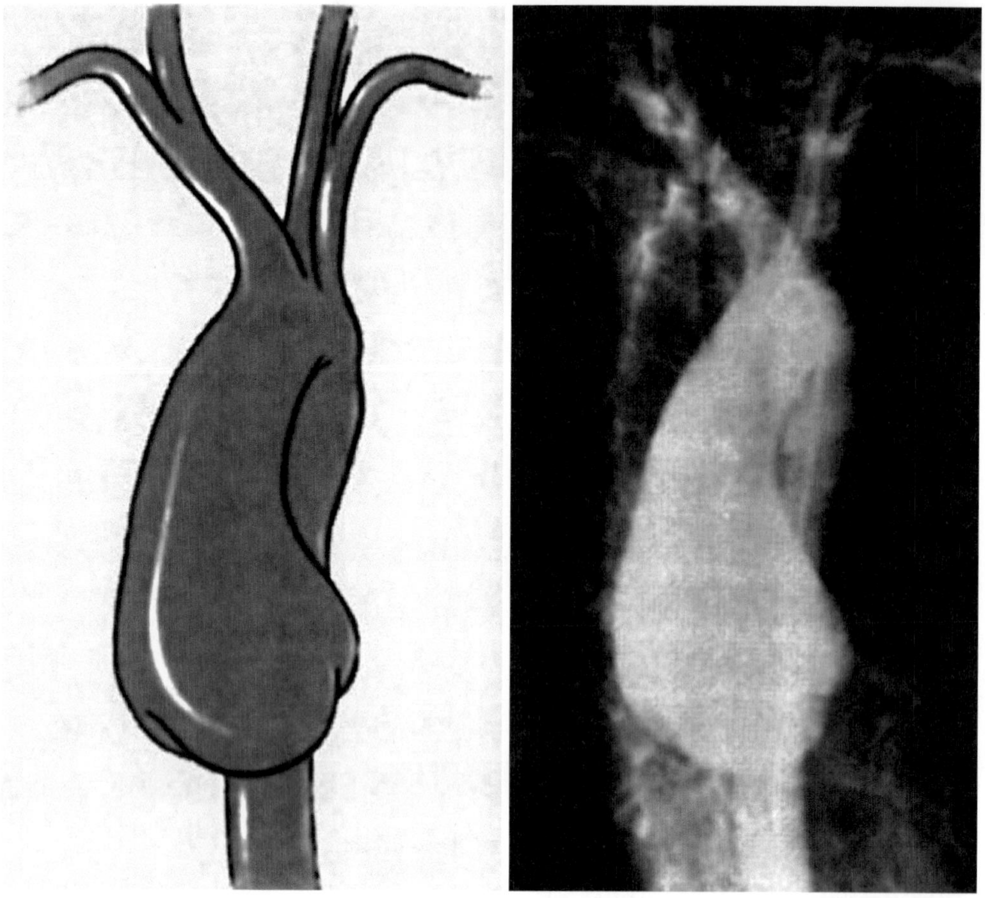

Fig. 4.1 Illustration and aortogram of an aneurysm of the ascending aorta. From Milewicz [5], reprinted with permission from Springer Nature

and the David procedure is considered the "reimplantation" technique [10, 11]. Both procedures are options for almost all patients with aortic root aneurysms, as long as the aortic valve is structurally normal. In addition, for both techniques, patient survival is excellent, and complications are rare.

Some patients with MFS develop a dissection through the medial layer of the aortic wall. Most of these are type I dissections (DeBakey classification), which also involve the descending thoracic aorta. Dissections involving the ascending aorta can occur in patients who have minimal to no enlargement of the ascending aorta. Most of these dissections occur in the absence of systemic hypertension. Angiography, transesophageal echocardiography, and magnetic resonance imaging are useful techniques for diagnosing aortic dissections. Beta blockers, when tolerated, are used for treatment.

Mitral valve prolapse is present in 70–90% of patients with MFS. Associated mitral regurgitation occurs in up to half of these patients, but serious mitral regurgitation is rare. Mitral valve prolapse can be associated with chest pain and palpitations.

Skeletal and Ocular Manifestations

The skeletal features of the disorder include increased height and arm span; anterior chest wall deformities (pectus excavatum or carinatum); long fingers and toes (arachnodactyly); mild-to-moderate joint laxity; a narrow, highly arched palate and crowding of the frontal teeth; pes planus (flat feet); protrusio acetabuli; and vertebral column abnormalities (scoliosis and thoracic lordosis). The skeletal manifestations of MFS are the most outwardly striking features of the disorder and are often the features that trigger the initial evaluation. Patients usually have a tall stature, primarily due to having long, thin legs, which is reflected in a decreased ratio of the upper body segment (height minus the lower segment) to the lower body segment (top of pubic ramus to the floor). They also generally have an arm span that is greater than their height. The reduced upper-to-lower segment ratio can be further exaggerated by scoliosis and kyphosis.

Marfan syndrome can also affect the eyes. In approximately 50% of the people with MFS, the lenses of the eyes are dislocated (ectopia lentis). Myopia is also common in patients with MFS, but retinal detachment is a rare complication.

Diagnosis

Diagnosing MFS is a complicated clinical decision. The diagnostic criteria for MFS were initially established by an international consortium of clinicians in 1986. The Ghent

Table 4.1 Revised Ghent criteria for diagnosing Marfan syndrome and related conditions

In the absence of family history:
1. Ao ($Z \geq 2$) AND EL = MFS[a]
2. Ao ($Z \geq 2$) AND *FBN1* = MFS
3. Ao ($Z \geq 2$) AND Syst (≥7 pts) = MFS[a]
4. EL AND *FBN1* with known Ao = MFS
EL with or without Syst AND with an *FBN1* not known with Ao or no *FBN1* = ELS
Ao ($Z < 2$) AND Syst (≥5 with at least one skeletal feature) without EL = MASS
MVP AND Ao ($Z < 2$) AND Syst (<5) without EL = MVPS
In the presence of family history (FH):
5. EL AND FH of MFS (as defined above) = MFS
6. Syst (≥7 pts) AND FH of MFS (as defined above) = MFS[a]
7. Ao ($Z \geq 2$ above 20 years old, ≥3 below 20 years) + FH of MFS (as defined above) = MFS[a]

Ao aortic diameter at the sinuses of Valsalva above indicated *Z*-score or aortic root dissection, *EL* ectopia lentis, *ELS* ectopia lentis syndrome, *FBN1* fibrillin-1 mutation, *FBN1* not known with Ao, *FBN1* mutation that has not previously been associated with aortic root aneurysm/dissection, *FBN1* with known Ao, *FBN1* mutation that has been identified in an individual with aortic aneurysm, *LDS* Loeys-Dietz syndrome, *MASS* myopia, mitral valve prolapse, borderline ($Z < 2$) aortic root dilatation, striae, skeletal findings phenotype, *MFS* Marfan syndrome, *MVPS* mitral valve prolapse syndrome, *SGS* Shprintzen-Goldberg syndrome, *Syst* systemic score, *vEDS* vascular form of Ehlers-Danlos syndrome, *Z* Z-score

From Loeys et al. [13]. Reprinted with permission from BMJ Publishing Group Ltd.

[a]Caveat: without discriminating features of SGS, LDS, or vEDS AND after *TGFBR1/2*, collagen biochemistry, *COL3A1* testing, if indicated. Other conditions/genes will emerge with time

criteria for diagnosing MFS were introduced in 1996 [12] and revised in 2010 [13]. The 2010 Ghent criteria focus on two cardinal features of MFS: aortic root aneurysm/dissection and ectopia lentis (Table 4.1). The presence of both of these features should be sufficient to diagnosis MFS. When the patient has no family history of MFS and has only one of these features, then the diagnosis is guided by genetic testing results or a "systemic score" that is based on other cardiovascular and ocular manifestations of MFS, as well as findings in other organ systems, such as the skeleton, dura, skin, and lungs (Table 4.2). When the patient has a family history of MFS, then the diagnosis can be made if the patient has one of the two cardinal features of MFS or a high systemic score (i.e., ≥7 points). However, the revised Ghent criteria also provide a caveat regarding the presence of unexpected findings that could be suggestive of an alternative diagnosis, such as Shprintzen-Goldberg syndrome, Loeys-Dietz syndrome, or the vascular form of Ehlers-Danlos syndrome.

Genetic Mutations

It has been clearly established that MFS can be caused by defects in the fibrillin gene (*FBN1*) on chromosome 15. A number of mutations in *FBN1* have been identified in affected individuals and families. An analysis of *FBN1* mutations responsible for MFS has indicated that in almost every case, the mutations are private—that is, every family or sporadically affected individual has a different mutation [14]. The majority of mutations are missense mutations that alter a single amino acid. In addition, a second locus for MFS, called the *MFS2* locus, has been mapped to 3p24-25 [15]. Furthermore, mutations in transforming growth factor-β (TGF-β) receptor type II (*TGFBR2*) have recently been described in patients with MFS [16].

Table 4.2 Scoring of systemic features of Marfan syndrome

• Wrist AND thumb sign—3 (wrist OR thumb sign—1)
• Pectus carinatum deformity—2 (pectus excavatum or chest asymmetry—1)
• Hindfoot deformity—2 (plain pes planus—1)
• Pneumothorax—2
• Dural ectasia—2
• Protrusio acetabuli—2
• Reduced US/LS AND increased arm/height AND no severe scoliosis—1
• Scoliosis or thoracolumbar kyphosis—1
• Reduced elbow extension—1
• Facial features (3/5)—1 (dolichocephaly, enophthalmos, downslanting palpebral fissures, malar hypoplasia, retrognathia)
• Skin striae
• Myopia >3 diopters—1
• Mitral valve prolapse (all types)—1

Maximum total: 20 points; score ≥7 indicates systemic involvement; *US/UL* upper segment/lower segment ratio

From Loeys et al. [13]. Reprinted with permission from BMJ Publishing Group Ltd.

Future Therapies

One direction for future therapies will be to prevent the steps that lead from a deficiency in fibrillin-1-containing microfibrils to the aortic wall pathology observed in MFS patients (fragmentation and degradation of the elastic fibers and loss of the smooth muscle cells in the medial layer). Another possible avenue for therapy is based on the findings that fibrillin-1 and microfibrils regulate the TGF-β family of growth factors (cytokines), which influence many aspects of cellular performance, including differentiation, proliferation, protein production, and survival [17].

Relapsing Polychondritis

Relapsing polychondritis is a rare disorder of unknown etiology that is characterized by inflammation and destruction of various cartilaginous structures [18, 19]. Circulating antibodies to type II collagen have been found in some patients [20]. Disease onset is usually in middle age, with men and women showing no difference in age of onset. Bilateral auricular chondritis (Fig. 4.2) is the most common symptom at presentation, followed by laryngotracheal involvement or saddle nose deformity (Fig. 4.3), arthritis, fever, and neurosensory hearing loss [22]. Approximately 15% of patients have systemic vasculitis affecting the medium or large arteries [22], and approximately 24% of patients have cardiovascular complications; the most common of these are aortic regurgitation, followed by mitral regurgitation, pericarditis, and myocardial ischemia [18, 22]. Patients may also develop aortic or large-artery aneurysms, which may thrombose or rupture.

The treatment used depends on the disease severity and the organs involved. Corticosteroids are usually required. Immunosuppressive agents may be effective in patients with steroid resistance or intolerance. Cardiac valve replacement is sometimes necessary [22].

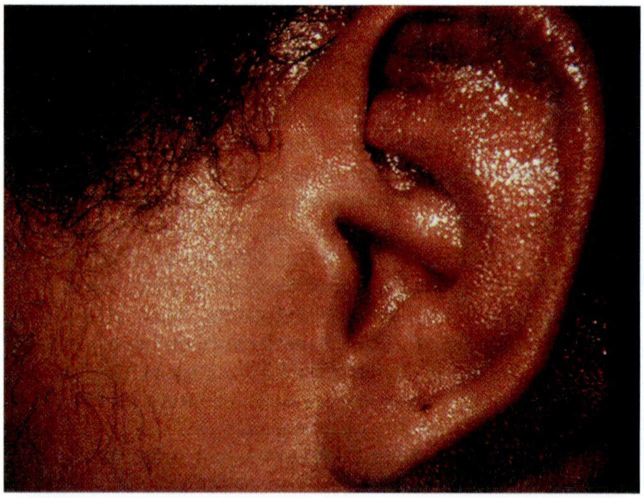

Fig. 4.2 Inflammation and partial collapse of the auricular cartilage in a patient with relapsing polychondritis. From Arnett and Willerson [21], reprinted with permission from Springer Nature

Seronegative Spondyloarthritis

Seronegative spondyloarthritis is a group of diseases that includes ankylosing spondylitis, reactive arthritis (formerly called Reiter's disease), psoriatic arthritis, and the arthritis associated with the idiopathic inflammatory bowel diseases ulcerative colitis and Crohn's disease [23]. These chronic arthritides are now known to be clinically, epidemiologically, and genetically separate entities; moreover, patients with these conditions do not have rheumatoid factor or antinuclear antibodies (ANAs).

Joint and Ocular Manifestation

All of these diseases are characterized by a sterile inflammatory process that affects the spinal or peripheral joints, as well as the tendons and ligamentous insertions (enthesitis), which often leads to bony fusion. In ankylosing spondylitis, the axial skeleton is predominantly involved. Joint fusion typically begins in the sacroiliac joints and then progressively ascends into the lumbar, dorsal, and cervical segments, resulting in a rigid and often deformed spine. Radiographs characteristically show sacroiliitis (Fig. 4.4), squaring of the vertebrae, and ossification of the spinal ligaments between the vertebrae (syndesmophytes), giving the spine a "bamboo" appearance (Fig. 4.5). Reactive arthritis and psoriatic arthritis primarily affect the peripheral joints, but similar spinal changes, especially sacroiliitis, occur in 20% of these patients (Fig. 4.6). Peripheral arthritis is a complication in 20% of inflammatory

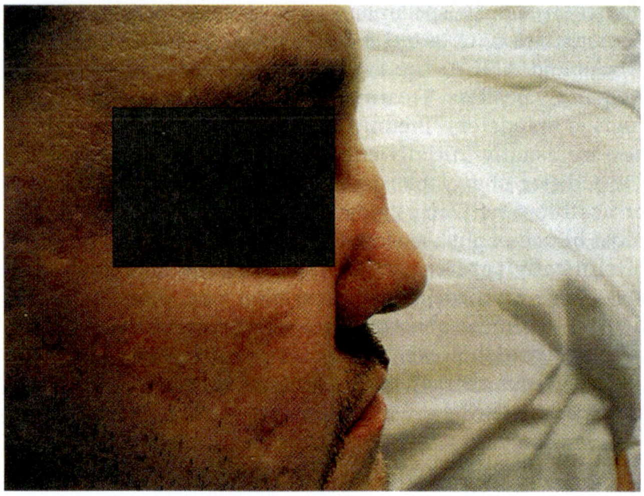

Fig. 4.3 Typical "saddle nose" deformity, which is caused by destruction and collapse of the nasal cartilage in patients with Wegener's granulomatosis or relapsing polychondritis. From Arnett and Willerson [21], reprinted with permission from Springer Nature

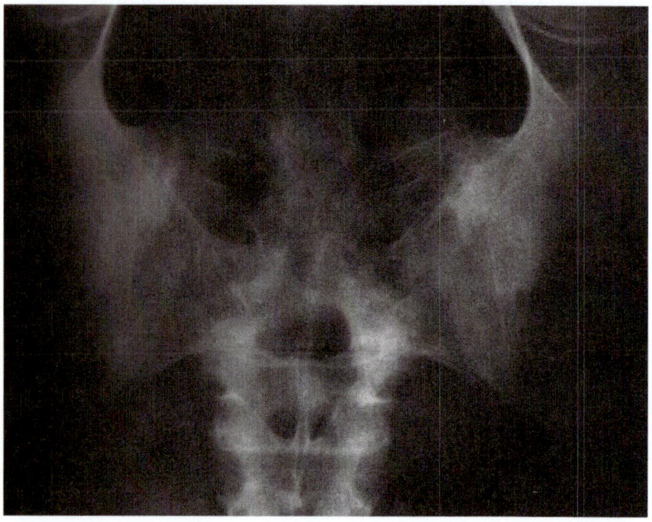

Fig. 4.4 Pelvic radiograph showing bilateral fusion of the sacroiliac joints (sacroiliitis) in a patient with a spondyloarthritis. From Arnett and Willerson [21], reprinted with permission from Springer Nature

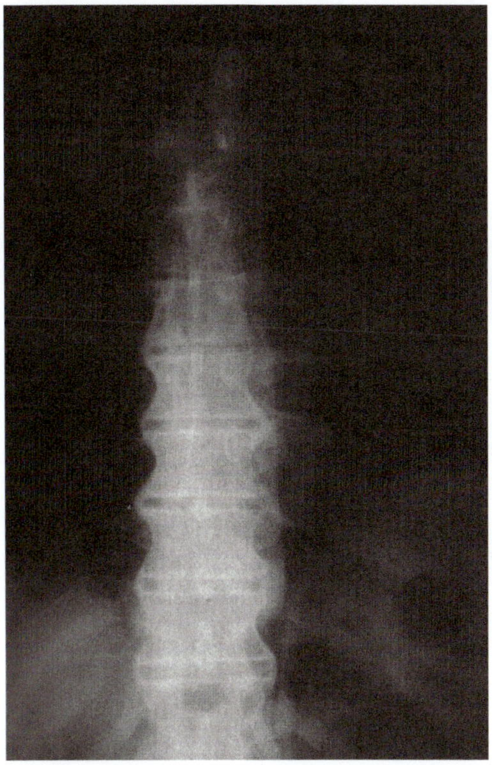

Fig. 4.5 Thoracolumbar radiograph showing calcified ligaments (syndesmophytes) bridging across intervertebral disks of a "bamboo" spine in a patient with ankylosing spondylitis. From Arnett and Willerson [21], reprinted with permission from Springer Nature

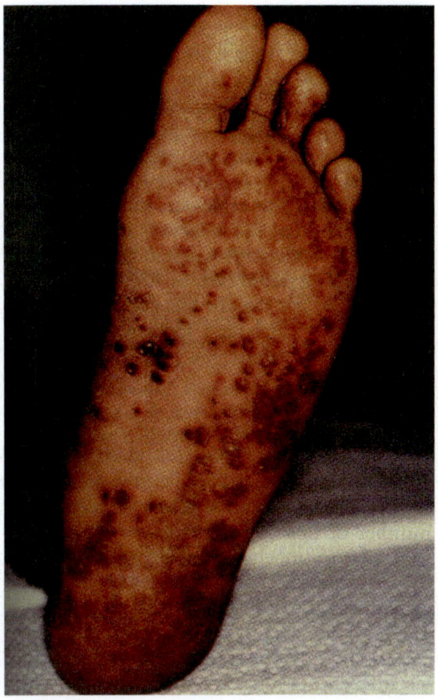

Fig. 4.6 The typical pustular rash (keratoderma blennorrhagica) of a patient with reactive arthritis. From Arnett and Willerson [21], reprinted with permission from Springer Nature

bowel disease cases, and spondylitis is a complication in 10% of these patients. Acute anterior uveitis occurs in approximately 25% of patients with a spondyloarthritis.

Cardiac Manifestations

A specific cardiac lesion is found in patients with spondyloarthritides. This lesion is aortic regurgitation, atrioventricular or bundle branch conduction defects, or, rarely, mitral regurgitation (Fig. 4.7) [24–31]. Dilatation and thickening

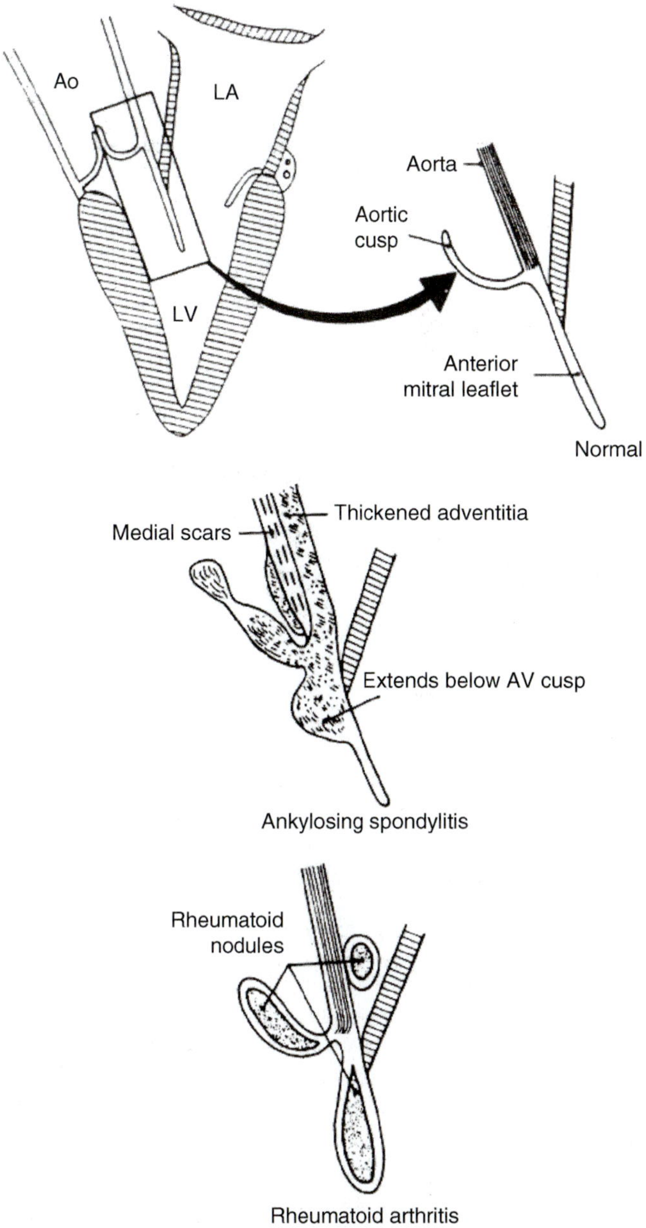

Fig. 4.7 Schematic representation of the typical cardiac lesions of ankylosing spondylitis contrasted with those of rheumatoid arthritis. *Ao* aorta, *AV* atrioventricular, *LA* left atrium, *LV* left ventricle. From Arnett and Willerson [21], reprinted with permission from Springer Nature

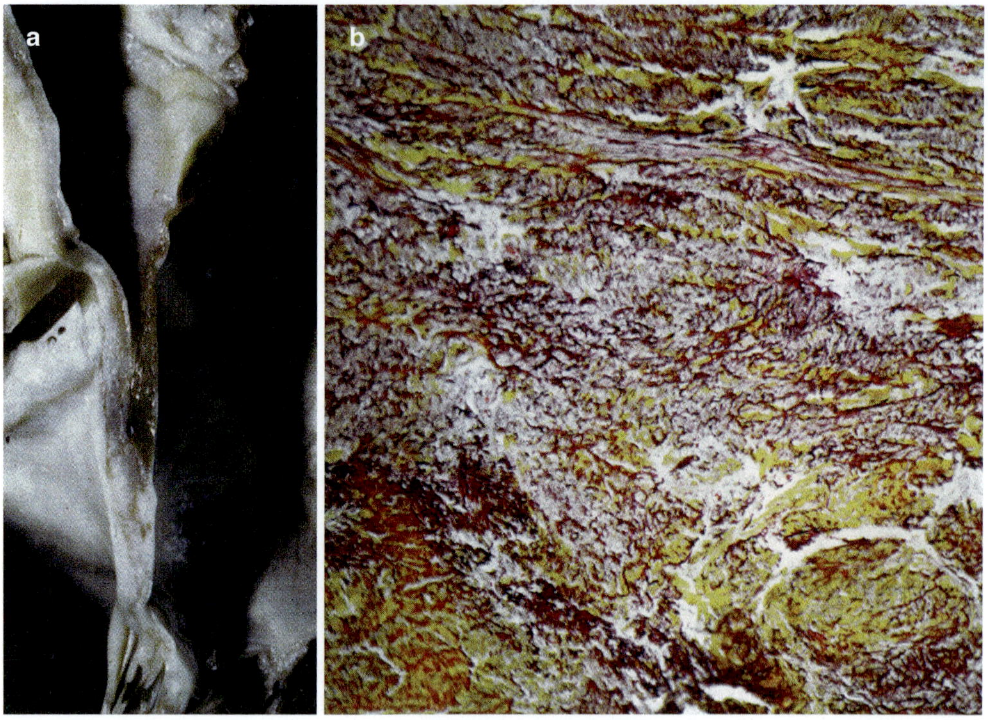

Fig. 4.8 Necropsy specimens from a patient with ankylosing spondylitis and aortic regurgitation. (**a**) Gross section through the aortic valve and interventricular septum showing thickening of these structures. (**b**) Histopathology of the same region showing fibrous thickening. From Arnett and Willerson [21], reprinted with permission from Springer Nature

of the walls of the proximal aortic root, especially behind and immediately above the sinus of Valsalva, have been shown histopathologically, along with thickening and shortening of the aortic valve cusps and the development of a fibrous mass (or bump) below the aortic valve (Figs. 4.7 and 4.8) [25–31]. Surrounding the vasa vasorum are collections of plasma cells and lymphocytes [26]. Mitral regurgitation occurs because of a similar fibrous thickening at the basal portion of the anterior mitral leaflet and dilatation of the left ventricle from aortic regurgitation. Bundle branch block and complete heart block occur as the fibrosing process extends from the membranous ventricular septum into the muscular septum, where it interrupts or destroys the conducting fibers in the atrioventricular bundle or proximal bundle branches [26, 32].

In approximately 5% of ankylosing spondylitis cases and in rare cases of reactive arthritis, the patient develops spondylitic heart disease [30, 33, 34]. In the reported cases of spondylitic heart disease, HLA-B27 positivity is usually found. This complication usually occurs after many years of having arthritis. First-degree atrioventricular block and aortic regurgitation have been reported in the early stages of the disease [35–37], even before the appearance of arthritis symptoms [35, 37]. Clinically inapparent aortic involvement may be found with echocardiography. Using two-dimensional transthoracic echocardiography, LaBresh et al. [38] found subaortic fibrous ridging or marked valvular leaflet thickening in 11 of 36 men with ankylosing spondylitis or chronic reactive arthritis, but not in any of the 29 normal, age-matched control men. In a study by Arnason et al. [39], transesophageal echocardiography showed aortic valve insufficiency in 10 of 29 men with ankylosing spondylitis, as well as the aortic and valvular thickening seen pathologically. Studies of men who required cardiac pacemakers for complete heart block have shown that these men had high frequencies of underlying spondyloarthritis (often occult) or HLA-B27 positivity. Bergfeldt and colleagues [40, 41] found clinical or radiographic evidence of spondyloarthritis in 28 (12.6%) of 223 men with permanent cardiac pacemakers, 85% of whom were HLA-B27 positive. They also showed that of 83 pacemaker recipients who had no clinical or radiographic stigmata of spondylitis, 17% were HLA-B27 positive, which was a significantly higher frequency than in normal controls (6%) [42]. In another group comprising 91 patients with aortic regurgitation, 15–20% of the patients were found to have B27-associated arthritis [25]. Furthermore, 88% of the male patients who had aortic regurgitation combined with severe conduction system abnormalities were HLA-B27 positive.

Aortic regurgitation and, less often, mitral regurgitation progress relatively rapidly. In most patients with these conditions, prosthetic valve replacement is required in less than 5 years [26, 27, 31, 40]. Patients with complete heart block should receive permanent cardiac pacemakers. There is no evidence that traditional anti-inflammatory or immunosuppressive drugs alter the course of spondylitic heart disease [43].

Rare cardiac features of ankylosing spondylitis and reactive arthritis include pericarditis, myocarditis, and giant cell valvulitis [34, 44]. Several echocardiographic studies have shown global ventricular dysfunction in patients with ankylosing spondylitis, reactive arthritis, or psoriatic arthritis, but the clinical significance of these finding is unclear [45, 46]. However, subtle aortic valve dysfunction may lead to left ventricular dysfunction in these patients [47–49].

Systemic Lupus Erythematosus

Systemic lupus erythematosus (SLE) is a multisystem autoimmune disease characterized by inflammatory lesions in many organs [50]. The disease occurs in people of any age or race, but young women in the childbearing years are most susceptible, especially Africans, Hispanics, and Asians [51]. Although the etiology of SLE is unknown, SLE is believed to be a complex and heterogeneous disease in which multiple genes (each with modest effects) [52–56] interact with various environment stimuli (e.g., ultraviolet light or viral infections), resulting in apoptosis [55] and acceleration of autoantigen presentation to the immune system [53, 57]. The strongest genetic effects appear to be related to hereditary deficiencies in the complement system and to certain class II HLA genes (HLA-DR2, -DR3, and -DR8 haplotypes) [52, 58].

Autoantibodies

Autoantibodies to intracellular nuclear constituents, such as double-stranded DNA (dsDNA), ribonucleoproteins (including Smith [Sm], RNP, Ro/SSA, and La/SSB), and histones, are characteristically found in SLE patients and account for the positive ANA tests in more than 98% of these patients [52, 59]. Autoantibodies to dsDNA, Sm, and ribosomal P are the most specific for this disease, but they are found in only a minority of the patients. Additional autoantibodies are also common, including those to cellular elements (e.g., red blood cells, lymphocytes, platelets, neurons, and endothelial cells) and plasma components (e.g., IgG, phospholipids, and clotting factors) [59]. Individual patients with SLE have their own distinctive autoantibody profiles, which remain relatively constant over time. Many of these autoantibodies are associated with and probably are the cause of specific clinical manifestations resulting from either the deposition of antigen-antibody immune complexes or antibody-mediated tissue damage. Associations or causal relationships have been established between specific autoantibodies and certain cardiac manifestations. Examples include associations between anti-Ro (SS-A) and La (SS-B) antibodies and congenital heart block [60] and between antiphospholipid antibodies and valvular heart disease (Libman-Sacks endocarditis), other cardiac lesions, and intravascular thromboses [61–63].

Prognosis

The spectrum of SLE effects, including the cardiac manifestations and prognosis of the disease, has changed considerably over the last 50 years [64]. With the advent of more sophisticated serologic tests, it is now possible to diagnose milder cases and those at earlier stages. Treatment with corticosteroids and other immunosuppressive agents, as well as the use of antibiotics, antihypertensives, and other drugs, when appropriate, has improved patient survival from less than 50% at 5 years in the 1950s to more than 90% at 10 years currently [51, 65]. Concomitantly, the prevalence of lupus carditis has decreased markedly; in the precorticosteroid era, lupus carditis was nearly universally present in patients with SLE, especially at autopsy, but the prevalence decreased to 55% in 1954, to 38% in 1971, and to 18% in 1978 [64].

Pathology

Any cardiac structure can be involved in SLE (Table 4.3) [64, 66–69]. However, the presence and extent of the pathologic cardiac lesions correlate poorly with other clinical

Table 4.3 Cardiac complications of systemic lupus erythematosus

Pericardium	Endocardium	Coronary artery disease	Other
Acute pericarditis supraventricular arrhythmias	Libman-Sacks endocarditis	Premature atherosclerosis	Pulmonary hypertension
Pericardial effusions	Valvular thickening, regurgitation, and/or stenosis	Arteritis	Congenital heart block in fetuses
Pericardial tamponade	Intrachamber thrombi	Thrombosis	
Constrictive pericarditis	Aortic arch syndrome		
Myocarditis Focal inflammatory lesions (immune complexes) Cardiac "myositis" Diffuse, small-vessel thromboses			

From Arnett and Willerson [21], reprinted with permission from Springer Nature manifestations. Acute and healed inflammatory lesions have been found scattered focally or diffusely throughout the pericardium, myocardium, valves, and coronary vasculature [64, 70]. Immunofluorescence studies showed extensive granular deposits of immunoglobulins and C3 in the heart, which correlated with the histopathologic changes seen [71]. Therefore, the major cause of lupus carditis is believed to be immune complex-mediated injury, rather than autoantibodies directly targeting cardiac tissues [72]. Another major pathogenetic mechanism is in situ thrombotic events on cardiac valves, other endocardial surfaces, and extracardiac vascular surfaces due to antiphospholipid antibodies [61–63, 73, 74]. There has been increasing evidence that premature atherosclerosis, including coronary atherosclerosis, is a complication of immunologic damage, systemic inflammation, long-term corticosteroid therapy, and other factors [64, 75, 76].

Cardiovascular Manifestations

Pericarditis is the most common cardiac complication in SLE patients, occurring in 19–48% of patients, and is the presenting feature in 1–2% of cases [64, 67, 75]. Clinical features include the typical substernal, position-related, pleuritic chest pain, which is sometimes associated with a pericardial rub and diffuse ST-segment elevation on the electrocardiogram (ECG). Atrial arrhythmias, including flutter and fibrillation, may be found due to the close proximity of the sinoatrial node to the pericardium, whereas ventricular ectopy is rare. Echocardiography often reveals a small pericardial effusion; however, large fluid accumulations with tamponade may occur and can be life threatening (Fig. 4.9). Constrictive pericarditis is rare [77].

Pericardial fluid from SLE patients shows a mild to moderate inflammatory exudate, is occasionally bloody, has white blood cell counts usually in the 2000–5000/mm^3 range, and has a mildly elevated protein level but normal glucose levels. Lupus erythematosus (LE) cells or ANAs may be found in the pericardial fluid of seropositive patients, but these cannot be used to discriminate lupus effusions from those due to other causes. Complement levels are typically low in these patients, and immune complexes have been found [64, 78, 79]. Prompt removal of pericardial fluid may be lifesaving when cardiac tamponade occurs and may be diagnostically necessary when infectious pericarditis is suspected.

The therapy for lupus pericarditis should be determined on the basis of its severity. For mild symptomatic pericarditis, especially that without significant pericardial effusion or other serious disease manifestations, indomethacin (75–150 mg/day, divided into three doses) may be effective. Alternatively, other nonsteroidal anti-inflammatory drugs may be used at doses recommended for arthritis. Some patients, however, require corticosteroids at a low-to-moderate dose (10–40 mg prednisone equivalent per day) to relieve the symptoms or resolve the effusions. Large effusions or pericardial tamponade should result in the prompt administration of high-dose intravenous corticosteroids (60–80 mg prednisone equivalent per day in two divided doses) (Fig. 4.9).

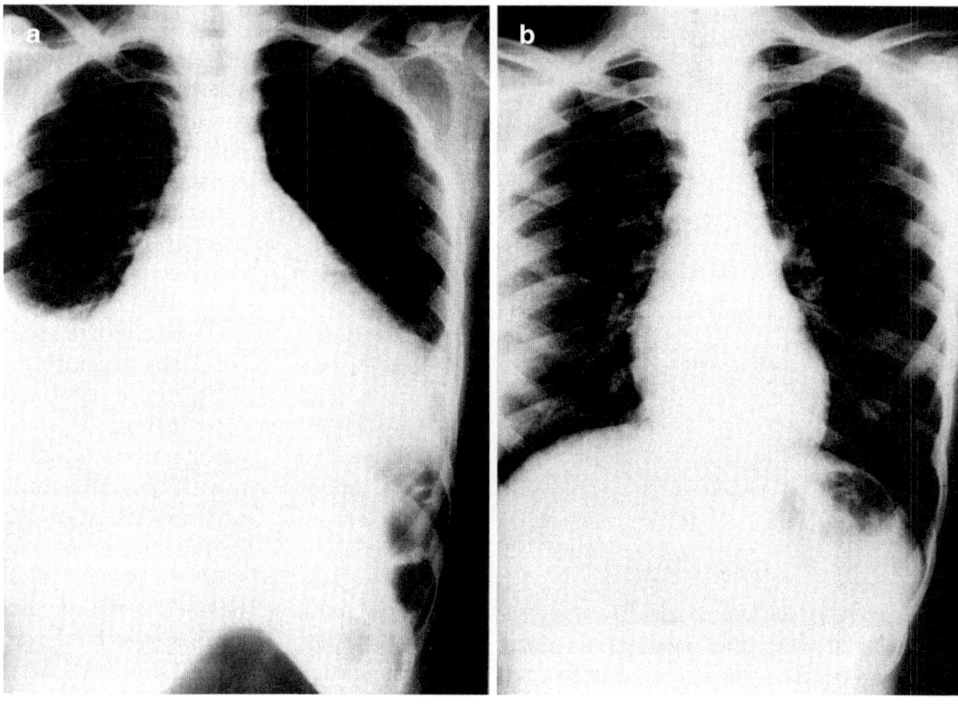

Fig. 4.9 Chest radiographs of a patient with SLE showing massive pericardial effusion and bilateral pleural effusions (**a**) and complete resolution of the effusions 4 weeks after treatment with corticosteroids (**b**). From Arnett and Willerson [21], reprinted with permission from Springer Nature

Myocardial involvement is clinically evident in 8–25% of reported series [64, 79, 80]. Several pathologic forms have been recognized, including diffuse small-vessel obliteration and myocyte destruction. They are probably the result of immune complex deposition [64, 81], myocardial cell degeneration and lymphocyte infiltration associated with skeletal myositis, anti-RNP antibodies [82], and global myocardial ischemia and dysfunction or acute myocardial infarction due to coronary artery thrombi associated with antiphospholipid antibodies [62, 83–85].

The earliest clinical manifestations of myocarditis include resting tachycardia, atypical chest discomfort, a third heart sound, and nonspecific ST-T wave changes on ECG. More overt signs include cardiomegaly in the absence of pericardial fluid or other causes of cardiac enlargement, congestive heart failure, and arrhythmias. Troponin levels are elevated. Echocardiography usually reveals multichamber enlargement, global myocardial dyskinesis, and a reduced ejection fraction. Transendocardial biopsy of the myocardium may be necessary to make the diagnosis and to determine the type and activity of the disease process [81]. The differential diagnosis should include secondary causes of myocardial dysfunction, such as hypertension, diabetes mellitus, premature atherosclerotic heart disease, and a rare form of vacuolar cardiomyopathy associated with the use of chloroquine and other antimalarials for treating SLE [86]. Active myocarditis requires aggressive corticosteroid therapy, along with appropriate measures to control arrhythmias and congestive heart failure [62, 66, 79, 80]. Prednisone (60–100 mg/day in two divided doses) should be given immediately, and the patient's cardiac status should be closely monitored clinically. Congestive heart failure should be treated as necessary with appropriate drugs. Serious atrial and ventricular arrhythmias should be suppressed pharmacologically. Anticoagulation should be used to prevent mural thrombi, especially when antiphospholipid antibodies, which promote intravascular thrombosis, are present. Once the signs of active myocarditis have resolved, the prednisone dose should be tapered slowly over weeks to months, and the patient should be closely monitored (as above) for clinical recurrences.

Premature atherosclerosis is an important cause of morbidity and mortality in SLE patients [76]. There are well-documented cases of SLE patients in their twenties having a myocardial infarction; often this is seen when the disease onset occurred in childhood [87, 88]. The prevalence of myocardial infarction in SLE patients has ranged from 4% to 45% in multiple series [32, 89–92]. In a case-control study that used electron beam computed tomography to detect coronary artery calcifications, calcifications were found in 33% of the patients younger than 50 years [93].

The cause of premature atherosclerosis in SLE patients is multifactorial (Fig. 4.10). Lupus itself appears to play a major role, the effects of which are mediated by antiphospholipid and other autoantibodies and by endothelial dysfunction. In addition, traditional cardiovascular disease risk factors appear to play a contributing role. Thus, aggressive control of disease activity, along with close monitoring and treatment of elevated low-density lipoprotein levels, hyperglycemia, and hypertension, are essential in the management of SLE [76, 94]. Coronary artery occlusion resulting from an active vasculitis occurs in SLE patients [85, 95]. Coronary arteriography may also prove to be helpful diagnostically when a beaded pattern or small aneurysms are seen in the coronary artery system. Treatment requires high-dose corticosteroids.

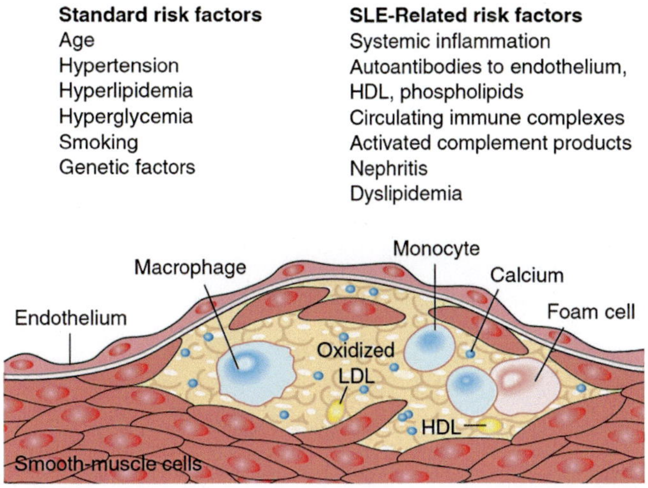

Fig. 4.10 The standard risk factors for atherosclerosis and those specifically related to SLE. The figure shows an arterial wall undergoing plaque formation and calcification and indicates multiple factors that accelerate the atherosclerosis process. *HDL* high-density lipoprotein, *LDL* low-density lipoprotein. From Arnett and Willerson [21], reprinted with permission from Springer Nature

It has been recognized that SLE patients can have spontaneous coronary artery thrombosis secondary to the presence of antiphospholipid antibodies [96, 97]. As with the atheromatous disease, the patient may have no other symptoms of active SLE. A positive test for antiphospholipid antibodies should raise clinical suspicion. Agents to lyse the coronary thrombus should be given promptly, followed by appropriate anticoagulation.

Valvular involvement has long been recognized in SLE patients, especially at autopsy [64]. In 1924, Libman and Sacks [98] first described a sterile verrucous endocarditis that usually affected the underside of the mitral valve leaflets (Fig. 4.11). Necropsy studies have since shown that approximately 43% of lupus patients have Libman-Sacks endocarditis, with the mitral valve being involved in 24% of cases, the aortic valve being involved in 5% of cases, the tricuspid valve being involved in 5% of cases, and the pulmonic valve being involved in 3% of cases [75, 76, 99]. The vegetations usually appear as small, flat or slightly raised projections adhered to the valve margins, commissures of the leaflets,

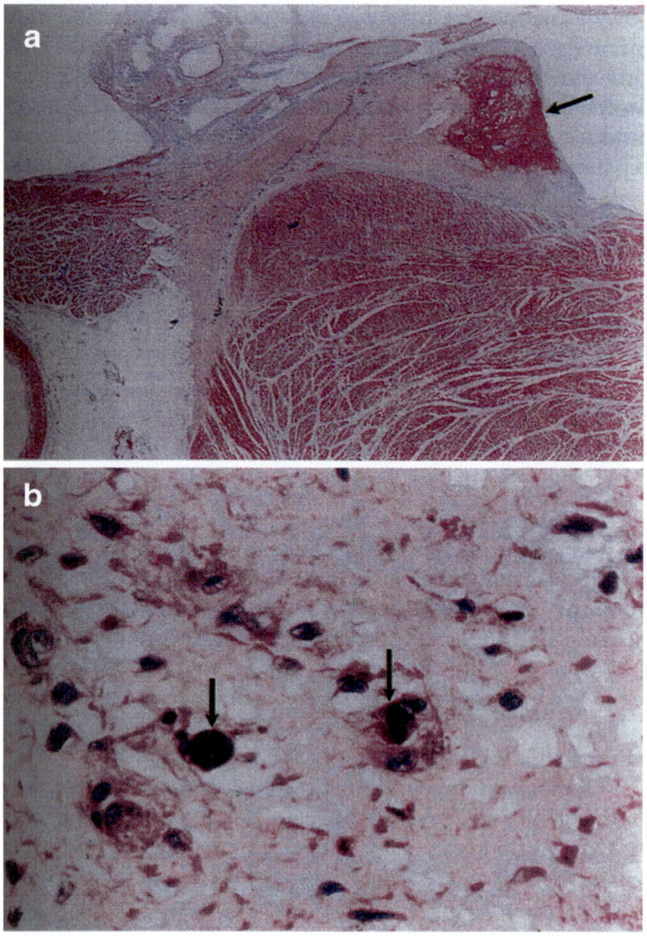

Fig. 4.11 (**a**) Low-power photomicrograph of the mitral valve and adjacent myocardium of a patient with SLE who had atypical verrucous endocarditis (Libman-Sacks endocarditis). A sterile vegetation consisting of an organizing thrombus (arrow) was located behind the mitral valve leaflet and was involved in producing adhesions between the mitral leaflet and the adjacent mural endocardium. (**b**) Image at higher magnification showing that the vegetation of atypical verrucous endocarditis contained distinctive hematoxylin bodies (arrows), which are also called lupus erythematosus (LE) bodies. From Arnett and Willerson [21], reprinted with permission from Springer Nature

chordae tendineae, and papillary muscles. As shown histologically, the vegetations are composed of lymphocytes, plasma cells, fibrous tissue, fibrin, and platelet thrombi, and hematoxylin bodies are occasionally observed (Fig. 4.11) [75, 99, 100]. The pathological findings associated with these vegetations are thought to be due to the subsequent organization of thrombi on the valve. Ultimately, valvular thickening and fusion of the commissures may lead to either valvular regurgitation or stenosis. Although clinical reports usually describe mitral regurgitation or aortic regurgitation, stenosis of both valves has occurred [94, 101]. Occasionally, emboli to the coronary or cerebral circulations have been reported [94, 102].

Multiple prospective cohort and case-control studies have conclusively demonstrated that a high percentage of SLE patients (approximately 50%) have verrucous endocarditis or valvular thickening with regurgitation or stenosis; these findings are significantly associated with having circulating antiphospholipid antibodies. During several years of follow-up, almost half of these patients in one study [74] and 22% in another [103] required surgical treatment, especially those with significant valvular regurgitation.

Antiphospholipid Antibody Syndrome

Approximately 30% of SLE patients test positive for antiphospholipid antibodies directly, and approximately 7–15% test positive for lupus anticoagulant when various coagulation assays are used [104–107]. These antibodies may prolong clotting indices, especially the partial thromboplastin time (thus the term lupus anticoagulant); however, they promote intravascular clotting in vivo. It is important to note that a lupus anticoagulant cannot be measured if the patient is receiving heparin therapy. Patients who have antiphospholipid antibodies may develop spontaneous venous or arterial thromboses, including superficial or deep venous clots with pulmonary embolization, cerebrovascular clots with strokes or other neurologic syndromes, digital or extremity ischemia, or a variety of other thrombotic phenomena, including involvement of the cardiac valves (Libman-Sacks endocarditis) (Table 4.4). In addition, antiphospholipid antibodies have been associated with recurrent spontaneous abortions, the skin abnormality livedo reticularis (Fig. 4.12), and thrombocytopenia.

Treatment

Other than the surgical repair of severely damaged cardiac valves, no other therapeutic strategies have been developed to prevent valvular damage [106, 108]. However, studies have shown that other thrombotic complications of antiphospholipid antibodies can be significantly reduced by chronic anticoagulation with warfarin, which maintains the international normalized ratio at 2–3 [109, 110]. There is

Table 4.4 Cardiac manifestations of antiphospholipid antibodies

Verrucous endocarditis (Libman-Sacks)   Embolization to coronary arteries or extracardiac sites (rare)
Valvular thickening and contracture   Aortic and/or mitral regurgitation and/or stenosis

Coronary vessel thromboses
  Myocardial infarction
  Global ventricular dysfunction

Mural thrombi (atrial or ventricular)
Aortic arch syndrome

From Arnett and Willerson [21], reprinted with permission from Springer Nature

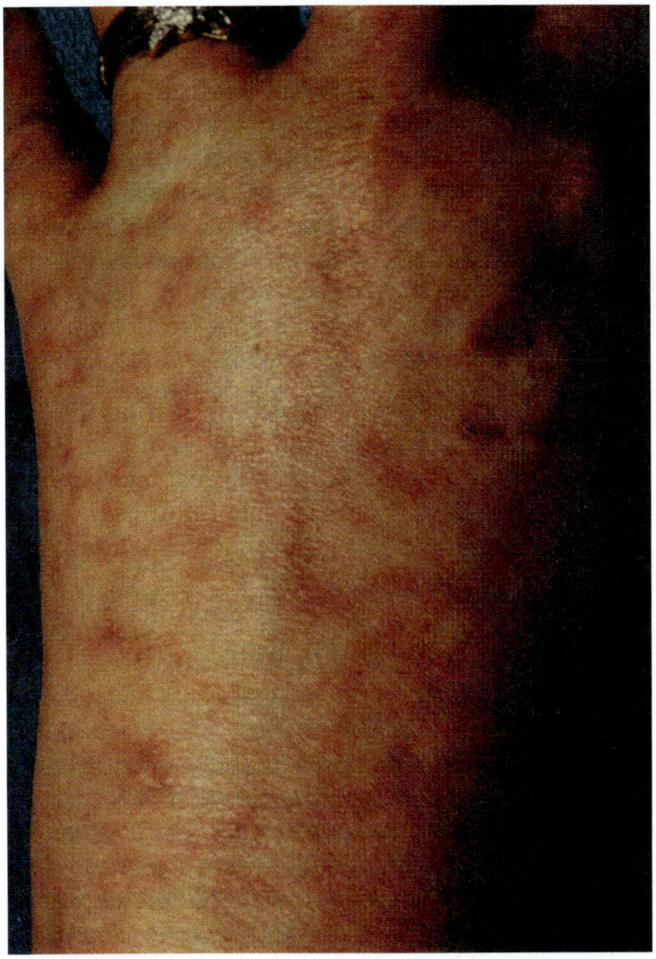

Fig. 4.12 Livedo reticularis in a patient with primary antiphospholipid syndrome. A biopsy of this skin rash would reveal thrombosis in the capillaries and small vessels. From Arnett and Willerson [21], reprinted with permission from Springer Nature

also probably merit in using low-dose aspirin (80 mg/day) in conjunction with warfarin in patients who have had a thrombotic event or as the one prophylactic drug in patients who have antiphospholipid antibodies but have not had a thrombotic event. Antimalarials, such as hydroxychloroquine (200 mg/day), may be useful for lowering antiphospholipid antibody levels. It is probably not helpful to use corticosteroids for treating isolated valvular disease.

Cardiovascular Manifestations

A primary antiphospholipid antibody syndrome has been described in patients who have had a clinical thrombotic event, including valvular heart disease, and have tested positive for anticardiolipin antibodies or lupus anticoagulants but who have not had any other features of SLE [111, 112]. In echocardiographic studies, 36% of these patients were found to have cardiac valvular lesions similar to those of SLE patients [113, 114]. A 5-year follow-up study found no benefit to using Coumadin anticoagulation to promote vegetation regression or prevent new valve lesions [115].

Patients with SLE, as well as those with primary antiphospholipid antibody syndrome, may present with acute coronary artery thromboses or global myocardial dysfunction due to diffuse, small-vessel clotting [83, 84]. Mural thrombi mimicking atrial myxoma have also been described, as well as the aortic arch syndrome [116, 117]. Therapy should include the use of thrombolytics and anticoagulants, including low-dose aspirin (80 mg/day) and warfarin. Whether corticosteroids are effective is unknown, but they should be avoided in patients with acute myocardial infarction for at least 2–3 weeks.

Takayasu's Arteritis

The clinical features of Takayasu's arteritis are described in Table 4.5 and shown in Fig. 4.13. Takayasu's arteritis was first noted by a Japanese ophthalmologist, Mikito Takayasu, who described a young woman with cataracts and arteriovenous anastomoses surrounding the optic papillae [119]. Subsequently, others called attention to two additional patients with similar ocular findings and no radial pulses. This syndrome also became known as pulseless disease or aortic arch syndrome [119–135]. The cause of Takayasu's arteritis is unknown, although Takayasu's arteritis is often preceded by an illness characterized by fever, malaise, weight loss, arthralgias, pleuritic pain, and fatigue. The majority of evidence suggests that Takayasu's arteritis has an autoimmune cause.

Pathology

The anatomic alterations found in patients with Takayasu's arteritis are marked intimal proliferation with fibrosis, scarring, and degeneration of the elastic fibers of the media with mononuclear cell infiltration. Fibrosis predominates over an inflammatory reaction. Arterial specimens contain giant cells. The intima and adventitia become thickened, injuring the vasa vasorum. Proliferative changes lead to narrowing of the aorta and the origins of the involved arteries. Late in the process, there is localized aneurysm formation, poststenotic dilatation, and calcification in the aorta and the involved arterial walls. The most significant changes occur at the points where the arteries originate from the aorta.

Vascular Manifestations

Takayasu's arteritis primarily involves the aortic arch and its major branches. The pulmonary artery may also be affected.

Table 4.5 Proposed criteria for the clinical diagnosis of Takayasu's arteritis

Criterion	Definition
Obligatory criterion	
Age ≤40 years	Age ≤40 years at diagnosis or at onset of "characteristic signs and symptoms" of 1-month duration in patient
Two major criteria	
1. Left midsubclavian artery lesion	The most severe stenosis or occlusion present in the midportion from the point 1 cm proximal to the left vertebral artery orifice to the point 3 cm distal to the orifice, as determined by angiography
2. Right midsubclavian artery lesion	The most severe stenosis or occlusion present in the midportion from the right vertebral artery orifice to the point 3 cm distal to the orifice, as determined by angiography
Nine minor criteria	
1. High erythrocyte sedimentation rate (ESR)	Unexplained persistent high ESR ≥20 mm/h (Westergren) at diagnosis or presence of the evidence in patient history
2. Carotid artery tenderness	Unilateral or bilateral tenderness of common carotid arteries by physician palpation; neck muscle tenderness is unacceptable
3. Hypertension	Persistent blood pressure ≥140/90 mmHg brachial or ≥160/90 mmHg popliteal at age ≤40 years or presence of the history at age ≤40 years
4. Aortic regurgitation or annuloaortic ectasia	By auscultation, Doppler echocardiography, or angiography By angiography or two-dimensional echocardiography
5. Pulmonary artery lesion	Lobar or segmental arterial occlusion or equivalent determined by angiography or perfusion scintigraphy; or presence of stenosis, aneurysm, luminal irregularity, or any combination in pulmonary trunk or in unilateral or bilateral pulmonary arteries, as determined by angiography
6. Left mid-common carotid lesion	Presence of the most severe stenosis or occlusion in the midportion of 5 cm in length from the point 2 cm distal to its orifice, as determined by angiography
7. Distal brachiocephalic trunk lesion	Presence of the most severe stenosis or occlusion in the distal third, as determined by angiography
8. Descending thoracic aortic lesion	Narrowing, dilation or aneurysm, luminal irregularity, or any combination, as determined by angiography; tortuosity alone is unacceptable
9. Abdominal aortic lesion	Narrowing, dilatation or aneurysm, luminal irregularity, or any combination and absence of lesion in aortoiliac region consisting of 2 cm of terminal aorta and bilateral common iliac arteries, as determined by angiography; tortuosity alone is unacceptable

In addition to the obligatory criterion, the presence of two major criteria, or one major and two or more minor criteria, or four or more minor criteria suggests a high probability of the presence of Takayasu's disease

From Ishikawa [118]. Reprinted with permission from Elsevier Science and Technology Journals

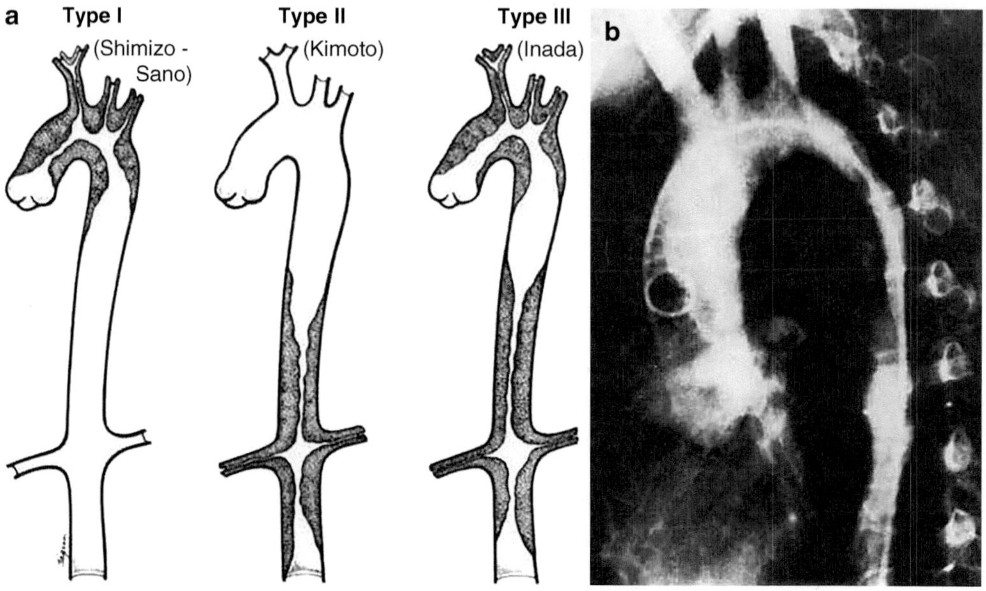

Fig. 4.13 (**a**) Figure showing the sites of inflammation in the aorta and branch vessels for the three types of Takayasu's arteritis. (**b**) Aortogram showing narrowing of the descending thoracic aorta in a patient with Takayasu's arteritis. The rapid tapering of the descending aorta has been likened to a "rat's tail" appearance. From Willerson et al. [147]. Reprinted with permission from Springer Nature

In the order of frequency, the most commonly involved arteries in patients studied in the United States were a subclavian artery (90%), a carotid artery (45%), a vertebral artery (25%), and a renal artery (20%) [131]. However, the mesenteric arteries and abdominal aorta may also be involved [136].

Ueno and associates [136] have classified Takayasu's arteritis into three types, depending on the arterial site of involvement (Fig. 4.13). Type I arteritis involves the aortic arch and its branches, type II involves the thoracoabdominal aorta and its branches, and type III involves both the aortic arch and the thoracoabdominal aorta and branches. A fourth category, involving the pulmonary artery, has been suggested (type IV) [125].

The occlusive disease usually progresses slowly over a period of months to years. The morbidity and mortality rates depend on the presence or absence of critical narrowing of the arteries in organs such as the heart, kidneys, and brain. The reported 5–7-year survival rates have been greater than 90% in patients without major complications, but less than 60% in patients with complications, such as those described earlier [122, 129].

Epidemiology and Clinical Presentation

Takayasu's arteritis affects women more frequently than men, at a ratio of 8:1, with the clinical onset of the disease typically occurring during the teenage years. In the majority of reported cases, the patients have been from Asia or Africa, and most large series have consisted of Asian women [125]. Often, there is an initial systemic illness characterized by fever, anorexia, malaise, weight loss, night sweats, arthralgias, pleuritic pain, and fatigue. Localized pain and tenderness occur over the affected arteries. Subsequently, patients report signs and symptoms related to the narrowing of major blood vessels. In most patients, the pulses become diminished or absent, and bruits develop over the involved vessels. Some patients develop systemic arterial hypertension, and occasionally heart failure occurs. The retinopathy described by Takayasu is found in only one-fourth of patients, and it is usually associated with carotid artery involvement. The ocular process may lead to blindness. Patients with type I or type III Takayasu's arteritis demonstrate the most classic findings of the disease (i.e., absent or diminished upper body pulses and difficult-to-measure blood pressure in one or both arms). Patients with type II Takayasu's arteritis often develop hypertension because of the renal artery involvement, but it may be difficult to recognize because of the reduced pulses in the arms. Heart failure, when it occurs, is generally associated with systemic arterial hypertension or aortic valve regurgitation. Ostial and proximal segments of the coronary arteries may be affected, leading to angina or myocardial infarction. Coronary artery aneurysms develop in some patients [120, 121, 123, 124, 128, 132, 135].

The laboratory abnormalities usually found in individuals with Takayasu's arteritis are an elevated sedimentation rate, mild anemia, an increase in the white blood cell count, and elevations in the serum immunoglobulins G or M. Matsuyama and colleagues [126] have reported that matrix metalloproteinase-2 (MMP-2), MMP-3, and MMP-9 levels are elevated in patients with Takayasu's arteritis and that MMP-3 and MMP-9 levels positively correlate with disease activity score.

Chest radiographs often show an enlarged heart in patients with hypertension, severe coronary artery disease, or significant aortic valvular insufficiency. Arteriography shows stenosis of the aorta or one of its major branches, saccular aneurysms, or complete occlusion of the major branch arteries arising from the aorta. The thoracic aorta in these patients often has a "rat-tail" appearance when viewed with angiography [124].

Diagnosis

Table 4.5 lists the major criteria used to make the diagnosis of Takayasu's arteritis. Takayasu's arteritis would be the probable diagnosis for a young (<40 years old) Asian woman who, after an inflammatory illness, has reduced subclavian and radial artery pulses and blood pressure.

Treatment

Adrenal steroids have been used to treat Takayasu's arteritis because they reduce fever, malaise, fatigue, and the elevated sedimentation rate [122, 131]. Cyclophosphamide has also been used at a dosage of 2 mg/kg/day, although the dosage may need to be adjusted to maintain the white blood cell count above 3000/mm^2. More recently, immunoglobulin has been administered to patients with Takayasu's arteritis and has been shown to provide some benefits, especially a more rapid resolution of the inflammatory process and protection against the development of coronary artery aneurysms. Antiplatelet agents and anticoagulants, including Coumadin and aspirin, have been administered to treat ischemic symptoms. Angiotensin-converting enzyme inhibitors are helpful in the treatment of systemic arterial hypertension.

Occasionally, a patient may require a surgical procedure to reestablish blood flow, such as a bypass procedure for obstructed arteries or excision and replacement of an aneurysmal segment. Miyata and colleagues [127] performed a retrospective review of 106 consecutive patients with Takayasu's arteritis who underwent surgical treatment at the University of Tokyo during the prior 40 years. The cumulative survival rate at 20 years was 73.5%, but a serious long-term complication was anastomotic aneurysm. Surgery appeared to increase the survival rate of the patients with the most extensive arteritis (type III), but conservative therapy appeared preferable in patients with less extensive disease. Percutaneous transluminal angioplasty has also been used to relieve discrete stenotic lesions involving the carotid, subclavian, renal, and mesenteric arteries [122, 129]. Operative treatment is graft replacement using techniques appropriate for the involved segment [137, 138].

Giant Cell Arteritis

Giant cell arteritis involves medium-sized arteries [139–144]; the aorta and its major branches are involved in only a minority of cases. Synonymous terms used to describe this entity are granulomatous, cranial, and temporal arteritis.

Middle-aged and older patients reporting diffuse muscle aches and stiffness and arthralgias may have a connective tissue disease known as polymyalgia rheumatica [139]. Some of these patients have giant cell arteritis, which may be identified by tender and swollen temporal arteries and a markedly elevated sedimentation rate, often greater than 70 mm/h. These patients are at risk of losing their vision if the disorder is not recognized and treated promptly with moderately large doses of steroids.

Pathology

The characteristic histologic lesion of giant cell arteritis is a granulomatous inflammation of medium-sized arteries, especially the arteries of the head and neck, most specifically the temporal arteries. An inflammatory infiltrate composed of plasma cells, eosinophils, and other mononuclear cells is usually found in the involved artery; this may occasionally lead to obstruction. The aortic wall may be altered by the inflammatory process, leading to localized aneurysm formation, aortic annular dilatation, and aortic regurgitation.

Epidemiology and Clinical Presentation

Typically, giant cell arteritis occurs in women 50 years of age and older, and it may be more common in black women [141]. Many of these patients also have polymyalgia rheumatica (i.e., diffuse muscle aches and arthralgias). The classic presentation consists of severe headaches, marked malaise, and a fever in association with a markedly elevated sedimentation rate. The headaches are often intense and occur over the temporal arteries and occipital regions. The temporal arteries are sensitive to pressure, and patients with this disease may not be able to rest their head against a pillow, wear a hat, or comb their hair. A large number of patients experience claudication in the jaw muscles while chewing; this symptom is suggestive of this diagnosis. Patients with giant cell arteritis may develop sudden blindness due to involvement of an ophthalmic artery, and the blindness may be irreversible. Other visual symptoms seen in some patients include blurring of vision and diplopia.

When the aorta and its major branches are involved, the symptoms and signs of giant cell arteritis are similar to those of Takayasu's arteritis. These symptoms include claudication of the upper extremities, paresthesia, Raynaud's phenomenon, myocardial ischemia, transient cerebral ischemic attacks, and, occasionally, ischemia of the lower extremities and abdominal angina. Rarely, aortic aneurysms, aortic regurgitation, and aortic dissection occur [144]. Renal artery involvement is rare with giant cell arteritis, whereas it is relatively common with Takayasu's arteritis.

Fever is present in many patients with giant cell arteritis. The involved arteries are thickened and tender. In addition, pulses may be lost, and bruits may occur over sites of arterial narrowing.

Diagnosis

The diagnosis of giant cell arteritis is made with a biopsy of an involved artery, usually the temporal artery. Arteriography may be helpful for differentiating granulomatous arteritis from arteriosclerosis by showing tapering stenosis alternating with segments of normal or even slightly increased arterial diameter; the absence of ulcerated atheromatous plaques; and the typical anatomic distribution of arteritis, including the subclavian, axillary, and brachial arteries [140].

Treatment

High-dose steroid therapy (60–80 mg of prednisone daily) should be administered to patients with granulomatous arteritis, especially patients with temporal arteritis. Steroids should be given in a single dose early in the morning. In patients with temporal arteritis, beginning steroid therapy is a relative emergency to prevent blindness. The sedimentation rate may be used as a guide to determine the effectiveness of the steroids and to indicate when the dosage may be reduced. After a period of high-dose steroid therapy, the steroid dosage is typically reduced gradually to a maintenance dosage of 5–15 mg/day for 1–2 years. Most patients improve, and their symptoms eventually resolve completely. Occasionally, the disease does not respond adequately to steroids, and other immunosuppressive therapy may be necessary.

Syphilitic Aortitis

When left untreated, syphilis can reach the tertiary phase, which is characterized by neurological and cardiovascular manifestations, such as syphilitic aortitis. The classic clinical findings in patients with syphilitic aortitis are a large saccular ascending aortic aneurysm, with or without aortic regurgitation, and coronary ostial stenosis. Figure 4.14 is a representative example of the hallmark findings with an otherwise normal coronary bed. Progressive aneurysm enlargement may lead to erosion of the sternum, pseudoaneurysm formation, or aortic dissection. Intramural hematoma of the ascending aorta has also been reported in patients with syphilis [146]. Although there has been a marked reduction in the incidence of syphilis, drug use, sexual promiscuity, and migration of the workforce in a globalized world have created opportunities for the disease to spread.

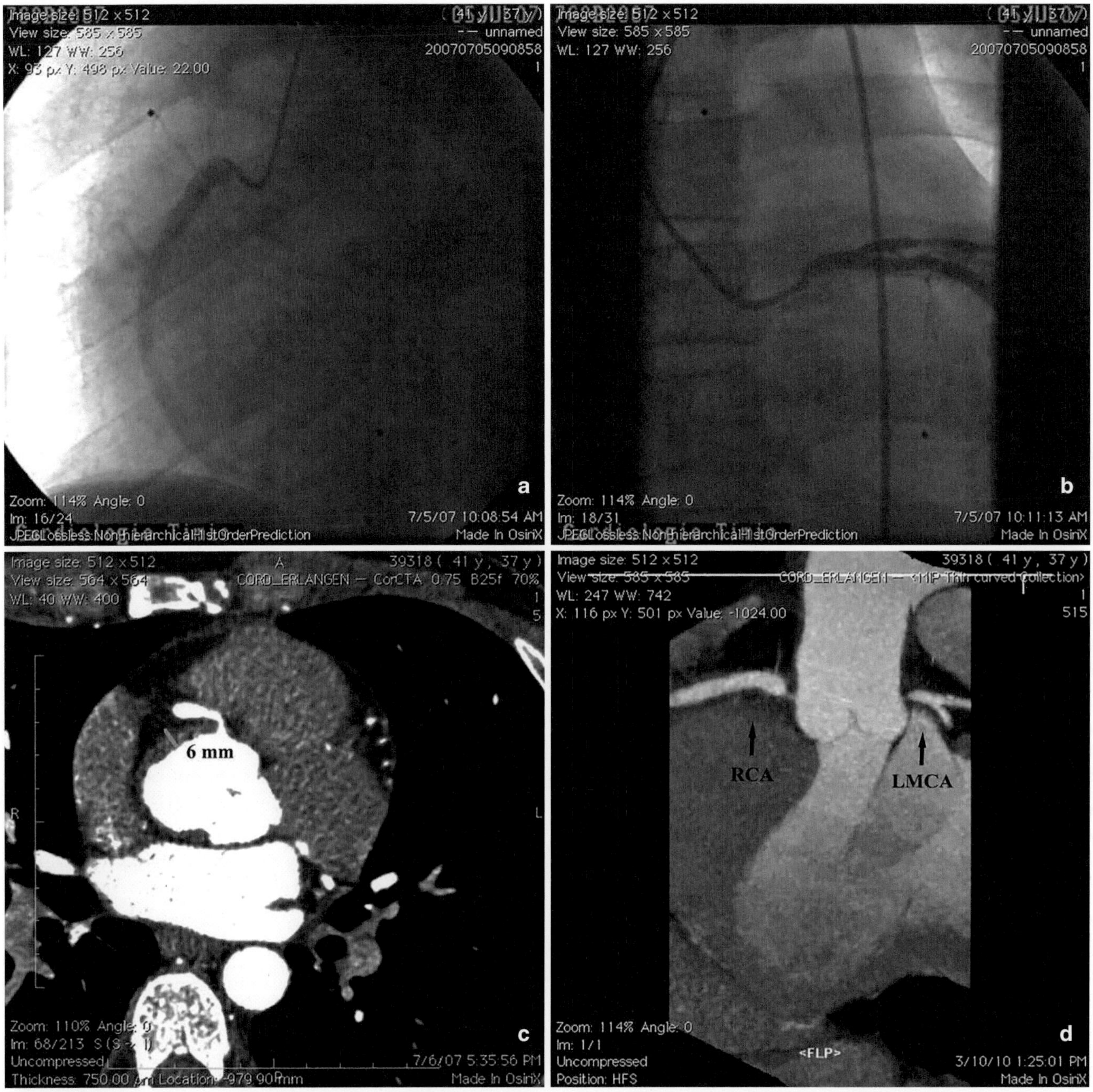

Fig. 4.14 Images from a patient with syphilis. (**a**, **b**) Coronary angiography showing ostial stenosis of the right (**a**) and left (**b**) coronary arteries. (**c**) Computed tomographic scan revealing a thickened aortic wall (6 mm), an irregular intima at the level of the aortic root, and right coronary ostial stenosis. (**d**) Ostial stenosis of the right coronary artery (RCA) and left main coronary artery (LMCA). From Feier et al. [145]. Reprinted with permission from Wolters Kluwer Health, Inc.

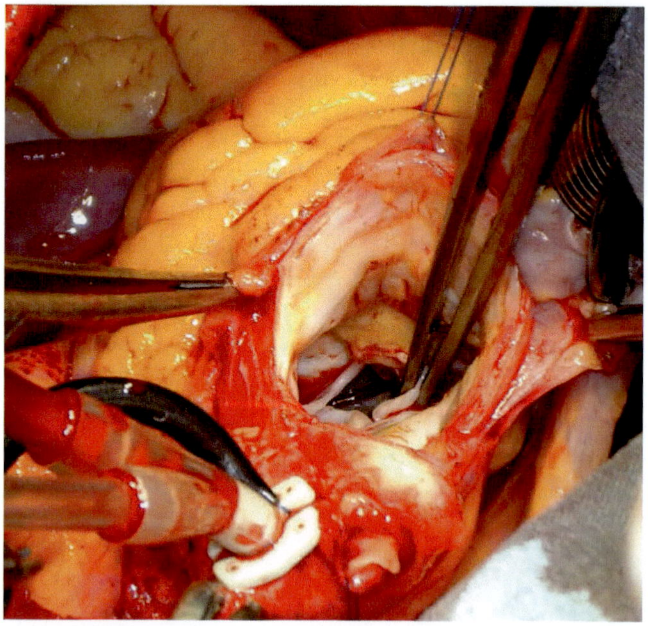

Fig. 4.15 Intraoperative view of the ascending aorta in a patient with syphilis. Tree barking of the intima and fibrosis and retraction of the aortic cusps are shown. From Feier et al. [145]. Reprinted with permission from Wolters Kluwer Health, Inc.

Pathology

The pathological findings of syphilitic aortitis include endarteritis obliterans of the vasa vasorum with a chronic inflammatory infiltrate of plasma cells and lymphocytes (Figs. 4.15 and 4.16) and disruption of the elastic fibers, tree barking of the intima of the ascending aorta (also seen in SLE and some other inflammatory diseases) (Fig. 4.15), and aortic regurgitation resulting from fibrosis and retraction of the aortic valve cusps and dilatation of the sinotubular junction. Patients may die suddenly due to rupture of an aortic aneurysm, or death may occur as a consequence of chronic heart failure associated with severe aortic regurgitation or myocardial infarction.

When surgery is performed, the ascending aorta has a hyperemic, inflammatory adventitia that adheres firmly to the surrounding structures. There is a markedly thickened wall with extensive longitudinal wrinkling into the aortic root, deforming and narrowing the coronary ostia (Fig. 4.15). The aortic valve leaflets are usually thickened and retracted, resulting in severe central aortic valve incompetence. Microscopic examination of the aortic tissue shows endarteritis obliterans of the vasa vasorum, a chronic inflammatory infiltrate in the medial layer with disruption of the elastic fibers, and a severely thickened intima (Fig. 4.16a, b).

Diagnosis

The diagnosis of syphilis can be made by identifying living spirochetes in tissue samples with the polymerase chain reaction assay or by using indirect (Venereal Disease Research Laboratory test) or direct *Treponema pallidum* hemagglutination test methods.

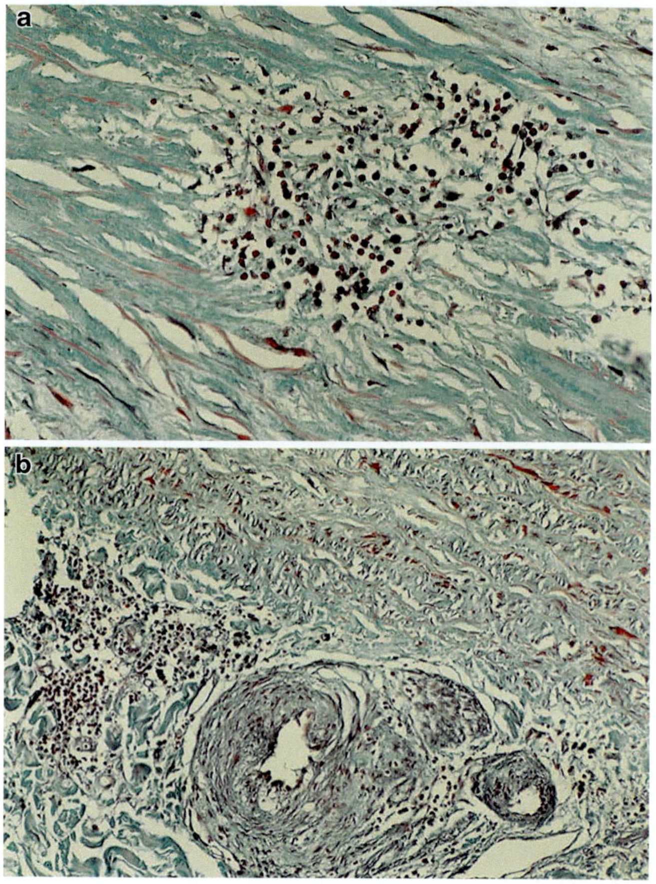

Fig. 4.16 Histologic sections from a patient with syphilis. (**a**) Chronic lymphocytic and plasmacytic inflammatory infiltrate of the medial layer with disruption of the elastic fibers (Masson's trichrome stain). (**b**) Endarteritis obliterans of the vasa vasorum (Masson's trichrome stain, magnification 200×). From Feier et al. [145]. Reprinted with permission from Wolters Kluwer Health, Inc.

Acknowledgement Portions of the chapter are adapted from *Cardiovascular Medicine, 3rd Edition*, Willerson J., Cohen F., Wellens H., Holmes Jr. D. (eds). 2014, and from chapters in this textbook: Arnett F. and Willerson J. "Connective Tissue Disease and the Heart," Chapter 10, and Milewicz D. "Inherited Disorders of Connective Tissues," Chapter 121. ©Springer-Verlag London Limited 2007.

References

1. Milewicz DM, Dietz HC, Miller DC. Treatment of aortic disease in patients with Marfan syndrome. Circulation. 2005;111: e150–7.
2. Murdoch JL, Walker BA, Halpern BL, Kuzma JW, McKusick VA. Life expectancy and causes of death in the Marfan syndrome. N Engl J Med. 1972;286:804–8.
3. Finkbohner R, Johnston D, Crawford ES, Coselli J, Milewicz DM. Marfan syndrome. Long-term survival and complications after aortic aneurysm repair. Circulation. 1995;91:728–33.

4. Silverman DI, Burton KJ, Gray J, et al. Life expectancy in the Marfan syndrome. Am J Cardiol. 1995;75:157–60.
5. Milewicz DM. Inherited disorders of connective tissue. In: Willerson JT, Cohn JN, Wellens HJJ, Holmes Jr DR, editors. Cardiovascular medicine. 3rd ed. London: Springer; 2007. p. 2557–66.
6. Davies RR, Goldstein LJ, Coady MA, et al. Yearly rupture or dissection rates for thoracic aortic aneurysms: simple prediction based on size. Ann Thorac Surg. 2002;73:17–27; discussion 27–8.
7. Gott VL, Greene PS, Alejo DE, et al. Replacement of the aortic root in patients with Marfan's syndrome. N Engl J Med. 1999;340:1307–13.
8. David TE, Feindel CM. An aortic valve-sparing operation for patients with aortic incompetence and aneurysm of the ascending aorta. J Thorac Cardiovasc Surg. 1992;103:617–21; discussion 622.
9. Sarsam MA, Yacoub M. Remodeling of the aortic valve anulus. J Thorac Cardiovasc Surg. 1993;105:435–8.
10. Birks EJ, Webb C, Child A, Radley-Smith R, Yacoub MH. Early and long-term results of a valve-sparing operation for Marfan syndrome. Circulation. 1999;100:II29–35.
11. de Oliveira NC, David TE, Ivanov J, et al. Results of surgery for aortic root aneurysm in patients with Marfan syndrome. J Thorac Cardiovasc Surg. 2003;125:789–96.
12. De Paepe A, Devereux RB, Dietz HC, Hennekam RC, Pyeritz RE. Revised diagnostic criteria for the Marfan syndrome. Am J Med Genet. 1996;62:417–26.
13. Loeys BL, Dietz HC, Braverman AC, et al. The revised Ghent nosology for the Marfan syndrome. J Med Genet. 2010;47:476–85.
14. Milewicz DM. Identification of defects in the fibrillin gene and protein in individuals with the Marfan syndrome and related disorders. Tex Heart Inst J. 1994;21:22–9.
15. Collod G, Babron MC, Jondeau G, et al. A second locus for Marfan syndrome maps to chromosome 3p24.2-p25. Nat Genet. 1994;8:264–8.
16. Mizuguchi T, Collod-Beroud G, Akiyama T, et al. Heterozygous TGFBR2 mutations in Marfan syndrome. Nat Genet. 2004;36:855–60.
17. Neptune ER, Frischmeyer PA, Arking DE, et al. Dysregulation of TGF-beta activation contributes to pathogenesis in Marfan syndrome. Nat Genet. 2003;33:407–11.
18. McAdam LP, O'Hanlan MA, Bluestone R, Pearson CM. Relapsing polychondritis: prospective study of 23 patients and a review of the literature. Medicine (Baltimore). 1976;55:193–215.
19. Trentham DE, Le CH. Relapsing polychondritis. Ann Intern Med. 1998;129:114–22.
20. Foidart JM, Abe S, Martin GR, et al. Antibodies to type II collagen in relapsing polychondritis. N Engl J Med. 1978;299:1203–7.
21. Arnett FC, Willerson JT. Connective tissue diseases and the heart. In: Willerson JT, Cohn JN, Wellens HJJ, Holmes Jr DR, editors. Cardiovascular medicine. 3rd ed. London: Springer; 2007. p. 2331–56.
22. Michet CJ Jr, McKenna CH, Luthra HS, O'Fallon WM. Relapsing polychondritis. Survival and predictive role of early disease manifestations. Ann Intern Med. 1986;104:74–8.
23. Arnett FC. Seronegative spondyloarthropathies. In: Dale DC, Federman DD, editors. ACP medicine, 2004–2005, vol. 2. New York: WebMD Professional Publishing; 2004. p. 2860.
24. Ansari A, Maron BJ. Images in cardiovascular medicine. Cardiovascular disease in ankylosing (Marie-Strumpell) spondylitis. Circulation. 1997;95:2585–6.
25. Bergfeldt L, Insulander P, Lindblom D, Moller E, Edhag O. HLA-B27: an important genetic risk factor for lone aortic regurgitation and severe conduction system abnormalities. Am J Med. 1988;85:12–8.
26. Bulkley BH, Roberts WC. Ankylosing spondylitis and aortic regurgitation. Description of the characteristic cardiovascular lesion from study of eight necropsy patients. Circulation. 1973;48:1014–27.
27. Paulus HE, Pearson CM, Pitts W Jr. Aortic insufficiency in five patients with Reiter's syndrome. A detailed clinical and pathologic study. Am J Med. 1972;53:464–72.
28. Roberts WC, Hollingsworth JF, Bulkley BH, Jaffe RB, Epstein SE, Stinson EB. Combined mitral and aortic regurgitation in ankylosing spondylitis. Angiographic and anatomic features. Am J Med. 1974;56:237–43.
29. Ruppert GB, Lindsay J, Barth WF. Cardiac conduction abnormalities in Reiter's syndrome. Am J Med. 1982;73:335–40.
30. Zvaifler NJ, Weintraub AM. Aortitis and aortic insufficiency in the chronic rheumatic disorders--a reappraisal. Arthritis Rheum. 1963;6:241–5.
31. Bergfeldt L, Edhag O, Rajs J. HLA-B27-associated heart disease. Clinicopathologic study of three cases. Am J Med. 1984;77:961–7.
32. El-Magadmi M, Bodill H, Ahmad Y, et al. Systemic lupus erythematosus: an independent risk factor for endothelial dysfunction in women. Circulation. 2004;110:399–404.
33. Arnett FC. Incomplete Reiter's syndrome: clinical comparisons with classical triad. Ann Rheum Dis. 1979;38:73–8.
34. Csonka GW. Workshop I. Features and prognosis of Reiter's syndrome. Clinical aspects of Reiter's syndrome. Ann Rheum Dis. 1979;38:4–7.
35. Lee SJ, Im HY, Schueller WC. HLA-B27 positive juvenile arthritis with cardiac involvement preceding sacroiliac joint changes. Heart. 2001;86:E19.
36. Machado H, Befeler B, Morales AR, Letter VA. Rapidly progressive aortic insufficiency in Reiter's syndrome. Ann Intern Med. 1974;81:121–2.
37. Stewart SR, Robbins DL, Castles JJ. Acute fulminant aortic and mitral insufficiency in ankylosing spondylitis. N Engl J Med. 1978;299:1448–9.
38. LaBresh KA, Lally EV, Sharma SC, Ho G Jr. Two-dimensional echocardiographic detection of preclinical aortic root abnormalities in rheumatoid variant diseases. Am J Med. 1985;78:908–12.
39. Arnason JA, Patel AK, Rahko PS, Sundstrom WR. Transthoracic and transesophageal echocardiographic evaluation of the aortic root and subvalvular structures in ankylosing spondylitis. J Rheumatol. 1996;23:120–3.
40. Bergfeldt L. HLA B27-associated rheumatic diseases with severe cardiac bradyarrhythmias. Clinical features and prevalence in 223 men with permanent pacemakers. Am J Med. 1983;75:210–5.
41. Bergfeldt L, Edhag O, Vedin L, Vallin H. Ankylosing spondylitis: an important cause of severe disturbances of the cardiac conduction system. Prevalence among 223 pacemaker-treated men. Am J Med. 1982;73:187–91.
42. Bergfeldt L, Moller E. Complete heart block—another HLA B27 associated disease manifestation. Tissue Antigens. 1983;21:385–90.
43. Reveille JD, Arnett FC. Spondyloarthritis: update on pathogenesis and management. Am J Med. 2005;118:592–603.
44. Podell TE, Wallace DJ, Fishbein MC, Bransford K, Klinenberg JR, Levine S. Severe giant cell valvulitis in a patient with Reiter's syndrome. Arthritis Rheum. 1982;25:232–4.
45. Crowley JJ, Donnelly SM, Tobin M, et al. Doppler echocardiographic evidence of left ventricular diastolic dysfunction in ankylosing spondylitis. Am J Cardiol. 1993;71:1337–40.
46. Gould BA, Turner J, Keeling DH, Hickling P, Marshall AJ. Myocardial dysfunction in ankylosing spondylitis. Ann Rheum Dis. 1992;51:227–32.
47. Hannu T, Nieminen MS, Swan H, Leirisalo-Repo M. Cardiac findings of reactive arthritis: an observational echocardiographic study. Rheumatol Int. 2002;21:169–72.
48. Jimenez-Balderas FJ, Garcia-Rubi D, Perez-Hinojosa S, et al. Two-dimensional echo Doppler findings in juvenile and adult onset ankylosing spondylitis with long-term disease. Angiology. 2001;52:543–8.

49. Saricaoglu H, Gullulu S, Bulbul Baskan E, Cordan J, Tunali S. Echocardiographic findings in subjects with psoriatic arthropathy. J Eur Acad Dermatol Venereol. 2003;17:414–7.
50. Wallace DJ, Hahn BH. Dubois' lupus erythematosus. 6th ed. Baltimore, MD: Lippincott Williams & Wilkins; 2002.
51. Alarcon GS, McGwin G Jr, Roseman JM, et al. Systemic lupus erythematosus in three ethnic groups. XIX. Natural history of the accrual of the American College of Rheumatology criteria prior to the occurrence of criteria diagnosis. Arthritis Rheum. 2004;51:609–15.
52. Arnett FC, Reveille JD. Genetics of systemic lupus erythematosus. Rheum Dis Clin N Am. 1992;18:865–92.
53. Koutouzov S, Jeronimo AL, Campos H, Amoura Z. Nucleosomes in the pathogenesis of systemic lupus erythematosus. Rheum Dis Clin N Am. 2004;30:529–58, ix.
54. Shen N, Tsao BP. Current advances in the human lupus genetics. Curr Rheumatol Rep. 2004;6:391–8.
55. Sheriff A, Gaipl US, Voll RE, Kalden JR, Herrmann M. Apoptosis and systemic lupus erythematosus. Rheum Dis Clin N Am. 2004;30:505–27, viii–ix.
56. Tsao BP. Update on human systemic lupus erythematosus genetics. Curr Opin Rheumatol. 2004;16:513–21.
57. Pisetsky DS. DNA as a marker of cell death in systemic lupus erythematosus. Rheum Dis Clin N Am. 2004;30:575–87, x.
58. Graham RR, Ortmann WA, Langefeld CD, et al. Visualizing human leukocyte antigen class II risk haplotypes in human systemic lupus erythematosus. Am J Hum Genet. 2002;71:543–53.
59. Sherer Y, Gorstein A, Fritzler MJ, Shoenfeld Y. Autoantibody explosion in systemic lupus erythematosus: more than 100 different antibodies found in SLE patients. Semin Arthritis Rheum. 2004;34:501–37.
60. Scott JS, Maddison PJ, Taylor PV, Esscher E, Scott O, Skinner RP. Connective-tissue disease, antibodies to ribonucleoprotein, and congenital heart block. N Engl J Med. 1983;309:209–12.
61. Leung WH, Wong KL, Lau CP, Wong CK, Liu HW. Association between antiphospholipid antibodies and cardiac abnormalities in patients with systemic lupus erythematosus. Am J Med. 1990;89:411–9.
62. Nayak AK, Komatireddy G. Cardiac manifestations of the antiphospholipid antibody syndrome: a review. Mo Med. 2002;99:171–8.
63. Straaton KV, Chatham WW, Reveille JD, Koopman WJ, Smith SH. Clinically significant valvular heart disease in systemic lupus erythematosus. Am J Med. 1988;85:645–50.
64. Stevens MB. Systemic lupus erythematosus and the cardiovascular system. In: Lahita RG, editor. Systemic lupus erythematosus. 1st ed. New York: Wiley; 1987. p. 673–90.
65. Reveille JD, Bartolucci A, Alarcon GS. Prognosis in systemic lupus erythematosus. Negative impact of increasing age at onset, black race, and thrombocytopenia, as well as causes of death. Arthritis Rheum. 1990;33:37–48.
66. Bijl M, Brouwer J, Kallenberg GG. Cardiac abnormalities in SLE: pancarditis. Lupus. 2000;9:236–40.
67. Hejtmancik MR, Wright JC, Quint R, Jennings FL. The cardiovascular manifestations of systemic lupus erythematosus. Am Heart J. 1964;68:119–30.
68. James TN, Rupe CE, Monto RW. Pathology of the cardiac conduction system in systemic lupus erythematosus. Ann Intern Med. 1965;63:402–10.
69. Shearn MA. The heart in systemic lupus erythematosus. Am Heart J. 1959;58:452–66.
70. Lin CC, Ding HJ, Chen YW, Wang JJ, Ho ST, Kao A. Usefulness of technetium-99m sestamibi myocardial perfusion SPECT in detection of cardiovascular involvement in patients with systemic lupus erythematosus or systemic sclerosis. Int J Cardiol. 2003;92:157–61.
71. Bidani AK, Roberts JL, Schwartz MM, Lewis EJ. Immunopathology of cardiac lesions in fatal systemic lupus erythematosus. Am J Med. 1980;69:849–58.
72. Das SK, Cassidy JT. Antiheart antibodies in patients with systemic lupus erythematosus. Am J Med Sci. 1973;265:275–80.
73. Bulckaen HG, Puisieux FL, Bulckaen ED, et al. Antiphospholipid antibodies and the risk of thromboembolic events in valvular heart disease. Mayo Clin Proc. 2003;78:294–8.
74. Galve E, Candell-Riera J, Pigrau C, Permanyer-Miralda G, Garcia-Del-Castillo H, Soler-Soler J. Prevalence, morphologic types, and evolution of cardiac valvular disease in systemic lupus erythematosus. N Engl J Med. 1988;319:817–23.
75. Bulkley BH, Roberts WC. The heart in systemic lupus erythematosus and the changes induced in it by corticosteroid therapy. A study of 36 necropsy patients. Am J Med. 1975;58:243–64.
76. Hahn BH. Systemic lupus erythematosus and accelerated atherosclerosis. N Engl J Med. 2003;349:2379–80.
77. Jacobson EJ, Reza MJ. Constrictive pericarditis in systemic lupus erythematosus. Demonstration of immunoglobulins in the pericardium. Arthritis Rheum. 1978;21:972–4.
78. Hunder GG, Mullen BJ, McDuffie FC. Complement in pericardial fluid of lupus erythematosus. Studies in two patients. Ann Intern Med. 1974;80:453–8.
79. Kao AH, Manzi S. How to manage patients with cardiopulmonary disease? Best Pract Res Clin Rheumatol. 2002;16:211–27.
80. Wijetunga M, Rockson S. Myocarditis in systemic lupus erythematosus. Am J Med. 2002;113:419–23.
81. Berg G, Bodet J, Webb K, et al. Systemic lupus erythematosis presenting as isolated congestive heart failure. J Rheumatol. 1985;12:1182–5.
82. Borenstein DG, Fye WB, Arnett FC, Stevens MB. The myocarditis of systemic lupus erythematosus: association with myositis. Ann Intern Med. 1978;89:619–24.
83. Gur H, Keren G, Averbuch M, Levo Y. Severe congestive lupus cardiomyopathy complicated by an intracavitary thrombus: a clinical and echocardiographic followup. J Rheumatol. 1988;15:1278–80.
84. Kattwinkel N, Villanueva AG, Labib SB, et al. Myocardial infarction caused by cardiac microvasculopathy in a patient with the primary antiphospholipid syndrome. Ann Intern Med. 1992;116:974–6.
85. Nanke Y, Kotake S, Shimamoto K, Fukasawa C, Hara M, Kamatani N. Systemic lupus erythematosus with myocardial dysfunction due to microvasculopathy. Lupus. 2000;9:464–7.
86. Ratliff NB, Estes ML, Myles JL, Shirey EK, McMahon JT. Diagnosis of chloroquine cardiomyopathy by endomyocardial biopsy. N Engl J Med. 1987;316:191–3.
87. Homcy CJ, Liberthson RR, Fallon JT, Gross S, Miller LM. Ischemic heart disease in systemic lupus erythematosus in the young patient: report of six cases. Am J Cardiol. 1982;49:478–84.
88. Spiera H, Rothenberg RR. Myocardial infarction in four young patients with SLE. J Rheumatol. 1983;10:464–6.
89. Bessant R, Hingorani A, Patel L, MacGregor A, Isenberg DA, Rahman A. Risk of coronary heart disease and stroke in a large British cohort of patients with systemic lupus erythematosus. Rheumatology (Oxford). 2004;43:924–9.
90. Bruce IN, Urowitz MB, Gladman DD, Ibanez D, Steiner G. Risk factors for coronary heart disease in women with systemic lupus erythematosus: the Toronto Risk Factor Study. Arthritis Rheum. 2003;48:3159–67.
91. Kao AH, Sabatine JM, Manzi S. Update on vascular disease in systemic lupus erythematosus. Curr Opin Rheumatol. 2003;15:519–27.
92. Vlachoyiannopoulos PG, Kanellopoulos PG, Ioannidis JP, Tektonidou MG, Mastorakou I, Moutsopoulos HM. Atherosclerosis in premenopausal women with antiphospholipid syndrome and systemic lupus erythematosus: a controlled study. Rheumatology (Oxford). 2003;42:645–51.
93. Asanuma Y, Oeser A, Shintani AK, et al. Premature coronary-artery atherosclerosis in systemic lupus erythematosus. N Engl J Med. 2003;349:2407–15.

94. Pritzker MR, Ernst JD, Caudill C, Wilson CS, Weaver WF, Edwards JE. Acquired aortic stenosis in systemic lupus erythematosus. Ann Intern Med. 1980;93:434–6.
95. Korbet SM, Schwartz MM, Lewis EJ. Immune complex deposition and coronary vasculitis in systemic lupus erythematosus. Report of two cases. Am J Med. 1984;77:141–6.
96. Asherson RA, Mackay IR, Harris EN. Myocardial infarction in a young man with systemic lupus erythematosus, deep vein thrombosis, and antibodies to phospholipid. Br Heart J. 1986;56: 190–3.
97. Maaravi Y, Raz E, Gilon D, Rubinow A. Cerebrovascular accident and myocardial infarction associated with anticardiolipin antibodies in a young woman with systemic lupus erythematosus. Ann Rheum Dis. 1989;48:853–5.
98. Libman E, Sacks B. A hitherto undescribed form of valvular and mural endocarditis. Arch Intern Med. 1924;33:701–37.
99. Ropes MW. Systemic lupus erythematosus. 1st ed. Cambridge: Harvard University Press; 1976.
100. Shapiro RF, Gamble CN, Wiesner KB, et al. Immunopathogenesis of Libman-Sacks endocarditis. Assessment by light and immunofluorescent microscopy in two patients. Ann Rheum Dis. 1977;36:508–16.
101. Lerman BB, Thomas LC, Abrams GD, Pitt B. Aortic stenosis associated with systemic lupus erythematosus. Am J Med. 1982;72:707–10.
102. Morelli S, Bernardo ML, Viganego F, et al. Left-sided heart valve abnormalities and risk of ischemic cerebrovascular accidents in patients with systemic lupus erythematosus. Lupus. 2003;12:805–12.
103. Roldan CA, Shively BK, Crawford MH. An echocardiographic study of valvular heart disease associated with systemic lupus erythematosus. N Engl J Med. 1996;335:1424–30.
104. Asherson RA, Cervera R, Piette JC, et al. Catastrophic antiphospholipid syndrome. Clinical and laboratory features of 50 patients. Medicine (Baltimore). 1998;77:195–207.
105. Love PE, Santoro SA. Antiphospholipid antibodies: anticardiolipin and the lupus anticoagulant in systemic lupus erythematosus (SLE) and in non-SLE disorders. Prevalence and clinical significance. Ann Intern Med. 1990;112:682–98.
106. Petri M. The clinical syndrome associated with antiphospholipid antibodies. J Rheumatol. 1992;19:505–7.
107. Roubey RA. Immunology of the antiphospholipid antibody syndrome. Arthritis Rheum. 1996;39:1444–54.
108. Fluture A, Chaudhari S, Frishman WH. Valvular heart disease and systemic lupus erythematosus: therapeutic implications. Heart Dis. 2003;5:349–53.
109. Crowther MA, Ginsberg JS, Julian J, et al. A comparison of two intensities of warfarin for the prevention of recurrent thrombosis in patients with the antiphospholipid antibody syndrome. N Engl J Med. 2003;349:1133–8.
110. Khamashta MA, Cuadrado MJ, Mujic F, Taub NA, Hunt BJ, Hughes GR. The management of thrombosis in the antiphospholipid-antibody syndrome. N Engl J Med. 1995;332:993–7.
111. Asherson RA. The catastrophic antiphospholipid syndrome. J Rheumatol. 1992;19:508–12.
112. Asherson RA, Khamashta MA, Ordi-Ros J, et al. The "primary" antiphospholipid syndrome: major clinical and serological features. Medicine (Baltimore). 1989;68:366–74.
113. Galve E, Ordi J, Barquinero J, Evangelista A, Vilardell M, Soler-Soler J. Valvular heart disease in the primary antiphospholipid syndrome. Ann Intern Med. 1992;116:293–8.
114. Niaz A, Butany J. Antiphospholipid antibody syndrome with involvement of a bioprosthetic heart valve. Can J Cardiol. 1998;14:951–4.
115. Zavaleta NE, Montes RM, Soto ME, Vanzzini NA, Amigo MC. Primary antiphospholipid syndrome: a 5-year transesophageal echocardiographic followup study. J Rheumatol. 2004;31:2402–7.
116. Ferrante FM, Myerson GE, Goldman JA. Subclavian artery thrombosis mimicking the aortic arch syndrome in systemic lupus erythematosus. Arthritis Rheum. 1982;25:1501–4.
117. Leventhal LJ, Borofsky MA, Bergey PD, Schumacher HR Jr. Antiphospholipid antibody syndrome with right atrial thrombosis mimicking an atrial myxoma. Am J Med. 1989;87:111–3.
118. Ishikawa K. Diagnostic approach and proposed criteria for the clinical diagnosis of Takayasu's arteriopathy. J Am Coll Cardiol. 1988;12:964–72.
119. Takayasu M. Case with unusual changes of the central vessels in the retina. Acta Soc Ophthal Jpn. 1908;12:554–5.
120. Cipriano PR, Silverman JF, Perlroth MG, Griepp RB, Wexler L. Coronary arterial narrowing in Takayasu's aortitis. Am J Cardiol. 1977;39:744–50.
121. Gronemeyer PS, deMello DE. Takayasu's disease with aneurysm of right common iliac artery and iliocaval fistula in a young infant: case report and review of the literature. Pediatrics. 1982;69:626–31.
122. Hall S, Barr W, Lie JT, Stanson AW, Kazmier FJ, Hunder GG. Takayasu arteritis. A study of 32 North American patients. Medicine (Baltimore). 1985;64:89–99.
123. Hashimoto Y, Numano F, Maruyama Y, et al. Thallium-201 stress scintigraphy in Takayasu arteritis. Am J Cardiol. 1991;67:879–82.
124. Lande A, Rossi P. The value of total aortography in the diagnosis of Takayasu's arteritis. Radiology. 1975;114:287–97.
125. Lupi-Herrera E, Sanchez-Torres G, Marcushamer J, Mispireta J, Horwitz S, Vela JE. Takayasu's arteritis. Clinical study of 107 cases. Am Heart J. 1977;93:94–103.
126. Matsuyama A, Sakai N, Ishigami M, et al. Matrix metalloproteinases as novel disease markers in Takayasu arteritis. Circulation. 2003;108:1469–73.
127. Miyata T, Sato O, Koyama H, Shigematsu H, Tada Y. Long-term survival after surgical treatment of patients with Takayasu's arteritis. Circulation. 2003;108:1474–80.
128. Morooka S, Saito Y, Nonaka Y, Gyotoku Y, Sugimoto T. Clinical features and course of aortitis syndrome in Japanese women older than 40 years. Am J Cardiol. 1984;53:859–61.
129. Nakao K, Ikeda M, Kimata S, Niitani H, Niyahara M. Takayasu's arteritis. Clinical report of eighty-four cases and immunological studies of seven cases. Circulation. 1967;35:1141–55.
130. Numano F, Isohisa I, Egami M, Ohta N, Sasazuki T. HLA-DR MT and MB antigens in Takayasu disease. Tissue Antigens. 1983;21:208–12.
131. Shelhamer JH, Volkman DJ, Parrillo JE, Lawley TJ, Johnston MR, Fauci AS. Takayasu's arteritis and its therapy. Ann Intern Med. 1985;103:121–6.
132. Talwar KK, Chopra P, Narula J, et al. Myocardial involvement and its response to immunosuppressive therapy in nonspecific aortoarteritis (Takayasu's disease)—a study by endomyocardial biopsy. Int J Cardiol. 1988;21:323–34.
133. Thorsen MK, San Dretto MA, Lawson TL, Foley WD, Smith DF, Berland LL. Dissecting aortic aneurysms: accuracy of computed tomographic diagnosis. Radiology. 1983;148:773–7.
134. Volkman DJ, Mann DL, Fauci AS. Association between Takayasu's arteritis and a B-cell alloantigen in North Americans. N Engl J Med. 1982;306:464–5.
135. Wu YJ, Martin B, Ong K, Klein NC, Cunha BA. Takayasu's arteritis as a cause of fever of unknown origin. Am J Med. 1989;87:476–7.
136. Ueno A, Awane Y, Wakabayashi A, Shimizu K. Successfully operated obliterative brachiocephalic arteritis (Takayasu) associated with the elongated coarctation. Jpn Heart J. 1967;8:538–44.
137. Cooley DA. Techniques in cardiac surgery. 2nd ed. Philadelphia, PA: W.B. Saunders Co.; 1984.

138. Robbs JV, Human RR, Rajaruthnam P. Operative treatment of nonspecific aortoarteritis (Takayasu's arteritis). J Vasc Surg. 1986;3:605–16.
139. Alestig K, Barr J. Giant-cell arteritis. A biopsy study of polymyalgia rheumatica, including one case of Takayasu's disease. Lancet. 1963;1:1228–30.
140. Ghose MK, Shensa S, Lerner PI. Arteritis of the aged (giant cell arteritis) and fever of unexplained origin. Am J Med. 1976;60:429–36.
141. Gonzalez EB, Varner WT, Lisse JR, Daniels JC, Hokanson JA. Giant-cell arteritis in the southern United States. An 11-year retrospective study from the Texas Gulf Coast. Arch Intern Med. 1989;149:1561–5.
142. Healey LA, Wilske KR. Manifestations of giant cell arteritis. Med Clin North Am. 1977;61:261–70.
143. Klein RG, Hunder GG, Stanson AW, Sheps SG. Large artery involvement in giant cell (temporal) arteritis. Ann Intern Med. 1975;83:806–12.
144. Salisbury RS, Hazleman BL. Successful treatment of dissecting aortic aneurysm due to giant cell arteritis. Ann Rheum Dis. 1981;40:507–8.
145. Feier H, Cioata D, Teodorescu-Branzeu D, Gaspar M. Coronary ostial stenosis in a young patient. Circulation. 2012;125:e367–8.
146. Roberts WC, Ko JM, Vowels TJ. Natural history of syphilitic aortitis. Am J Cardiol. 2009;104:1578–87.
147. Willerson JT, Coselli JS, LeMaire SA, et al. Diseases of the aorta. In: Willerson JT, Cohn JN, Wellens HJJ, Holmes Jr DR, editors. Cardiovascular medicine. 3rd ed. London: Springer; 2007. p. 1623–61.

5 Comprehensive Approach to Aortic Valve Disease

Blase A. Carabello, Haziam Alwair, and Rajasekhar Nekkanti

Aortic Stenosis

Etiology

While it was once viewed as a "degenerative" disease, it is now clear that aortic stenosis (AS) develops from an active inflammatory process with histopathologic features similar to coronary artery disease (CAD) [1]. Indeed the initial plaque of AS resembles the coronary plaque as shown in Fig. 5.1. Further, the AS valve is inflamed with some areas of the valve measurably hotter than other areas. These hotter areas are infiltrated with lymphocytes consistent with an inflammatory process [2]. Because of this similarity to CAD, statins, so effective in treating CAD, have been tested in AS in hope of retarding disease progression [3–5]. Unfortunately, these trials failed, probably because of the differences in the mechanisms by which plaques cause harm in the two diseases. In CAD, statins presumably stabilize the plaque (perhaps by enhancing calcification) preventing plaque rupture [6]. However, in AS, in which many valves harbor not just calcium but also true bone, this same enhancement of calcification could worsen leaflet immobility canceling out the beneficial effects of the agents [7]. Nonetheless it is this change in the etiology of AS in developed countries from rheumatic fever to an atherosclerosis-like disease that kindles a search for the pathways leading to calcification. This search is likely to find new pharmacologic targets for preventing the disease or retarding its progression. A possible future target is the proprotein convertase subtilisin/kexin type 9 system (PCSK9). PCSK9 activates the removal of LDL receptors, increasing LDL and LP(a) both implicated in the pathogenesis of AS [8]. Inhibitors of PCSK9 decrease both LDL and LP(a), a reduction that could forestall AS progression.

About 1–2% of the US population is born with a bicuspid instead of a tricuspid aortic valve. Possibly because of less favorable hemodynamics causing increased shear stress, bicuspid valves become stenotic a decade or two earlier in life than do tricuspid aortic valves. Or it may be that the NOTCH 2 gene which plays a role in both cusp development and calcification is involved [9].

Rheumatic fever and subsequent rheumatic heart disease are a rare cause of AS in developed countries but are a much more common cause in the developing world. When rheumatic heart disease is the etiology, the mitral valve is almost always involved. These and other rarer causes of AS are listed below.

Causes of aortic stenosis

1. Calcific atherosclerotic disease
2. Rheumatic heart disease
3. Post radiation
4. Carcinoid syndrome
5. Serotonergic drugs: ergotamine, pergolide, cabergoline, fenfluramine
6. Ochronosis
7. Paget's disease

Bicuspid Aortic Valve and Aortic Root Dilatation

Bicuspid aortic valve may also be associated with aortopathy leading to aortic root or ascending aorta dilatation, more commonly with joined right and left cusps than with other

B. A. Carabello (✉)
Cardiology Division, Brody School of Medicine, East Carolina University, Greenville, NC, USA

Department of Cardiovascular Sciences, Vidant Medical Center, Greenville, NC, USA
e-mail: carabellob16@ecu.edu

H. Alwair
Division of Cardiac Surgery, Department of Cardiovascular Sciences, East Carolina Heart Institute, Greenville, NC, USA

R. Nekkanti
Department of Cardiovascular Sciences, Vidant Medical Center, Greenville, NC, USA

B. A. Carabello (ed.), *Valvular Heart Disease*, Cardiovascular Medicine, https://doi.org/10.1007/978-1-4471-2840-3_5

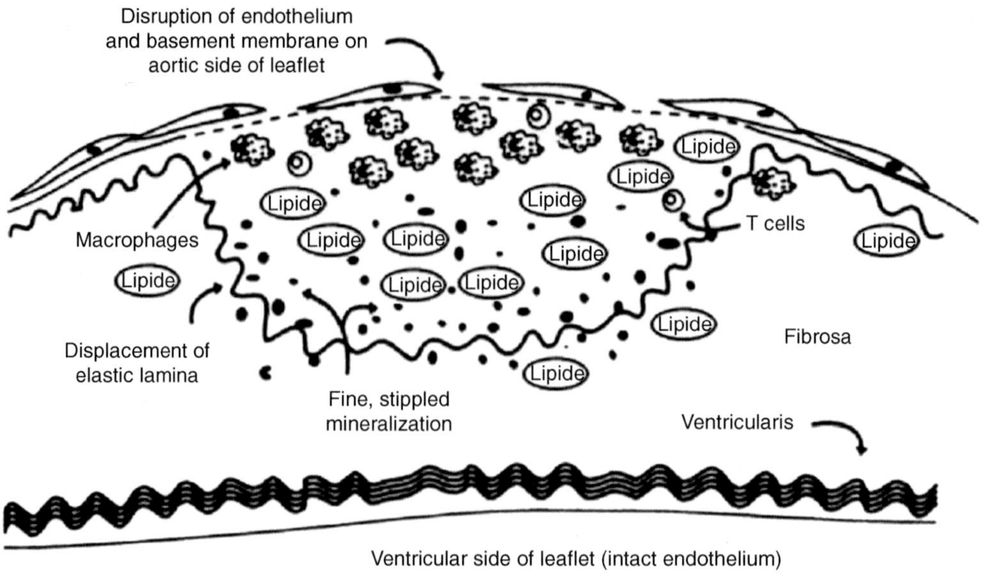

Fig. 5.1 A cartoon of the histology of the initial plaque of aortic stenosis is demonstrated. There is a remarkable similarity to the atherosclerotic plaque of coronary artery disease with a lipid laden core infiltrated with inflammatory cells. Taken form Ref. [1]. From Otto CM, et al. [1]. Reprinted with permission from Wolters Kluwer Health, Inc.

patterns of bicuspidization [10, 11]. Root enlargement occurs in AS but is more prominent in aortic regurgitation. The cause of this dilatation is debated between two major theories [12–14]: (1) bicuspid valve is part of a syndrome associated with a genetic predisposition to aortic root dilatation distinct from other aortic syndromes (Marfan, Loeys Dietz, etc.); (2) abnormal flow exiting the misshapen aortic valve impinges on the aorta, increasing wall stress at the impingement points, causing aortic dilatation [12]. In fact, matrix metalloproteinases (MMPs) appear to be activated in areas of jet impingement supporting the flow hypothesis [12, 14]. However other areas of the aorta not impacted by flow impingement also show root dilatation. It may be that both mechanisms play a role in bicuspid valve-associated aortopathy. A broader discussion of this topic is found in Chap. 4.

Pathophysiology and Its Relationship to Symptoms

As derived by Ross and Braunwald (Fig. 5.2a) and confirmed by randomized trials [15–17], the presence or absence of symptoms in patients with AS remains a demarcation point in the disease, with symptomatic patients having a much worse prognosis than asymptomatic patients. Thus understanding the pathophysiology of AS symptoms is a key to understanding the disease. Narrowing of the aortic orifice to one-half its normal 3.0 cm^2 area causes little obstruction to outflow (Table 5.1). However further stenosis requires progressively greater left ventricular (LV) pressure to drive blood past the narrowed opening. At an aortic valve area (AVA) of 1.0 cm^2 there is typically a 25 mmHg mean pressure gradient between the LV and the aorta. Further narrowing to 0.7 cm^2 causes a 50 mm HG gradient while a decrease to 0.5 cm^2 leads to a 100 mmHg transvalvular gradient.

The LV response to this pressure overload is the development of concentric hypertrophy (LVH) and/or concentric remodeling. Pressure overload in some way triggers the addition of sarcomeres in parallel so that each myocyte becomes thicker, in turn leading to increased wall thickness, and, if total mass increases, left ventricular hypertrophy (LVH). In some cases, ventricular geometry changes in such a way that LV radius decreases as wall thickness increases so that there is not true hypertrophy but rather concentric remodeling. Left ventricular hypertrophy is usually viewed as a double-edged sword, with both beneficial and pathologic consequences. Afterload, the force that opposes contraction is often described as wall stress (σ), where $\sigma = P \times r/2h$ and P = systolic pressure, r = LV radius, and h = wall thickness. Increased thickness in the denominator (concentric hypertrophy) offsets increased pressure in the numerator, thus maintaining normal stress (afterload) helping to maintain normal ejection and thus is beneficial [18, 19]. Unfortunately pathologic LVH contributes to the causes of angina, heart failure and syncope. Left ventricular hypertrophy impairs coronary blood flow reserve that normally accompanies the increased oxygen demands of increased stroke work [20, 21]. Impaired reserve may stem from diminished capillary ingrowth insufficient to meet the increase in muscle mass [22]. Reserve is further decreased from increased LV filling pressure due to impaired diastolic relaxation. Increased LV filling pressure reduces the pressure gradient for coronary flow (aortic diastolic pressure minus LV diastolic pressure) especially to the subendocardium, further contributing to potential exercise induced ischemia [21]. Increased wall thickness and increased collagen deposition also impair diastolic filling leading to heart failure symptoms [23–25]. Eventually LVH also causes systolic dysfunction, the exact mechanisms of which are still debated but ischemia, impaired calcium handling, excess afterload, and

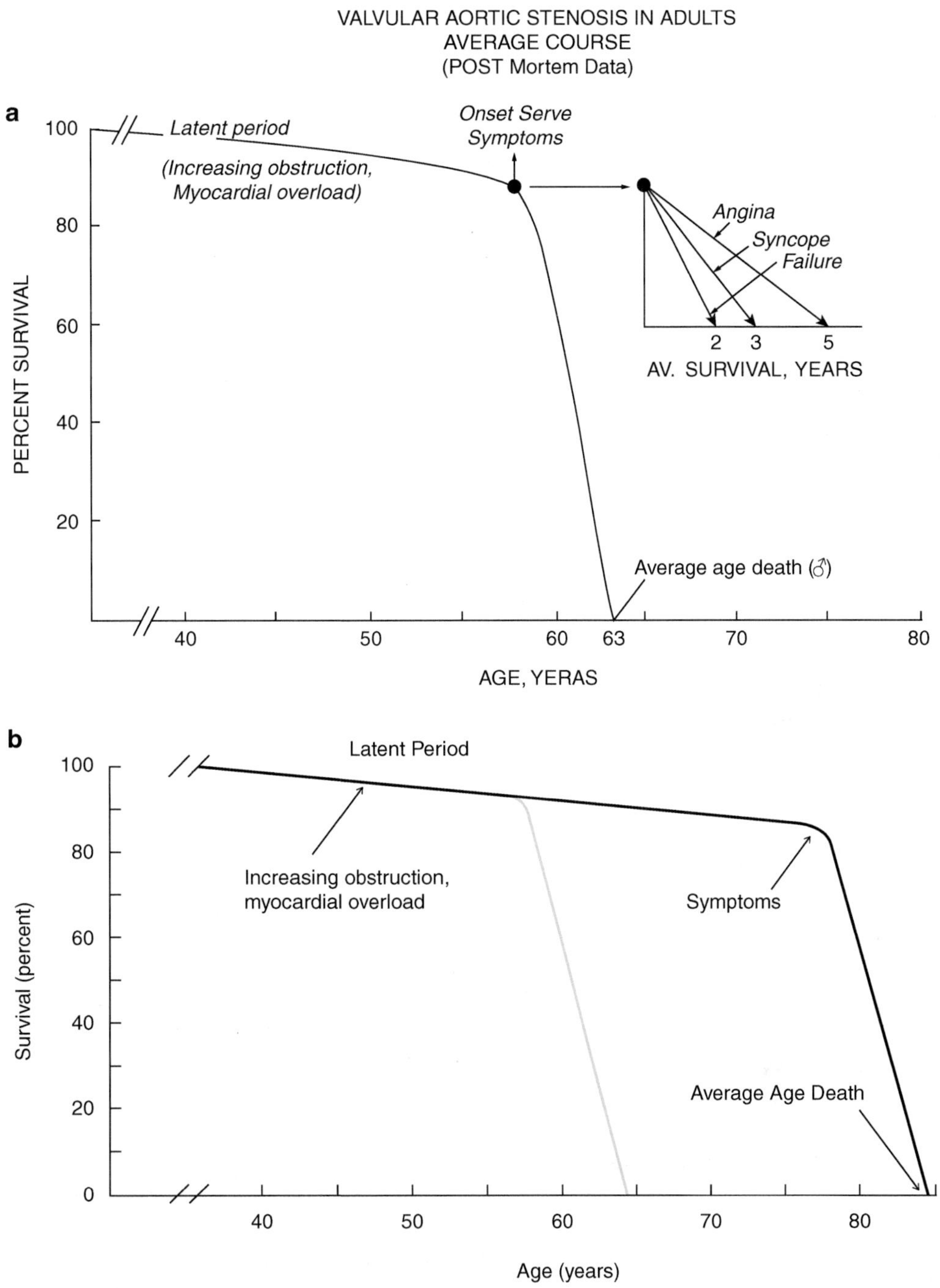

Fig. 5.2 (**a**) The natural history of aortic stenosis from mid-twentieth century is demonstrated. Following a long latent period where survival is nearly normal, the onset of symptoms of angina, syncope and heart failure heralds a dramatic worsening in prognosis. Adopted form Ref. [15]. From Ross JR, Braunwald E [15]. Reprinted with permission from Wolters Kluwer Health, Inc. (**b**) The natural history of aortic stenosis in the twenty-first century as depicted by Bonow and confirmed by randomized trials finds the same impact of symptoms but with onset 10–20 years later in life owing to a change in etiology of the disease. From Carabello BA [29]. Reprinted with permission from Wolters Kluwer Health, Inc.

Table 5.1 Aortic valve area and transvalvular gradient

AVA (cm^2)	Mean gradient (mmHg)
1.5	11
1.2	17
1.0	25
0.7	51
0.5	100
0.4	156

AVA aortic valve area. Data developed from the Gorlin formula assuming a cardiac output of 6 L/min, a heart rate of 80 and a systolic ejection period of 340 ms

apoptosis play a role [21, 26–28]. LVH by diminishing LV cavity volume reduces stroke volume and cardiac output contributing to hypotension and syncope during activity.

Evolution of the Natural History of Aortic Stenosis

The data compiled to develop Fig. 5.2a came from relatively young patients with rheumatic or congenital AS. At the time (1968), echocardiography was in its infancy and Doppler

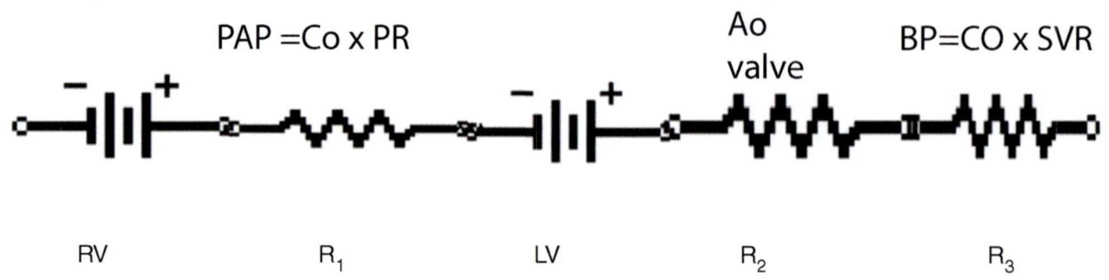

Fig. 5.3 The heart in aortic stenosis modeled as an electrical circuit where RV = right ventricle, R_1 = the pulmonary vascular resistance, LV = left ventricle, R_2 = the resistance offered by the stenotic aortic valve and R_3 the total peripheral resistance. Earlier detection and treatment of aortic stenosis has caused R_2 to lessen over the past 50 years while onset of aortic stenosis later in life occurs when more patients have hypertension increasing the importance of R_3. From Carabello BA [31]. Reprinted with permission from Wolters Kluwer Health, Inc.

interrogation of jet velocity was not yet available. Thus valve severity could only be studied invasively, during cardiac catheterization, a procedure reserved for clearly symptomatic patients with advanced disease. Today patients are older as etiology has changed from rheumatic to atherosclerotic-calcific disease and noninvasive evaluation has become both perfected and routine [29]. As a consequence, patients are detected with severe disease but less severe and with milder symptoms than when invasive techniques were required for diagnosis. And they are older (Fig. 5.2b) and more prone to hypertension. Today, as depicted in Fig. 5.3, the resistance offered by the aortic valve (R_2) is less while the resistance offered by the periphery (R_3) is more than it was 40 years ago. Accordingly, therapy must be directed at treating not just the stenotic aortic valve but also at treating systemic hypertension when it is present [30, 31].

The Stages of AS and Grading of Severity

The stages of VHD are listed in Table 5.2 [32]. As they apply to AS, stage A, at risk for AS, might be represented by a patient with a bicuspid valve. Stage B, progressive disease, is represented by a patient with mild or moderate AS. There is a modest transvalvular gradient of 10–20 mmHg, mild LVH, and no measurable clinical consequences. Class C_1 is asymptomatic severe compensated AS in which the patient has severe AS, no symptoms, and normal LV function. It must be noted that the current definition of "severe" AS has significant limitations. "Severe" AS is defined in the ACC/AHA Guidelines [32] by an aortic valve area of ≤1.0 cm², a peak transaortic jet velocity of ≥4.0 m/s, a mean aortic gradient of ≥40 mmHg, or and indexed AVA of 0.6 cm²/m². However as shown in Fig. 5.4, there often is internal inconsistency in these definitions in which some patients would be classified as having severe AS by one criterion but moderate by another [33]. In such cases all data including the physical exam, the echocardiographic appearance of the valve, and the hemodynamics must be taken together to ascertain AS severity. Further some patients appear to be intolerant of pressure

Table 5.2 Stages of valvular heart disease

Stage	Definition	Description
A	At risk	Patients with risk factors for development of VHD
B	Progressive	Patients with progressive VHD (mild-to-moderate severity and asymptomatic)
C	Asymptomatic severe	Asymptomatic patients who have the criteria for severe VHD: C_1: Asymptomatic patients with severe VHD in whom the left or and right ventricles remains compensated C_2: Asymptomatic patients with severe VHD with decompensation of the left or right ventricle
D	Symptomatic severe	Patients who have developed symptoms as a result of VHD

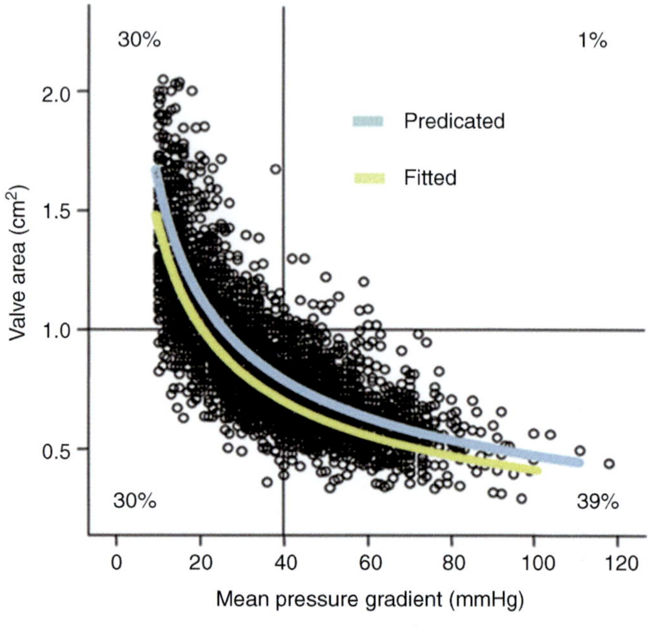

Fig. 5.4 Valve area and mean gradient from over 3400 patients with aortic stenosis are plotted against each other. The data fit (yellow line) closely to that predicted by the Gorlin formula (blue line). Importantly in 30% of patients (lower left quadrant) the data are discordant with valve area in the "severe" range while gradient only predicts moderate disease. From Minners J, et al. [33]. Reprinted with permission from Oxford University Press

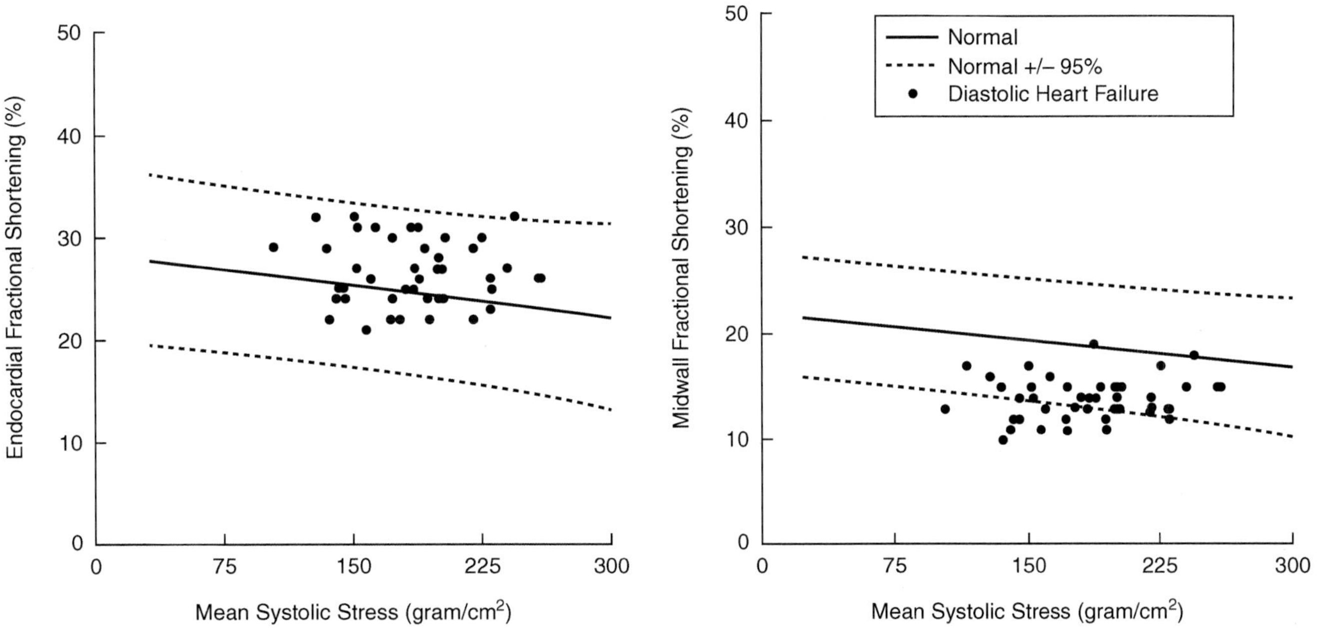

Fig. 5.5 Endocardial left ventricular shortening (left) and mid-wall shortening (right) are plotted against systolic stress (afterload) for patients with left ventricular hypertrophy. Dotted lines represent the boundaries for normal subjects. Mid-wall shortening that better reflects total myocardial function across the left ventricular wall is low normal or abnormal in aortic stenosis patients, performance not reflected when only examining endocardial events, i.e., ejection fraction. From Baicu CF, et al. [36]. Reprinted with permission from Wolters Kluwer Health, Inc.

overload, developing symptoms and LV dysfunction with relatively small gradients and at aortic valve areas larger than defined by current guidelines [34, 35]. Management of symptomatic patients currently defined as having less than severe AS awaits further study.

Class C_2 is represented by the asymptomatic patient with severe AS and LV dysfunction. Such patients are rare and are asymptomatic usually because of a sedentary lifestyle, with reduced cardiac demand. This class of patient requires aortic valve replacement (AVR) even though they are asymptomatic since further delay leads to worsening and irrevocable LV damage. At issue however is what defines LV dysfunction in AS. With the concentric LVH present in AS, the extra sarcomeres present can contract subnormally yet still thicken enough to maintain a normal ejection fraction (Fig. 5.5) [36]. Recent data suggest that while normal ejection fraction is often defined as ≥50%, in AS survival may be reduced if EF falls below 60% [35], which may be a better demarcator for the definition of LV dysfunction. Class D is composed of symptomatic patients with severe AS. As noted above, the prognosis for such patients is dire without AVR.

Disease Progression

AS is caused by an active inflammatory process and as such is predictably a progressive disease, with the degree of stenosis worsening over time. While the disease is seldom static, the rate of progression is remarkably variable from patient to patient. Jet velocity on average increases 0.2–0.4 m/s/year, mean gradient 7–20 mmHg/year and AVA decreases 0.1–0.2 cm²/year [3, 5, 37–40]. These data are useful in determining the interval between patient follow-up visits. Every patient should be educated to look for the development of the classic symptoms of AS and advised to alert the provider if they occur. However knowledge that the disease is entering the severe phase serves to focus increased scrutiny onto the patient, questioning him/her closely about symptomatic status. To this end, periodic echocardiography helps define the progression of disease specific to the patient being followed. Considering the data noted above, it would be highly unlikely that a patient with mild disease (jet velocity <2.5 m/s) would progress to severe disease in 1–2 years so that echocardiography every 2–3 years should provide sufficient surveillance unless there is a change in symptom status. On the other hand, patients with more advanced disease require more frequent echocardiographic observation, every 1–2 years for jet velocity 2.5–3.0 m/s and yearly for jet velocity >3.0 m/s. The above suggestions presume normal LV stroke volume and must be modified if stroke volume is abnormally low.

Diagnosis

Physical Exam

The diagnosis of AS is often first suspected when a murmur is detected during routine physical examination. Typically

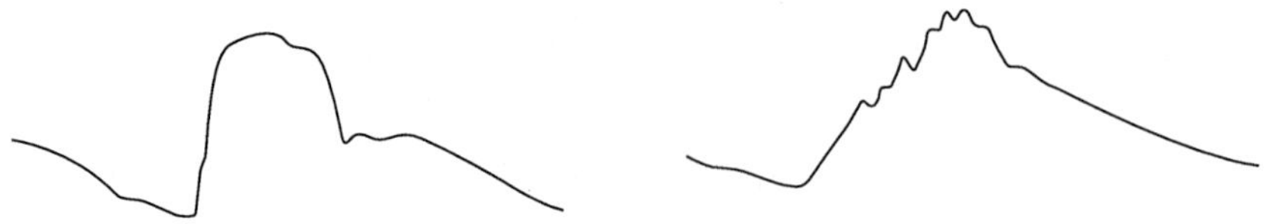

Fig. 5.6 Carotid pulse tracings similar to the pulse felt during physical examination for a normal subject (left) and the delayed pulse of a patient with aortic stenosis (right) is shown. From Carabello BA [41]. Reprinted with permission from Lange Medical Books/McGraw Hill

the murmur of AS is a raspy systolic ejection murmur that radiates to the neck. In mild disease the murmur peaks in mid-systole creating a crescendo-decrescendo murmur. However as stenosis increases, peak intensity occurs progressively later in systole and peaks at end systole in severe disease. In some cases the murmur is heard loudest in the aortic area, diminishes over the sternum, and is heard loudly again at the LV apex, misleading the examiner to believe that two murmurs (aortic and mitral) are present (Gallavardin's phenomenon). The intensity of the murmur is often inversely related to disease severity because in advanced AS reduced stroke volume decreases the loudness of the murmur. Thus a soft late peaking systolic ejection murmur may indicate severe disease. If the patient experiences variation in R–R interval during the exam, either due to premature beats or atrial fibrillation, murmur intensity increases after longer R–R intervals because stroke volume increases. This finding helps distinguish the murmur from that of mitral regurgitation where murmur intensity does not change following longer pauses.

The carotid upstrokes are typically reduced in volume and delayed in timing (parvus et tardus, Fig. 5.6) [41] because the stenosis takes momentum from the blood stream as it exits the valve. There is often an S_4 reflecting the poor compliance of the hypertrophied LV. Because the aortic valve neither opens nor closes well, the A_2 component of the second heart sound is often lost yielding a soft single second sound. This finding seems less common today than it was decades ago when the disease was detected later in its course.

Imaging

The EKG may exhibit criteria for the presence of LVH and the chest X-ray may demonstrate a boot-shaped heart consistent with concentric LVH but echocardiography forms the mainstay of diagnosis. The 2-D images assess LV function and the extent of LVH. In severe AS the aortic valve is heavily calcified and nearly immobile. If tricuspid valve regurgitation is present, right ventricular and peak pulmonary artery pressure can be estimated and may reflect LV filling pressure. Doppler interrogation of the valve demonstrates acceleration of blood as it passes through the stenotic valve because velocity must increase to maintain flow through a narrowed orifice [flow = area (A) × velocity (V)]. Using the modified Bernoulli equation, the pressure gradient (g) across the valve is calculated as $g = 4V^2$. Because flow must be equal on either side of the valve (continuity), ($A_1 \times V_1 = A_2 \times V_2$). In turn $CSA_1 \times VTI_1 = CSA_2 \times VTI_2$ so that $CSA_2 = CSA_1 \times VTI_1/VTI_2$, where CSA_1 = aortic outflow tract (LVOT) cross-sectional area, VTI_1 = aortic outflow tract time-velocity integral, VTI_2 = aortic valve time-velocity integral, and CSA_2 = aortic valve area. Because peak transvalvular jet velocity is directly measured primary data, not relying on calculation form other data, it has become the foundation of AS severity assessment when LV function and stroke volume are normal. However, because stroke volume generates flow velocity, AS severity may be underestimated in low flow states. In these cases, valve area that assesses gradient and velocity in the context of flow assumes greater importance in severity assessment. Obtaining these data is subject to several pitfalls of which the clinician must be aware.

Challenges and Pitfalls

1. The maximum aortic velocity and the mean gradient can be grossly underestimated if the continuous Doppler beam is not aligned parallel or near parallel to the stenotic jet. As such the insonification angle between the Doppler beam and the jet should be maintained at less than 30°. However the stenotic jet can be eccentric and the aorta can be unwound making this technically challenging (Fig. 5.7). In such cases, a transesophageal echocardiogram may help to obtain the maximum velocities by careful manipulation of the probe using multiple planes (Figs. 5.8, 5.9, and 5.10).

Challenges When Using the Continuity Equation for Assessment of Aortic Stenosis

Based on the principle of conservation of mass, the aortic valve area is derived from the continuity equation noted above. Deriving the area of the LVOT is crucial to the accuracy of the calculation.

Assuming the LVOT is a circular structure, the LVOT area is calculated from the following equation:

$$\text{LVOT area} = \pi \times \frac{\text{Diameter of LVOT}^2}{4}$$

Thus, if the diameter of the LVOT is not measured diligently using multiple attempts and in "ZOOM" view, overestimation or underestimation of the severity of aortic stenosis may occur. This is by far the most common reason for underestimating aortic valve area.

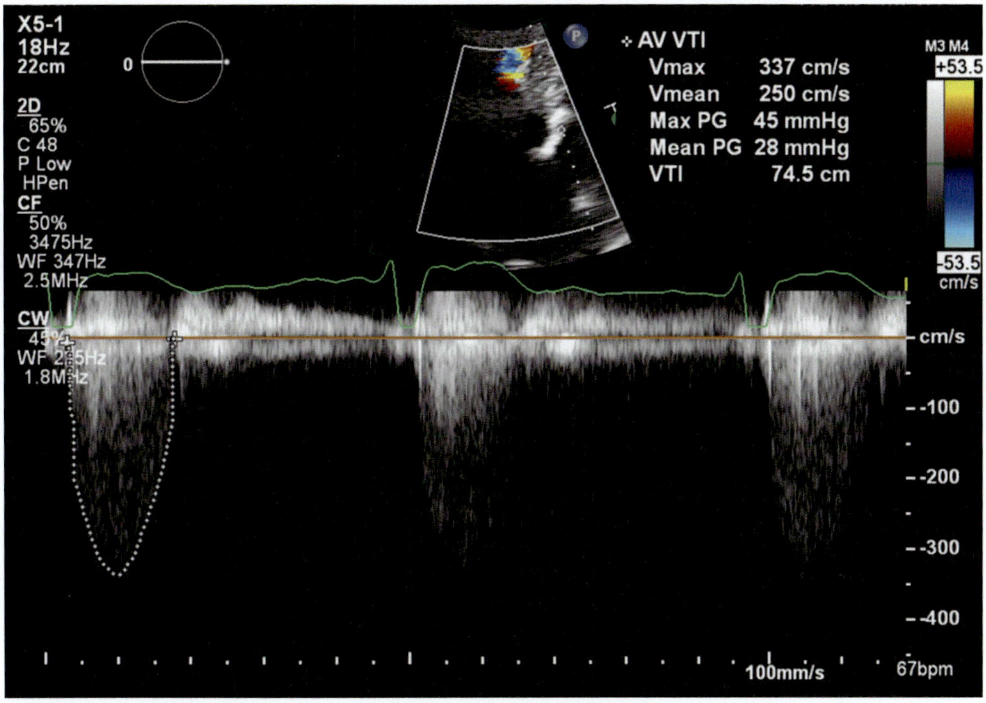

Fig. 5.7 Continuous wave Doppler of the aortic stenosis jet in a patient with uncontrolled chronic systemic hypertension resulting in an unwound aorta. This anatomy constrains the ability to obtain the best Doppler angle of insonification resulting in underestimation of the maximum velocities. The mean gradient appears to be 28 mmHg and the maximum velocity is estimated to be 3.5 m/s

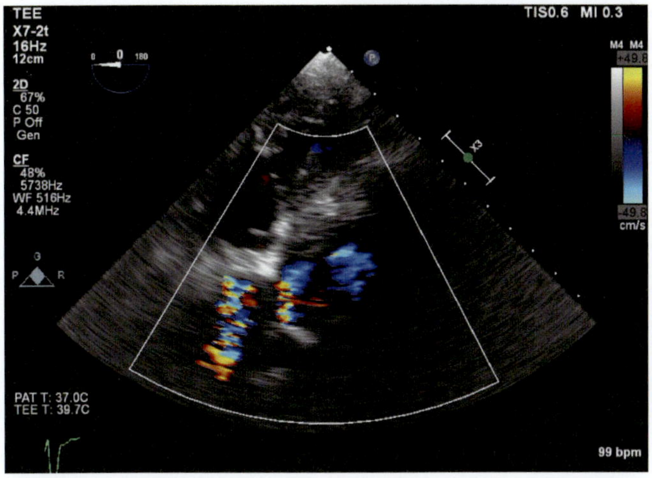

Fig. 5.8 In this case the eccentric aortic stenosis jet causes the inability to align the Doppler beam to obtain the maximum aortic velocity as shown below

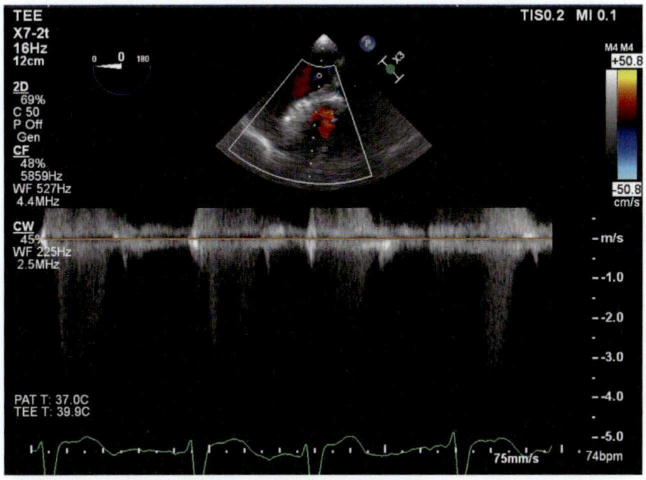

Fig. 5.9 Note the faint spectral Doppler envelopes from the deep trans gastric TEE views. The Doppler envelope is poorly defined giving an unreliable estimate the mean gradient and the peak velocity is underestimated

Technique for Proper Measurement of LVOT Diameter

The following caveats should be followed to maintain reproducibility and reliability of the measurement of LVOT diameter:

1. Always use the "ZOOMED" view and acquire a cine loop in the left parasternal long axis view.

   Measure at the "hinge points'—inner edge to inner edge in mid-systole as shown in Fig. 5.11.

   In the left PLAX view, the lateral resolution is better and the risk of underestimating the LVOT diameter is reduced. Moreover the left PLAX view offers axial resolution which is always better than lateral resolution in echocardiography. The measurement should be made in mid-systole as there conformational change in the aortic root during the cardiac cycle and the annulus assumes a more circular shape during this phase.
2. Always measure at the "hinge points" where the cuspal insertion is noted and, in a plane, parallel to the LVOT (Fig. 5.12). A parallel view gives a more accurate measurement than an oblique view. If the measurement is made from the apparent (virtual) annulus as shown in Fig. 5.13, it may overestimate the LVOT dimension.

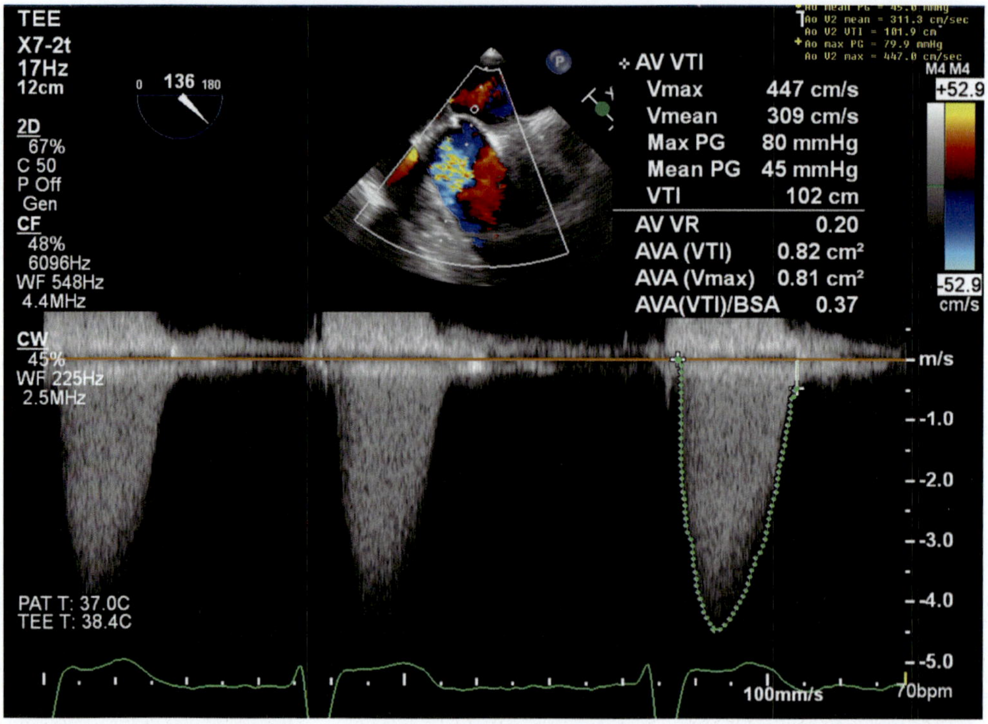

Fig. 5.10 In the same patient withdrawal of the probe to a mid-esophageal location and sampling the flow with continuous Doppler yields a higher aortic velocity with a dense spectral envelope. This case illustrates the importance of using multiple planes and views to obtain the highest velocities, avoiding underestimation of the severity of aortic stenosis. The true mean gradient was 45 mmHg and the maximum velocity was 4.5 m/s

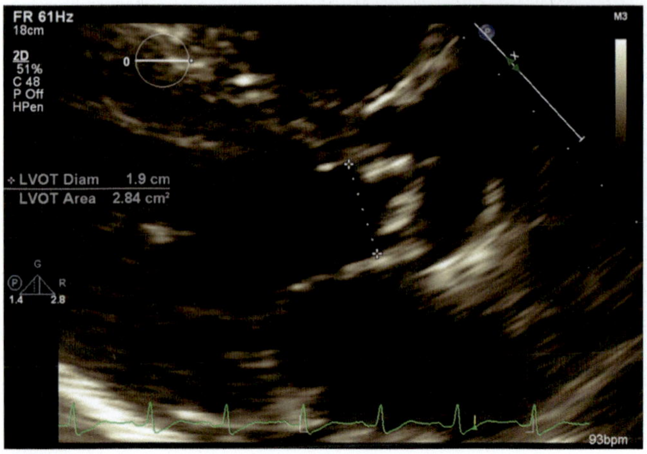

Fig. 5.11 The "zoomed" view for proper measurement of the aortic annulus is shown

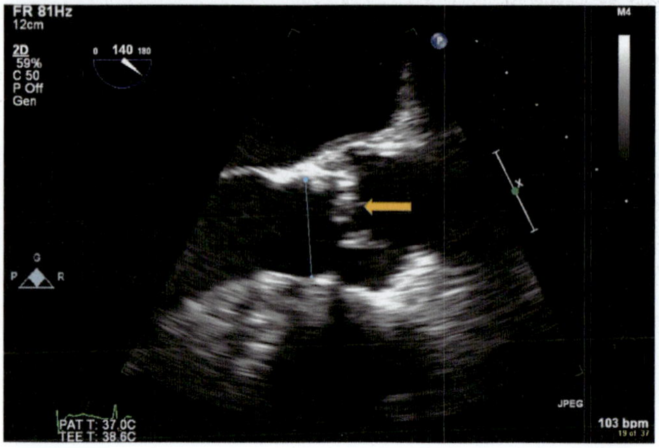

Fig. 5.12 TEE study with measurement taken from the "hinge points" between the cusps at the "virtual annulus" estimates the diameter of the LVOT at 2.2 cm. The arrow points to the cuspal separation during systole

3. Once a parallel view is confirmed, rotate/angulate the transducer till the largest diameter of the LVOT is obtained. This can be noted by dissecting the plane through the right coronary cusp anteriorly and the inter-leaflet triangle between the left coronary and the noncoronary cusp posteriorly. If the two leaflets are visualized anteriorly and posteriorly, the largest diameter has not been obtained (Figs. 5.14 and 5.15).
4. Morphological changes in the subaortic location that may hinder accurate measurement of the LVOT diameter such as the bulky calcium protrusion shown in Fig. 5.16 but can be excluded for greater accuracy as shown in Fig. 5.17.
5. Septal hypertrophy. Septal hypertrophy is frequently seen in patients with aortic stenosis (Fig. 5.18). Care should be taken to identify the aortic annulus and measurements should be done at proper location so that the diameter is not underestimated. This can be corrected by using the zoomed view and careful alignment parallel to the LVOT (Fig. 5.19).
6. Technical limitations
   (a) Body habitus

   Poor acoustic windows in a patient with COPD or morbid obesity, the aortic root may not be well

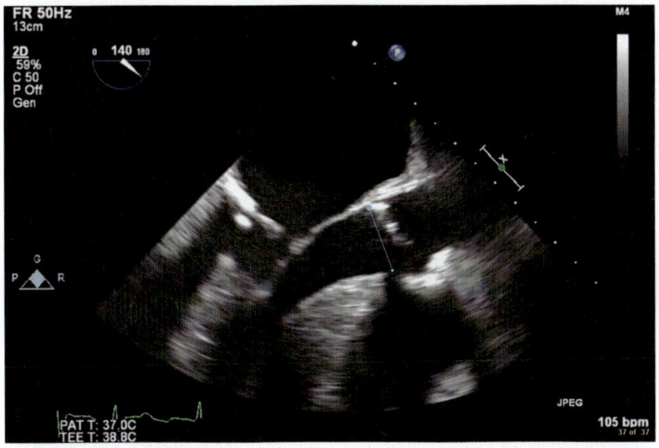

Fig. 5.13 TEE study with measurement taken from the commissure between the left and noncoronary cusp to the right cusp at the "virtual annulus" overestimates the diameter of the LVOT at 2.4 cm

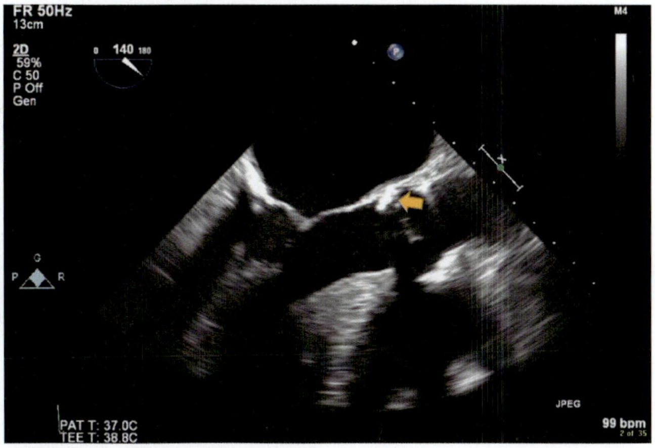

Fig. 5.16 A bulky calcium deposit (arrow) blocks proper annulus measurement

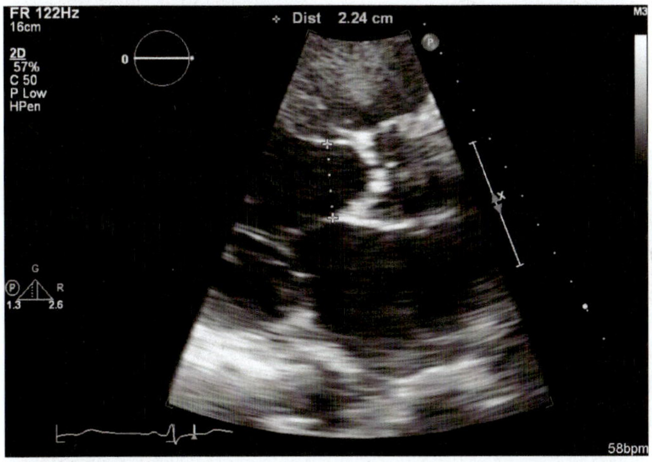

Fig. 5.14 The right coronary cusp (RCC) and the posterior cusp are both well-defined and the LVOT dimension measures 2.2 cm

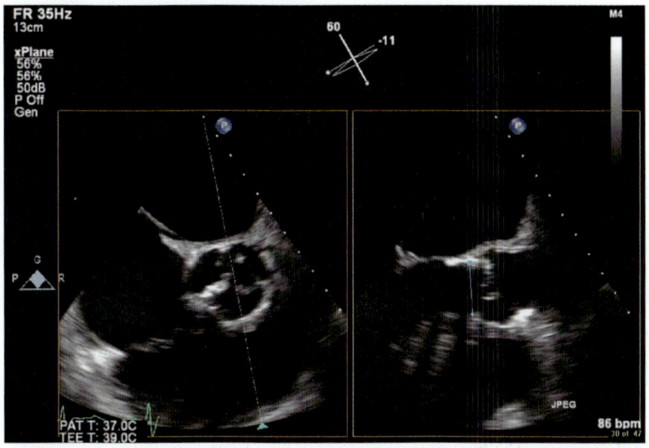

Fig. 5.17 Using biplane TEE, the mass seen in Fig. 5.16 was excluded, the "hinge points" were clearly defined and the annular size is more accurately estimated at 2.2 cm

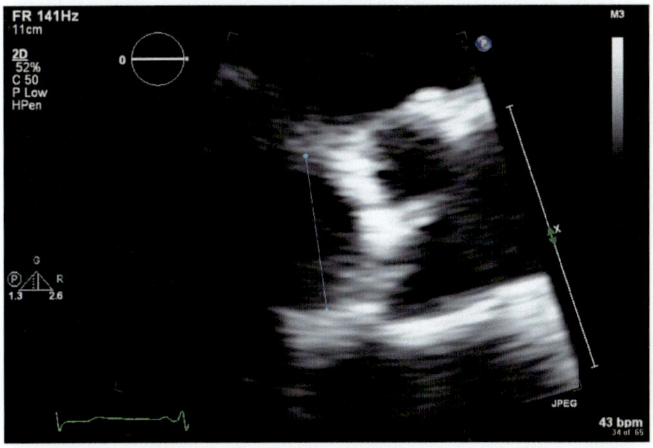

Fig. 5.15 The RCC is well visualized but the posterior RCC is not well visualized and the LVOT dimension is overestimated at 2.4 cm

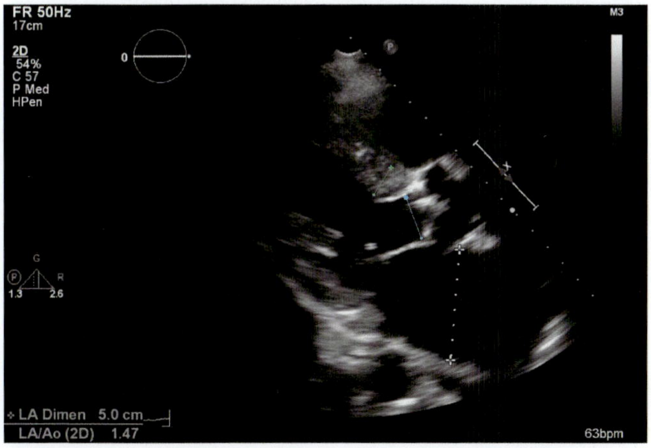

Fig. 5.18 The green line indicates septal wall thickness measured at 1.5 cm. The blue line indicates LVOT measurement which has been underestimated at 1.9 cm

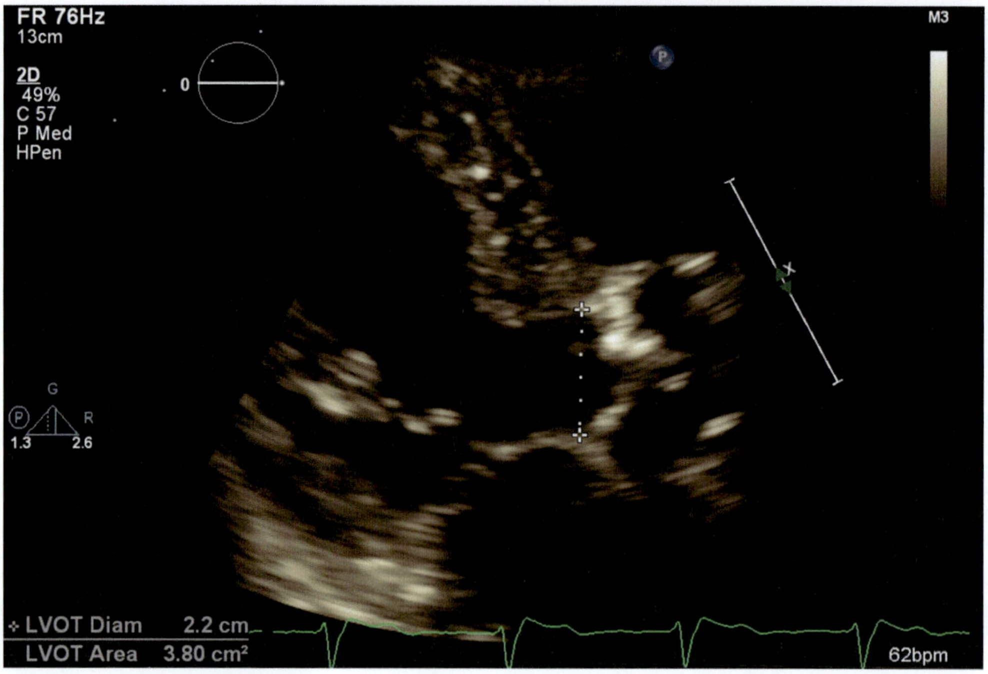

Fig. 5.19 Using zoomed views from the case noted in Fig. 5.18 and more careful alignment in parallel to the LVOT, the measurement of the AV annulus is now 2.2 cm

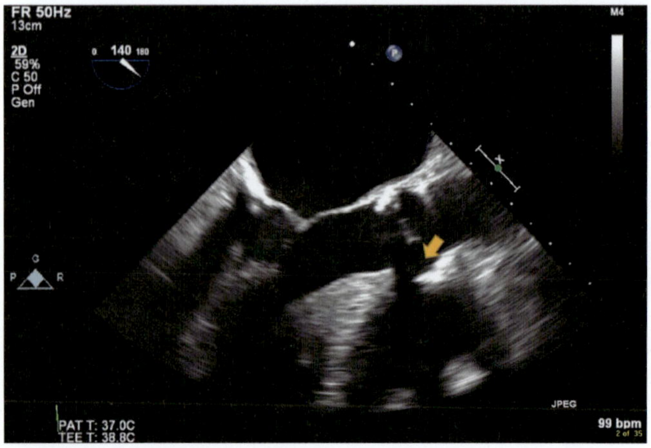

Fig. 5.20 The arrow points to the acoustic shadowing from the subaortic calcification that results in poor definition of the aortic valve annulus

visualized. Alternate methods of imaging such as TEE can be used for estimation of the LVOT diameter.

(b) Acoustic shadowing from calcified aortic valve and aortic root as shown in Fig. 5.20 may cause inaccurate measurement of the LVOT.

(c) Diligent attention must be paid to the gain and the use of focalization to improve image optimization.

Other Imaging Modalities

Because calcification is a key bodily response to tissue damage, it is logical that the degree of calcification of the aortic valve would correlate with AS severity. Indeed valve calcification measured using multidetector CT scanning correlates with valve area [42–44]. Thus valve calcification may be a useful adjunct in deciding AS severity in borderline cases or when standard measures of assessment are discordant with one another.

Cardiac Catheterization

Prior to the advances made in echocardiography, invasive hemodynamic evaluation was the gold standard for AS severity assessment. Both noninvasive and invasive techniques use the same principle to define valve area (A) where $A = F/V$ and F = flow and V = flow velocity. During echocardiography, velocity is measured directly. Invasively, velocity is calculated using Torricelli's equation $v = 2\sqrt{gh}$, where g is the velocity due to gravity (converting force to mmHg) and h = the mean pressure gradient. Valve area is determined by the Gorlin formula [45], AVA = $F/2\sqrt{gh}$ where flow is determined by thermodilution or Fick methods and the gradient obtained by directly measuring pressure proximal (left ventricle) and distal (aorta) to the aortic valve. Invasive technique is used when there are discrepancies between the clinical presentation and echocardiography or when body habitus precludes obtaining clear echocardiographic data. Thus when invasive AVA determination is made, it is assumed that the data must be of the highest quality in order to resolve the diagnostic dilemma at hand. As such there must be fastidious attention paid to pressure recording and cardiac output determination. Pulse delay makes recording from the femoral artery inaccurate and should not be used. Cardiac output today is often made using an assumed value for oxygen consumption in the Fick equation potentially leading to large errors in its determination [46] and as a consequence large errors in calculating valve area.

Medical Therapy

Aortic stenosis is a mechanical problem with only a mechanical solution, i.e., aortic valve replacement. No medical therapy has been demonstrated to alter the natural history of the disease. Because most patients today are elderly and because the incidence of hypertension increases with age, many AS patients also have systemic hypertension. There is a natural concern that antihypertensive agents that cause vasodilatation might lead to hypotension because fixed valve obstruction to flow could impair cardiac output. Thus any antihypertensive agent should be used on a "start low and go slow" basis. However there are several reports of the use of vasodilators to treat both hypertension and acute heart failure in AS [47–50], although no antihypertensive regimen has been shown superior in the treatment of AS patients with hypertension. If heart failure has intervened and AVR is contraindicated because of the presence of severe comorbidities, diuretics can be used to relieve symptoms. Because standard heart failure therapy has not been tested in AS in any large randomized trial, there is no evidence that such therapy would be beneficial nor is there any defined mechanism by which heart failure therapy might prolong life in AS.

Indications for Surgery

Symptomatic AS

Suggested by Ross and Braunwald [15] and confirmed by recent clinical trials [16, 17], symptomatic AS, untreated by AVR, has one of the highest mortality rates in medicine, about 2% per month or 75% at 3 years (Fig. 5.2). Conversely AVR restores life expectancy to or toward that of an unaffected population especially after the age of 70 (Fig. 5.21) [51]. Thus AVR is mandatory in symptomatic AS patients unless the presence of severe comorbidities makes AVR impossible. It should be noted that while AVR greatly improves prognosis compared to no therapy, Fig. 5.21 demonstrates that the earlier in life that AVR is required, the greater is the deficit between normal age-matched survival and actual survival. That is, AVR does not restore life span to normal in young patients. This might be because prosthetic valves have their own inherent risks (see below) or because AS may cause permanent LV dysfunction not reversed by AVR. It may be hoped that earlier AVR or AVR with more perfect prostheses might improve post-AVR survival but this remains conjecture for now.

Asymptomatic Severe AS

Less certain is the therapy for patients with asymptomatic severe AS (Class C_1). The risk of sudden death in truly asymptomatic patients is about 1% per year [52] (Fig. 5.22), similar to the operative mortality rate in experienced centers. However assessing symptomatic status is problematic. Some patients may deny or fail to recognize their symptoms. Many AS patients are elderly and often ascribe their fatigue or dyspnea to "getting old." When a 78-year-old patient notes that they tire or become breathless more easily than a few years ago, this could in fact truly represent aging or, conversely, the onset of AS symptoms. In this regard exercise testing may be very useful in establishing objective evidence of dyspnea on exertion and the hemodynamic response to stress [53, 54]. Patients who fail to achieve age-predicted exercise tolerance or who fail to exhibit a normal rise in blood pressure during exercise should probably undergo early AVR (Fig. 5.23). Likewise, patients with very high jet velocities (>5.0 m/s) and who have very severe AS (AVA <0.6 cm^2) probably benefit from AVR prior to the onset of overt AS

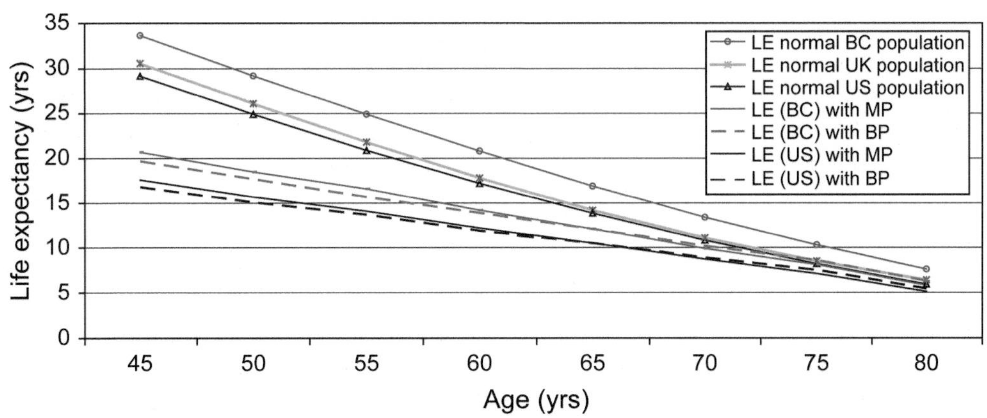

Fig. 5.21 Life expectancy (LE) for British Columbia (BC), for the United Kingdom (UK), and the United States (US) is plotted for normal subjects and those with bioprosthetic aortic valves (BP), and patients with mechanical prosthetic valves (MP). On average, normal 50-year-old patients are expected to live another 28 years while patients with valve prostheses are projected to live only 18 years longer. The difference narrows with age, in part because death is inevitable and in part because the prosthesis is present for fewer years. From van Geldorp MWA, et al. [51]. Reprinted with permission from Elsevier

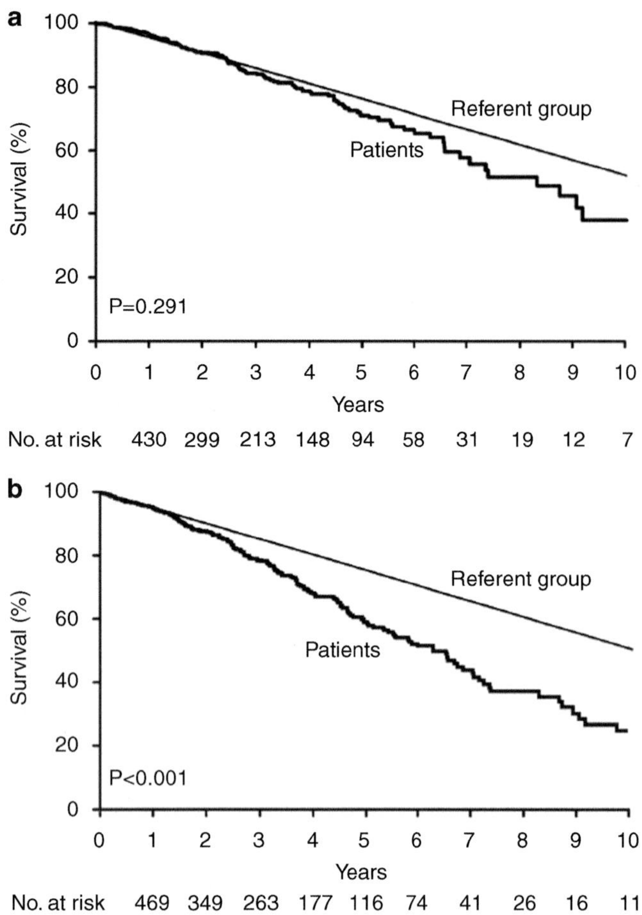

Fig. 5.22 Life expectancy is shown for a normal matched population and for asymptomatic patients with severe aortic stenosis censored at the onset of symptoms (**a**) or when valve replacement was performed (**b**). Asymptomatic patients have an excellent prognosis as indicted in Fig. 5.2a. However the worse prognosis when assessed at aortic valve replacement (**b**) suggests that there is delay from symptom onset to definitive therapy with patients dying in the interim. From Pellikka PA, et al. [52]. Reprinted with permission from Wolters Kluwer Health, Inc.

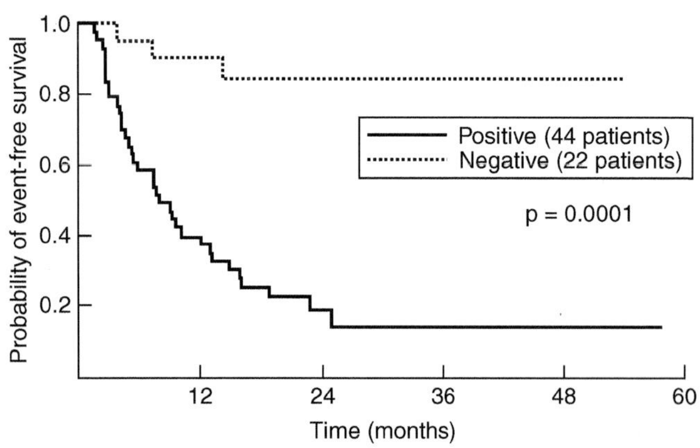

Fig. 5.23 Prognosis in severe aortic stenosis is stratified according to results of exercise testing. The difference in event-free survival between patients with a negative versus positive exercise test is striking. From Amato MC, et al. [54]. Reprinted with permission from BMJ Publishing Group Ltd.

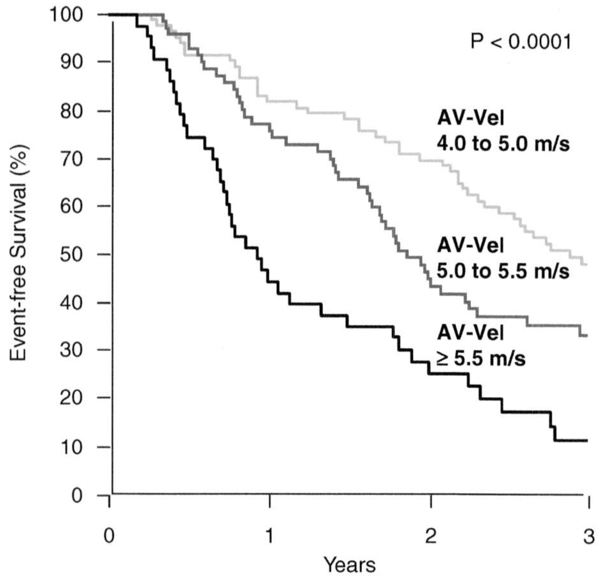

Patients with AV-Vel from 4.0 to 5.0 m/s
Pts. at risk: 82 69 59 38
Patients with AV-Vel from 5.0 to 5.5 m/s
Pts. at risk: 72 53 29 18
Patients with AV-Vel from ≥ 5.5 m/s
Pts. at risk: 44 20 11 5

Fig. 5.24 The impact of transaortic jet velocity on patients with aortic stenosis is demonstrated. The higher the jet velocity the more likely that an event (symptoms or death) will occur with jet velocity exceeding 5 m/s being particularly ominous. From Rosenhek R, et al. [55]. Reprinted with permission from Wolters Kluwer Health, Inc.

symptoms (Fig. 5.24) because symptom onset and its attendant risk of sudden death is immanent [55, 56]. In such patients the overt onset of symptoms is almost certain to occur within 1–2 years, during which time the patient may be lost to follow-up or encounter other serious medical conditions so that there may be little gained by delaying AVR further.

Biomarkers also play a role in assessment of the asymptomatic AS patient. Increased levels of brain natriuretic hormone (BNP) and troponin presage a worsened outcome for AS patients. While no specific level of these markers that might trigger AVR is agreed upon, elevated BNP seems to be a promising biomarker helpful in timing AVR [57–61]. Some of the uncertainty regarding the level of BNP that is prognostic stems for failure to normalize BNP for age and sex. In fact the ratio of patient BNP to the normal value for that patient's age and sex has had independent prognostic importance in AS patients (Fig. 5.25) [61].

An issue often arises concerning the aortic valve management of patients with only moderate AS (and asymptomatic from the AS itself) who are undergoing cardiac surgery addressing another cardiac issue, usually coronary revascularization. As noted above, AS is a progressive disease.

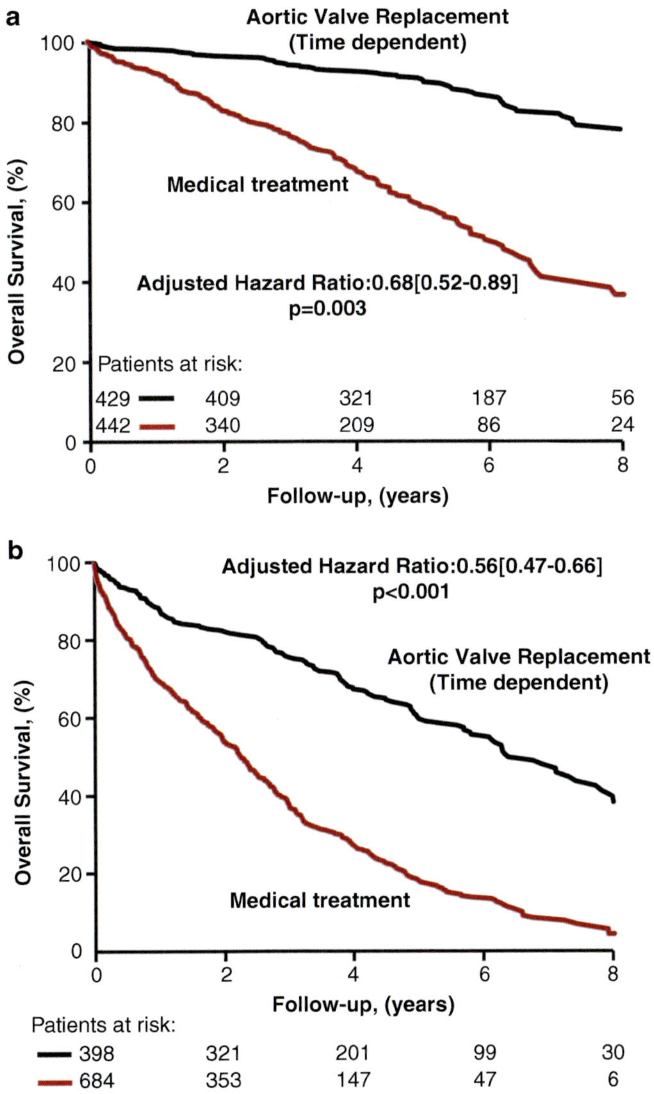

Fig. 5.25 Prognosis in patients with severe aortic stenosis according to brain type natriuretic hormone is demonstrated. Patients with a BNP/normal ratio of >2 (**b**) is compared to that of patients with a ratio <2 (**a**) for patients treated surgically (black line) or "medically" (red line). Patients with high BNP fared worse with both types of therapies. From Clavel MA, et al. [61]. Reprinted with permission from Elsevier

Bypass surgery leaving moderate AS untreated could result in symptomatic AS developing in 2–3 years, necessitating AVR during a second operation. While TAVR might be reasonable in that situation, currently, most heart teams would elect to perform AVR at the time of bypass surgery in patients with moderate AS. While there are no randomized trials addressing this issue, data support better long-term outcomes when AVR accompanies such operations [62].

Of note a recent study of propensity matched pairs demonstrated benefit for patients undergoing AVR prior to symptom onset [63]. However almost two-thirds of these patients had one of the indications noted above for undergoing early AVR and over 30 patients who developed symptoms did not undergo AVR. The issue may be settled by the results of an ongoing randomized trial comparing TAVR to observation in asymptomatic patients with severe AS (Edwards Early TAVR Trial).

Mechanical Therapy: SAVR and TAVR

Valve replacement is the only definitive therapy for AS and can be accomplished either at cardiac surgery (SAVR) or through transcatheter techniques (TAVR). The decision regarding which approach is best for a given patient is decided by the Heart Team composed of structural cardiologists, general cardiologists, imagers, heart surgeons, anesthesiologists and most importantly the patient (TAVR is covered extensively in Chap. 10). The decision will in part be based upon LV function, the need for other cardiac procedures, comorbidities, surgical history, age, patient preference, social considerations and the risk calculated from the STS database. As an example of the factors involved in decision-making, consider an 80-year-old woman who is healthy except for aortic stenosis but uses a walker for mobility due to severe knee and hip problems and has no family or other local support. Although her mortality is low for SAVR, a TAVR might be recommended because the patient would have trouble adhering to sternal precautions post-operatively and bed rest postoperatively might worsen her immobility. On the other hand, a patient with a high predicted mortality from AVR but who also has severe coronary disease not amenable to percutaneous intervention might be recommended for a surgical valve so that the associated coronary disease can be addressed at the time of surgery.

Surgical Therapy (SAVR)

Aortic Valve Anatomy for the Surgeon: Avoiding Injury to Vital Structures

The aortic valve is usually trileaflet and the leaflets are recognized by their relationship to the coronary arteries: left, right, and noncoronary. The noncoronary leaflet abuts the anterior leaflet of the mitral valve. The Bundle of His lies adjacent to the commissure between the right and the noncoronary cusp. An aortic valve annular stitch that inadvertently sews into mitral tissue can cause mitral dysfunction postoperatively. If calcium is debrided too deeply, heart block can result from direct injury to the His Bundle; if not enough calcium is debrided from the annulus, compression of the His bundle may also cause heart block.

Type of Valve Replacement: Mechanical vs. Bioprosthetic

Once a decision has been made that a patient should undergo surgical aortic valve replacement, the type of replacement valve must be addressed. For most patients the two options are either a bioprosthetic or mechanical valve. Bioprosthetic valves are made from precisely cut pieces of bovine or porcine pericardium although some are actual pig allograft aortic valves secured inside a reinforced fabric suture ring. Human homografts are still used in some centers but difficulty in obtaining them reduces their usefulness. While enhanced durability was expected from homografts, it is not clear that homografts are more durable than other tissue valves. Mechanical valves are made of pyrolytic carbon, a graphite material that has extremely smooth surfaces and are designed with "washing jets" that prevent clot formation on the hinges. The valves are so smooth that metal instruments touching the valve during the operation damage them; instead, plastic tools must be used to manipulate mechanical valves.

The strengths and weaknesses of each valve type are well known and well summarized [64]. Mechanical valves require vitamin K antagonist (VKA) anticoagulation to reduce the risk of thromboembolism while tissue valves carry the risk of structural deterioration requiring reoperation. Mechanical valves generally function well for the lifetime of the patient although they are not entirely free of structural failure because valve obstruction can occur from thrombus or pannus ingrowth of fibrous tissue. This risk is low, probably less than 1% per year [65]. Unfortunately the risk of major bleeding from anticoagulation is 1–2% per year. A patient receiving a mechanical valve in his/her 20s carries a 50–80% lifetime risk of bleeding or thromboembolic complications [64]. In some cases the clicking sound of mechanical valves is so bothersome to the patient that the valve may have to be removed. Tissue valves on the other hand require no anticoagulation. The risk of deterioration varies according to the age of the patient at implantation. In patients older than 70, 95% of tissue valves function well at 10 years and 90% function well at 15 years. In patients younger than 50, 50% of bioprostheses deteriorate in 5–10 years [64]. It is unclear why bioprosthetic valves deteriorate more rapidly in younger patients, but it is thought that it might be due to differences in calcium metabolism. Bioprosthetic deterioration is accelerated in patients on dialysis [66].

Older age, bleeding risk (history of bleeding, exposure to trauma in the workplace, frequent falls) and patient preference for avoiding anticoagulation favor bioprosthetic AVR and avoidance of anticoagulation. Young age and a second disease requiring anticoagulation such as atrial fibrillation favor AVR with a mechanical valve. While it had been hoped that newer non VKA anticoagulants might make anticoagulation easier and thus make mechanical valves more attractive, this hope has not yet been realized [67].

Aortic Valve Autografts: The Ross Procedure

In the Ross procedure the patient's pulmonary valve is transplanted into the aortic position while a homograft replaces the pulmonic valve. The principle of the Ross procedure is that the native pulmonic valve functions durably in the aortic position while the homograft has enhanced durability (compared to placement in the aortic position) in the low-pressure pulmonary position. This procedure is advantageous in young patients who wish to avoid the complications of anticoagulation from mechanical valves or the almost certain need for reoperation for standard bioprosthetic valves. Freedom from reintervention for the Ross procedure in properly selected patients can be comparable long term to that for mechanical aortic valves. Reoperation rate on the autograft in adults is 1.0% per year and on the homograft 0.65% per year [68]. In a randomized trial, the Ross procedure was superior to homograft AVR [69]. The Ross procedure is a technically demanding operation that has generated controversy and a wide disparity in outcome. It trades disease of one valve for potential disease in two. Candidates for the Ross should be referred to surgeons who specifically specialize in the operation and who have outcome records that prove success.

Operative Planning

Predicting Valve Size

Preoperative planning is integral to the success of the procedure and many issues must be considered prior surgery. Data needed for preoperative planning is obtained largely through preoperative imaging at echocardiography and cardiac catheterization. Standard bioprostheses and mechanical valves are inherently stenotic; while they have a larger effective orifice area than the diseased valve being removed, their orifice area is still smaller than a normal native valve. Patient-prosthetic mismatch wherein the replaced valve is too small for the cardiac demands of the patient in which it is placed, worsens postoperative outcome [70]. Thus every effort is made to insert the largest valve possible. Several factors affect this practice. Valve size can be estimated preoperatively from echocardiographic or CT images of the aortic annulus and outflow tract. Sizing will be confirmed at surgery but it is helpful to predict sizing beforehand. General practice is to insert at least a 23 mm valve which will help avoid patient prosthetic mismatch and will facilitate valve-in-valve TVAR later if the SAVR valve fails (see Chap. 10). If the aortic annulus is small, root enlargement may be necessary which complicates the procedure and increases cross-clamp ischemic time. Generally 2.5 h of cross clamp time with the heart arrested and ischemic is well tolerated by patients with preserved cardiac function. In this context, root enlargement takes about 30 min, the aortic valve replacement itself takes an hour, each bypass graft takes an additional 15 min or longer if using arterial grafts or if the targets are difficult. A maze procedure takes 30 min. Patients with a low ejection fraction or pulmonary hypertension tolerate long clamp times poorly occasionally necessitating mechanical support postoperatively.

Planning for Myocardial Protection

The advent of cardioplegia during surgery reduced intraoperative ischemic myocardial damage and greatly improved outcomes, making delivery of adequate cardioplegia a key to success. However many factors can interfere with proper myocardial protection and should be anticipated before the operation.

- *Left ventricular hypertrophy*. Patients with aortic stenosis have LVH that may require greater doses of cardioplegia to cool and arrest the heart and may require multiple attempts at defibrillation when the heart is reperfused after the aortic cross clamp is removed.
- *Right heart protection*. Cardioplegia can be administered both antegrade into the coronary arteries and retrograde through the coronary sinus. Retrograde cardioplegia is very effective for the left ventricle but less so for the right. Protecting the right ventricle (RV) is further complicated because the right ventricle is more subject to warming due to room light, ambient air, and blood returning to the right atrium. Protecting the right ventricle is made more difficult when the right coronary is stenotic or occluded as demonstrated by the preoperative coronary arteriogram. In a patient with a chronically occluded right coronary, also undergoing coronary grafting, an effective strategy is to perform the right coronary distal anastomosis immediately and then administer cardioplegia into the vein graft. Right heart protection is even more of a concern if the patient suffers from preoperative RV dysfunction. Patients with RV dysfunction may require epinephrine and milrinone during separation from cardiopulmonary bypass and these drugs are often administered before weaning from cardiopulmonary bypass in such cases, an eventuality that can be anticipated preoperatively.
- *Aortic regurgitation*. If greater than mild aortic regurgitation is present, the heart may not arrest effectively when antegrade cardioplegia is administered to the coronaries indirectly through the aortic root. In this case, a retrograde cardioplegia cannula is placed into the coronary sinus and cardioplegia is administered to arrest the heart immediately. Next, after aortotomy, cardioplegia is delivered directly into the coronary ostia. Thus the presence and severity of aortic regurgitation must be assessed preoperatively during echocardiography.

Mitral Involvement: Calcium Extent

Occasionally the aortic calcium extends into the anterior leaflet of the mitral valve in complete continuity with the calcium involving the annulus along the noncoronary leaflet. Usually this calcium can be removed without affecting mitral function. However calcium along the right coronary-noncoronary commissure can be more difficult to deal with as it can extend all the way into the ventricular septum risking a ventricular septal defect before reaching good tissue. (This often anticipated from the preoperative echocardiogram). In this case, enough calcium will be debrided from the aortic annulus to allow the valve to sit inside the annulus and sutures are placed from the outside of the aorta to secure the valve. Sometimes there are large deposits of calcium located beneath the annulus in the left ventricular outflow tract and while these may not affect seating of the valve they can interfere with the opening and closing of mechanical valve leaflets so the calcium may need to be removed.

Obviously it is better to consider the all above issues prior to surgery so that the surgeon is prepared to ameliorate them during the operation.

The Operation

The usual AVR begins with a sternotomy. The mammary artery is harvested if a bypass operation is planned. Heparin is administered and a cannula is placed in the aorta. A large venous cannula is placed through the right atrium and directed into the inferior vena cava or bicaval cannulation is performed if there is a reason to open the right atrium. Cardiopulmonary bypass is initiated and blood is drained from the right side of the heart and pumped with constant flow into the aorta to maintain mean blood pressure. A left ventricular vent is placed through the right superior pulmonary vein and blood is pumped out of the left ventricle and into the cardiopulmonary bypass reservoir along with the venous blood from the cava and/or right atrium. This allows the surgeon to work in a dry field and keeps the heart decompressed. Left ventricular decompression is particularly important in surgery for aortic stenosis because most patients have concomitant concentric LVH that increases myocardial oxygen consumption. A key determinant of myocardial oxygen consumption is wall tension and maintaining decompression reduces wall tension and myocardial ischemia. A retrograde cardioplegia cannula is placed into the coronary sinus through a small right atriotomy. An antegrade cardioplegia cannula is usually placed into the ascending aorta and serves to decompress the ascending aorta, facilitates administration of cardioplegia, and helps de-air the heart at the end of the operation. An alternative to placing an antegrade cardioplegia cannula is to open the aorta immediately after applying the cross clamp, directly cannulating the coronaries to administer antegrade cardioplegia.

Regardless of what other procedures are planned, the aortic valve is usually removed first and the annulus is sized. Once the valve is removed, the distal coronary anastomoses are performed if coronary bypass is planned. If a mitral operation is also being performed, that procedure is performed before the aortic valve is inserted because the mitral valve is very difficult or impossible to visualize with a prosthetic aortic valve in place.

The aortic annulus size, estimated prior to surgery is confirmed with plastic sizers that mimic the shape of the valve.

With optimal sizing, the valve should fit easily within the annulus without any slack but should not be so tight that it causes excessive tension which can result in disruption of the annulus and valve dehiscence. If the annulus is too small for placement of an adequate sized prosthesis, there are several options. The valve can be tilted above the annulus on the noncoronary side allowing for placement of a valve one size greater than could be placed without this maneuver. If aortic enlargement is necessary to accommodate an adequate prosthesis size, the annulus is enlarged by cutting thru its middle at the noncoronary leaflet between the trigones. A pericardial or Dacron patch closes the defect. The annular enlargement can be extended into the anterior leaflet of the mitral valve if needed.

Sutures are placed circumferentially around the annulus to secure the valve. The number of sutures is counted and a decision is made on how to distribute the sutures on the prosthetic valve suture ring. The sutures beneath the left coronary are tied first because it is very difficult to place additional sutures in this area if there is a perivalvular leak. A probe is used to make sure the valve is seated securely in the annulus and that there are no holes that could become a perivalvular leak, causing postoperative hemolysis. Seating the valve properly into the annulus can encounter two problems. First, there can be calcium deposits that can prevent valve seating. Secondly, the prosthetic valve is circular while the aortic annulus is scalloped causing gaps between the valve and the annulus.

Once the aorta is closed, the cross clamp is removed, reperfusing the heart and the patient is weaned from cardiopulmonary bypass. A transesophageal echo is used to evaluate function and to look for perivalvular leak. Heparin and Coumadin are begun on day 3 for patients receiving mechanical valves.

Complications

The most common major complication from aortic valve replacement is heart block requiring pacemaker placement after AVR in 5% of patients. The Bundle of His lies beneath the aortic annulus at the right-noncoronary commissure in the ventricular septum. Stitches mooring the valve must be placed through the annulus deep enough to secure the valve but not so deep that they injure conduction system, problematic because the conduction system is not visible to the surgeon.

Perivalvular leaks are rare but may cause hemolysis when they do occur. They usually can be observed with expectation that they will enlarge enough that they no longer cause hemolysis yet not become so large that they are hemodynamically significant. If frequent transfusions are required postoperatively, redo surgery or percutaneous intervention is indicated.

Aortic valve replacement carries a stroke risk of about 2% [71]. The calcium deposits around the aortic annulus have the consistency wet sand once the intima overlying the calcium is exposed and every effort is made to prevent calcium embolization. The ventricle is aggressively irrigated to remove any calcium that may have been unseen. However despite these efforts, some small pieces of calcium may embolize and by way of prevention, carotid protection devices are being investigated to prevent intraoperative stroke [72].

Postoperative Course

Aortic valve replacement acutely reduces LV afterload, enhancing LV ejection, potentially reducing filling pressure and increasing stroke volume. Accordingly, even patients in advanced preoperative heart failure may enjoy a surprisingly uneventful postoperative course. However several caveats must be considered especially relating to postoperative hypotension and hypertension.

- *Hypotension*. Concentric LVH almost invariably causes diastolic dysfunction that persists well into the postoperative period. As such higher than average filling pressure (volume expansion) may be necessary to maintain adequate preload and forward output. Reduced afterload may also predispose to LV cavity obliteration and systolic anterior motion (SAM) of the mitral valve causing LV outflow obstruction unless LV cavity volume is maintained. Inotrope administration and/or balloon counterpulsation, usual treatments for postoperative hypotension, will serve only to worsen SAM thereby reducing cardiac output. Conversely patients with severe preoperative LV dysfunction may be resistant to inotropic support for low output postoperatively and thus require high dosed inotropes and/or balloon counterpulsation.
- *Hypertension*. Blood pressure = cardiac output × total peripheral resistance. AVR may lead to improved forward output into the stiff aortae of elderly patients causing hypertension, necessitating antihypertensive therapy [73]. Failure to control postoperative hypertension may result in greater LV afterload than was present when the stenotic valve was still in place.

Special Cases

Low Flow, Low Gradient Low Ejection Fraction Aortic Stenosis

Reduced ejection fraction in AS is caused by three mechanisms—increased afterload, impaired contractility or some combination of both [74]. Excess afterload in AS occurs when pressure overload exceeds the ability of hypertrophy to compensate for the load, i.e., the pressure term in the numerator of the Laplace equation (above) exceeds the thickness term in the denominator. Thus systolic wall stress increases, depressing ejection fraction [75]. In such cases, when AVR relieves the pressure overload, ejection fraction returns to or toward normal as the afterload excess is removed. In other cases, EF is depressed because innate contractility is impaired [28]. Such patients have both low ejection fraction and a low transvalvular gradient. Many consider this condition to be present when the EF IS <0.40 and the mean transvalvular gradient is <40 mmHg. However especially problematic patients are those patients with reduced EF whose transmural gradients are <20 mmHg wherein there is extremely depressed contractility [28, 76]. When reduced EF is due to impaired contractility, outcome following AVR is less optimistic than when there is simply afterload mismatch. Mortality rate in this condition can exceed 30% [28, 76–78]. Patients who demonstrate inotropic reserve by increasing stroke volume by >20% with dobutamine infusion have a reasonable surgical mortality of about 10% while AVR mortality may exceed 30% in those who fail to show inotropic reserve (Fig. 5.26) [79] exemplified in Figs. 5.27, 5.28 and 5.29. However for those reserve-negative patients who survive AVR, postoperative EF may improve substantially making decision-making in this group extremely fraught [80] as it would be unfortunate to deny them AVR because of failed inotropic reserve. In such patients a trial of balloon valvotomy (BAV) may be warranted. Following BAV there is only a modest reduction in pressure gradient and only a modest increase in AVA. Yet, in some patients these slight improvements can lead to marked clinical improvement suggesting that AVR might be of benefit although the exact use of BAV as a therapeutic trial is still uncertain [81, 82].

In question is whether patients with low gradient and low flow transition from a high flow high gradient, normal ejection fraction state or had some predisposition to low flow, low ejection to begin with. It appears that the latter condition is more prevalent. Experimental data suggest a predetermined tendency regarding hypertrophy extent and function [83, 84] and as noted above patients with this condition have lower initial ejection fraction and LV dysfunction even when the disease is not yet “severe” by current definitions [34, 35].

In still other patients a severely reduced aortic valve area may be calculated at rest but when cardiac output is

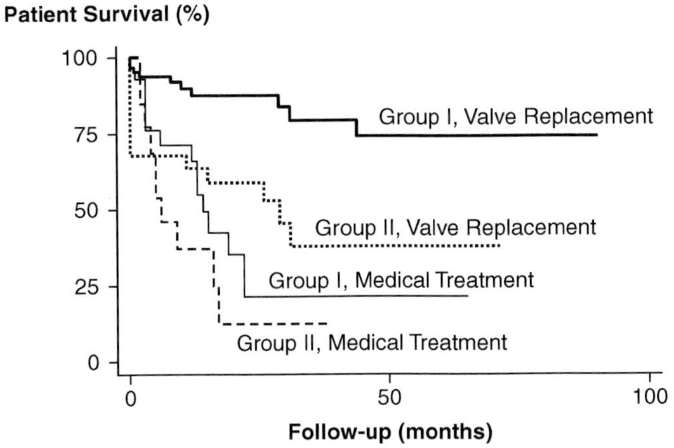

Fig. 5.26 Survival after aortic valve replacement is shown for patients with severe aortic stenosis and low ejection fraction with low transvalvular gradient. Patients that augmented stroke volume ≥20% with dobutamine infusion (group I) had better outcome with valve replacement than patients without inotropic reserve (group II). From Monin JL, et al. [79]. Reprinted with permission from Wolters Kluwer Health, Inc.

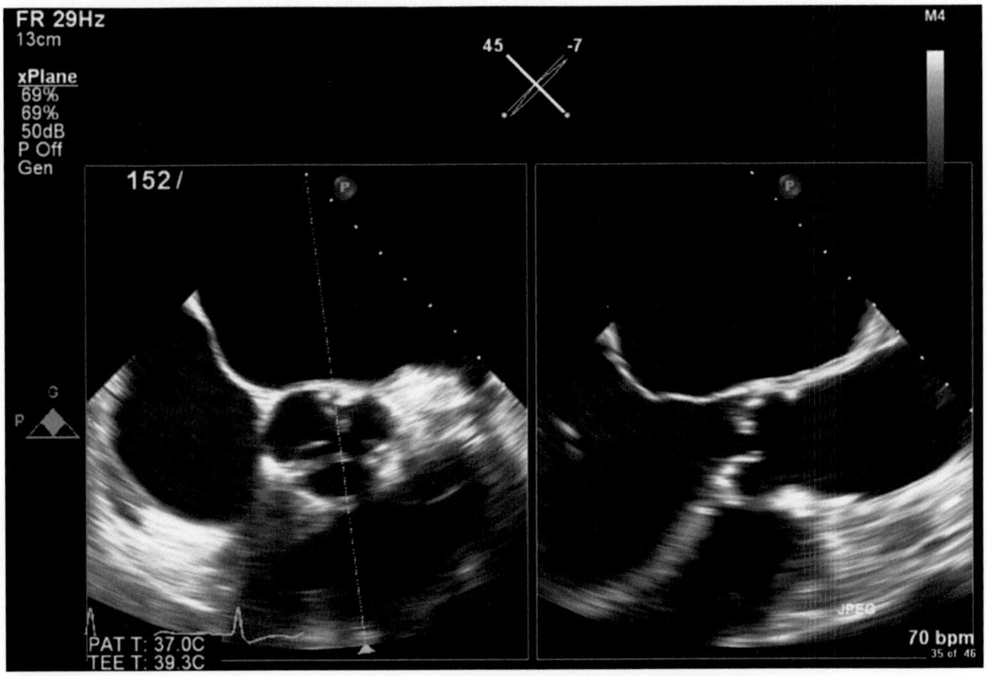

Fig. 5.27 A patient with low gradient low EF AS is shown in this figure, and in Figs. 5.28 and 5.29. In this figure the *X*-plane TEE views of the aortic valve are shown in short axis (left panel) and long axis (right panel) demonstrating severe AS

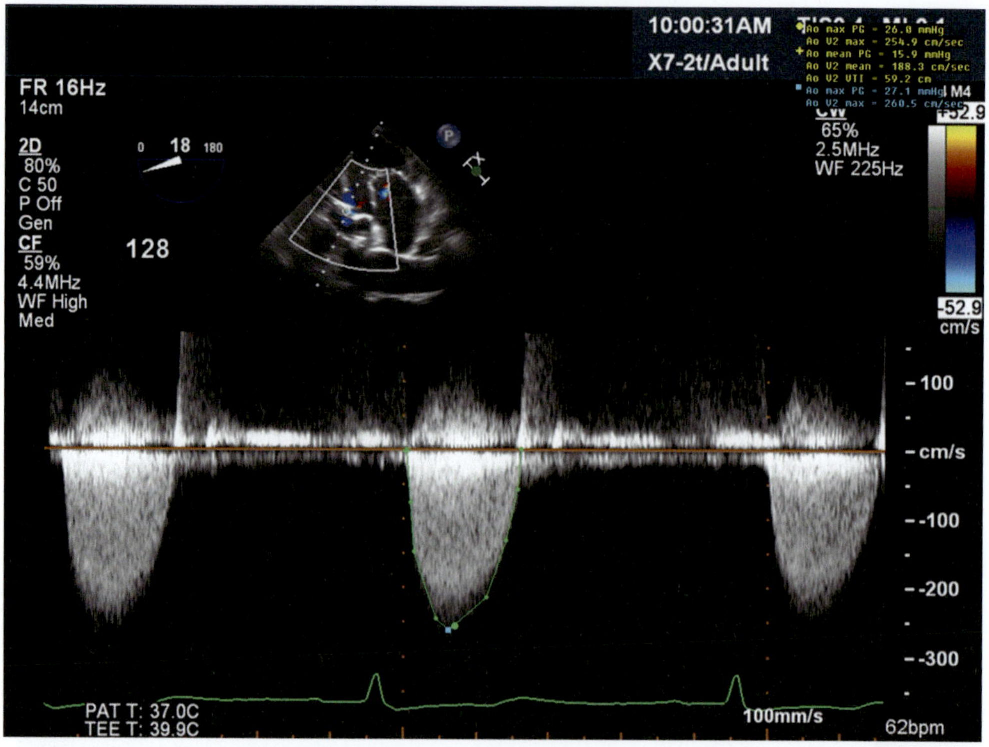

Fig. 5.28 Continuous wave Doppler of the aortic jet estimating a mean gradient of 16 mm and peak velocity of 2.5 m/s not meeting criteria for "severe" AS

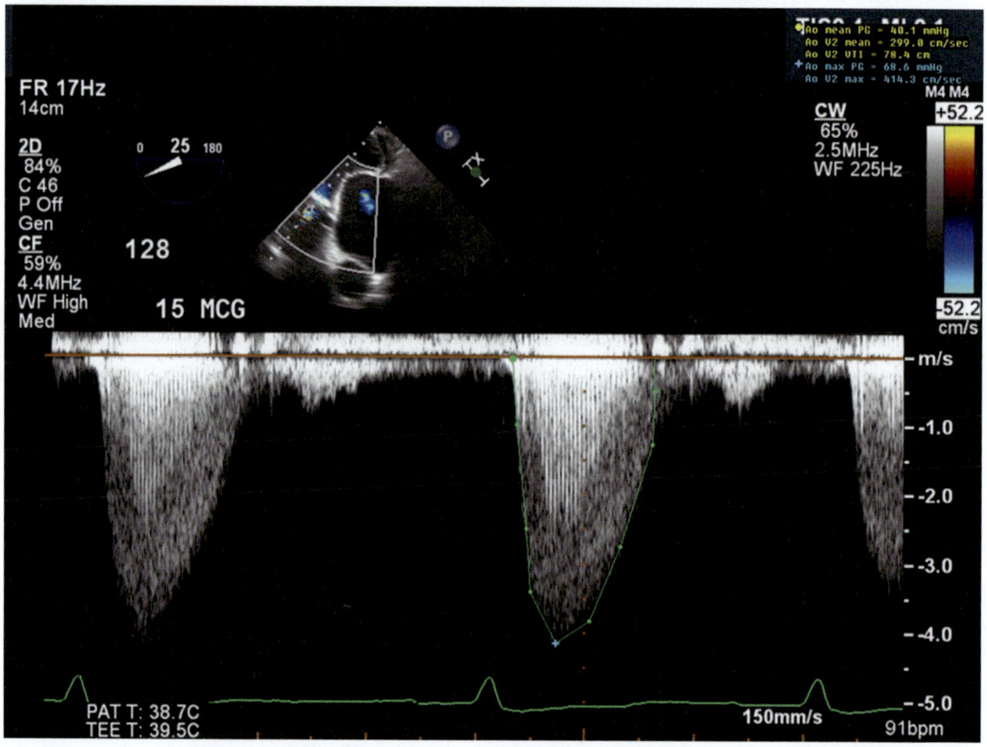

Fig. 5.29 After administration of 15 mcg/kg/min dobutamine infusion, the peak velocity increased to 4 m/s with a mean gradient of 40 mmHg. LV ejection fraction increased from 25% to 40%

increased by inotropic infusion, the valve opens more widely, gradient increases only slightly so that a much larger valve area is calculated [85–87]. In such patients there is pseudo aortic stenosis, i.e., an apparently small orifice when flow is reduced but a much larger opening when contractile force and flow are increased [87]. Such patients have a primary cardiomyopathy and require therapy for that condition rather than AVR [88]. However it is unknown whether some patients with pseudo AS might still benefit from the modest afterload reduction offered by AVR especially when performed with the less invasive TAVR approach.

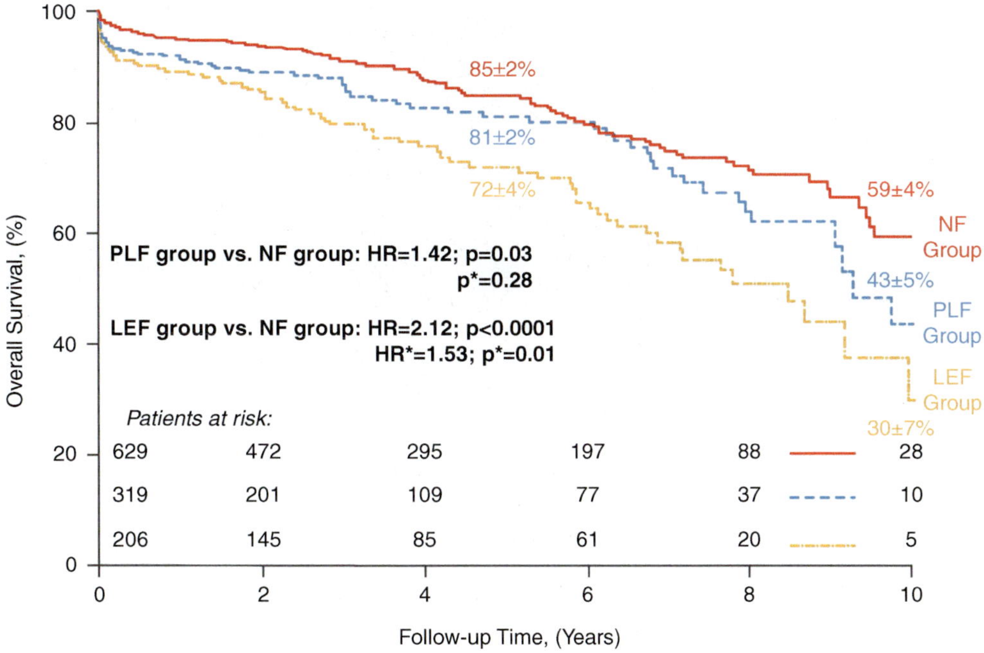

Fig. 5.30 Prognosis following aortic valve replacement is shown for aortic stenosis patients with normal stroke volume (NF), for patients with reduced stroke volume despite normal ejection fraction (PLF), and for patients with low stoke volume and low ejection fraction (LEF). From Clavel MA, et al. [92]. Reprinted with permission from Elsevier

Low Flow, Low Gradient Normal Ejection Fraction Aortic Stenosis

In some AS patients there is reduced stroke volume (and thus reduced gradient) despite normal ejection fraction, a condition sometimes referred to as paradoxic low flow AS, paradoxic because there is low stroke volume despite preserved EF [89]. In many such cases there is extreme concentric LVH that in turn reduces LV volume so that a normal ejection fraction of a small end diastolic volume produces reduced stroke volume and reduced transvalvular gradient. The low gradient in turn may mislead the clinician into believing that the AS is not severe. However when this group of patients develops symptoms, their prognosis is impaired and they benefit from AVR [89–93]. Prognosis after AVR is not as hopeful as it is for patients with normal stroke volume (Fig. 5.30) [91] but it still exceeds that for so-called “medical” therapy which for practical purposes in nonexistent. It must be noted that this syndrome has led to much confusion regarding its diagnosis and therapy. Faulty measurement of the outflow tract diameter may cause underestimation of valve area. Thus valve area alone should not be used to judge AS severity in these cases. Rather physical examination, gradient, valve area, and valve calcification should be integrated to make the correct diagnosis. When this procedure is followed it is clear that this syndrome is a verified entity requiring appropriate therapy (Figs. 5.31 and 5.32) [94].

Guideline Summary

The algorithm for the treatment of aortic stenosis as summarized from the AHA/ACC guidelines [32] for the management of valvular heart disease is shown in Fig. 5.33.

Aortic Regurgitation

Etiology

Aortic regurgitation (AR) occurs when pathology of either the aortic root or of the aortic valve leaflets cause failure of leaflet coaptation [96].

Etiology of aortic regurgitation

Leaflet causes

- Rheumatic Valve Disease
- Infective Endocarditis
- Bicuspid aortic valve
- Myxomatous valve disease
- Serotonergic drugs
- Valve Trauma
- Radiation
- Collagen Vascular Disease
- Marantic (noninfectious) endocarditis

Aortic root causes

- Marfan Syndrome
- Hypertension
- Ehlers-Danlos Syndrome
- Loeys Dietz Syndrome
- Syphilis
- Dissecting aneurysm
- Annulo-aortic Ectasia
- Ankylosing Spondylitis
- Giant Cell arteritis

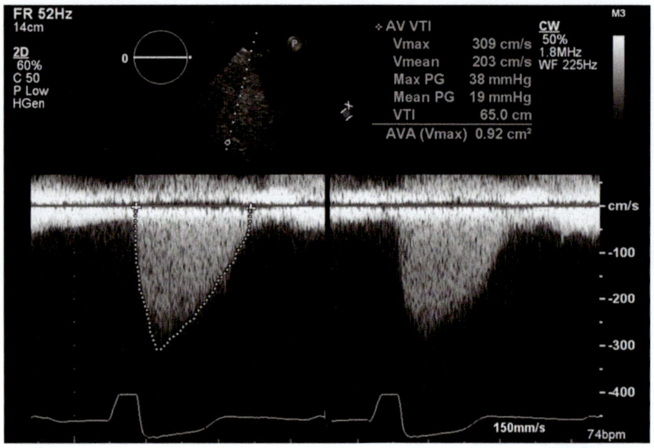

Fig. 5.31 Low mean gradient was noted in a patient with severe aortic stenosis yet the valve area was calculated to be 0.9 cm^2 categorizing it as severe. Severity was supported by leaflet immobility and heavy calcification shown in Fig. 5.32

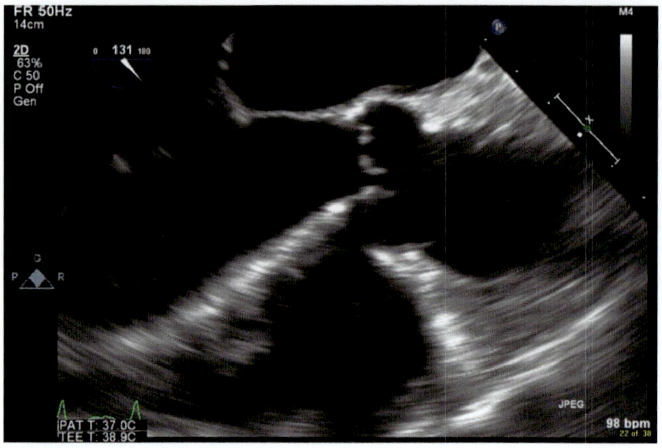

Fig. 5.32 TEE view of the left ventricular outflow tract from the patient shown in Fig. 5.31 demonstrating severe restriction of the aortic valve. Global LV systolic function was preserved with LVEF of 55–60% at rest. The hemodynamic profile is consistent with paradoxical low flow–low gradient aortic stenosis with normal left ventricular systolic function

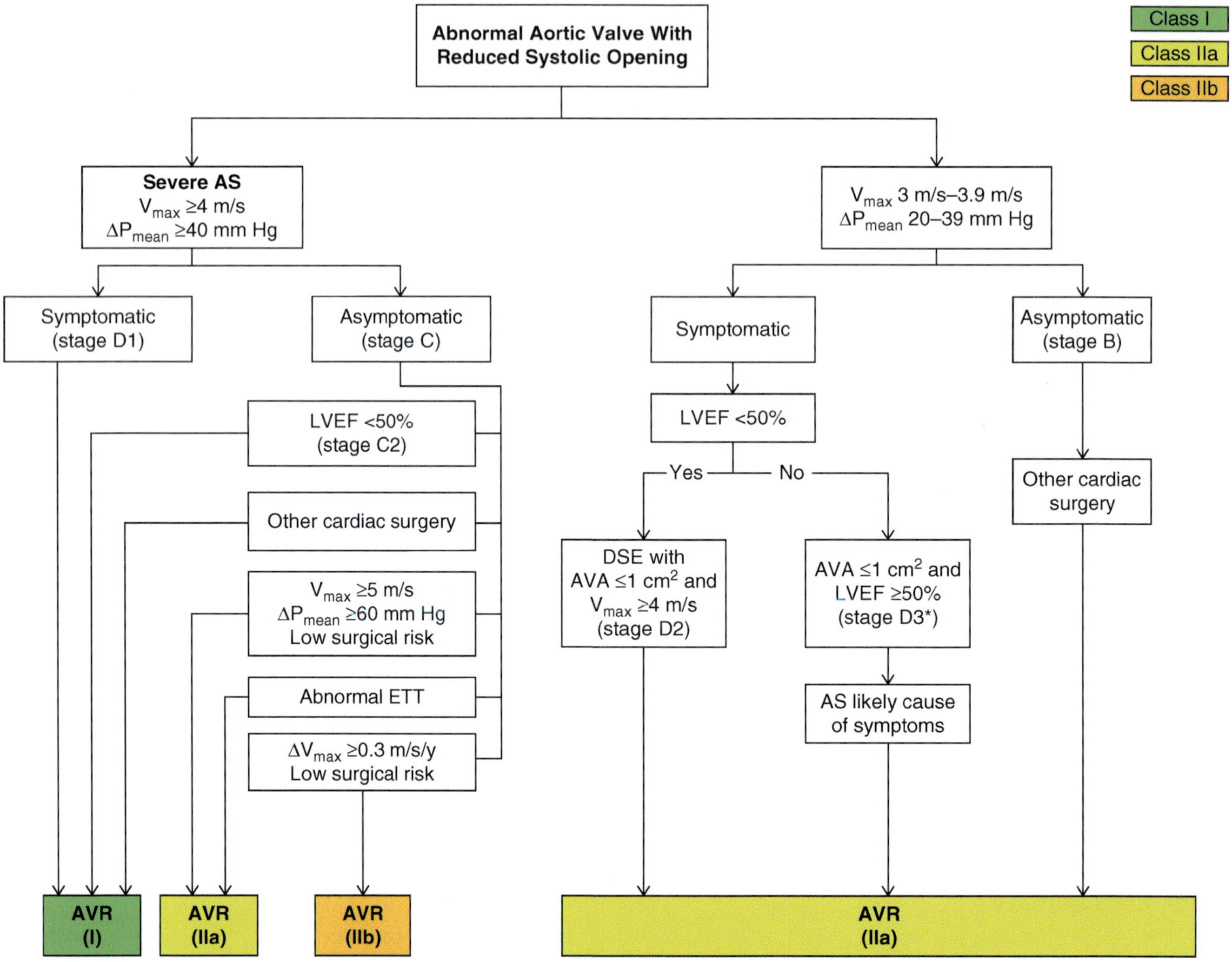

Fig. 5.33 The algorithm for the treatment of AS patients according to the 2014 AHA/ACC guidelines is shown. From Nishimura RA, et al. [32]. Reprinted with permission from Wolters Kluwer Health, Inc.

The most common leaflet abnormality leading to AR is bicuspid aortic valve (see above) [10–14]. In some cases, there is clear valve pathology with leaflet retraction while in other cases the aortic root dilatation, sometimes associated with bicuspid valve, pulls the leaflets away from their coaptation point. Other leaflet pathologies causing AR include infective endocarditis, collagen vascular disease (primarily systemic lupus erythematous), rheumatic heart disease, advanced stage cancer (marantic endocarditis), and trauma. Aortic root pathologies leading to AR include Marfan syndrome, aortic dissection, syphilis, giant cell arteritis, hypertension, and Ehlers-Danlos syndrome [95].

Pathophysiology and Its Relation to Symptoms

Formerly classified as a volume overload lesion, AR causes both increased preload and afterload (Fig. 5.34) [96]. Unquestionably, the volume lost to regurgitation is compensated by LV dilatation in order to increase total stroke volume thereby offsetting the regurgitant volume. However in AR the large total stroke volume is discharged into the aorta in turn causing a widened pulse pressure and, as a consequence, increased systolic pressure. Increased systolic

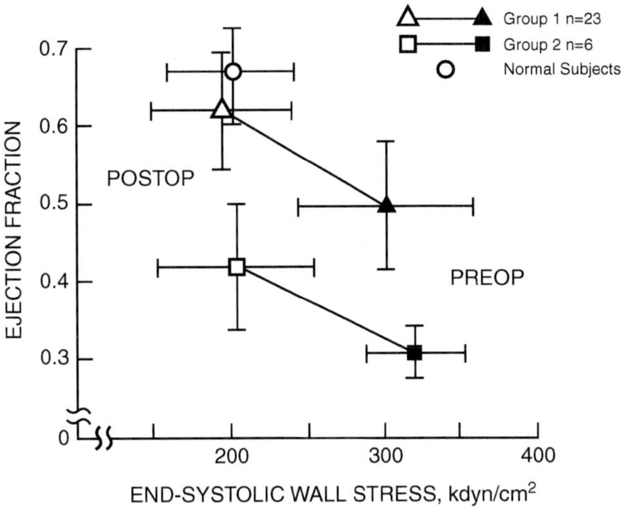

Fig. 5.35 Wall stress (afterload) and ejection fraction (EF) are plotted before (preop) and after (postop) aortic valve replacement for severe aortic regurgitation. Even patients with depressed preoperative EF improved after surgery that reduces afterload. From Taniguchi K, et al. [97]. Reprinted with permission from Elsevier

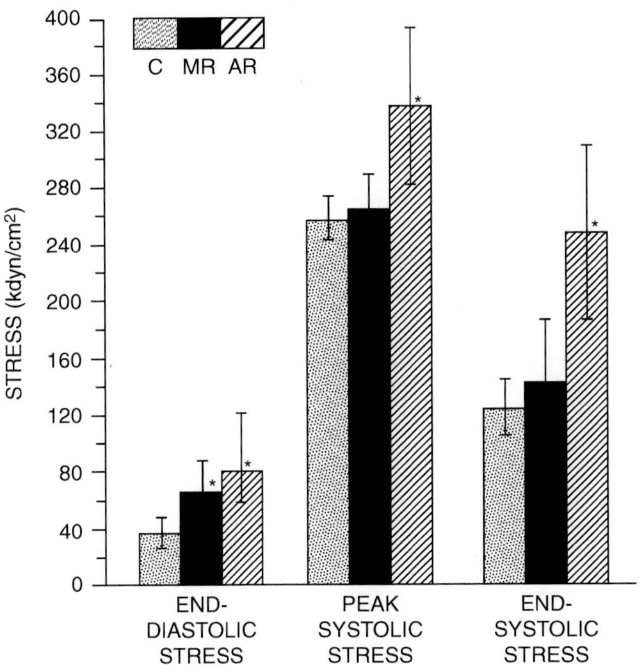

Fig. 5.34 Wall stress for normal subjects is compared to that of patients with mitral regurgitation (MR, white bars) and patients with matched severity of aortic regurgitation (AR, cross hatched bars). Diastolic stress is increased in both volume overloading lesions but systolic stress (afterload) is increased only in AR, indicating that this lesion represents both volume and pressure overload. From Wisenbaugh T, et al. [96]. Reprinted with permission from Elsevier

pressure, together with the increased left ventricular radius in the Laplace equation, greatly increases systolic wall stress (afterload). Indeed, afterload in the patient with AR can be as high as that seen in the classic pressure overload lesion, AS [97]. Ventricular remodeling occurs in accordance with loading conditions. Left ventricular volumes are increased to compensate flow lost to regurgitation but LV wall thickness is also increased in response to increased LV pressure [98]. In a way afterload excess is "beneficial" in that depressed preoperative ejection fraction often returns to normal following surgery as afterload is reduced (Fig. 5.35) [97]. However prolonged, severe AR eventually leads to severe LV enlargement, increased collagen deposition and increases in other elements of the extracellular matrix. These changes displace contractile elements, leading to contractile dysfunction and heart failure [99, 100]. Thus the most common symptoms of AR are those of left sided heart failure and include exercise intolerance and dyspnea on exertion and in more advanced disease, orthopnea, PND and edema.

The rapid runoff of flow returning to the LV during diastole decreases aortic diastolic pressure. A modest decrease is well tolerated but severe diastolic hypotension may cause reduced coronary perfusion and angina and/or reduced cerebral perfusion and syncope. However angina and syncope are much rarer in AR than in AS. Other symptoms reported in severe AR include episodes of chest pain associated with peripheral dilatation and flushing (pseudo Nothnagel attacks) and occasionally an unpleasant awareness of the arterial pulsations especially in the neck.

Diagnosis

Physical Exam

The physical examination of the patient with severe chronic AR can be one of the most dramatic in cardiology. Blood pressure measurement finds a widened pulse pressure and in severe AR, Korotkoff sounds may be heard at very low pressures, in some cases representing LV end diastolic pressure. The enlarged LV causes the hyperdynamic apical impulse to be shifted down and to the left and is often easily visible even on casual inspection of the chest. The typical murmur of AR is a high pitched diastolic blow best heard along the left sternal border with the patient sitting up and leaning forward. The length of the murmur represents the length of diastolic backward flow; thus longer murmurs usually indicate more severe AR. Impingement of the AR jet onto the mitral valve causes it to partially close and to vibrate, in turn producing a diastolic rumble similar to that of mitral stenosis (Austin Flint murmur), almost always indicating that the AR is severe. The widened pulse pressure produces a myriad of signs including Corrigan's pulse (a brisk upstroke and rapid decline of the carotid pulse) bobbing of the head (de Musset's sign), systolic plethora and diastolic blanching of the nail bed when traction is placed on the nail (Quincke's pulse), a to and fro murmur in the femoral artery when pressure is placed on the femoral artery with the bell of the stethoscope (Duroziez's sign), and an augmentation of systolic blood pressure in the leg over brachial pressure by >40 mmHg (Hill's sign).

Imaging

The EKG usually demonstrates the criteria diagnostic for LVH. The chest X-ray demonstrates an enlarged heart. However as with all valvular heart disease, echocardiography forms the mainstay of diagnosis.

Echocardiography plays a vital role in delineation of the aortic valve pathology, mechanism of aortic regurgitation and aides in quantification by using color and spectral Doppler variables. In addition, 3D transesophageal echocardiography offers supplemental anatomic information. However, there are pitfalls in each modality that must be considered in order to avoid misdiagnosing the lesion severity.

Spectral Doppler Methods

1. Pressure Half-time

   Pressure half time (PHT) is the time required for the pressure gradient to decay to half its original value. Larger orifices permit a more rapid equilibration of pressure on either side or the orifice. Therefore pressure decay is more rapid and pressure half-time shorter.

   As shown in the above schematic (Fig. 5.36), the pressure half time method to estimate valve area in mitral stenosis is dependent on the flow between two chambers one of which is a chamber with a single-outlet and the other is a receiving chamber with a single inlet. Unfortunately factors other than orifice size affect PHT. Compliance of the two chambers also affects the rate of pressure decay. In a stenotic lesion like mitral stenosis, this theoretical construct works well provide the compliance of the emptying and receiving chambers is not altered acutely. Accuracy of the PHT method depends on the recording and measuring the initial peak velocity to avoid under or overestimation of valve areas.

   In aortic regurgitation there is a double inlet (the return from the pulmonary veins and from the regurgitant aortic valve). Thus, PHT is affected not only by AR severity but also by afterload (systemic blood pressure and vascular resistance which affect the amount of AR), regurgitant orifice size, and left ventricular compliance. Patients with higher LV filling pressure tend to have the shortest PHT and steepest slope for any given angiographic grade.

   To avoid over or underestimation of PHT, there must be a well-defined spectral Doppler envelope of the aortic regurgitant flow. Only a part of the AR jet may be recorded in situations where there is change in the direction of the jet. The upper part of the AR jet is difficult to record in 14–31% of the patients as shown in Figs. 5.37 and 5.38. However as shown in Fig. 5.39, there is a clearer demarcation of the regurgitant velocity envelope. Because of these vagaries PHT should not be used to precisely quantify the severity of chronic aortic regurgitation, but it can distinguish mild from severe aortic regurgitation.

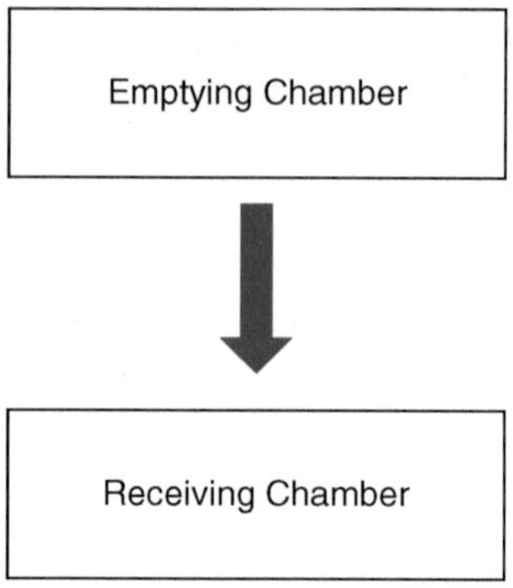

Fig. 5.36 Pressure half time is determined by the rate of emptying and the equalization of pressure between the emptying chamber and the receiving chamber

2. Diastolic mitral regurgitation

Diastolic mitral regurgitation can be observed by either color Doppler or spectral Doppler methods and is an indicator of severe aortic regurgitation because severe AR forces flow across the open mitral valve in diastole (Fig. 5.40).

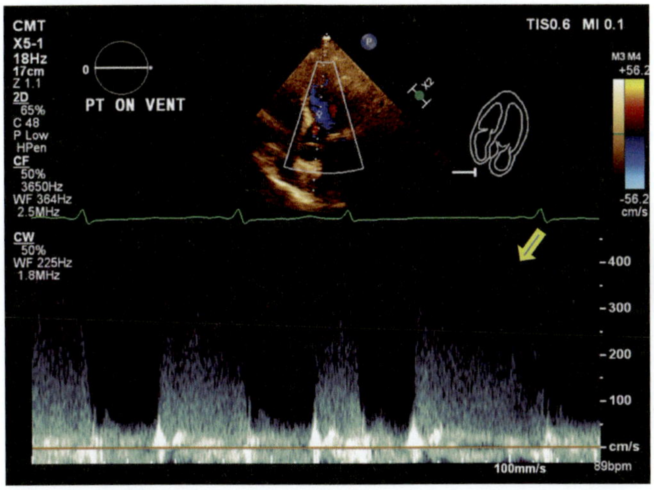

Fig. 5.37 Spectral Doppler envelope of the aortic regurgitant flow. The arrow points the faint upper part of the envelope. Note, the rhythm is atrial fibrillation and the deceleration slope is therefore variable and the peak aortic regurgitant velocity is difficult to discern

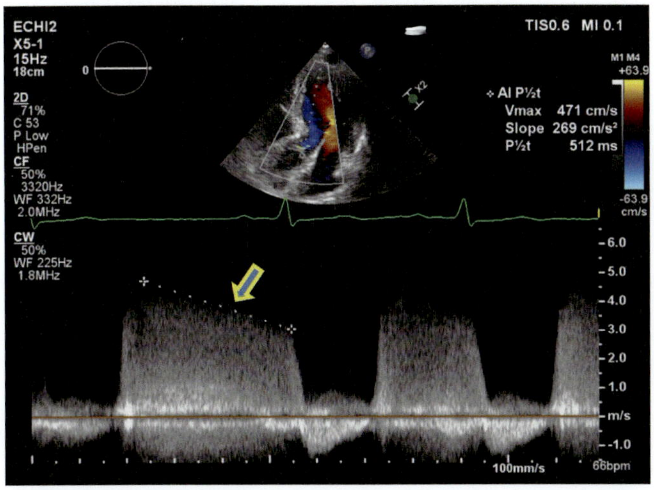

Fig. 5.38 The upper part of the slope (arrow) is well defined, but the peak velocity on which the computation of the PHT is dependent is still difficult to determine

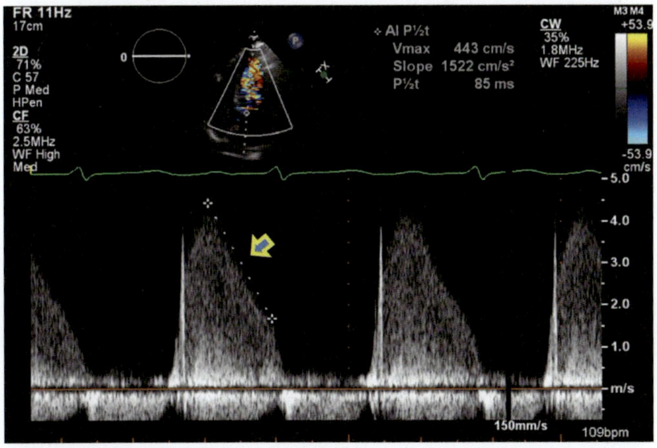

Fig. 5.39 A well-defined Doppler envelope is demonstrated. The arrow points to the steep slope in severe acute aortic regurgitation. Pressure half time is 85 ms

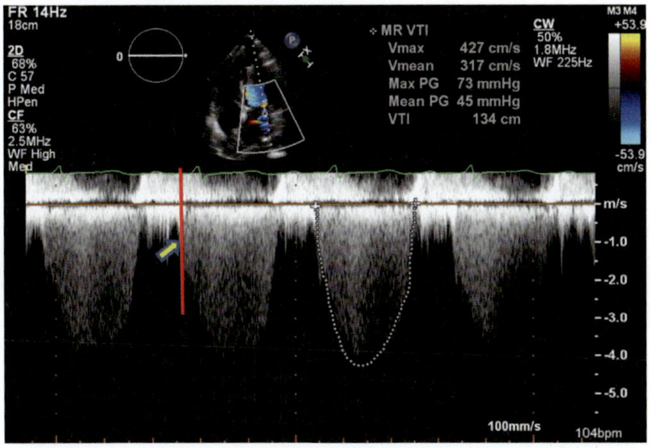

Fig. 5.40 The arrow points to the onset of mitral regurgitation before the start of ventricular systole. Notice the onset of mitral regurgitation before the inscription of QRS on the ECG (red line)

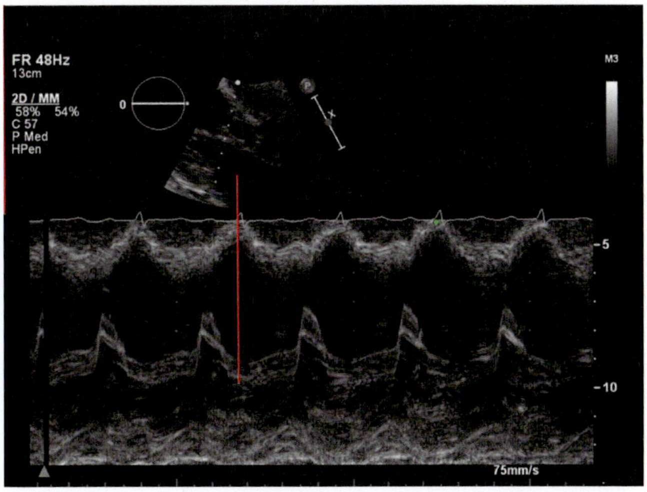

Fig. 5.41 Type A early diastolic closure of mitral valve is shown for a patient with severe aortic regurgitation

M-Mode Echocardiography

Premature closure of the mitral valve (Fig. 5.41) in the setting of severe (and usually acute) aortic regurgitation is classified into Type A (mitral A wave is suppressed but closure occurs before the onset of ventricular systole) or Type B where there is absence of the mitral A wave and closure occurs in mid-diastole.

Tachycardia should be excluded as a cause of mitral E and A fusion before attributing the absence of A wave to severe aortic regurgitation. Early diastolic closure of the mitral valve has been shown to correlate with angiographic grade 3+ or 4+ aortic regurgitation.

Color M-Mode Echocardiography

A simple semiquantitative method of estimating the severity of aortic regurgitation is color m-mode of the origin of the jet (Fig. 5.42). A jet diameter greater than or equal to 12 mm identifies a regurgitant fraction greater than or equal to 40% with a sensitivity of 88.2% and a specificity of 95.2%.

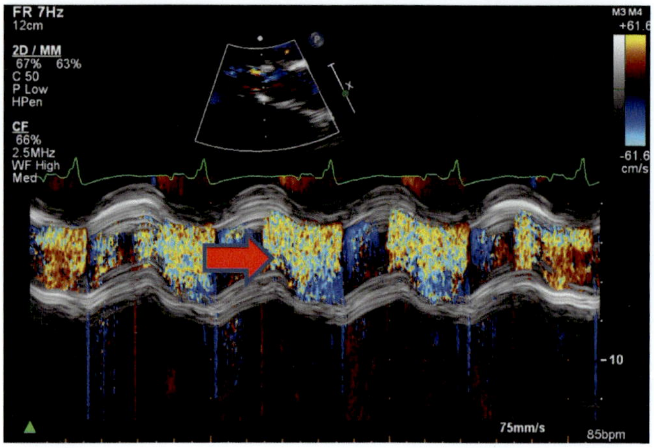

Fig. 5.42 Color M-mode is shown for a patient with severe aortic regurgitation due to leaflet perforation. The regurgitant flow (arrow) fills most of the left ventricular outflow tract throughout diastole

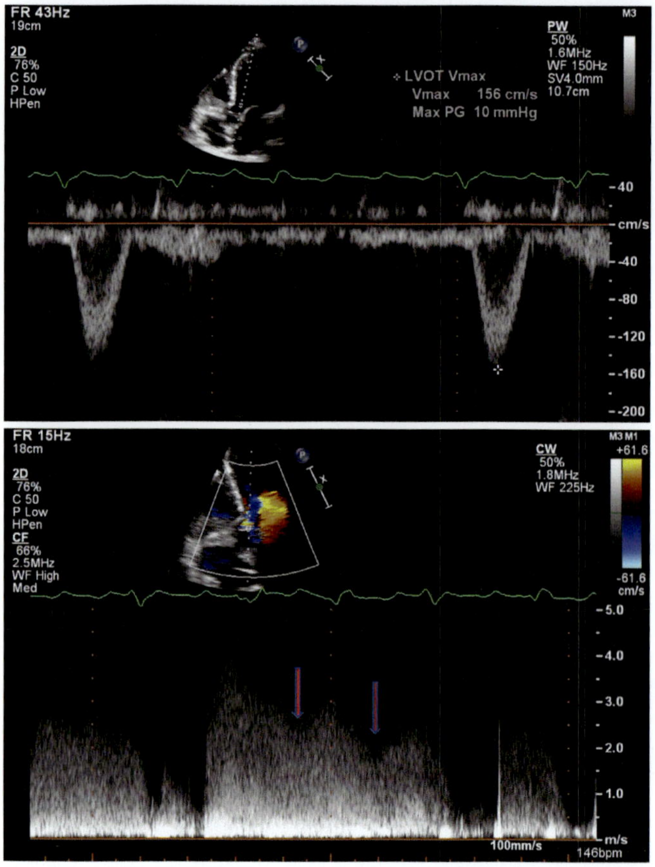

Fig. 5.43 Upper panel. Note the absence of LVOT flow despite the presence of QRS complexes on the EKG. Rhythm is atrial flutter. Lower panel. The arrows point to the "a" dip caused by flutter waves in the setting of elevated left atrial and left ventricular pressures and systemic hypotension

3D Echocardiography

3D echocardiography offers supplemental information regarding the mechanism of aortic valve regurgitation. Defects like perforations are sometimes difficult to visualize by 2D echocardiograms while 3D *en face* views from the aortic root can help in detecting valve perforations.

Systolic Aortic Regurgitation

Aortic regurgitation is usually a diastolic phenomenon, but systolic regurgitation has been noted when there is decreased preload and ineffective ventricular systole resulting in continued regurgitation through a closed aortic valve in both systole and diastole as shown in Fig. 5.43.

Medical Therapy

For the patient with AR who develops hypertension, standard therapy for hypertension should be employed. Concern is raised about the use of beta-blockers which slow heart rate thereby increasing diastolic regurgitant time. While beta-blockers are not first-line therapy for hypertension, it appears they can be used with caution in AR [101]. Because AR causes an increase in afterload, afterload reducing therapy has been employed in an effort to forestall the need for surgery. However this approach has met with disparate and confusing results; thus no firm recommendation can be made to advocate using afterload reduction to forestall the need for AVR [102–104]. The therapeutic goal in treating patients with AR is to provide valve replacement or repair before heart failure ensues. If the patient has already developed heart failure standard guideline directed heart failure therapy is warranted prior to surgery or in place of surgery if surgery is precluded by other medical conditions or personal preference.

Indications for Surgery

Severe AR is often tolerated for years (Fig. 5.44) [105–107] but eventually this mechanical problem must be treated with a mechanical solution, usually AVR but occasionally aortic valve repair. As noted above, valve replacement with a mechanical valve subjects the patient to the need for vitamin K antagonist anticoagulation with its inherent risks of thromboembolism or hemorrhage; if a bioprostheses is implanted, there is inherent risk of structural valve deterioration necessitating reoperation.

Because of these risks and because AR is tolerated relatively well, surgery is timed to be late enough in the course of the disease to avoid these complications but early enough to avoid irreversible LV damage and heart failure. Because the onset of symptoms marks a downturn in prognosis (Fig. 5.45) AVR is provided at the onset of cardiac symptoms, usually dyspnea on exertion and exercise intolerance [108]. Excessive cardiac enlargement and/or a fall in LV systolic performance are indications for AVR even if the patient remains asymptomatic [109, 110]. Thus surgery is indicated when EF falls toward 0.50 or when end systolic dimension approaches 50–55 mm or when end diastolic dimension approaches 70–75 mm. However a recent study (Fig. 5.46) suggests that patients might benefit from AVR much earlier, at an end systolic dimension as small as 40 mm [111]. The progression toward these endpoints which trigger surgery occurs at the rate of about 4% per year [105].

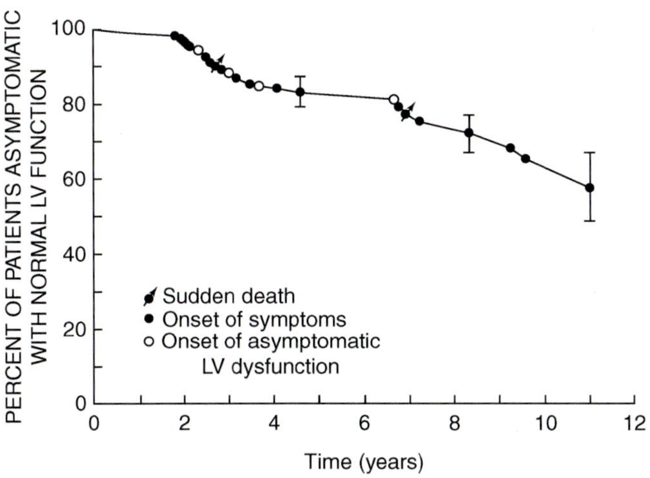

Fig. 5.44 The natural history or aortic regurgitation is demonstrated. Sudden death is rare and the onset of symptoms or asymptomatic left ventricular dysfunction occurs at a slow rate, about 4% per year. From Bonow RO, et al. [105]. Reprinted with permission from Wolters Kluwer Health, Inc.

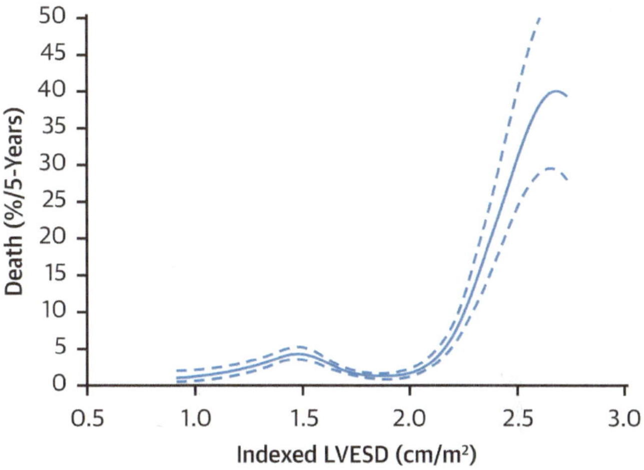

Fig. 5.46 The probability of survival for patients with severe aortic regurgitation worsened when indexed end systolic dimension exceeded 2.0. Considering an average body surface area of 2.0, an end systolic dimension of 4.0 cm could be a trigger for valve replacement. From Mentias A, et al. [111]. Reprinted with permission from Elsevier

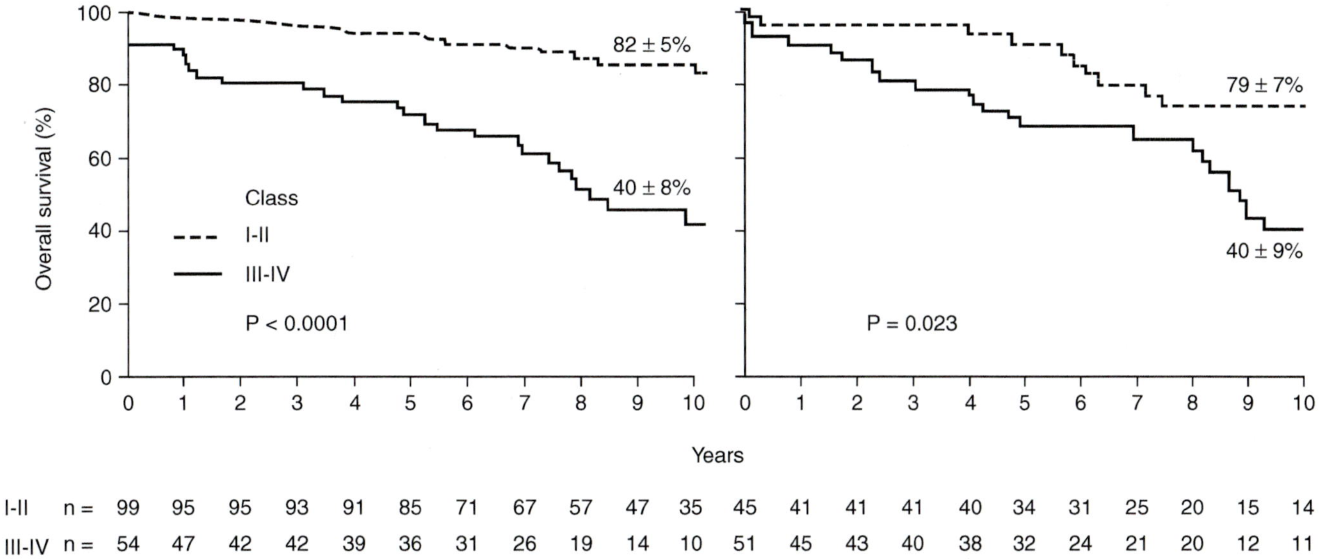

Fig. 5.45 The impact of severe (NYHA class III or IV) symptoms is marked whether the patient has normal ejection fraction (left panel) or reduced ejection fraction (right panel). From Klodas E, et al. [108]. Reprinted with permission from Elsevier

Mechanical Therapy

The majority of patients with AR are treated surgically with the valve replacements noted above for aortic stenosis. TAVR is employed almost exclusively for patients with AS because the annular calcification, so prominent in that disease but usually absent in AR, is used to anchor the TAVR. However TAVR valves apt for the treatment of AR are currently under development and are likely to become available in the near future [112].

Valve repair, the mainstay for the therapy of primary mitral regurgitation is in its relative infancy for the aortic valve. However aortic repair techniques are being perfected. Techniques used to correct AR include shortening of the free edge of a prolapsing leaflet (plication), patching holes and or retracted leaflet edges with pericardium, tricuspidization of bicuspid valves, and aortic plication when root dilatation is the cause of the AR [113]. A meta-analysis of almost 3000 patients undergoing aortic valve repair found a 12% reoperation rate at 5 years [114].

Acute Severe Aortic Regurgitation

Pathophysiology

Acute AR, often caused by valve disruption from infective endocarditis, impacts a left ventricle unprepared for an acute severe volume overload. As noted in Fig. 5.47, in chronic AR the LV gradually enlarges to accommodate the volume overload as AR increases over time [115]. However in acute severe AR there has been no time for eccentric hypertrophy to develop. The small unprepared LV receives the extra volume from regurgitation with high filling pressure (Fig. 5.48) [87], pulmonary congestion and decreased forward stroke volume. Aortic diastolic pressure falls and LV diastolic pressure increases so that they become equal toward end diastole (Fig. 5.48) abolishing the pressure gradient driving coronary blood flow potentially causing subendocardial ischemia and LV dysfunction. Mean arterial pressure falls both from the reduced diastolic pressure from run off into the LV and from reduced forward cardiac output. High LV diastolic pressure may exceed left atrial pressure, closing the mitral valve in diastole instead of systole (Fig. 5.41). This action may help protect the lungs from extreme left atrial pressure but also limits forward mitral flow.

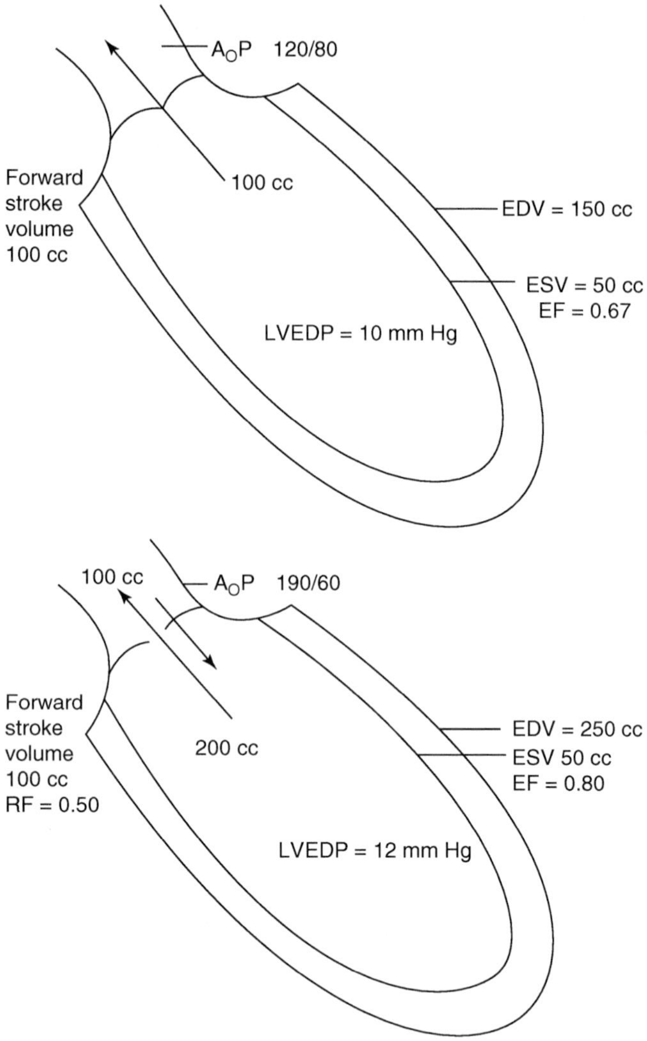

Fig. 5.47 (**a**, **b**) Compare normal physiology (**a**) with that of chronic compensated severe aortic regurgitation. In (**b**) there has been dilatation of the left ventricle allowing for normal forward stroke volume and filling pressure despite severe regurgitation. *AoP* aortic pressure, *EDV* end diastolic volume, *EF* ejection fraction, *ESV* end systolic volume, *LVEDP* left ventricular end diastolic pressure, *RF* regurgitant fraction. From Carabello BA. Aortic Valve Disease. In: Willerson J.T., Wellens H.J.J., Cohn J.N., Holmes D.R. (eds) Cardiovascular Medicine. Springer, London, ©2007. Reprinted with permission

Presentation

The patient may experience sudden dyspnea or the symptoms of heart failure may develop more insidiously.

The dramatic physical exam of chronic AR is absent in acute AR, potentially leading the clinician to miss the

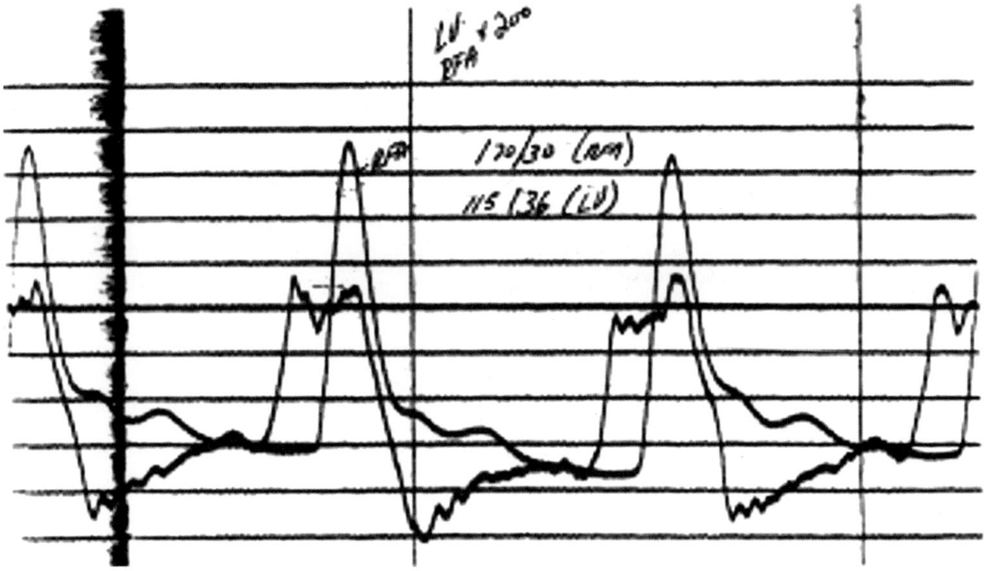

Fig. 5.48 Pressure tracings from a patient with severe acute aortic insufficiency are shown. Systolic aortic pressure (Ao) is augmented (Hills sign) while there is early diastasis between aortic diastolic and left ventricular diastolic pressure. From Carabello BA, et al. [87]. Reprinted with permission from John Wiley & Sons

diagnosis. There may be a modest tachycardia and reduced diastolic blood pressure. However because the LV is normal in volume, the total stroke volume is not increased as it is in chronic AR. Therefore the signs of severe chronic AR are absent in acute AR. The AO-LV gradient is present only in early diastole (Fig. 5.48) thus the diastolic murmur is short and often unimpressive. Preclosure of the mitral valve causes S1 to be soft. Thus the exam is misleadingly unimpressive. A subtle increase in pulse and respiratory rate, a modest decrease in diastolic blood pressure, a soft S1 and a short diastolic murmur may be the only clues that acute severe AR is present. This relatively benign exam may be consistent with a dire outcome. Reduced cardiac output, high LV filling pressures and reduced coronary blood flow may lead to a rapid downhill course and death in the absence of prompt surgical intervention.

Management

Prompt recognition leading to diagnostic imaging and prompt aortic valve replacement is the only effective course of therapy [116]. Attempts to temporize with medical therapy are rarely helpful. Vasodilators that may improve forward flow but lower blood pressure and may cause shock. Pressor agents worsen the aortic regurgitation as does intra-aortic balloon counterpulsation which is contraindicated. While there is fear that a prosthetic valve will become re-infected this occurs less than 5% of the time [117]. Thus surgery should not be delayed for the purpose of longer antibiotic exposure. Adequate care of the patient with acute severe AR due to infective endocarditis requires a multispecialty team composed of expert cardiologists, imagers, infectious disease experts and cardiac surgeons.

Guideline Summary

The algorithm for the treatment of aortic regurgitation as summarized from the AHA/ACC guidelines [32] for the management of valvular heart disease is shown in Fig. 5.49.

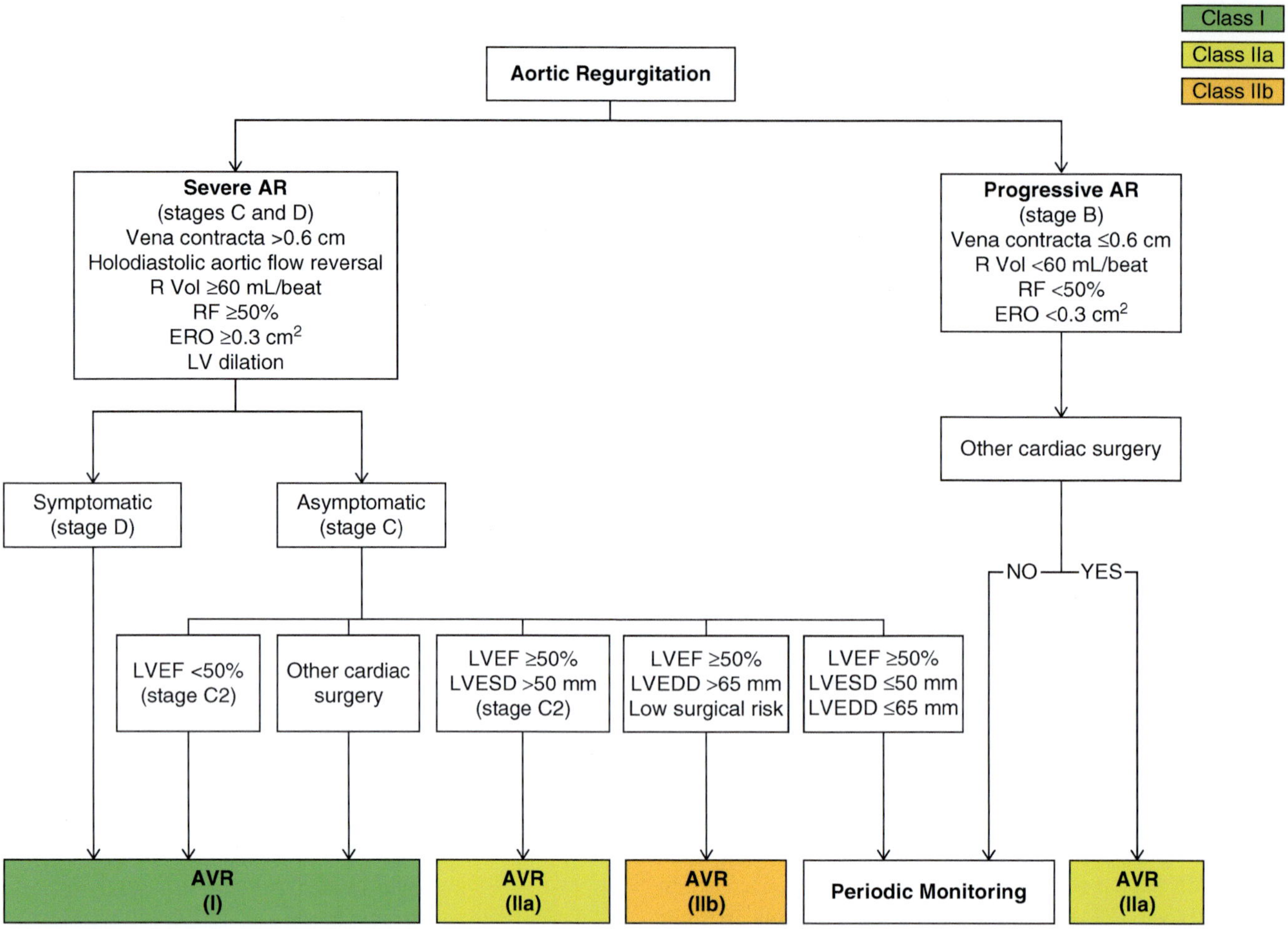

Fig. 5.49 The algorithm for the treatment of AS patients according to the 2014 AHA/ACC guidelines is shown. From Nishimura RA, et al. [32]. Reprinted with permission from Wolters Kluwer Health, Inc.

References

1. Otto CM, Kuusisto J, Reichenbach DD, Gown AM, O'Brien KD. Characterization of the early lesion of 'degenerative' valvular aortic stenosis: histological and immunohistochemical studies. Circulation. 1994;90:844–53.
2. Toutouzas K, Drakopoulou M, Synetos A, Tsiamis E, et al. In vivo aortic valve thermal heterogeneity in patients with nonrheumatic aortic valve stenosis the: first in vivo experience in humans. J Am Coll Cardiol. 2008;52(9):758–63.
3. Cowell SJ, Newby DE, Prescott RJ, Bloomfiend P, Reid J, Northridge DB, Boon NA, Scottish Aortic Stenosis and Lipid Lowering Trial, Impact on Regression (SALTIRE) Investigators. A randomized trial of intensive lipid-lowering therapy in calcific aortic stenosis. N Engl J Med. 2005;352:2389–97.
4. Rossebo AB, Pederson TR, Bowan K, Brudi P, et al. SEAS Investigators. Intensive lipid lowering with simvastatin and ezetimibe in aortic stenosis. N Engl J Med. 2008;359:1343–56.
5. Chan KL, Teo K, Dumsnil JG, Ni A Tam J, Investigators ASTRONOMER. Effect of lipid lowering with rosuvastatin on progression of aortic stenosis: results of the aortic stenosis progression observation: measuring effects of rosuvastatin (ASTRONOMER) trial. Circulation. 2010;121:306–14.
6. Puri R, Nocholls SJ, Shao M, Kataoka Y, et al. Impact of strains on serial coronary calcification during atheroma progression and regression. J Am Coll Cardiol. 2015;65(13):1273–82.
7. Wu B, Elmariah S, Kaplan FS, Cheng G, Mohler ER III. Paradoxical effects of statins on aortic valve myofibroblasts and osteoblasts: implications for end-stage valvular heart disease. Arterioscler Thromb Vasc Biol. 2005;25:592–7.
8. Kamstrup PR, Tybjaerg-Hansen A, Nordestgaard BG. Elevated lipoprotein(a) and risk of aortic valve stenosis in the general population. J Am Coll Cardiol. 2014;63(5):470–7.
9. Wirrig EE, Yutzey KE. Conserved transcriptional regulatory mechanisms in aortic valve development and disease. Arterioscler Thromb Vasc Biol. 2014;34(4):737–41.
10. Ikonomidis JS, Ruddy JM, Benton SM Jr, Arroyo J, et al. Aortic dilatation with bicuspid aortic valves: cusp fusion correlates to matrix metalloproteinases and inhibitors. Ann Thorac Surg. 2012;93:457–63.
11. Russo CF, Cannata A, Lanfranconi M, Vitali E, Garatti A, Bonacina E. Is aortic wall degeneration related to bicuspid aortic valve anatomy in patient with valvular disease? J Thorac Cardiovasc Surg. 2008;136:937–42.
12. Guzzardi DG, Barker AJ, van Ooij P, Malaisrie SC, et al. Valve-related hemodynamics mediate human bicuspid aortopathy: insights from wall shear stress mapping. J Am Coll Cardiol. 2015;66:892–900.

13. Siu SC, Silversides CK. Bicuspid aortic valve disease. J Am Coll Cardiol. 2010;55:2789–800.
14. Spinale FG, Bolger A. Fate versus flow. Wall shear stress in the aortopathy associated with bicuspid aortic valves. J Am Coll Cardiol. 2015;66:901–4.
15. Ross J Jr, Braunwald E. Aortic stenosis. Circulation. 1968;38:61–7.
16. Leon MB, Smith CR, Mack M. Miller DC, Moses JW, et al. PARTNER Trial Investigators. Transcatheter aortic-valve implantation for aortic stenosis in patient who cannot undergo surgery. N Engl J Med. 2010;363(71):1597–607.
17. Adams DH, Popma JJ, Reardon MJ, Yakubov SJ, et al. U.S. CoreValve Clinical Investigators. Transcatheter aortic valve replacement using a self-expanding bioprosthesis in patients with severe aortic stenosis at extreme risk for surgery. N Engl J Med. 2014;370(19):1790–8.
18. Grossman W, Jones D, McLaurin LP. Wall stress and patterns of hypertrophy in the human left ventricle. J Clin Invest. 1975;56:56–64.
19. Kupari M, Turto H, Lommi J. Left ventricular hypertrophy in aortic valve stenosis: preventive or promotive of systolic dysfunction and heart failure. Eur Heart J. 2005;26:1790–6. Epub 2005 Apr 28.
20. Marcus ML, Doty DB, Hiratzka LF, Wright CB, Easham CL. Decreased coronary reserve: a mechanism for angina pectoris in patients with aortic stenosis and normal coronary arteries. N Engl J Med. 1982;307:1362–6.
21. Nakano K, Corin WJ, Spann JFJ, Biederman RW, Denslow S, Carabello BA. Abnormal subendocardial blood flow in pressure overload hypertrophy is associated with pacing-induced subendocardial dysfunction. Circ Res. 1989;65:155–64.
22. Breisch EA, White FC, Bloor CM. Myocardial characteristics of pressure overload hypertrophy: a structural and functional study. Lab Investig. 1984;51:333–42.
23. Zile MR, Brutsaert DL. New concepts in diastolic dysfunction and diastolic heart failure: part II—causal mechanisms and treatment. Circulation. 2002;105:1503–8.
24. Hess OM, Ritter M, Schneider J, Grimm J, Turina M, Krayenbuehl HP. Diastolic stiffness and myocardial structure in aortic valve disease before and after valve replacement. Circulation. 1984;69:85–65.
25. Weidemann F, Herrmann S, Stork S, Niemann M, et al. Impact of myocardial fibrosis in patients with symptomatic severe aortic stenosis. Circulation. 2009;120:577–84.
26. Ito K, Yan X, Feng X, Manning WJ, Dillman WH, Lorell BH. Transgenic expression of sarcoplasmic reticulum Ca++ ATPase modifies the transition from hypertrophy to early heart failure. Circ Res. 2001;89:422–9.
27. Olivetti G, Abbi R, Quaini F, et al. Apoptosis in the falling human heart. N Engl J Med. 1997;336:1131–41.
28. Carabello BA, Green LH, Grossman W, Cohn LH, Koster JK, Collins JJ Jr. Hemodynamic determinants of prognosis of aortic valve replacement in critical aortic stenosis and advanced congestive heart failure. Circulation. 2980;62:42–8.
29. Carabello BA. Compendium: introduction to aortic stenosis. Circ Res. 2013;113(2):179–85.
30. Kadem L, Dumesnil JG, Rieu R, Durand LG, Garcia D, Pibarot P. Impact of systemic hypertension on the assessment of aortic stenosis. Heart. 2005;91(3):354–61.
31. Carabello BA. Georg Ohm and the changing character of aortic stenosis: it's not your grandfather's Oldsmobile. Circulation. 2012;125:2295–7.
32. Nishimura RA, Otto CM, Bonow RO, Carabello BA, Erwin JP 3rd, Guyton RA, O'Gara PT, Ruiz CE, Skubas NJ, Sorajja P, Sundt TM 3rd, Thomas JD, American College of Cardiology/American Heart Association Task Force on Practice Guidelines. 2014 AHA/ACC guideline for the management of patients with valvular heart disease: executive summary: a report of the American College of Cardiology/American Heart Association Task Force on Practice Guidelines. J Am Coll Cardiol. 2014;63(22):2438–88.
33. Minners J, Allgeier M, Gohlke-Baerwolf C, Kienzle RP, Neumann FJ, Jander N. Inconsistencies of echocardiographic criteria for the grading of aortic valve stenosis. Eur Heart J. 2008;29(8):1043–8.
34. Herrmann S, Fries B, Liu D, Hu K, Stoerk S, Voelker W, Ruppert C, Lorenz K, Ertl G, Weidemann F. Differences in natural history of low- and high-gradient aortic stenosis from nonsevere to severe stage of the disease. J Am Soc Echocardiogr. 2015;28(11):1270–82.
35. Ito S, Miranda WR, Nkomo VT, et al. Reduced left ventricular ejection fraction in patients with aortic stenosis. J Am Coll Cardiol. 2018;71:1313–21.
36. Baicu CF, Zile MR, Aurigemma GP, Gaasch WH. Left ventricular systolic performance, function, and contractility in patients with diastolic heart failure. Circulation. 2005;111(18):2306–12.
37. Brener SJ, Duffy CI, Thomas JD, Stewart WJ. Progression of aortic stenosis in 394 patients: relation to changes in myocardial and mitral valve dysfunction. J Am Coll Cardiol. 1995;25(2): 305–10.
38. Otto CM, Pearlman AS, Gardner CL. Hemodynamic progression of aortic stenosis in adults assessed by Doppler echocardiography. J Am Coll Cardiol. 1989;13(3):545–50.
39. Rosenhek R, Rader F, Loho N, Gabriel H, Heger M, Klaar U, Schemper M, Binder T, Maurer G, Baumgartner H. Statins but not angiotensin-converting enzyme inhibitors delay progression of aortic stenosis. Circulation. 2004;110(10):1291–5.
40. Moura LM, Ramos SF, Zamorano JL, Barros IM, Azevedo LF, Rocha-Gonçalves F, Rajamannan NM. Rosuvastatin affecting aortic valve endothelium to slow the progression of aortic stenosis. J Am Coll Cardiol. 2007;49(5):554–61.
41. Carabello BA. Aortic stenosis. In: Crawford MH, editor. Current diagnosis and treatment in cardiology. New York: Appleton & Lange; 1995. p. 87–98.
42. Clavel MA, Messika-Zeitoun D, Pibarot P, et al. The complex nature of discordant severe calcified aortic valve disease grading: new insights from combined Doppler echocardiographic and computed tomographic study. J Am Coll Cardiol. 2013;62(24):2329–38.
43. Clavel MA, Malouf J, Messika-Zeitoun D, et al. Aortic valve area calculation in aortic stenosis by CT and Doppler echocardiography. JACC Cardiovasc Imaging. 2015;8(3):248–57.
44. Aggarwal SR, Clavel MA, Messika-Zeitoun D, et al. Sex differences in aortic valve calcification measured by multidetector computed tomography in aortic stenosis. Circ Cardiovasc Imaging. 2013;6(1):40–7.
45. Gorlin R, Gorlin SG. Hydraulic formula for calculation of the area of the stenotic mitral valve, other cardiac valves, and central circulatory shunts. I. Am Heart J. 1951;41(1):1–29.
46. Dehmer GJ, Firth BG, Hillis LD. Oxygen consumption in adult patients during cardiac catheterization. Clin Cardiol. 1982;49:1860–7.
47. Khot UN, Novaro GM, Popovic ZB, Mills RM, Thomas JD, Tuzcu EM, Hammer D, Nissen SE, Francis GS. Nitroprusside in critically ill patients with left ventricular dysfunction and aortic stenosis. N Engl J Med. 2003;348:1756–63.
48. Lindman BR, Zajarias A, Madrazo JA, Shah J, et al. Effects of phosphodiesterase type 5 inhibition on systemic and pulmonary hemodynamics and ventricular function in patients with severe symptomatic aortic stenosis. Circulation. 2012;125:2353–62.
49. Eleid MF, Nishimura RA, Sorajja P, Borlaug BA. Systemic hypertension in low-gradient severe aortic stenosis with preserved ejection fraction. Circulation. 2013;128:1349–53.
50. Nadir MA, Wei L, Elder DH, Libianto R, et al. Impact of renin-angiotensin system blockade therapy on outcome in aortic stenosis. J Am Coll Cardiol. 2011;58:570–6.

51. van Geldorp MWA, Jamieson WRE, Kappetein AP, Ye J, et al. Patient outcome after aortic valve replacement with a mechanical or biological prosthesis: weighing lifetime anticoagulant-related event risk against reoperation risk. J Thorac Cardiovasc Surg. 2009;137:881–6.
52. Pellikka PA, Sarano ME, Nishimura RA, Malouf JS, Bailey KR, Scott CG, Barnes ME, Tajik AJ. Outcome of 622 adults with asymptomatic, hemodynamically significant aortic stenosis during prolonged follow-up. Circulation. 2005;111:3290–5.
53. Das P, Rimington H, Chambers J. Exercise testing to stratify risk in aortic stenosis. Eur Heart J. 2005;26:1309–13. Epub 2005 Apr 8.
54. Amato M, Moffa PJ, Werner KE, Ramires JA. Treatment decision in asymptomatic aortic valve stenosis: role of exercise testing. Heart. 2001;86:381–6.
55. Rosenhek R, Zilberszac R, Schemper M, Czerny M, Mundigler G, Graf S, Bergler-Klein J, Grim M, Gabiel H, Maurer G. Natural history of very severe aortic stenosis. Circulation. 2010;121(1):151–6.
56. Otto CM, Burwash IG, Legget ME, et al. Prospective study of asymptomatic valvular aortic stenosis. Clinical, echocardiographic, and exercise predictors of outcome. Circulation. 1997;95(9):2262–70.
57. Bergler-Klein J, Klaar U, Heger M, Rosenhek R, Mundigler G, Gabriel H, Binder T, Pacher R, Maurer G, Baumgartner H. Natriuretic peptides predict symptom-free survival and postoperative outcome in severe aortic stenosis. Circulation. 2004;109:2302–8.
58. Nessmith MG, Fukuta H, Brucks S, Little WC. Usefulness of an elevated B-type natriuretic peptide in predicting survival in patients with aortic stenosis treated without surgery. Am J Cardiol. 2005;96:1445–8. Epub 2005 Oct 3.
59. Lim P, Monin JL, Monchi M, Garot J, Pasquet A, Hittinger L, Vanoverschelde JL, Carayon A, Gueret P. Predictors of outcome in patients with severe aortic stenosis and normal left ventricular function: role of B-type natriuretic peptide. Eur Heart J. 2004;25:2048–53.
60. Steadman CD, Ray S, Ng LL, McCann GP. Natriuretic peptides in common valvular heart disease. J Am Coll Cardiol. 2010;55:2034–48.
61. Clavel MA, Malouf J, Michelena HI, Suri RM, Jaffe AS, Mahoney DW, Enriquez-Sarano M. B-type natriuretic peptide clinical activation in aortic stenosis: impact on long-term survival. J Am Coll Cardiol. 2014;63(19):2016–25.
62. Pereira JJ, Balaban K, Lauer MS, Lytle B, Thomas JD, Garcia MJ. Aortic valve replacement in patients with mild or moderate aortic stenosis and coronary bypass surgery. Am J Med. 2005;118:735–42.
63. Taniguchi T, Morimoto T, Shiomi H, Ando K, et al. CURRENT AS Registry Investigators. Initial surgical versus conservative strategies in patients with asymptomatic severe aortic stenosis J Am Coll Cardiol. 2015;66(25):2827–38.
64. Rahimtoola SH. Choice of prosthetic heart valve in adults an update. J Am Coll Cardiol. 2010;55(22):2413–26.
65. Dangas GD, Weitz JI, Giustino G, Makkar R, Mehran R. Prosthetic heart valve thrombosis. J Am Coll Cardiol. 2016;68(24):2670–89.
66. Phan K, Zhao DF, Zhou JJ, Karagaratnam A, Phan S, Yan TD. Bioprosthetic versus mechanical prostheses for valve replacement in end-stage renal disease patients: systematic review and meta-analysis. J Thorac Dis. 2016;8(5):769–77.
67. Eikelboom JW, Connolly SJ, Brueckmann M, Granger CB, et al. Dabigatran versus warfarin in patients with mechanical heart valves. N Engl J Med. 2013;369(13):1206–14.
68. Charitos EI, Takkenberg JJ, Hanke T, Gorski A, et al. Reoperations on the pulmonary autograft and pulmonary homograft after the Ross procedure: an update on the German Dutch Ross Registry. J Thorac Cardiovasc Surg. 2012;144(4):813–21, discussion 821–3.
69. El-Hamamsy I, Eryigit Z, Stevens LM, Sarang Z, et al. Long-term outcomes after autograft versus homograft aortic root replacement in adults with aortic valve disease: a randomised controlled trial. Lancet. 2010;376:524–31.
70. Pibarot P. Prosthesis-patient mismatch: definition, clinical impact, and prevention. Heart. 2006;92(8):1022–9.
71. Reardon MJ, Van Mieghem NM, Popma JJ, Kleiman NS, et al. SURTAVI Investigators. Surgical or transcatheter aortic-valve replacement in intermediate-risk patients. N Engl J Med. 2017;376(14):1321–31.
72. Mack MJ, Acker MA, Gelijns AC, Overbey JR, et al. Cardiothoracic Surgical Trials Network (CTSN). Effect of cerebral embolic protection devices on CNS infarction in surgical aortic valve replacement: a randomized clinical trial. JAMA. 2017;318(6):536–47.
73. Perlman GY, Loncar S, Pollak A, Gilon D, Alcalai R, Planer D, Lotan C, Danenberg HD. Post-procedural hypertension following transcatheter aortic valve implantation: incidence and clinical significance. JACC Cardiovasc Interv. 2013;6:472–8.
74. Huber D, Grimm J, Koch R, Krayenbuehl HP. Determinants of ejection performance in aortic stenosis. Circulation. 1981;64:126–34.
75. Gunther S, Grossman W. Determinants of ventricular function in pressure-overload hypertrophy in man. Circulation. 1979;59(4):679–88.
76. Tribouilloy C, Levy F, Rusinaru D, Guéret P, et al. Outcome after aortic valve replacement for low-flow/low-gradient aortic stenosis without contractile reserve on dobutamine stress echocardiography. J Am Coll Cardiol. 2009;53:1865–73.
77. Brogan WC, Grayburn PA, Lange RA, Hillis LD. Prognosis after valve replacement in patients with severe aortic stenosis and a low transvalvular pressure gradient. J Am Coll Cardiol. 1993;21:1657–60.
78. Connolly HM, Oh JK, Schaff HV, Roger VL, Osborn SL, Hodge DO, Tajik AJ. Severe aortic stenosis with low transvalvular gradient and severe left ventricular dysfunction: result of aortic valve replacement in 52 patients. Circulation. 2000;101:1940–6.
79. Monin JL, Monchi M, Petit H, Baleynaud S, et al. Low-gradient aortic stenosis: operative risk stratification and predictors for long-term outcome: a multicenter study using dobutamine stress hemodynamics. Circulation. 2003;108:319–24.
80. Quere JP, Monin JL, Levy F, Petit H, et al. Influence of preoperative left ventricular contractile reserve on postoperative ejection fraction in low-gradient aortic stenosis. Circulation. 2006;113:1738–44.
81. Nwaejike N, Mills K, Stables R, Field M. Balloon aortic valvuloplasty as a bridge to aortic valve surgery for severe aortic stenosis. Interact Cardiovasc Thorac Surg. 2015;20(3):429–35.
82. Kefer J, Gapira JM, Pierard S, De Meester C, Gurne O, Chenu P, Renkin J. Recovery after balloon aortic valvuloplasty in patients with aortic stenosis and impaired left ventricular function: predictors and prognostic implications. J Invasive Cardiol. 2013;25:235–41.
83. Buermans HPJ, Redout EM, Schiel AE, Musters RJ, et al. Microarray analysis reveals pivotal divergent mRNA expression profiles early in the development of either compensated ventricular hypertrophy or heart failure. Physiol Genomics. 2005;21:314–223.
84. Koide M, Nagatsu M, Zile MR, Hamawaki M, et al. Premorbid determinants of left ventricular dysfunction in a novel model of gradually induced pressure overload in the adult canine. Circulation. 1997;95(6):1601–10.
85. Casale PN, Palacios IF, Abascal VM, Harrell L, Davidoff R, Weyman AE, Fifer MA. Effects of dobutamine on Gorlin and continuity equation valve areas and valve resistance in valvular aortic stenosis. Am J Cardiol. 1992;70(13):1175–9.
86. Nishimura RA, Grantham JA, Connolly HM, Schaff HV, Higano ST, Holmes DR Jr. Low-output, low-gradient aortic stenosis in

patients with depressed left ventricular systolic function: the clinical utility of the dobutamine challenge in the catheterization laboratory. Circulation. 2002;106:809–13.
87. Carabello BA, Ballard WL, Gazes PC, Sahn SA, Heffner JF. Cardiology pearls. Philadelphia, PA: Hanley & Belfus; 1994.
88. Fougeres E, Tribouilloy C, Monchi M, Petit-Eisenmann H, et al. Outcomes of pseudo-severe aortic stenosis under conservative treatment. Eur Heart J. 2012;33(19):2426–33.
89. Dumesnil JG, Pibarot P, Carabello BA. Paradoxical low flow and/or low gradient severe aortic stenosis despite preserved left ventricular ejection fraction: implication for diagnosis and treatment. Eur Heart J. 2010;31:281–9.
90. Hachicha Z, Dumensnil JG, Bogaty P, Pibarot P. Paradoxical low flow, low gradient severe stenosis despite preserved ejection fraction is associated with higher afterload and reduced survival. Circulation. 2007;115:2856–64.
91. Clavel MA, Dumesnil JG, Capoulade R, Mathieu P, Senchal M, Pibarot P. Outcome of patients with aortic stenosis, small valve area and low-flow, low-gradient despite preserved left ventricular ejection fraction. J Am Coll Cardiol. 2012;60:1259–67.
92. Clavel MA, Berthelot-Richer M, Le Ven F, Capoulade R, Dahou A, Dumesnil JG, Mathieu P, Pibarot P. Impact of classic and paradoxical low flow on survival after aortic valve replacement for severe aortic stenosis. J Am Coll Cardiol. 2015;65(7):645–53.
93. Herrmann S, Störk S, Niemann M, Lange V, et al. Low-gradient aortic valve stenosis myocardial fibrosis and its influence on function and outcome. J Am Coll Cardiol. 2011;58(4):402–12.
94. Dayan V, Vignolo G, Magne J, Clavel MA, Mohty D, Pibarot P. Outcome and impact of aortic valve replacement in patients with preserved LVEF and low-gradient aortic stenosis. J Am Coll Cardiol. 2015;66(23):2594–603.
95. Waller BF, Howard J, Fess S. Pathology of aortic valve stenosis and pure aortic regurgitation: a clinical morphologic assessment—part II. Clin Cardiol. 1994;17:150–6.
96. Wisenbaugh T, Spann JF, Carabello BA. Differences in myocardial performance and load between patients with similar amounts of chronic aortic versus chronic mitral regurgitation. J Am Coll Cardiol. 1984;3(4):916–23.
97. Taniguchi K, Nakano S, Hirose H, Matsuda H, Shirakura R, Sakai K, Kawamoto T, Sakaki S, Kawashima Y. Preoperative left ventricular function: minimal requirement for successful late results of valve replacement for aortic regurgitation. J Am Coll Cardiol. 1987;10(3):510–8.
98. Feiring AJ, Rumberger JA. Ultrafast computed tomography analysis of regional radius-to-wall thickness ratios in normal and volume-overloaded human left ventricle. Circulation. 1992;85(4):1423–32.
99. Schwarz F, Flameng W, Schaper J, Langebartels F, Sesto M, Hehrlein F, Schlepper M. Myocardial structure and function in patients with aortic valve disease and their relation to postoperative results. Am J Cardiol. 1978;41(4):661–9.
100. Krayenbuehl HP, Hess OM, Monrad ES, Schneider J, Mall G, Turina M. Left ventricular myocardial structure in aortic valve disease before, intermediate, and late after aortic valve replacement. Circulation. 1989;79(4):744–55.
101. Sampat U, Varadarajan P, Turk R, Kamath A, Khandhar S, Pai RG. Effect of beta-blocker therapy on survival in patients with severe aortic regurgitation results from a cohort of 756 patients. J Am Coll Cardiol. 2009;54:452–7.
102. Scognamiglio R, Rahimtoola S, Faoli G, Nistri S, Dalla Volta S. Nifedipine in asymptomatic patients with severe aortic regurgitation and normal left ventricular function. N Engl J Med. 1994;331:689–94.
103. Evangelista A, Tornos P, Samola A, Permanyer-Miralda G, Soler-Soler J. Long-term vasodilator therapy in patients with severe aortic regurgitation. N Engl J Med. 2005;353:1342–9.
104. Greenberg B, Massie B, Bristow JD, Cheitlin M, Siemienczuk D, Topic N, Wilson RA, Szlachcic J, Thomas D. Long-term vasodilator therapy of chronic aortic insufficiency. A randomized double-blinded, placebo-controlled clinical trial. Circulation. 1988;78(1):92–103.
105. Bonow RO, Lakatos E, Maron BJ, Epsstein SE. Serial long-term assessment of the natural history of asymptomatic patients with chronic aortic regurgitation and normal left ventricular systolic function. Circulation. 1991;84(4):1625–35.
106. Bonow RO, Dodd JT, Maron BJ, O'Gara PT, White GG, McIntosh CL, Clark RE, Epstein SE. Long-term serial changes in left ventricular function and reversal of ventricular dilatation after valve replacement for chronic aortic regurgitation. Circulation. 1988;78(5 Pt 1):1108–20.
107. Borer JS, Bonow RO. Contemporary approach to aortic and mitral regurgitation. Circulation. 2003;108:2432–8.
108. Klodas E, Enriquez-Sarano M, Tajik AJ, Mullany CJ, Bailey KR, Seward JB. Optimizing timing of surgical correction in patients with severe aortic regurgitation: role of symptoms. J Am Coll Cardiol. 1997;30:746–52.
109. Henry WL, Bonow RO, Rosing DR, Epstein SE. Observations on the optimum time for operative intervention for aortic regurgitation. II. Serial echocardiographic evaluation of asymptomatic patients. Circulation. 1980;61(3):484–92.
110. Chaliki HP, Mohty D, Avierinos JF, Scott CG, Schaff HV, Tajik AJ, Enriquez-Sarano M. Outcomes after aortic valve replacement in patients with severe aortic regurgitation and markedly reduced left ventricular function. Circulation. 2002;106:2687–93.
111. Mentias A, Feng K, Alashi A, Rodriguez LL, et al. Long-term outcomes in patients with aortic regurgitation and preserved left ventricular ejection fraction. J Am Coll Cardiol. 2016;68(20):2144–53.
112. Silaschi M, Conradi L, Wendler O, Schlingloff F, et al. The JUPITER registry: one-year outcomes of transapical aortic valve implantation using a second generation transcatheter heart valve for aortic regurgitation. Catheter Cardiovasc Interv. 2018;91(7):1345–51.
113. Komya TA. Aortic valve repair update. Gen Thorac Cardiovasc Surg. 2015;63(6):309–19.
114. Saczkowski R, Malas T, Kerchove L, El Khoury G, Boodhwanim M. Systematic review of aortic valve preservation and repair. Ann Cardiothorac Surg. 2013;2:3–9.
115. Carabello BA. Aortic regurgitation: hemodynamic determinants of prognosis. In: Cohn LC, DiSesa VJ, editors. Aortic regurgitation. New York: Marcel Dekker; 1986. p. 89–104.
116. Funakoshi S, Kaji S, Yamamuro A, Tani T, Kinoshita M, Okada Y, Furukawa YJ. Impact of early surgery in the active phase on long-term outcomes in left-sided native valve infective endocarditis. Thorac Cardiovasc Surg. 2011;142(4):836–42.
117. Klieverik LM, Yacoub MH, Edwards S, Bekkers JA, Roos-Hesselink JW, Kappetein AP, Takkenberg JJ, Bogers AJ. Surgical treatment of active native aortic valve endocarditis with allografts and mechanical prostheses. Ann Thorac Surg. 2009;88(6):1814–21.

Comprehensive Assessment of Primary Mitral Valve Disease: Clinical Presentation, Diagnosis, Medical and Surgical Therapy

6

Brian R. Lindman, Spencer J. Melby, Nishath Quader, Marc A. Sintek, and Marc R. Moon

Introduction

Primary mitral valve disease encompasses those entities where disease of the valve itself causes the pathophysiology leading to clinical impairment. Primary mitral valve disease comprises a variety of pathologies that lead to valvular regurgitation or stenosis. In the developed world, clinicians most often encounter patients with mitral regurgitation (MR). Advances in echocardiography, particularly 3D, have substantially improved the diagnosis of mitral valve pathology and quantification of lesion severity. Currently no medical therapy directed at primary MR improves the natural history of the disease, but significant progress has been made in the surgical management of primary MR where better repair techniques have decreased operative mortality and improved durability.

Clinical Presentation

Mitral Regurgitation

Acute MR is relatively uncommon, but may occur due to disruption of various parts of the mitral apparatus, including a perforated leaflet (infective endocarditis), torn chord (myxomatous disease), or ruptured papillary muscle (myocardial infarction). In the context of a left atrium (LA) and left ventricle (LV) that have not undergone adaptive changes to volume overload, this sudden substantial increase in volume is associated with a rapid increase in LV end-diastolic and LA pressure leading to pulmonary edema and respiratory distress. Reflex tachycardia helps maintain forward flow, but cardiac output is often inadequate and associated with hypotension and shock. As such, patients with acute MR can present suddenly in a severely decompensated state requiring urgent supportive care and intervention.

The key to the diagnosis of all valvular disease is the auscultation of a typical murmur on physical examination. However because of the rapid rise in LA pressure in acute MR, the typical holosystolic murmur of MR is often shortened, occurring only in early systole and also may be relatively low in intensity.

Myxomatous degeneration of the mitral valve is the leading cause of primary MR in developed countries and often is first noted on physical exam as a mid-systolic click (as the redundant valve tissue and chordae snap as the valve closes) followed by a late systolic murmur as the leaflets extend past their coaptation point. Maneuvers that decrease LV volume, i.e., Valsalva, becoming upright, etc., cause the click to occur earlier in systole and the murmur to become louder and more holosystolic. The opposite occurs with maneuvers that increase LV volume such as squatting. As the disease progresses, the murmur becomes progressively more holosystolic and when regurgitation is severe may be followed by an S3 owing to the rapid filling of the large volume of blood stored in the LA during systole.

Chronic primary MR, however, can progress slowly over many years and symptoms may develop insidiously [1]. The development of symptoms is due to a number of factors including the regurgitant volume, compensation of the LV in terms of size and systolic function, and whether there is associated pulmonary hypertension or an atrial arrhythmia. Commonly, the initial symptom is dyspnea with considerable exertion that becomes more limiting over time with less exercise. These early symptoms may be missed in older patients who are more sedentary or dismissed as attributable to aging.

B. R. Lindman (✉) · N. Quader · M. A. Sintek
Vanderbilt Medical school, Nashville, USA
e-mail: blindman@dom.wustl.edu

S. J. Melby
Cardiothoracic Surgery Division, Department of Surgery, Washington University School of Medicine, St. Louis, MO, USA

M. R. Moon
Cardiovascular Disease, Cardiothoracic Surgery, Barnes-Jewish Hospital, St. Louis, MO, USA

B. A. Carabello (ed.), *Valvular Heart Disease*, Cardiovascular Medicine, https://doi.org/10.1007/978-1-4471-2840-3_6

Mitral Stenosis

The most common cause of symptomatic mitral stenosis (MS) is rheumatic carditis, which has decreased in prevalence markedly in the developed world with the widespread availability of antibiotics [2, 3]. However this decrease began prior to antibiotic usage implicating improved socioeconomic factors in the decline in incidence. The process of inflammation, fibrosis, and calcification that occurs after rheumatic fever causes a progressive narrowing of the mitral orifice over decades. Symptom onset is insidious and related to the severity of orifice obstruction, severity of pulmonary vascular remodeling and hypertension, and patient activity level. Patients generally present with decreased exercise capacity, dyspnea on exertion, and fatigue. Other symptoms may include orthopnea, palpitations (from associated atrial arrhythmias), hemoptysis, and chest pain [3]. A systemic embolism may be the first presenting sign. Physiologic states that either increase transvalvular flow or decrease diastolic filling time (e.g., exercise, pregnancy, fever, hyperthyroidism, atrial arrhythmia) can precipitate or worsen symptoms due to increased LA pressure and transvalvular gradient. Extreme left atrial enlargement may impinge upon the left recurrent laryngeal nerve causing hoarseness (Ortners syndrome) or may cause dysphagia from compression of the esophagus.

The typical murmur of MS is a soft diastolic rumble heard best with the patient in the left lateral decubitus position. It may be accompanied by a diastolic thrill. S1 is typically loud as the valve, held open by the transmitral gradient throughout diastole, closes from the fully open (albeit stenotic) position. In very severe disease valve movement may be so limited that S1 is soft instead of loud. The diastolic rumble is usually preceded by an opening snap (OS). The interval between S2 and OS is a good guide to MS severity. In severe disease, high LA pressure opens the valve sooner than in mild disease producing a narrow S2–OS interval. If pulmonary hypertension has intervened, the pulmonic component of S2 has increased intensity and an RV lift may be palpated.

Disease Staging

The 2014 AHA/ACC guidelines on valvular heart disease shifted away from classifying the severity of valve disease into categories of mild, moderate, and severe [4, 5]. The emphasis, instead, is on a more integrative assessment of the stages of the valve disease that are more patient-centered with implications for the timing of intervention. These stages incorporate qualitative and quantitative hemodynamic assessment of the valve lesion, the response of the left and/or right ventricle to the volume or pressure overload, the effect of the valve lesion on the pulmonary circulation and heart rhythm, and patient symptoms [5]. With respect to mitral valve disease, stage A represents patients with risk factors for mitral valve disease (a history of rheumatic fever for instance); stage B represents patients with progressive mitral valve disease that is asymptomatic and not yet severe; stage C1 represents patients with severe mitral valve disease but compensated right and left ventricles, no or minimal pulmonary hypertension and no symptoms; stage C2 may be characterized by progressive ventricular enlargement and/or systolic impairment, and/or increasing pulmonary pressure, but still no symptoms; and stage D is characterized by severe mitral valve disease accompanied by symptoms and usually some combination of atrial/ventricular enlargement, impaired systolic function, pulmonary hypertension, and atrial arrhythmia [5]. Table 6.1 shows the integration of these factors for the stages of primary MR. Similarly, Table 6.2 shows the stages of MS; these characteristics are focused on rheumatic MS and, compared to prior guidelines, reflect emphasis on the hemodynamics usually associated with symptom onset.

Etiology and Classification

Mitral Regurgitation

There is a fundamental distinction between ***primary*** and ***secondary*** *MR*. Primary MR was often referred to as organic MR, whereas secondary MR (addressed in Chap. 7) was commonly described as functional MR. The two diseases have different etiologies, pathophysiology, natural history, and a different response to and indications for medical, transcatheter, and surgical therapies. Primary MR is a disease of the valve, including the leaflets, chordae tendineae, papillary muscles, or annulus. Because valve abnormalities and the regurgitation they cause ***are*** the disease, treating the valve can be curative. The most common cause of primary MR, and the most common etiology leading to surgery, is mitral valve prolapse (MVP) [1, 6]. Abnormal elongation and redundancy of the leaflets accompanied by elongation of chordae and dilatation of the annulus leads to prolapse of the valve past its coaptation point causing MR. Primary MR presents as a spectrum of lesions [7]. On one end are older patients with fibroelastic deficiency, inadequate tissue and localized pathology of a single scallop or a single chord (Fig. 6.1). At the other end of the spectrum are younger patients with excess tissue, extensive, diffuse, and marked myxomatous changes of the leaflets and chordal apparatus associated with billowing leaflets, often referred to as Barlow's disease (Fig. 6.1).

Table 6.1 Stages of primary mitral regurgitation

Grade	Definition	Valve anatomy	Valve hemodynamics[a]	Hemodynamic consequences	Symptoms
A	At risk of MR	• Mild mitral valve prolapse with normal coaptation • Mild valve thickening and leaflet restriction	• No MR jet or small central jet area <20% LA on Doppler • Small vena contracta <0.3 cm	• None	• None
B	Progressive MR	• Severe mitral valve prolapse with normal coaptation • Rheumatic valve changes with leaflet restriction and loss of central coaptation • Prior IE	• Central jet MR 20–40% LA or late systolic eccentric jet MR • Vena contracta <0.7 cm • Regurgitant volume <60 mL • Regurgitant fraction <50% • ERO <0.40 cm^2 • Angiographic grade 1–2+	• Mild LA enlargement • No LV enlargement • Normal pulmonary pressures	• None
C	Asymptomatic severe MR	• Severe mitral valve prolapse with normal coaptation • Rheumatic valve changes with leaflet restriction and loss of central coaptation • Prior IE • Thickening of leaflets with radiation heart disease	• Central jet MR >40% LA or holosystolic eccentric jet MR • Vena contracta ≥0.7 cm • Regurgitant volume ≥60 mL • Regurgitant fraction ≥50% • ERO ≥0.40 cm^2 • Angiographic grade 3–4+	• Moderate or severe LA enlargement • LV enlargement • Pulmonary hypertension may be present at rest or with exercise • C1: LVEF >60% and LVESD <40 mm • C2: LVEF ≤60% and LVESD ≥40 mm	• None
D	Symptomatic severe MR	• Same as stage C	• Same as stage C	• Moderate or severe LA enlargement • LV enlargement • Pulmonary hypertension present	• Decreased exercise tolerance • Exertional dyspnea

Adapted from [5]
Abbreviations: *ERO* effective regurgitant orifice, *IE* infective endocarditis, *LA* left atrial, *LV* left ventricular, *LVEF* left ventricular ejection fraction, *LVESD* left ventricular end-systolic dimension, *MR* mitral regurgitation
[a]Several valve hemodynamic criteria are provided for assessment of MR severity, but not all criteria for each category will be present in each patient. Categorization of MR severity as mild, moderate, or severe depends on data quality and integration of these parameters in conjunction with other clinical evidence

Secondary MR is a disease of the LV that has led to abnormal shape/structure and function that cause displacement of one or both papillary muscles, leaflet tethering and inadequate coaptation, and often annular dilatation [8, 9]. Secondary MR may result from ischemic or nonischemic ventricular disease. Because the mitral valve itself is not the origin of the disease, therapy directed only at MR may reduce regurgitation but cannot cure the basic underlying pathology.

The Carpentier classification of the types of mitral valve pathologies is commonly used today (Fig. 6.2) [10]. Type I exhibits normal leaflet motion but annular dilation or leaflet perforation. Type II is leaflet prolapse. Type III describes leaflet restriction. Type III is further divided into IIIa (restricted opening) and IIIb (restricted closing).

Mitral Stenosis

Mitral stenosis most commonly occurs as a consequence of rheumatic fever, a history of which is noted in approximately 60% of patients with pure MS [3, 5]. Significant annular calcification causing calcific MS is the next most common cause, but relatively infrequently leads to obstruction severe enough to warrant valve replacement.

Diagnosis

Imaging Assessment

Mitral Regurgitation

Two-Dimensional Transthoracic Echocardiography

Transthoracic echocardiography (TTE) is readily available and usually the initial diagnostic test to evaluate MR. The mitral valve apparatus includes the leaflets, the chordae tendineae, annulus, papillary muscles, and the insertions into the LV wall [11]. Because the diseases are so different, it is

Table 6.2 Stages of mitral stenosis

Grade	Definition	Valve anatomy	Valve hemodynamics	Hemodynamic consequences	Symptoms
A	At risk of MS	• Mitral valve doming during systole	• Normal transmitral flow velocity	• None	• None
B	Progressive MS	• Rheumatic valve changes with commissural fusion and diastolic doming of the mitral valve leaflets • Planimetered MVA >1.5 cm^2	• Increased transmitral flow velocities • MVA >1.5 cm^2 • Diastolic pressure half-time <150 ms	• Mild-moderate LA enlargement • Normal pulmonary pressure at rest	• None
C	Asymptomatic severe MS	• Rheumatic valve changes with commissural fusion and diastolic doming of the mitral valve leaflets • Planimetered MVA ≤1.5 cm^2 • MVA ≤1.0 cm^2 with very severe MS	• MVA ≤1.5 cm^2 • MVA ≤1.0 cm^2 with very severe MS • Diastolic pressure half-time ≥150 ms • Diastolic pressure half-time ≥220 ms with very severe MS	• Severe LA enlargement • Elevated PASP >30 mmHg	• None
D	Symptomatic severe MS	• Same as stage C	• Same as stage C	• Same as stage C	• Decreased exercise tolerance • Exertional dyspnea

Adapted from [5]
Abbreviations: *LA* left atrial, *LV* left ventricular, *MS* mitral stenosis, *MVA* mitral valve area, *PASP* pulmonary artery systolic pressure

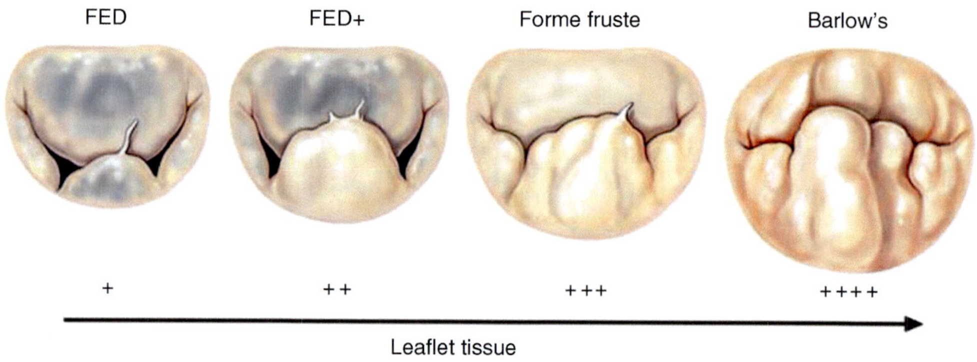

Fig. 6.1 Spectrum of degenerative/myxomatous mitral valve disease. From Adams DH, Rosenhek R, Falk V. Degenerative mitral valve regurgitation: best practice revolution. Eur Heart J. 2010;31(16):1958–1966. Reprinted with permission from Oxford University Press. *FED* fibroelastic deficiency disease

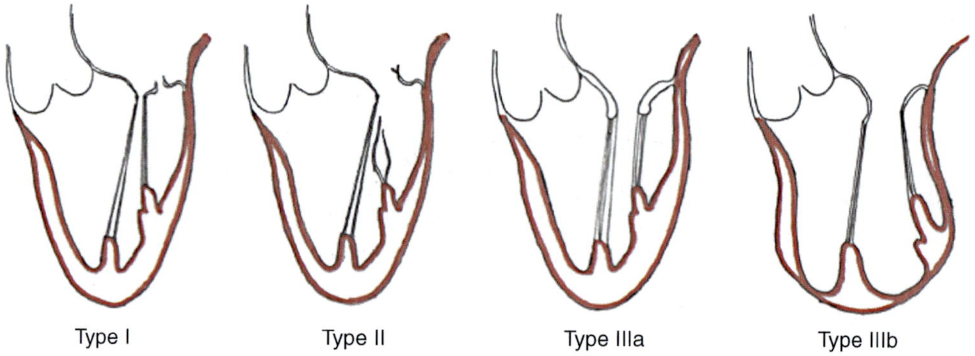

Fig. 6.2 Carpentier classification of mitral valve regurgitation. Type I exhibits normal leaflet motion but annular dilation or leaflet perforation. Type II is leaflet prolapse. Type III describes leaflet restriction. Type III is further divided into IIIa (restricted opening) and IIIb (restricted closing)

important to distinguish between primary and secondary MR, a distinction that can usually be made from two-dimensional (2D) TTE. In primary MR the diagnosis of prolapse is made on the TTE parasternal long view where the mitral leaflets are displaced >2 mm into the left atrium during systole [12]. Often, TTE can identify pathology of the specific scallops responsible for the leak. The six scallops of the mitral valve can be identified in the parasternal short axis view and color Doppler can then be used to confirm the origin of the MR jet and the scallops involved. In the parasternal long view, the A2 and P2 scallops can be visualized. The apical four chamber view allows for visualization of the A3, A2, and P1 scallops; while the TTE two chamber view displays P3, A2, P1 (Fig. 6.3). Unlike in primary MR where distinct valvular pathology is found, in secondary MR the valve itself is usually normal. Tethering of the valve by distorted LV geometry prevents leaflet coaptation causing a centrally directed jet.

TTE can provide guidance as to the feasibility of mitral valve repair by providing assessment of scallop anatomy or leaflet tethering and demonstrates the extent of mitral annular calcification. In addition to an assessment of the etiology and anatomy of the MR, TTE provides an accurate assessment of LA and LV size, LV function, and pulmonary artery pressures, all of which are important in clinical management.

Two-Dimensional Transesophageal Echocardiography

2D transesophageal echocardiography (TEE) can be used to evaluate the mitral valve apparatus and often adds important anatomical information in the assessment of mitral valve pathology in cases of moderate to severe MR. The echocardiographer should be familiar with mapping of the mitral valve using 2D TEE [13]. In the midesophageal four chamber view, typically at 0°, the tips of the leaflets are the A2 and P2 scallops. When the transducer is withdrawn slightly from the esophagus with the LV outflow tract in view, the A1 and P1 scallops are visualized. When the transducer is advanced further past the midesophageal view, the A3 and P3 scallops are then visualized. At the 60° view, also termed the bicommissural view, the scallops visualized are the P1, A2, and P3 scallops with the P1 scallop being closest to the left atrial appendage (LAA) and the P3 scallop the furthest from the LAA. Finally, at the 120° view, the A2 and P2 scallops are visualized (Fig. 6.4). Using this strategy the entire mitral valve can be visualized for the presence of prolapse and/or flail segments.

Three-Dimensional (3D) Echocardiography: Advantages and Pitfalls over 2D

Three-dimensional (3D) echocardiography has significantly improved the assessment of mitral valve disease [14]. With multiplane 2D TEE, the echocardiographer has to be familiar with the different mitral scallops and construct a map of the mitral valve to convey the valve pathology to surgeons or interventionalists. 3D TEE enables better communication between the surgeon and the echocardiographer by providing "the surgeon's view" of the mitral valve. In this view, the mitral valve is visualized from the LA perspective with the aortic valve at the 12 o'clock position (Fig. 6.5). Advances in 3D echocardiography allow for excellent spatial and temporal resolution so that a very accurate assessment of mitral valve structure, function, and dynamic changes can be recorded [15]. 3D echocardiography allows for better characterization of leaflet pathology compared to 2D TEE. Due to the saddle shape of the mitral annulus, distortion in the mitral anatomy can lead to misinterpretation of scallops with

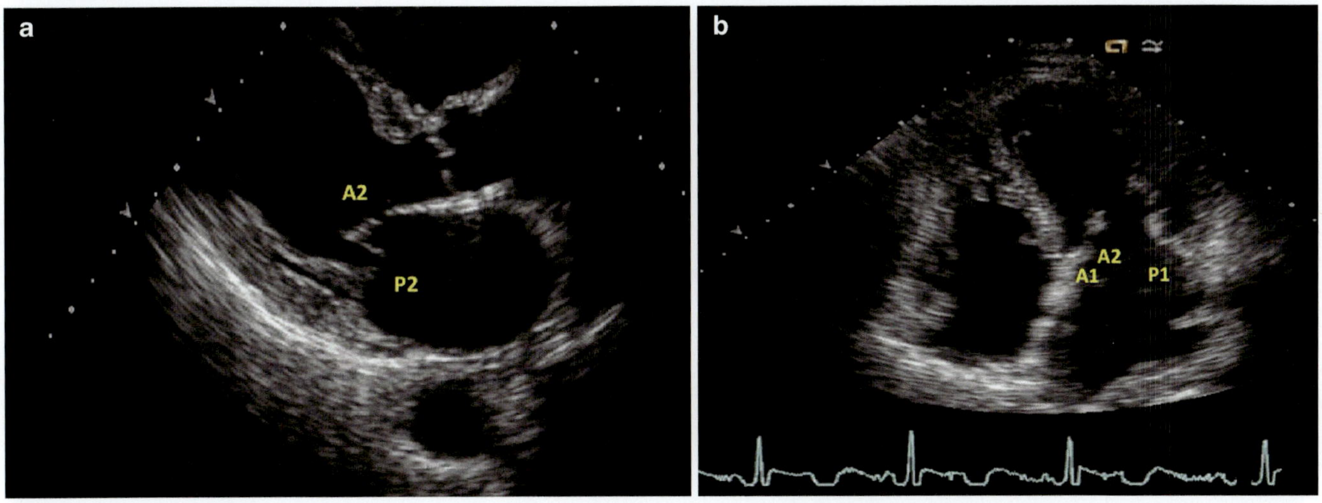

Fig. 6.3 Panel **a**: Transthoracic parasternal long axis view demonstrating the posterior leaflet prolapse. The scallops at the mitral leaflet tips are A2 and P2. Panel **b** is an apical four chamber view demonstrating the scallops seen in this view are A1, A2, and P1

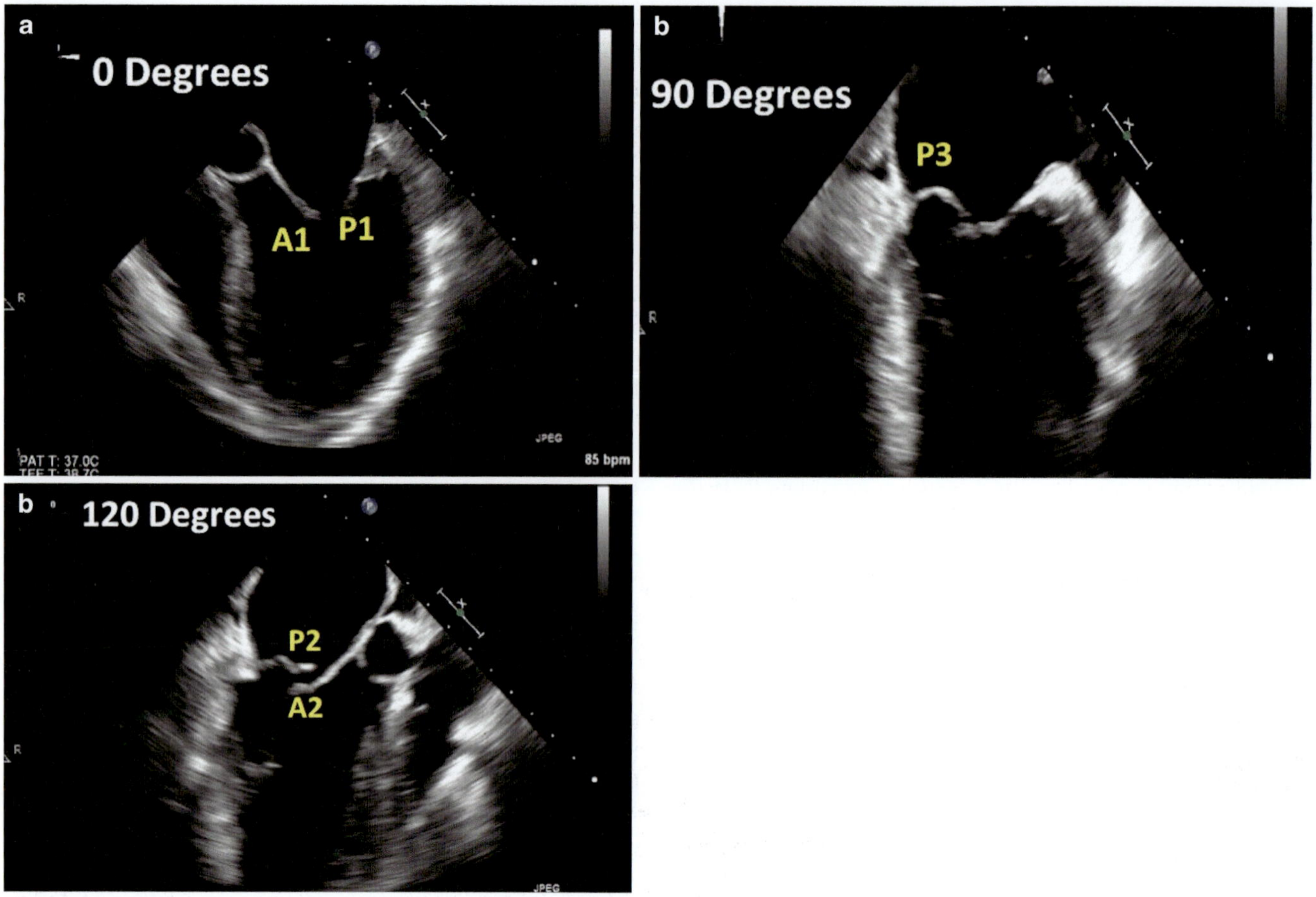

Fig. 6.4 Transesophageal echocardiogram (TEE) demonstrating the different mitral scallops. Panel **a**: at 0°, A1 and P1 scallops are seen in the high esophageal view with the left ventricular outflow tract in view. Panel **b**: at 90°, the P3 scallops is seen which appears to prolapse. Panel **c**: at 120°, A2 and P2 scallops are seen. P2 scallop is flail

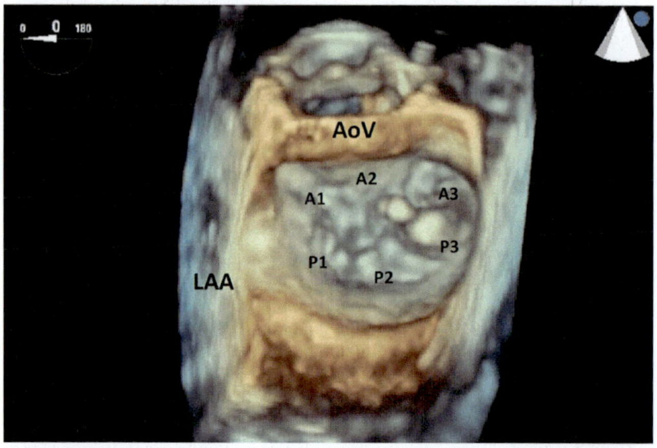

Fig. 6.5 3D echocardiogram demonstrating the mitral valve in the "surgeon's view" with the aortic valve (AoV) at the 12 o'clock location and left atrial appendage (LAA) on the lateral aspect. One can now visualize all six scallops of the mitral valve. Note that the P3 scallop prolapses and is flail

2D TEE (Fig. 6.6). In addition, 3D echocardiography allows for better characterization of lesions such as mitral clefts and commissural scallops which are not easily identifiable by 2D echocardiography alone (Fig. 6.7). Moreover 3D echo with color can identify the exact location of the regurgitant jet (Fig. 6.8).

However, 3D echocardiography has its limitations [15, 16]. It requires that the echocardiographer be familiar with image acquisition and manipulation. Errors in manipulation of the image can lead to misinterpretation of the lesions. The echocardiographer should routinely position the aortic valve at the 12 o'clock position relative to the mitral valve when using 3D TEE in mitral valve assessment. 3D echocardiography frequently involves combining several volumes of image sectors, so any patient movement or irregular heart rhythm can produce what is termed "stitch artifact" (Fig. 6.9). Finally, the echocardiographer has to be aware of image dropout, which may once again lead to misinterpretation of lesions (Fig. 6.10).

Computed Tomography and Magnetic Resonance Imaging in Assessment of Mitral Regurgitation

Computed tomography (CT) and magnetic resonance imaging (MRI) are infrequently utilized in the evaluation of the mitral valve, but can provide important, complementary

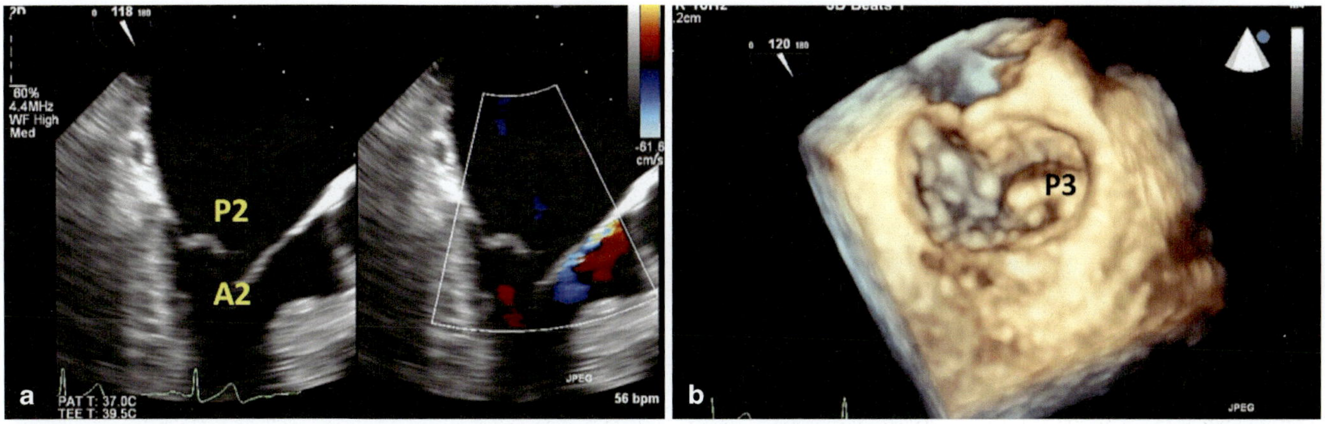

Fig. 6.6 Transesophageal echocardiogram (TEE) demonstrating that 2D TEE by itself may lead to misrepresentation of scallops. In panel **a** at 120°, the P2 scallop appears to be flail. However in panel **b** when 3D echocardiogram is utilized, it is actually the P3 scallop (which is very large) that prolapses rather than the P2 scallop

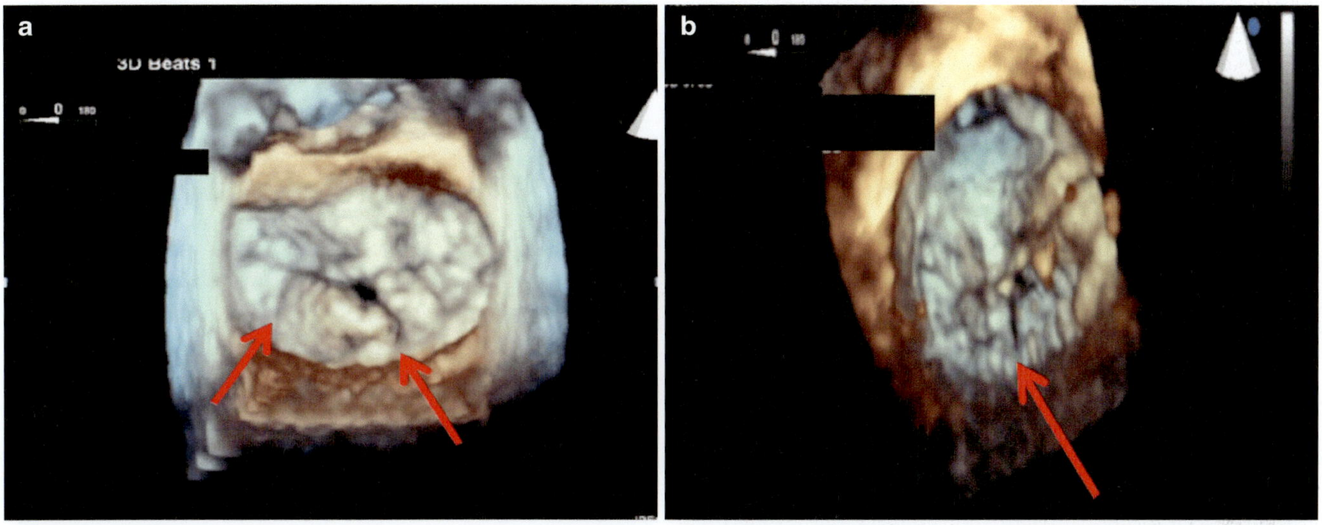

Fig. 6.7 3D echocardiography can be utilized to identify mitral clefts, which would not be seen on 2D TEE. Panel **a** demonstrates 3D of the mitral valve showing indentations between the mitral scallops (red arrows) that extend from the mitral leaflet tips to the annulus. Panel **b** demonstrates the clefts as seen from the ventricular aspect

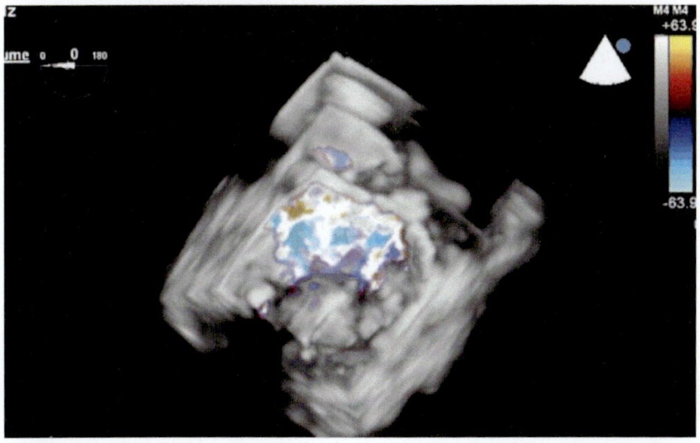

Fig. 6.8 3D echocardiography with color can be used to identify the origin of mitral regurgitation. Shown is an example of P2 prolapse. When 3D with color is used, one can visualize the mitral regurgitation originating from the P2 scallop and directed anteriorly

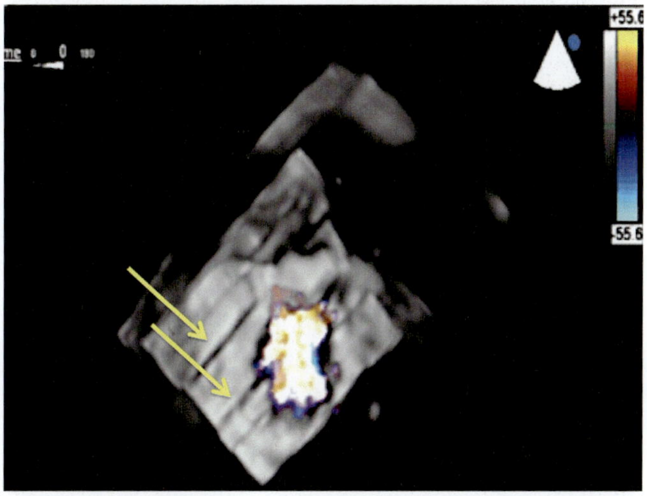

Fig. 6.9 "Stitch artifact" (yellow arrows) can occur in 3D images as a result of an irregular heart rhythm, patient movement or breathing

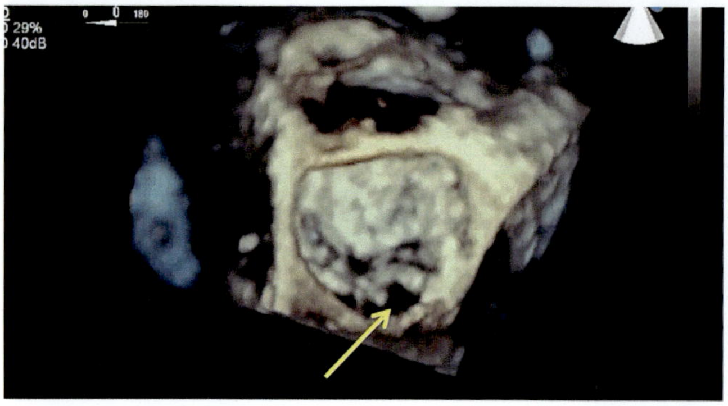

Fig. 6.10 When utilizing 3D echocardiography, the echocardiographer has to be able to differentiate echocardiographic drop out (yellow arrow) from true defects

information to echocardiography. CT can be utilized for diagnosis of mitral valve prolapse [17]. An advantage of CT over echocardiography is that it not only can help in the diagnosis of mitral valve prolapse, but also can concomitantly assess coronary anatomy [18], LV function [19, 20], and the presence of left atrial appendage thrombus [21]. CT can also be used to evaluate the extent of mitral annular calcification, which may help plan surgery and assess the feasibility of mitral repair. MRI is also useful for the assessment of MR, particularly in patients with poor echocardiographic views. MRI provides an assessment of mitral valve anatomy, quantification of MR severity, and accurate assessment of LV size and function [22].

Left Ventriculography in Assessment of Mitral Regurgitation

Left ventriculography can qualitatively assess severity of mitral regurgitation [23]. With regurgitation that is classified as mild (1+), contrast clears from the LA with one beat, and does not opacify the LA; 2+ regurgitation is classified as moderate, and contrast does not clear with one beat and faintly opacifies the entire LA; 3+ regurgitation is classified as moderate to severe, contrast opacifies the entire LA in one beat; 4+ regurgitation is classified as severe, and contrast densely opacifies the entire LA into the pulmonary veins (Fig. 6.11). The regurgitant volume can also be calculated by subtracting the stroke volume obtained by the Fick or thermodilution method from the difference between end diastolic volume and end systolic volume. Common pitfalls in the use of ventriculography in assessing MR are (1) induction of ventricular extrasystoles that can cause factitious MR and (2) injecting too little contrast to opacify both LA and LV (at least 50 cc should be injected), thereby underestimating MR severity.

Doppler Quantitation of Mitral Regurgitation

Qualitative and quantitative indices of MR severity are shown in Table 6.1 [5, 12, 24]. One of the more commonly used **qualitative** parameters is regurgitant jet area. Large jets represent a greater severity of MR than smaller jets but this method has several pitfalls. The Nyquist limit is often set too low, which (falsely) increases the jet area. Jet area may be deceptively underrepresented in acute severe MR where there is rapid rise in left atrial pressure diminishing the transvalvular driving gradient and confining MR to early systole. In addition, central jets usually appear larger than eccentric jets due to entrainment of red blood cells on either side of the jet. Thus the echocardiographer must use caution in interpreting highly eccentric jets when using color Doppler and jet area alone (Fig. 6.12).

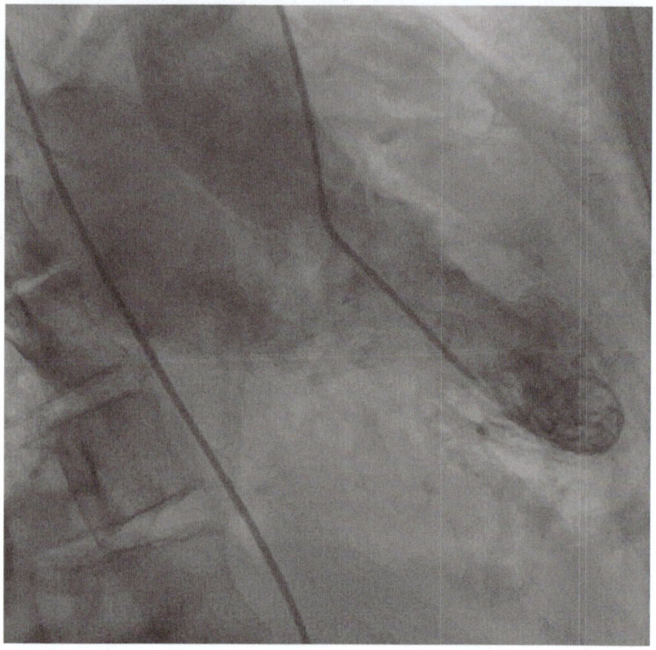

Fig. 6.11 A left ventriculogram demonstrating a hyperdynamic left ventricle with dense opacification of the left atrium in systole consistent with severe mitral regurgitation

Color Doppler can also be used to assess the size of the vena contracta, which is the narrowest portion or neck of the regurgitant jet as it crosses the mitral annular plane into the LA and reflects MR severity by implying the size of the regurgitant orifice (Fig. 6.13). One advantage of the vena contracta method is that it can be used in eccentric jets. The cutoff values for the different degrees of MR are listed in Table 6.1.

The proximal isovelocity surface area (PISA) or flow convergence method is utilized in the **quantitative** assessment of the severity of MR (Fig. 6.13). This method is based on the premise that as blood approaches a regurgitant orifice it forms hemispheric shells of increasing velocity and decreasing surface area [25]. If the Nyquist limit is known, then the area of the hemisphere, which provides an effective regurgitant orifice area (EROA), can be calculated using the formula [24, 25]:

$$\text{EROA} = \left(2\Pi r^2 * V_a\right) / \text{Pk}V_{\text{reg}}$$

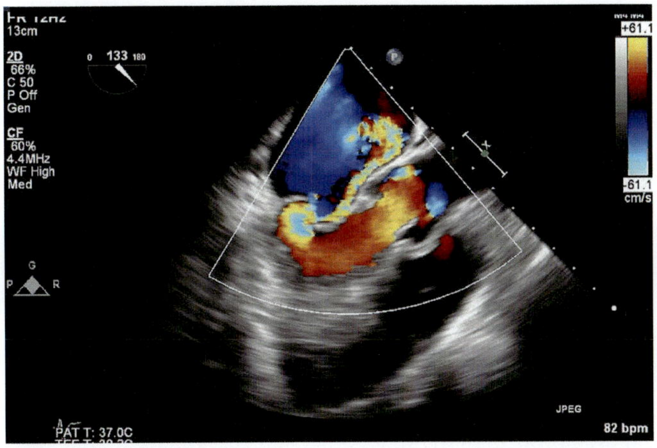

Fig. 6.12 Highly eccentric jets may lead to underestimation of the degree of mitral regurgitation not only by color Doppler but also by the PISA method. In this figure, there is a flail posterior leaflet leading to a highly eccentric jet of severe mitral regurgitation. However, color Doppler appears to underestimate the severity of MR

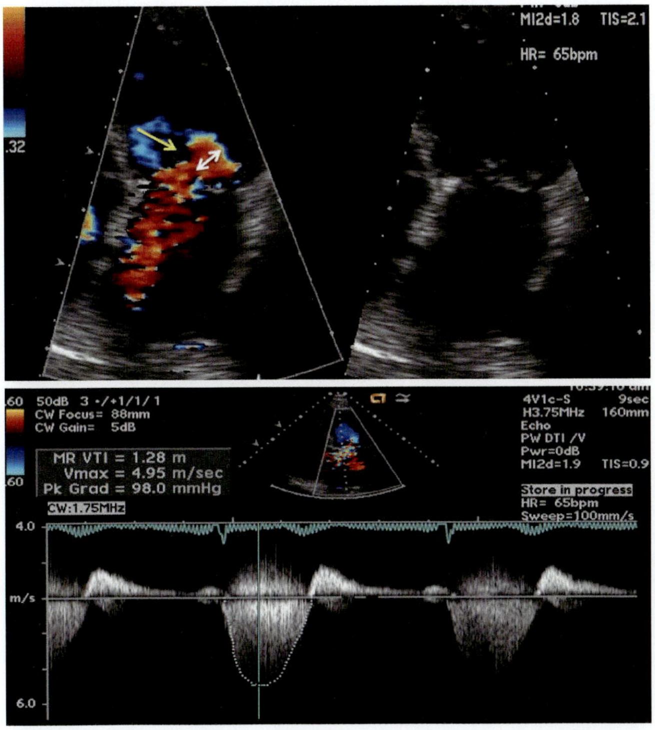

Fig. 6.13 Quantification of mitral regurgitation requires identification of the zone of flow convergence. One should identify the narrowest portion of the jet as demonstrated by the yellow arrow (vena contracta). Also, one should identify the PISA radius (white arrow) to allow for calculation of the effective regurgitant orifice area (EROA) using the PISA method. The echocardiographer should also obtain a continuous wave Doppler of the mitral regurgitation since the peak velocity and the velocity time integral are also used to calculate the EROA and the regurgitant volume

where r represents the radius of the hemisphere, V_a represents the velocity of the Nyquist limit, and PkV_{reg} represents the peak MR velocity obtained by continuous wave Doppler. A limitation of the PISA method is the need to use a correction factor if the base of the hemisphere is not a flat surface. In addition, in highly eccentric jets, 2D EROA may underestimate the severity of MR; thus, this method is more applicable to central jets. Because the true shape of the EROA may not actually be a hemisphere, 3D EROA maybe more useful in the true quantitative assessment of MR severity (Fig. 6.14) [26]. In addition, any error made in measurement of the PISA radius will lead to a substantial error in the EROA calculation because the radius is squared in the flow convergence equation.

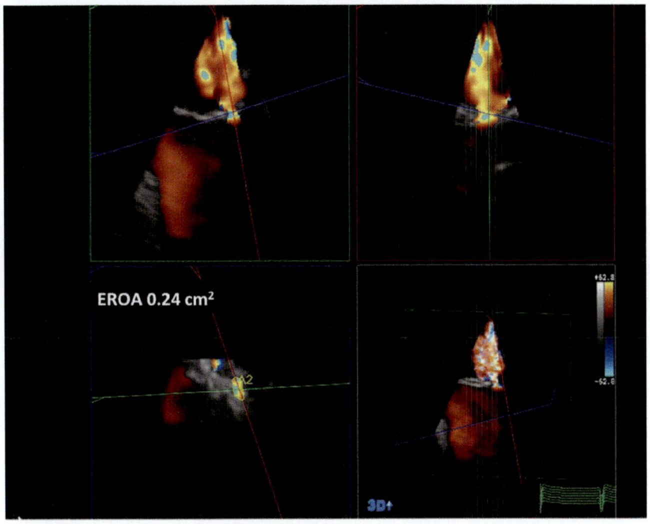

Fig. 6.14 3D echocardiography can be utilized to measure the EROA. One can align orthogonal planes to the regurgitant jet to identify the EROA. The EROA can then be traced. In this figure, the EROA can be visualized en face and reveals an area of 0.24 cm^2

Pulsed wave Doppler is another method to qualitatively assess MR severity [24]. In patients with severe MR, the E wave velocity is usually greater than 1.2 m/s; the presence of an A wave dominant mitral inflow pattern virtually excludes the presence of severe MR [27]. Pulsed wave Doppler can also be used to calculate the MR regurgitant volume and fraction using the continuity equation [25]. This method is useful when the MR jet is highly eccentric. However, since the annular measurement is a key component of the analysis, any error in its measurement can produce large errors in the calculation of the regurgitant volume and fraction.

Lastly, pulsed wave Doppler can be used to assess pulmonary vein flow. In patients with severe MR, forward systolic pulmonary vein flow can be reversed or blunted (Fig. 6.15). Caution should be used when using this method as the sole criteria for assessing MR severity since elevations in LA pressure and atrial fibrillation may also cause the systolic flow in the pulmonary vein to be blunted [25].

Common pitfalls in the echocardiographic assessment of MR severity are shown in Table 6.3.

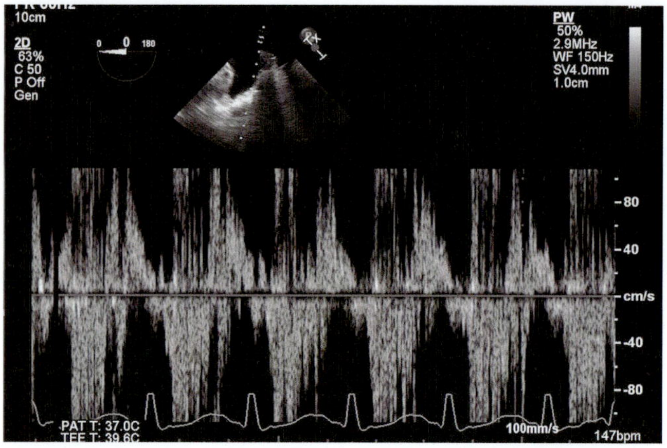

Fig. 6.15 One of the suggestive signs of severe mitral regurgitation is systolic reversal in pulmonary veins, shown here with flow below the baseline when pulse wave Doppler is placed in the pulmonary vein

Table 6.3 Common pitfalls in the echocardiographic assessment of MR severity

• Relying on color Doppler to assess the severity of MR, particularly when the Nyquist limit is too low
• Color Doppler is inadequate when jets are highly eccentric
• Quantification of MR severity can be limited with an eccentric jet or multiple jets
• Underestimating MR severity based on a TEE due to anesthesia and lower blood pressure
• EROA may not be a true hemisphere as previously thought
• Failure to recognize imaging artifacts (stitch, drop out, etc.) on 3D TEE
• Mitral gradients for MS can vary and are highly dependent on heart rate and cardiac output
• 2D TEE is limited in the diagnosis of mitral clefts or commissural scallops
• Color Doppler to assess MR severity may be deceptive in the setting of acute severe MR

Echocardiographic Evaluation of Mitral Stenosis

It is important to distinguish between calcific and rheumatic MS because it has implications for treatment strategies wherein balloon valvuloplasty is ineffective in calcific disease. Calcific MS mainly involves annular calcification and is seen in elderly patients, those with renal disease, hypertension, and atherosclerotic disease [28]. The commissures are usually spared in this disease and valve thickening, if present, predominates at the base of the leaflets while the leaflet tips are usually spared (Fig. 6.16a). This is in contrast to rheumatic MS where there is commissural fusion, chordal calcification, leaflet thickening, and calcification that predominates at the leaflet tips (Fig. 6.16b) [3].

Transthoracic Echocardiographic Evaluation of Mitral Stenosis

TTE is not only used to assess the etiology of MS (calcific versus rheumatic) but is also used to determine the severity and hemodynamic consequences of MS [25]. Continuous wave Doppler (CWD) should be used to assess peak and mean mitral gradients (Fig. 6.17). In addition, the heart rate at which the gradients are measured should be noted as tachycardia can increase the gradient. Anemia, hyperthyroidism, fever, pregnancy, or significant MR can also increase the transvalvular gradient due to increased flow.

The mitral valve area is commonly calculated from the pressure half-time ($T_{1/2}$), which is defined as the time required for the maximum pressure gradient to decrease by half of its original value. The pressure half-time is determined by measuring the slope of E wave obtained by CWD (Fig. 6.18). Mitral valve area can then be calculated by the formula [29]:

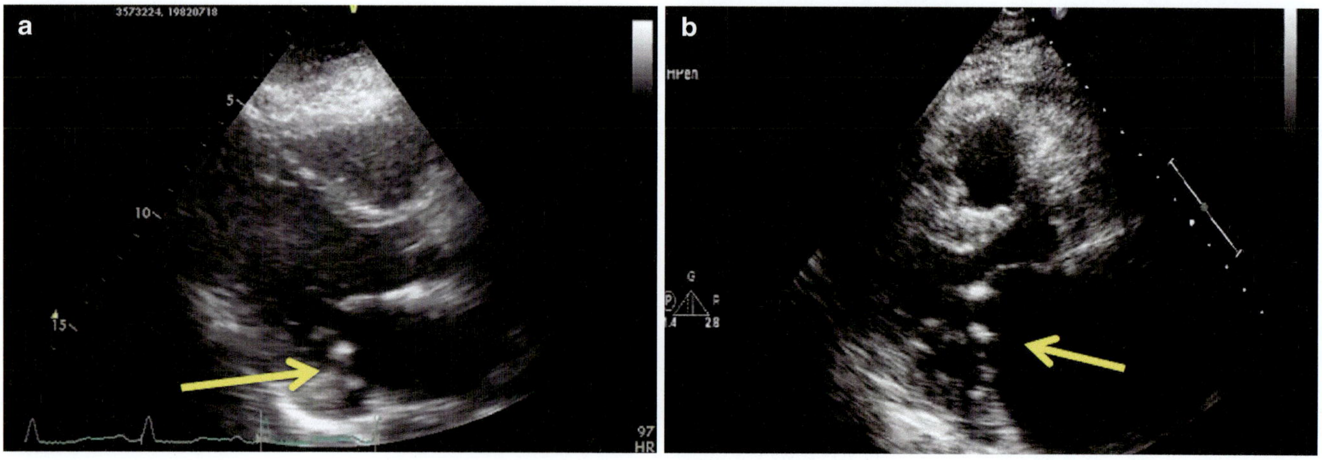

Fig. 6.16 Differentiating calcific mitral stenosis (MS) from rheumatic MS. Panel **a** demonstrates a patient with calcific MS. The arrow demonstrates the calcium at the mitral annulus which is classic for calcific MS where the leaflets are generally spared. Panel **b** demonstrates a patient with rheumatic MS with the calcification most prominent at the leaflet tips. The calcification may also extend into the subvalvular apparatus

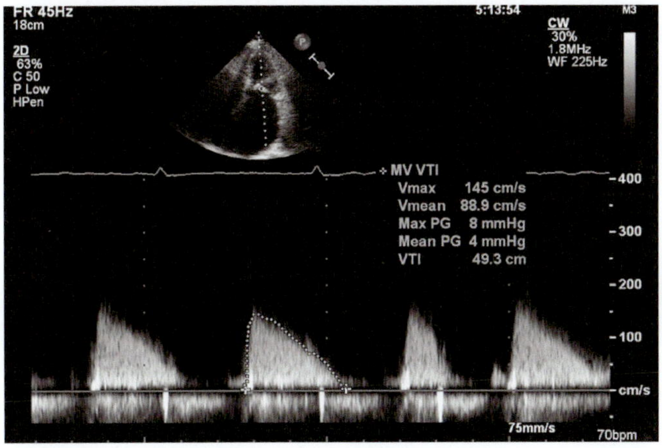

Fig. 6.17 Continuous wave Doppler should be utilized to assess mitral gradients. In this example, there was a mean mitral valve gradient of 4 mmHg

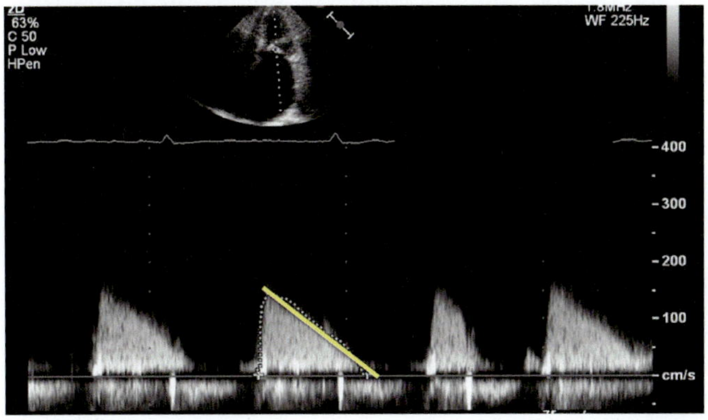

Fig. 6.18 The slope of the E wave can be measured (yellow line) which gives the deceleration time. This can be used to calculate the pressure half-time by multiplying the deceleration time by 0.29. The pressure half-time can then be used to calculate the mitral valve area

$$\mathrm{MVA} = 220 / T_{1/2}$$

where $T_{1/2}$ represents the pressure half-time. However, pressure half-time can be affected by changes in LV compliance and moderate or severe aortic regurgitation. Thus, pressure half-time should not be the sole criterion used to assess the severity of MS. In rheumatic MS, mitral valve area can also be determined by planimetry [25, 30], performed in the parasternal short axis view at the level of the mitral valve, taking care to measure at the leaflet tips (Fig. 6.19). The transmitral pressure gradient is determined by the modified Bernoulli equation and valve area can be determined using the continuity equation. This method is most accurate in the absence of mitral regurgitation. TTE is also used to assess pulmonary artery pressures since pulmonary hypertension is a known complication of significant MS.

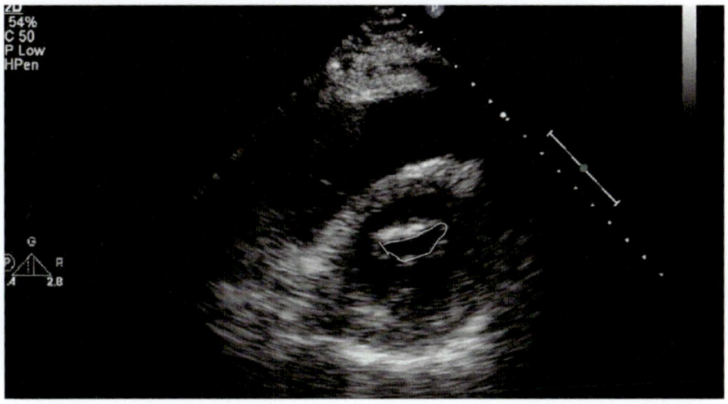

Fig. 6.19 The mitral valve area can be measured via planimetered in the parasternal short axis view

Transesophageal Echocardiography in Assessment of Mitral Stenosis

TEE is usually employed prior to balloon valvuloplasty to confirm the absence of an LA appendage thrombus, assess the degree of concomitant mitral regurgitation, better assess the degree of leaflet and subvalvular calcification and thickening [31], and develop the Wilkins score for predicting the outcome of percutaneous balloon mitral valvuloplasty [32]. In this evaluation, one to four points each is given according to ascending severity for leaflet mobility, leaflet calcification, leaflet thickening and subvalvular disease yielding a score ranging from 4–16. A score of 8 or less is predicts a suitable percutaneous valvuloplasty. In contrast, a valve with a score of 12 or more portends an unfavorable outcome. Contraindications for percutaneous balloon mitral valvuloplasty include the presence of moderate or more mitral regurgitation and the presence of a left atrial appendage thrombus. 3D TEE can also be used to assess the mitral orifice area and is more accurate than 2D planimetric measurements.

Strengths and limitations of various echocardiographic modalities for assessing MR and MS are shown in Table 6.4.

Hemodynamic Assessment

Invasive hemodynamics has been the cornerstone of our understanding of valvular heart disease [33] and has served as the gold standard for validation of modern noninvasive techniques [34]. However, given the advances in noninvasive imaging of the mitral valve and LV, hemodynamic assessment of mitral disease is performed infrequently today. Doppler echocardiography and 2D and 3D TTE and TEE are excellent for the evaluation of mitral valve pathologies and are currently considered the diagnostic tools of choice [5]. Nonetheless, invasive hemodynamic assessment of mitral valve pathologies should still be considered in patients when the clinical history and symptoms don't correlate with noninvasive assessments or when the various noninvasive modalities don't agree with each other. Invasive hemodynamics may also be of help when imaging is suboptimal or when the noninvasive hemodynamic estimates don't correlate with the visual interpretation of the echocardiographic images. Invasive hemodynamics help clarify the clinical significance of mitral valve pathology in a patient with shortness of breath and concomitant lung disease. Elevated LA and LV filling pressures support a cardiac cause of the patient's dyspnea while normal LA and LV filling pressures together with increased pulmonary artery pressure suggest a pulmonary cause. Additionally pharmacologic agents can be administered to assess reversibility of pulmonary hypertension in a patient with mitral stenosis. Because dyspnea usually occurs with exercise but not at rest, exercise hemodynamic studies can provide additional information regarding symptom causation, information that may be difficult to evaluate with noninvasive modalities. Lastly invasive studies are helpful immediately post procedure because noninvasive evaluation, especially Doppler pressure half-time derived mitral valve area, is inaccurate immediately post mitral balloon valvuloplasty [35].

Table 6.4 Strengths and limitations of various echocardiographic modalities for assessing mitral regurgitation and stenosis

	Strengths	Limitations
Mitral regurgitation		
2D TTE	• Quantify MR • Differentiate between primary and secondary MR • LA and LV size can be used as one of the parameters to assess MR severity and chronicity • Accurate assessment of LV function	• Quantification limited with eccentric jets • Quantification limited in the presence of multiple jets • Severity can be underestimated in acute severe MR • Detailed assessment of scallop/leaflet anatomy for primary MR is often not feasible
2D TEE	• Detailed assessment of scallop/leaflet anatomy for primary MR • Quantify MR if TTE views are poor	• More invasive procedure with sedation • Sedation ± lower blood pressure can misleadingly decrease the MR severity
3D TEE	• Integrated view of the valve pathology as a whole to guide surgical planning • Detection of mitral clefts	• Requires an experienced echocardiographer • Unreliable if 2D image quality is poor
Mitral stenosis		
2D TTE	• Differentiate rheumatic from calcific MS • Planimeter mitral valve area • Measure LA size • Measure transvalvular gradient and pulmonary pressure	• Excessive calcification and shadowing artifact may limit the assessment of leaflet and subvalvular thickness and calcification
2D TEE	• Accurate assessment of leaflet and subvalvular mobility, thickness, and calcification • Evaluate for LA thrombus and MR severity	• Sedation, hemodynamic changes, and angulation may alter the transvalvular mean gradient
3D TEE	• Planimeter mitral valve area more accurately than 2D	• Requires a stable rhythm; atrial fibrillation is a common occurrence in mitral stenosis

Abbreviations: *MR* mitral regurgitation, *LA* left atrium, *LV* left ventricle, *TTE* transthoracic echocardiography, *MS* mitral stenosis, *2D* two-dimensional

Mitral Stenosis

Mitral stenosis is probably the most common mitral valve pathology for which a clinician might pursue invasive hemodynamic assessment. Severe MS produces an LA/LV diastolic gradient without diastasis. The pulmonary capillary wedge pressure (PCWP) is commonly used as a surrogate for left atrial pressure and a pigtail catheter is used to cross the aortic valve to assess LV pressure (Fig. 6.20). These standard measurements provide the diastolic gradient from PCWP to LV and help judge stenosis severity with reasonable accuracy [36]. The gradient measurement from the LA to LV is critical to the calculation of the mitral valve area but using the PCWP as a surrogate for direct LA pressure measurement has pitfalls. PCWP waveforms are delayed by 40–120 ms relative to the LA waveforms and proper gradient assessment requires phase shifting the PCWP waveform back such that the V wave intersects the downslope of the LV pressure tracing (Fig. 6.20) [37].

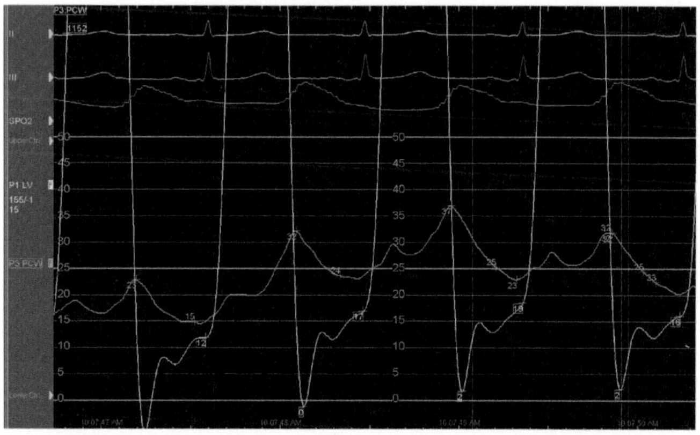

Fig. 6.20 Simultaneous LV (yellow) and PCWP (green) pressure tracings at 100 mm/s recording speed in a patient being evaluated for mitral stenosis. The PCWP pressure tracing has been phase shifted such that the V wave intersects the downslope of the LV pressure tracing. Note the absence of diastasis in the LV tracing and the significant gradient during diastole between the PCWP and the LV such that the PCWP is always higher than the LV pressure; both features of significant mitral stenosis

Operators should also obtain a blood aspirate demonstrating highly oxygenated LA blood from the catheter to prove that the catheter is truly wedged [36]. PCWP should not be used as a surrogate for LA pressure in cases of veno-occlusive disease or when there is any doubt about the quality of the PCWP tracing. In such cases the transvalvular gradient is evaluated by simultaneous measurement of the LV and LA via trans-septal puncture. Modern computer software computes the area delineated by the diastolic PCWP and LV waveforms to obtain the mean gradient; 5 cardiac cycles should be averaged for patients in sinus rhythm (Fig. 6.21). Atrial fibrillation is common in patients with MS and the variability in diastolic filling time greatly affects the mean gradient. Thus 10 cycles should be averaged in patients with atrial fibrillation (Fig. 6.22).

Traditionally, the Gorlin formula has been used to derive the mitral valve area and requires measurement of the diastolic filling period and the cardiac output (Table 6.5) [38, 39]. Hakki proposed a simpler formula to determine the area of a stenotic valve and showed an excellent correlation to mitral valve area calculated by the Gorlin formula (Table 6.5) [40]. Both formulas still rely on the planimetric assessment of the gradient between the LA and LV during diastole, which can be cumbersome without the aid of software programs. Cui proposed a simpler determination of the mean transvalvular gradient that estimates mean LV diastolic pressure as left ventricular end diastolic pressure/2 and showed excellent correlation with the gradient determined by the standard planimetric approach [41]. Additionally, this method allows for determination of mitral valve area by simple pullback from the LV to LA, potentially making arterial puncture unnecessary when trans-septal catheterization is employed. Importantly, the Cui method requires measurement of mean LA pressure and it should be used with caution in patients with tachycardia as this may violate the assumption of LV waveform morphology underlying Cui's simplification. However since invasive hemodynamics are usually employed only when the diagnosis is unclear and because an error in gradient calculation of as

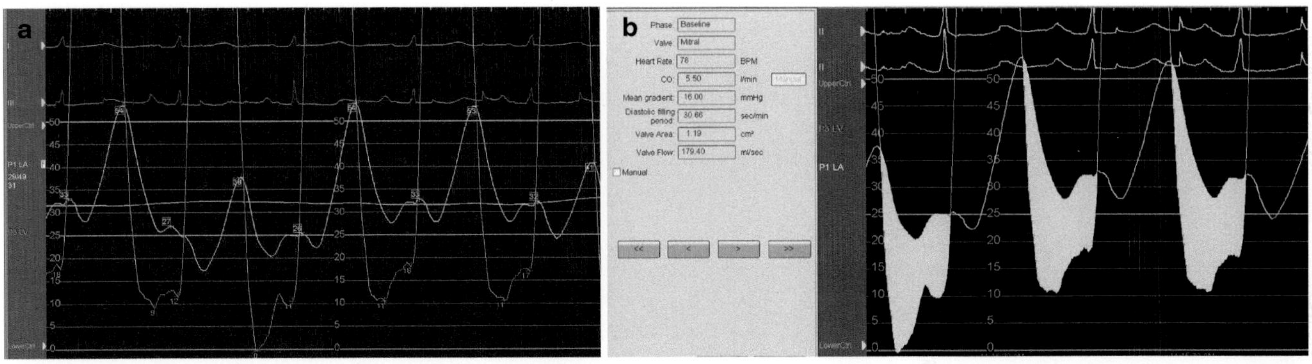

Fig. 6.21 Simultaneous LV (red) and LA (yellow) pressure tracings at 100 mm/s recording speed in a patient being evaluated for balloon mitral valvuloplasty. Gradient assessment using the Gorlin formula and computer software

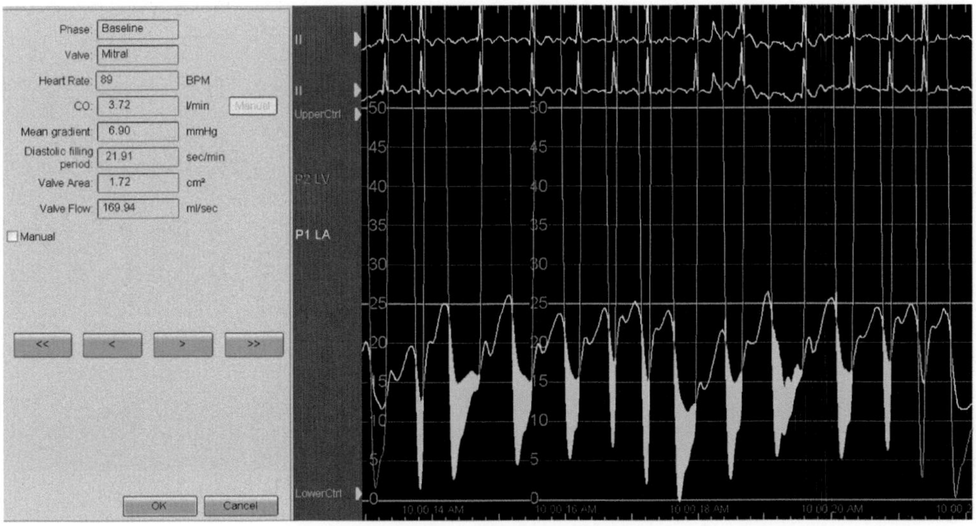

Fig. 6.22 Simultaneous LV (red) and LA (yellow) pressure tracings at 25 mm/s recording speed in a patient after balloon mitral valvuloplasty and in atrial fibrillation. Notice the significant difference in area for each traced diastole. All shaded diastolic areas were averaged and the valve area was calculated according to the Gorlin formula as shown

little as 3 mmHg might change management, all effort should be made to determine the actual LA-LV gradient.

Mitral Regurgitation

Although more common than MS, MR is not commonly evaluated with invasive hemodynamic measures. When non-invasive imaging of MR severity is not clear, left ventriculography in addition to hemodynamic assessments can be performed. Severe MR should be considered when a V wave noted in the PCWP or LA pressure tracing is two times the higher than the mean PCWP while a V wave three times the mean PCWP is specific for severe MR [42]. Ventricular afterload, LA compliance and LV dysfunction can all affect the size of the V wave independent of mitral valve pathology and, as such, the absence of a V wave should not be used to rule out significant MR [43]. The ratio of the V wave to the total LV diastolic area may also be helpful in grading mitral regurgitation but is largely unavailable outside the catheterization laboratory [44]. Figure 6.23 shows an LA pressure tracing before and after a MitraClip (Abbott Vascular) procedure where a prominent V wave nearly disappears after the MR is corrected. Although somewhat rare, a prominent V wave that subsides spontaneously should trigger an evaluation for ischemic papillary muscle dysfunction as transient MR may not be evident on noninvasive imaging unless ischemia is provoked. Finally, invasive hemodynamic evaluation can provide some insight into the chronicity of MR. Acute or decompensated MR usually produces a very prominent V wave and steep Y descent signaling a very high LA pressure. In contrast, chronic compensated MR may demonstrate elevated filling pressure but with a relatively small V wave as atrial compliance has had time to increase, compensating for the chronic volume load.

Table 6.5 Formulas for hemodynamic calculations for mitral stenosis

Gorlin formula	MVA = (CO/DFP) ∗ HR, where 37.6 = Gorlin's *K* constant (44.3) ∗ 0.85 37.6 ∗ $\sqrt{\text{MVG}}$
Hakki formula	MVA = CO/$\sqrt{\text{MVG}}$
Cui method	MVG = Mean LA pressure – (LVEDP/2)

MVA mitral valve area (cm^2), *MVG* mean mitral valve gradient (mmHg), *CO* cardiac output (L/min), *DFP* diastolic filling period/time from MV open to closure (s), *LA* left atrial (mmHg), *LV* left ventricle (mmHg)

Medical Therapy

Mitral Regurgitation

Acute severe MR generally requires urgent/emergent surgical therapy. As a temporizing measure, intravenous vasodilator therapy with nitroprusside or hydralazine may reduce the regurgitant volume (thus, reducing pulmonary edema) and improving forward flow [45–47]. Temporary percutaneous mechanical support with intra-aortic balloon counterpulsation or the Impella (Abiomed) catheter may also be considered to stabilize the patient prior to definitive treatment. For those with suspected infective endocarditis as the cause of the acute MR, antibiotics should be administered immediately after blood cultures have been obtained.

For chronic primary MR with preserved LV function, there is currently no indication for medical therapy directed at the MR to improve clinical outcomes. While it would seem reasonable that vasodilator therapy would lessen LV afterload resulting in a decreased MR, less LV volume overload, and presumably a more favorable natural history, small studies testing this hypothesis have shown little or no benefit [48–50]. Accordingly, vasodilator therapy is not indicated for normotensive asymptomatic patients with primary MR [5]. An early phase clinical study suggested potential benefits for LV func-

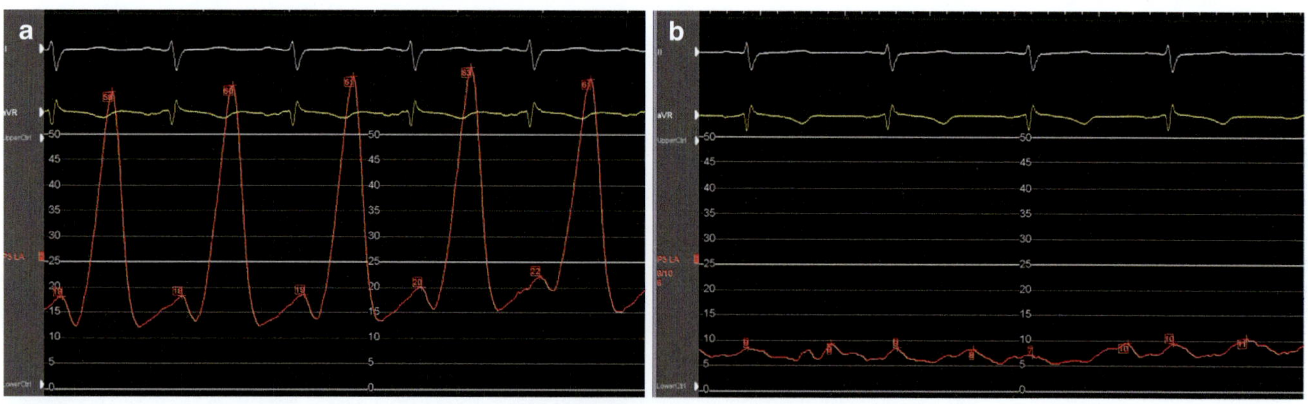

Fig. 6.23 The LA pressure tracing in a patient with a P3 flail mitral leaflet and severe MR. She underwent a successful MitraClip (Abbott Vascular) procedure with near resolution of her MR. As exhibited in the post clip tracing, the large V wave resolved and now resembles a more normal LA tracing

tion in patients with chronic MR treated with ß1-receptor blockade and a preclinical study raised the possibility of benefit from the phosphodiesterase type 5 inhibitor sildenafil [51, 52]. Further studies are needed to identify if medical therapy will slow the natural history and improve patient outcomes for those with significant primary MR. Despite the lack of a role for medical therapy for normotensive patients with chronic primary MR, hypertension should be treated per guideline recommendations given the known morbidity and mortality associated with uncontrolled hypertension.

Chronic secondary MR is characterized by LV dysfunction either due to myocardial infarction or nonischemic cardiomyopathy. As such, it is appropriate to treat such patients with guideline-directed medical therapy for heart failure, including ß-blockers, angiotensin converting enzyme inhibitors or angiotensin receptor blockers, and aldosterone antagonists [5].

Mitral Stenosis

Secondary prevention of rheumatic fever is indicated for patients with rheumatic MS (see Chap. 2 for details) [5]. Atrial arrhythmia occurs in 30–40% of patients with severe MS [3, 5]. Because of significant LA enlargement and fibrosis that can occur with severe MS, rhythm control is often ineffective and therapy is directed toward rate control. Atrial fibrillation with a rapid ventricular response can be particularly problematic for patients with MS as the decreased diastolic filling time increases LA pressure and causes or exacerbates shortness of breath. Negative dromotropic agents can be used to slow the ventricular response. Because of great stroke risk, anticoagulation with vitamin K antagonists is indicated for patients with MS and (1) an atrial arrhythmia (regardless of whether it is paroxysmal, persistent, or permanent); (2) prior embolic stroke; or (3) a LA thrombus [5].

Surgical Therapy

Indications for Mitral Valve Surgery

Mitral Regurgitation

As surgical outcome has improved over time, indications for surgery have become progressively more liberal. In the past when operative mortality for mitral valve replacement was high, patients were treated medically even for symptomatic MR. However today's mortality rates for patients with preserved LV function who undergo mitral valve repair for MR is less than 1% with 5-year mortality from cardiac causes less than 5% [53]. The AHA/ACC recommendations for surgical intervention for primary MR are shown in Table 6.6 [5]. Mitral valve surgery is indicated for symptomatic patients with chronic severe primary MR and LV ejection fraction >30%. Mitral valve surgery is recommended for asymptomatic patients with chronic severe primary MR and LV dysfunction or dilation (LV ejection fraction 30–60% and/or LV end-systolic dimension ≥40 mm). The guidelines emphasize the importance of valve repair over replacement for primary MR, recognizing that repair is much less satisfactory for rheumatic valvulopathy. They also emphasize the performance of mitral valve repair at centers of excellence by high volume surgeons

Table 6.6 ACC/AHA recommendations for surgical intervention for primary MR

Level I	• Symptomatic patients with chronic severe primary MR (stage D) and LVEF >30% • Asymptomatic patients with chronic severe primary MR and LV dysfunction (LVEF 30–60% and/or LVESD ≥40 mm, stage C2) • Repair is recommended in preference to replacement when surgical treatment is indicated for patients with chronic severe primary MR limited to the posterior leaflet • Repair is recommended in preference to MVR when surgical treatment is indicated for patients with chronic severe primary MR involving the anterior leaflet or both leaflets when a successful and durable repair can be accomplished • Concomitant MV repair or replacement is indicated in patients with chronic severe primary MR undergoing cardiac surgery for other indications
Level IIa	• Repair is reasonable in asymptomatic patients with chronic severe primary MR (stage C1) with preserved LV function (LVEF >60% and LVESD <40 mm) in whom the likelihood of a successful and durable repair without residual MR is >95% with an expected mortality rate of <1% when performed at a Heart Valve Center of Excellence • Repair is reasonable for asymptomatic patients with chronic severe nonrheumatic primary MR (stage C1) and preserved LV function in whom there is a high likelihood of a successful and durable repair with (1) new onset of AF or (2) resting pulmonary hypertension (PA systolic arterial pressure >50 mmHg) • Concomitant MV repair is reasonable in patients with chronic moderate primary MR (stage B) undergoing cardiac surgery for other indications
Level IIb	• May be considered in symptomatic patients with chronic severe primary MR and LVEF ≤30% (stage D) • Repair may be considered in patients with rheumatic mitral valve disease when surgical treatment is indicated if a durable and successful repair is likely or if the reliability of long-term anticoagulation management is questionable • Transcatheter MV repair may be considered for severely symptomatic patients (NYHA class III/IV) with chronic severe primary MR (stage D) who have a reasonable life expectancy but a prohibitive surgical risk because of severe comorbidities

Adapted from [5]

Abbreviations: *AF* atrial fibrillation, *COR* class of recommendation, *LV* left ventricular, *LVEF* left ventricular ejection fraction, *LVESD* left ventricular end-systolic dimension, *MR* mitral regurgitation, *MV* mitral valve, *MVR* mitral valve replacement, *NYHA* New York Heart Association, *PA* pulmonary artery who have a high successful valve repair rate at a low mortality rate. The skill and experience of the surgeon and center is particularly important for more complicated valve pathology (e.g., anterior or bileaflet prolapse). In excellent hands mitral repair returns survival to that of normal subjects [54]. However variability in repair rate can vary from 0% to 90% for individual surgeons [55].

Significant debate surrounds the question of whether to offer surgery to asymptomatic patients with severe primary MR and preserved LV function versus close observation and surgery when symptoms or early LV dysfunction is detected [56–59]. In this regard, the AHA/ACC guidelines indicate that performance of mitral repair is reasonable in the asymptomatic patient with severe primary MR and preserved LV function especially when there is new onset atrial fibrillation or pulmonary hypertension and when there is a high likelihood of successful and durable repair. The triggers for surgery connoting LV dysfunction are an ejection fraction of ≤60% and or an LV end systolic dimension of ≥40 mm [5]. However the 2017 ACC/AHA focused update of the valve guidelines indicates that it is not necessary to wait until these thresholds are reached to opt for surgery, especially if longitudinal studies indicate progression toward those triggers [60]. In the absence of new onset atrial fibrillation or pulmonary hypertension, the guidelines indicate that it is reasonable to perform mitral repair in the asymptomatic patient with severe primary MR when the likelihood of a successful and durable repair without residual MR is >95% with an expected mortality rate of <1% and when it is performed at a valve center of excellence [5, 60]. It must be emphasized that the guideline does not mean the center (or surgeon) must repair 95% of all mitral valves operated. It means that there is a 95% chance of repair of the particular valve in question by that specific surgeon, a highly likely outcome, for instance for P2 prolapse.

Mitral Stenosis

The first recorded surgery for an intra-cardiac correction was for MS, a relatively common condition in the late 1800s and early 1900s following rheumatic fever. Sir Thomas Lauder Brunton from Scotland, opined in 1902 that the mitral valve might be surgically repaired, and Dr. Elliott Cutler at Harvard Medical School in Boston accomplished the first recorded mitral operation in 1923 by using a neurosurgical tenotomy knife through a ventricular incision to open the fused commissures [61]. A few years later, in 1925, Henry Souttar, a British surgeon, successfully fractured the stenotic mitral valve using his finger through a hole in the LA appendage and relieved the stenosis of a young woman. His contemporary physicians did not think the procedure safe and he received no further referrals, despite the survival of his patient [62]. Subsequent attempts by the group at Harvard had only a single survivor (the first out of a sequence of 10) and the procedure was abandoned. It was not until 1948 when several surgeons independently employed the same or similar techniques to relieve mitral stenosis that the surgical world was transformed and cardiac surgery became a reality [63–66].

Mitral valve intervention is generally recommended for patients with severe MS (mitral valve area [MVA] ≤1.5 cm^2) and symptoms or, in the absence of symptoms, when cardiac surgery will be performed for another indication [5]. In the asymptomatic patient with MVA ≤1.5 cm^2, intervention would be reasonable when there is very severe MS (MVA ≤1.0 cm^2) or a concomitant atrial arrhythmia or significant pulmonary hypertension [5].

Today, for patients with rheumatic MS, standard corrective treatment follows the same principles as the earlier surgical commissurotomy although the approach is less invasive: percutaneous balloon valvuloplasty is now the primary mode of intervention for these patients when pathology is suitable for this approach (see Chap. 8) [5, 32, 67, 68]. When anatomy is not suitable for the percutaneous approach, or if a patient must undergo surgery for another cardiac pathology, open mitral valve commissurotomy or, more commonly, valve replacement is performed [5].

Mitral Valve Anatomy for the Surgeon

The two leaflet valve is a complex structure, and disturbance of any part of the apparatus can result in regurgitation. The components of the valve are: the two leaflets (anterior, posterior), the annulus, the chordae, the two papillary muscles, and the LV wall. The leaflets are scalloped into thirds, conventionally labeled A1, A2, and A3 for the anterior leaflet and P1, P2, and P3 for the posterior leaflet (Fig. 6.24), and these designations are used for operative planning and intervention. The fibrous trigone is a continuation of tissue of the anterior leaflet of the mitral valve and

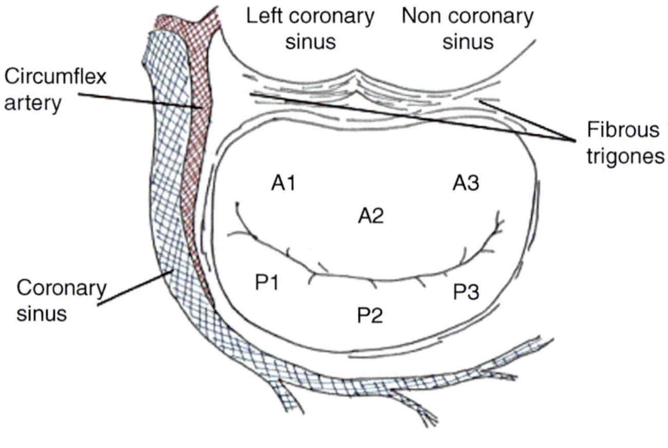

Fig. 6.24 Anatomy of the mitral valve

is contiguous with the aortic valve (including the left and non-coronary leaflets) and contributes importantly to the fibrous skeleton of the heart. Because of this fibrous construction, it has been widely held that this portion of the annulus is preserved from dilatation in pathologic states, which allows for successful annuloplasty with a partial ring or band. There is limited data which suggests that some dilatation may occur [69]. The left and right fibrous trigones are used to anchor sutures for annuloplasty or valve replacement superiorly. Approximately 40% of the annulus is accounted for by these trigones (contiguous with the mitral valve anterior leaflet) while the remaining 60% of the annulus is along the posterior leaflet attachment.

The chordae tendineae, string-like fibrous connective tissue which attach the leaflets to the ventricular wall, are important supporting structures consisting of both primary chordae (attached to the edge of the leaflet) and secondary chordae (attached to the underside of the leaflets between the edge and the annulus). Each of the papillary muscles (anterolateral and posteromedial) has chordae which attach to both leaflets. The surgeon can make use of the intact chordae from one leaflet to support a flail portion of the other by transferring a section of the leaflet with intact chordae (chordal transfer, almost exclusively from posterior leaflet to anterior leaflet). The posterior leaflet also has tertiary chordae which attach directly from the underside of the valve to the ventricular wall. The blood supply to the anterolateral papillary muscle typically comes from the left anterior descending and the circumflex arteries, while the posteromedial papillary muscle is usually supplied by only a posterior descending artery or branch of the circumflex, which makes it more susceptible to ischemia, infarction, and rupture.

Leaflet redundancy can cause increased leaflet stress and increased systolic movement into the atrium (prolapse) of the affected leaflet leading to decreased coaptation and regurgitation. The increased systolic stress on abnormal leaflets can cause rupture of weakened chordae worsening regurgitation. Any of these pathologic states may be present, requiring surgical attention to annular dilatation (usually addressed by annuloplasty), excess leaflet tissue (resection), and/or ruptured chordae (resection or chordal repair/replacement). Today, the mainstay of surgical intervention of myxomatous disease is repair (as opposed to replacement), as excellent outcomes have been achieved with advanced techniques. Even in valves with extensive myxomatous changes, or *Barlow's valves* [70, 71], good results from repair with resection of redundant valve tissue and chordal replacement can be achieved [72].

Important structures to be aware of (and avoided) for the surgeon also include the atrioventricular node superiomedially and aortic valve leaflets and root superiorly. Although not a part of the valve per se, the coronary sinus runs adjacent to the posterior annulus and the circumflex artery courses near A1, P1, and P2 (Fig. 6.24).

Mitral Valve Repair

As repair of the mitral valve should be accomplished in the vast majority of cases, the surgeon's understanding of the techniques and limitations is imperative. One of the most common indications for surgery in a patient with a myxomatous valve is isolated prolapse of the middle scallop of the posterior leaflet (P2) and a dilated annulus and the AHA/ACC guidelines note that planned mitral valve replacement of simple P2 prolapse is no longer acceptable therapy [5]. Quadrangular resection of the prolapsing segment (often found with a ruptured chordae on the segment) with ring or band annuloplasty has been the mainstay of treatment [73]. Simplification of the resection by substitution of a triangular resection (instead of quadrangular resection which requires leaflet advancement) is effective and eliminates the need for disconnection of the leaflet. In the majority of cases, this simple repair technique, coupled with an annuloplasty, will eliminate the mitral regurgitation (Fig. 6.25).

Ensuring that the coaptation area along the leaflets after repair is sufficient is key in eliminating MR; typically five

a

b

c

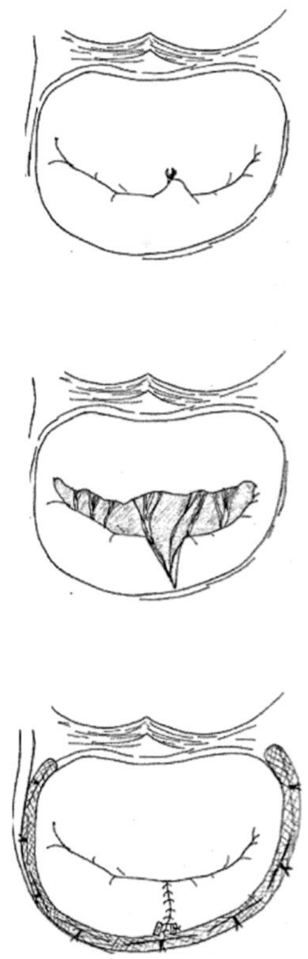

Fig. 6.25 Triangular resection and repair of a typical P2 prolapse. Prolapsed segment of P2 with typical chordal rupture (**a**). Resection of prolapsed segment (**b**). Completed repair with annuloplasty band (**c**)

millimeters will ensure an adequate area of support for the valve during systole. The surgeon must be facile with testing methods in the operating room after completion of the repair to ensure adequacy of repair and to help prevent unnecessary additional cross-clamp time for revision.

As annuloplasty became increasingly important in the repair of mitral valves, several devices became available to facilitate the procedure. Multiple choices exist but the most common include rigid or flexible full circumferential rings (buttressing the entire annulus) and rigid or flexible partial bands (buttressing the posterior annulus, leaving the fibrous trigone section untethered). Sizing of the ring is accomplished by measurement of the height or area of the anterior leaflet. Excellent results have been reported with both full and partial rings. The decision to implant a flexible versus rigid or full ring versus partial band is generally left up to the surgeon based on familiarity with the device and assessment of the fibrous trigone to predict the possibility of future annular enlargement.

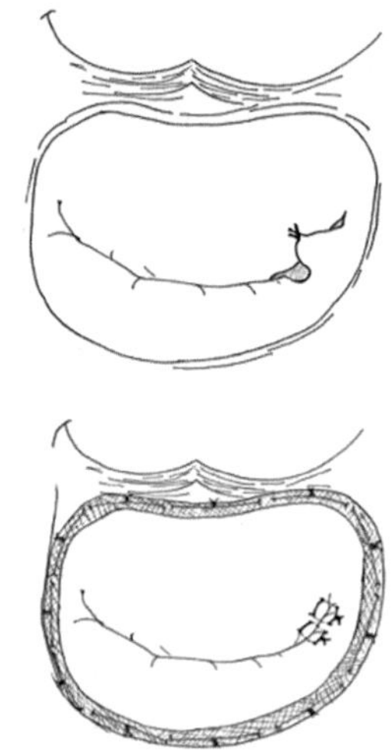

Fig. 6.26 P3 rupture repair. Typical flail P3 segment with chordal rupture (**a**). Repaired segment with edge to edge closure of defect and annuloplasty ring (**b**)

Complex Repairs: Chordal Replacement or Transfer

Replacement of chordae can be accomplished by creation of neochordae (typically using polytetrafluoroethylene, or PTFE sutures) or by chordal transfers. These methods are generally reserved for ruptured chordae other than P2 or elongated chordae. Measurement of adjacent chordae can be used to recreate the neo-chord optimal length or pre-measured lengths of suture material can be used. Both anterior and posterior chordae can be replaced. Likewise chordal transfer is a useful technique in instances where adjacent leaflet tissue can be resected (where it would not compromise valve function) and a chordae transferred to the pathologic leaflet. In this manner, the natural chordal length is ensured. The most common and effective chordal transfer involves moving an intact P2 chordae to an area of ruptured chordae on A2. Chordal shortening techniques have also been employed when chordae are intact but the leaflet edge is prolapsed, although most surgeons have gravitated toward chordal replacement in this setting based on the perception of improved durability. A typical P3 rupture can be repaired with or without resection of the posterior flail portion of the leaflet and closure of the portion of the commissure closest to the annulus with inversion of leaflet edges, followed by annuloplasty (Fig. 6.26).

Edge-to-Edge Apposition or "Alfieri" Stitch

The "Alfieri stitch" or "edge-to-edge" apposition stitch that sutures the bellies of the two leaflets together can be used when other methods fail [74]. This stitch creates a double orifice valve. Good results of this technique when coupled with annuloplasty have been reported, although long-term results of the technique without annuloplasty have been unsatisfactory [75, 76]. Concern for creating a non-physiologic state without maintenance of the normal bileaflet anatomy has precluded widespread use, and currently this procedure is limited to application in high-risk patients or as a rescue procedure when standard techniques fail. The Alfieri principle is the basis of percutaneous edge-to-edge repair [77, 78].

Intraoperative Echocardiography

Intraoperative echocardiography is essential for successful mitral surgery by defining the valve pathoanatomy, planning the operation and confirming the achievement of good results or the need for repair revision after native circulation has returned. TEE is indicated in every case unless contraindicated for esophageal anatomic reasons [5]. The decision to operate on the mitral valve is based upon preoperative assessment of MR under normal resting conditions. Because anesthesia greatly alters LV loading and MR severity, assessment of MR severity from intraoperative TEE should never override the preoperative decision that had been based on conscious pathophysiology.

Mitral Valve Replacement

Although mitral valve repair should supplant replacement in most cases of myxomatous disease, there are situations in which a valve replacement becomes necessary, especially in treating rheumatic valvulopathy. Replacement can be achieved by resection of the diseased leaflet tissue with preservation of the leaflet edge and primary chordal attachments, and incorporation of the leaflet tissue into the trans-annular sutures, which allows support of the papillary muscles and ventricular wall after the procedure. Maintenance of papillary-annular continuity is associated with improved LV function following mitral valve replacement [79–82]. Superior long-term outcomes in patients who had chord-sparing procedures versus those without has made it the standard of care in cases where replacement is necessary [83]. With severe rheumatic involvement, often the chordae are too foreshortened and thickened to permit preservation. In these circumstances, PTFE neochordae (as described above) can be inserted to maintain annular continuity to both papillary muscles.

Bioprosthetic vs. Mechanical

Mechanical valves have superior longevity but require anticoagulation, typically with warfarin. Bioprosthetic valves can be used to avoid the need for anticoagulation with warfarin (aspirin or another antiplatelet oral medication is sufficient) but can deteriorate and may require subsequent valve replacement. Age, ability to comply with long-term anticoagulation, risks of bleeding, and other patient factors including preference must be considered in the selection of valve type.

Special Considerations

Papillary Muscle Rupture

In cases of papillary muscle rupture that causes torrential MR, surgery should be undertaken emergently, as this condition is poorly tolerated. Even if there is a partial papillary muscle rupture with hemodynamic stability, urgent surgery is indicated because it may progress to complete papillary muscle rupture. In cases of ruptured chordae tendineae, mitral repair is usually feasible and preferred over replacement but with papillary muscle rupture, expedient replacement is generally preferred. The patient's overall condition must be considered and timing of surgery balanced with patient comorbidities and the possibility of optimization of concurrent problems prior to surgery (e.g., renal failure, sepsis, heart failure).

Atrial Fibrillation

As atrial fibrillation is a common sequela of mitral valve disease, correction of this arrhythmia in tandem with mitral surgery is usually warranted. Excellent results of the Cox-Maze IV procedure using bipolar radiofrequency ablation and cryoablation have been reported by several groups, with freedom from atrial fibrillation >90% after 1 year. Addition of the lesion set as described by Cox, Boineau, Schuessler et al. in the late 1980s yields the highest rates of freedom from atrial fibrillation [84]. Most of the incisions can be replaced with ablations (either bipolar radiofrequency or cryothermy) that create transmural lesions with similar excellent long-term outcomes (Fig. 6.27) [85]. In high-risk cases or in patients undergoing second or subsequent surgeries for mitral disease, a more limited set of lesions such as pulmonary vein isolation and an isthmus lesion may be warranted. These sub-sets of lesions uniformly have lower rates of success and patients should be made aware of the tradeoff of risks and benefits of a full Cox-Maze procedure versus a subset of equivalent lesions [86].

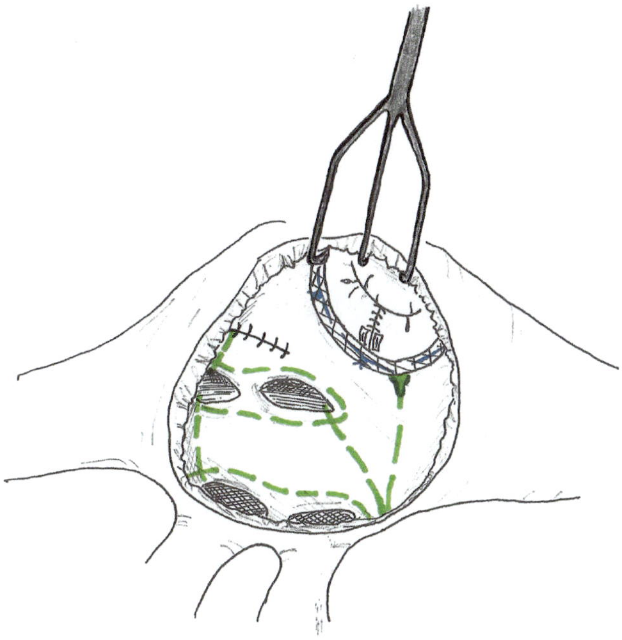

Fig. 6.27 Cox-Maze lesions in the left atrium (right atrial lesions not shown) for atrial fibrillation at the time of mitral valve repair. Standard left atriotomy with mitral valve visualized after repair. Ablations (green dashed lines) can be carried out with bipolar radiofrequency clamp or with cryo. Lesions encircling the pulmonary veins are connected along the back of the left atrium to isolate the entire posterior left atrium. An ablation is carried out from the inferior edge of the atriotomy to the mitral valve annulus. When this lesion is completed with bipolar radiofrequency, an additional cryo lesion on the valve annulus is necessary (green) along with an additional lesion on the exterior of the heart to ablate the coronary sinus (not shown). An additional lesion connecting the left superior pulmonary vein with the resected left atrial appendage is completed

Systolic Anterior Motion

Systolic anterior motion (SAM) of the mitral valve occurs when the anterior leaflet is captured in the left ventricular outflow tract during systole, which can precipitate outflow obstruction, hemodynamic compromise with hypotension, tachycardia, and death. In patients with hypertrophic cardiomyopathy, the risk increases for SAM after mitral repair. Several risk factors have been described, but elongated/redundant valve tissue with displacement of the coaptation point toward the left ventricular outflow tract (LVOT) clearly predisposes to SAM. Patients who undergo repair with annuloplasty are at risk, as leaflet tissue and the coaptation point may be moved posteriorly, and tissue leaflet may get caught up in the LVOT during systole. Initial therapy for intraoperative SAM include: (1) cessation of inotropes, (2) intravascular volume expansion, (3) beta blockade, and (4) augmentation of LV afterload. Surgical revision is rarely necessary [87].

Complications

Mitral Annular Calcification

Valves with extensive mitral annular calcification (often referred to as "MAC") may require debridement of the annular tissue near the posterior leaflet for both relief of stenosis and/or to create an area of suitability to place annular stitches to support a ring or new valve. In this condition, risk of a postoperative atrioventricular groove disruption can occur as pressurized blood from the ventricle can intercalate into the newly debrided area and create a highly morbid hematoma formation between the left atrium and ventricle. This condition usually progresses to hemorrhage and carries a very high mortality. Repair is often only achievable by emergent redo surgery with removal (and subsequent re-replacement) of the valve or ring and creation of a supporting patch over the area using ventricular muscle and atrial layers to support the patch and then the patch to support the replacement valve.

Coronary Artery Occlusion

Coronary artery occlusion can occur if care is not taken in the sutures placed in the annulus at A1, P1, and P2, as the circumflex artery courses near the annulus in this area (Fig. 6.24). Aortic valve injury can occur with stitches placed too deeply in one of the fibrous trigones of the anterior annulus.

Paravalvular Regurgitation

Paravalvular regurgitation or ring dehiscence can be seen if inadequate sutures are placed at the time of surgery, or if the tissue holding the suture is weakened by subsequent infection or other pathology. Severity of the regurgitation, heart failure symptoms, and the presence of hemolysis will guide the decision of whether a subsequent procedure to correct the problem is necessary.

Summary

Surgical techniques for mitral valve disease have improved dramatically over the last three decades. Current surgical techniques allow for the repair of the majority of degenerative valves with excellent results and very low operative mortality rates. Patients with mitral valve disease should be referred to a center of excellence with high volume mitral valve surgery to ensure optimal outcomes for patients.

Understanding and treatment of mitral valve disease continues to evolve. It is now recognized that primary and secondary MR are virtually two different diseases with different etiologies, pathophysiologies, therapies, and outcomes. The advances in echocardiography and mitral repair for primary MR allow for earlier and safer surgery without exposing the patient to the risks of prosthetic valve replacement. The biggest challenge in management is in the therapy for secondary MR where there is still no treatment for the advanced LV damage that usually accompanies the condition.

For the treatment of mitral stenosis, a disease becoming rare in developed countries because rheumatic fever has become rare, percutaneous balloon valvuloplasty has replaced surgery in most cases.

References

1. Otto CM. Clinical practice. Evaluation and management of chronic mitral regurgitation. N Engl J Med. 2001;345(10):740–6.
2. Ralph AP, Carapetis JR. Group a streptococcal diseases and their global burden. Curr Top Microbiol Immunol. 2013;368:1–27.
3. Wood P. An appreciation of mitral stenosis. I. Clinical features. Br Med J. 1954;1(4870):1051–63.
4. Bonow RO, Carabello BA, Chatterjee K, de Leon AC Jr, Faxon DP, Freed MD, Gaasch WH, Lytle BW, Nishimura RA, O'Gara PT, O'Rourke RA, Otto CM, Shah PM, Shanewise JS. 2008 focused update incorporated into the ACC/AHA 2006 guidelines for the management of patients with valvular heart disease: a report of the American College of Cardiology/American Heart Association Task Force on Practice Guidelines (Writing Committee to revise the 1998 guidelines for the management of patients with valvular heart disease). Endorsed by the Society of Cardiovascular Anesthesiologists, Society for Cardiovascular Angiography and Interventions, and Society of Thoracic Surgeons. J Am Coll Cardiol. 2008;52(13):e1–142.
5. Nishimura RA, Otto CM, Bonow RO, Carabello BA, Erwin JP 3rd, Guyton RA, O'Gara PT, Ruiz CE, Skubas NJ, Sorajja P, Sundt TM 3rd, Thomas JD. 2014 AHA/ACC Guideline for the management of patients with valvular heart disease: a report of the American College of Cardiology/American Heart Association Task Force on Practice Guidelines. Circulation. 2014;129(23):e521–643.
6. Deloche A, Jebara VA, Relland JY, Chauvaud S, Fabiani JN, Perier P, Dreyfus G, Mihaileanu S, Carpentier A. Valve repair with Carpentier techniques. The second decade. J Thorac Cardiovasc Surg. 1990;99(6):990–1001; discussion 1001–2.
7. Adams DH, Rosenhek R, Falk V. Degenerative mitral valve regurgitation: best practice revolution. Eur Heart J. 2010;31(16):1958–66.
8. Di Salvo TG, Acker MA, Dec GW, Byrne JG. Mitral valve surgery in advanced heart failure. J Am Coll Cardiol. 2010;55(4):271–82.
9. Levine RA, Schwammenthal E. Ischemic mitral regurgitation on the threshold of a solution: from paradoxes to unifying concepts. Circulation. 2005;112(5):745–58.
10. Carpentier A. Cardiac valve surgery—the "French correction". J Thorac Cardiovasc Surg. 1983;86(3):323–37.
11. Bonow RO, Mann DL, Zipes DP, Libby P. Braunwald's heart disease: a textbook of cardiovascular medicine. 9th ed. London: Elsevier; 2011.
12. Lancellotti P, Tribouilloy C, Hagendorff A, Popescu BA, Edvardsen T, Pierard LA, Badano L, Zamorano JL, Scientific Document Committee of the European Association of Cardiovascular I. Recommendations for the echocardiographic assessment of native valvular regurgitation: an executive summary from the European Association of Cardiovascular Imaging. Eur Heart J Cardiovasc Imaging. 2013;14(7):611–44.
13. Foster GP, Isselbacher EM, Rose GA, Torchiana DF, Akins CW, Picard MH. Accurate localization of mitral regurgitant defects using multiplane transesophageal echocardiography. Ann Thorac Surg. 1998;65(4):1025–31.
14. O'Gara P, Sugeng L, Lang R, Sarano M, Hung J, Raman S, Fischer G, Carabello B, Adams D, Vannan M. The role of imaging

in chronic degenerative mitral regurgitation. JACC Cardiovasc Imaging. 2008;1(2):221–37.
15. Tsang W, Lang RM. Three-dimensional echocardiography is essential for intraoperative assessment of mitral regurgitation. Circulation. 2013;128(6):643–52; discussion 652.
16. McCarthy PM. Three-dimensional echocardiography is not essential for intraoperative assessment of mitral regurgitation. Circulation. 2013;128(6):653–8; discussion 658.
17. Feuchtner GM, Alkadhi H, Karlo C, Sarwar A, Meier A, Dichtl W, Leschka S, Blankstein R, Gruenenfelder J, Stolzmann P, Cury RC. Cardiac CT angiography for the diagnosis of mitral valve prolapse: comparison with echocardiography1. Radiology. 2010;254(2):374–83.
18. Meijboom WB, Mollet NR, Van Mieghem CA, Kluin J, Weustink AC, Pugliese F, Vourvouri E, Cademartiri F, Bogers AJ, Krestin GP, de Feyter PJ. Pre-operative computed tomography coronary angiography to detect significant coronary artery disease in patients referred for cardiac valve surgery. J Am Coll Cardiol. 2006;48(8):1658–65.
19. Dewey M, Muller M, Eddicks S, Schnapauff D, Teige F, Rutsch W, Borges AC, Hamm B. Evaluation of global and regional left ventricular function with 16-slice computed tomography, biplane cineventriculography, and two-dimensional transthoracic echocardiography: comparison with magnetic resonance imaging. J Am Coll Cardiol. 2006;48(10):2034–44.
20. Wu YW, Tadamura E, Kanao S, Yamamuro M, Okayama S, Ozasa N, Toma M, Kimura T, Kita T, Marui A, Komeda M, Togashi K. Left ventricular functional analysis using 64-slice multidetector row computed tomography: comparison with left ventriculography and cardiovascular magnetic resonance. Cardiology. 2008;109(2):135–42.
21. Hur J, Kim YJ, Nam JE, Choe KO, Choi EY, Shim CY, Choi BW. Thrombus in the left atrial appendage in stroke patients: detection with cardiac CT angiography—a preliminary report. Radiology. 2008;249(1):81–7.
22. Cawley PJ, Maki JH, Otto CM. Cardiovascular magnetic resonance imaging for valvular heart disease: technique and validation. Circulation. 2009;119(3):468–78.
23. Moscucci M. Grossman and Baim's cardiac catheterization, angiography, and intervention. 8th ed. Philadelphia, PA: Lippincott, Williams, & Wilkins; 2013.
24. Zoghbi WA, Enriquez-Sarano M, Foster E, Grayburn PA, Kraft CD, Levine RA, Nihoyannopoulos P, Otto CM, Quinones MA, Rakowski H, Stewart WJ, Waggoner A, Weissman NJ. Recommendations for evaluation of the severity of native valvular regurgitation with two-dimensional and Doppler echocardiography. J Am Soc Echocardiogr. 2003;16(7):777–802.
25. Armstrong WF. Feigenbaum's echocardiography. 7th ed. Philadelphia, PA: Lippincott, Williams, & Wilkins; 2009.
26. Yosefy C, Levine RA, Solis J, Vaturi M, Handschumacher MD, Hung J. Proximal flow convergence region as assessed by real-time 3-dimensional echocardiography: challenging the hemispheric assumption. J Am Soc Echocardiogr. 2007;20(4):389–96.
27. Thomas L, Foster E, Schiller NB. Peak mitral inflow velocity predicts mitral regurgitation severity. J Am Coll Cardiol. 1998;31(1):174–9.
28. Wunderlich NC, Beigel R, Siegel RJ. Management of mitral stenosis using 2D and 3D echo-Doppler imaging. JACC Cardiovasc Imaging. 2013;6(11):1191–205.
29. Thomas JD, Weyman AE. Doppler mitral pressure half-time: a clinical tool in search of theoretical justification. J Am Coll Cardiol. 1987;10(4):923–9.
30. Baumgartner H, Hung J, Bermejo J, Chambers JB, Evangelista A, Griffin BP, Iung B, Otto CM, Pellikka PA, Quinones M. Echocardiographic assessment of valve stenosis: EAE/ASE recommendations for clinical practice. Eur J Echocardiogr. 2009;10(1):1–25.
31. Carabello BA. Modern management of mitral stenosis. Circulation. 2005;112(3):432–7.
32. Wilkins GT, Weyman AE, Abascal VM, Block PC, Palacios IF. Percutaneous balloon dilatation of the mitral valve: an analysis of echocardiographic variables related to outcome and the mechanism of dilatation. Br Heart J. 1988;60(4):299–308.
33. Mueller RL, Sanborn TA. The history of interventional cardiology: cardiac catheterization, angioplasty, and related interventions. Am Heart J. 1995;129(1):146–72.
34. Nishimura RA, Carabello BA. Hemodynamics in the cardiac catheterization laboratory of the 21st century. Circulation. 2012;125(17):2138–50.
35. Thomas JD, Wilkins GT, Choong CY, Abascal VM, Palacios IF, Block PC, Weyman AE. Inaccuracy of mitral pressure half-time immediately after percutaneous mitral valvotomy. Dependence on transmitral gradient and left atrial and ventricular compliance. Circulation. 1988;78(4):980–93.
36. Lange RA, Moore DM Jr, Cigarroa RG, Hillis LD. Use of pulmonary capillary wedge pressure to assess severity of mitral stenosis: is true left atrial pressure needed in this condition? J Am Coll Cardiol. 1989;13(4):825–31.
37. Kern M, Lim M, Goldstein J. Hemodynamic rounds: interpretation of cardiac pathophysiology from pressure waveform analysis. New York: Wiley-Blackwell; 2009.
38. Gorlin R, Gorlin SG. Hydraulic formula for calculation of the area of the stenotic mitral valve, other cardiac valves, and central circulatory shunts. I. Am Heart J. 1951;41(1):1–29.
39. Cohen MV, Gorlin R. Modified orifice equation for the calculation of mitral valve area. Am Heart J. 1972;84(6):839–40.
40. Hakki AH, Iskandrian AS, Bemis CE, Kimbiris D, Mintz GS, Segal BL, Brice C. A simplified valve formula for the calculation of stenotic cardiac valve areas. Circulation. 1981;63(5):1050–5.
41. Cui W, Dai R, Zhang G. A new simplified method for calculating mean mitral pressure gradient. Catheter Cardiovasc Interv. 2007;70(5):754–7.
42. Baim DS. Grossman's cardiac catheterization, angiography, and intervention. 7th edition: Philadelphia, PA: Lippincott Williams & Wilkins; 2006; pp. 642–3.
43. Fuchs RM, Heuser RR, Yin FC, Brinker JA. Limitations of pulmonary wedge V waves in diagnosing mitral regurgitation. Am J Cardiol. 1982;49(4):849–54.
44. Freihage JH, Joyal D, Arab D, Dieter RS, Loeb HS, Steen L, Lewis B, Liu JC, Leya F. Invasive assessment of mitral regurgitation: comparison of hemodynamic parameters. Catheter Cardiovasc Interv. 2007;69(2):303–12.
45. Goodman DJ, Rossen RM, Holloway EL, Alderman EL, Harrison DC. Effect of nitroprusside on left ventricular dynamics in mitral regurgitation. Circulation. 1974;50(5):1025–32.
46. Greenberg BH, Massie BM, Brundage BH, Botvinick EH, Parmley WW, Chatterjee K. Beneficial effects of hydralazine in severe mitral regurgitation. Circulation. 1978;58(2):273–9.
47. Yoran C, Yellin EL, Becker RM, Gabbay S, Frater RW, Sonnenblick EH. Mechanism of reduction of mitral regurgitation with vasodilator therapy. Am J Cardiol. 1979;43(4):773–7.
48. Dujardin KS, Enriquez-Sarano M, Bailey KR, Seward JB, Tajik AJ. Effect of losartan on degree of mitral regurgitation quantified by echocardiography. Am J Cardiol. 2001;87(5):570–6.
49. Harris KM, Aeppli DM, Carey CF. Effects of angiotensin-converting enzyme inhibition on mitral regurgitation severity, left ventricular size, and functional capacity. Am Heart J. 2005;150(5):1106.
50. Wisenbaugh T, Sinovich V, Dullabh A, Sareli P. Six month pilot study of captopril for mildly symptomatic, severe isolated mitral and isolated aortic regurgitation. J Heart Valve Dis. 1994;3(2):197–204.
51. Ahmed MI, Aban I, Lloyd SG, Gupta H, Howard G, Inusah S, Peri K, Robinson J, Smith P, McGiffin DC, Schiros CG, Denney T Jr, Dell'Italia LJ. A randomized controlled phase IIb trial of beta(1)-

receptor blockade for chronic degenerative mitral regurgitation. J Am Coll Cardiol. 2012;60(9):833–8.
52. Kim KH, Kim YJ, Ohn JH, Yang J, Lee SE, Lee SW, Kim HK, Seo JW, Sohn DW. Long-term effects of sildenafil in a rat model of chronic mitral regurgitation: benefits of ventricular remodeling and exercise capacity. Circulation. 2012;125(11):1390–401.
53. Bridgewater B, Hooper T, Munsch C, Hunter S, von Oppell U, Livesey S, Keogh B, Wells F, Patrick M, Kneeshaw J, Chambers J, Masani N, Ray S. Mitral repair best practice: proposed standards. Heart. 2006;92(7):939–44.
54. David TE, Armstrong S, McCrindle BW, Manlhiot C. Late outcomes of mitral valve repair for mitral regurgitation due to degenerative disease. Circulation. 2013;127(14):1485–92.
55. LaPar DJ, Ailawadi G, Isbell JM, et al. Mitral valve repair rates correlate with surgeon and institutional experience. J Thorac Cardiovasc Surg. 2014;148(3):995–1003.
56. Gillam LD, Schwartz A. Primum non nocere: the case for watchful waiting in asymptomatic "severe" degenerative mitral regurgitation. Circulation. 2010;121(6):813–21; discussion 821.
57. Suri RM, Vanoverschelde JL, Grigioni F, Schaff HV, Tribouilloy C, Avierinos JF, Barbieri A, Pasquet A, Huebner M, Rusinaru D, Russo A, Michelena HI, Enriquez-Sarano M. Association between early surgical intervention vs watchful waiting and outcomes for mitral regurgitation due to flail mitral valve leaflets. JAMA. 2013;310(6):609–16.
58. Rosenhek R, Rader F, Klaar U, Gabriel H, Krejc M, Kalbeck D, Schemper M, Maurer G, Baumgartner H. Outcome of watchful waiting in asymptomatic severe mitral regurgitation. Circulation. 2006;113(18):2238–2244.59.
59. Borer JS. Early surgery or watchful waiting for asymptomatic severe degenerative mitral regurgitation: is the answer now clear? J Am Coll Cardiol. 2014;63(22):2408–10.
60. Nishimura RA, Otto CM, Bonow RO, Carabello BA, et al. 2017 AHA/ACC focused update of the 2014 AHA/ACC guideline for the management of patients with valvular heart disease: a report of the American College of Cardiology/American Heart Association Task Force on Clinical Practice Guidelines. J Am Coll Cardiol. 2017;70(2):252–89.
61. Elliott C, Cutler SAL. Cardiotomy and valvulotomy for mitral stenosis: experimental observations and clinical notes concerning an operated case with recovery. Boston Med Surg J. 1929;188:1023.
62. Souttar HS. The surgical treatment of mitral stenosis. Br Med J. 1925;2(3379):603–6.
63. Crawford FA Jr. Horace Smithy: pioneer heart surgeon. Ann Thorac Surg. 2010;89(6):2067–7.
64. Harken DE, Ellis LB, et al. The surgical treatment of mitral stenosis; valvuloplasty. N Engl J Med. 1948;239(22):801–809.65.
65. Bailey CP. The surgical treatment of mitral stenosis (mitral commissurotomy). Dis Chest. 1949;15(4):377–97.
66. Baker C, Brock RC, Campbell M. Valvulotomy for mitral stenosis; report of six successful cases. Br Med J. 1950;1(4665):1283–93.
67. Lock JE, Khalilullah M, Shrivastava S, Bahl V, Keane JF. Percutaneous catheter commissurotomy in rheumatic mitral stenosis. N Engl J Med. 1985;313(24):1515–8.
68. Reyes VP, Raju BS, Wynne J, Stephenson LW, Raju R, Fromm BS, Rajagopal P, Mehta P, Singh S, Rao DP, et al. Percutaneous balloon valvuloplasty compared with open surgical commissurotomy for mitral stenosis. N Engl J Med. 1994;331(15):961–7.
69. McCarthy PM. Does the intertrigonal distance dilate? Never say never. J Thorac Cardiovasc Surg. 2002;124(6):1078–9.
70. Barlow JB, Bosman CK, Pocock WA, Marchand P. Late systolic murmurs and non-ejection ("mid-late") systolic clicks. An analysis of 90 patients. Br Heart J. 1968;30(2):203–18.
71. Barlow JB, Pocock WA. The significance of late systolic murmurs and mid-late systolic clicks. Md State Med J. 1963;12:76–7.
72. Jouan J, Berrebi A, Chauvaud S, Menasche P, Carpentier A, Fabiani JN. Mitral valve reconstruction in Barlow disease: long-term echographic results and implications for surgical management. J Thorac Cardiovasc Surg. 2012;143(4 Suppl):S17–20.
73. Perier P. Quadrangular resection for repair of posterior leaflet prolapse. Multimed Man Cardiothorac Surg. 2005;2005(1129):mmcts.2004.000893.
74. De Bonis M, Lapenna E, Buzzatti N, Taramasso M, Calabrese MC, Nisi T, Pappalardo F, Alfieri O. Can the edge-to-edge technique provide durable results when used to rescue patients with suboptimal conventional mitral repair? Eur J Cardiothorac Surg. 2013;43(6):e173–9.
75. De Bonis M, Lapenna E, Maisano F, Barili F, La Canna G, Buzzatti N, Pappalardo F, Calabrese M, Nisi T, Alfieri O. Long-term results (</=18 years) of the edge-to-edge mitral valve repair without annuloplasty in degenerative mitral regurgitation: implications for the percutaneous approach. Circulation. 2014;130(11 Suppl 1):S19–24.
76. De Bonis M, Lapenna E, Lorusso R, Buzzatti N, Gelsomino S, Taramasso M, Vizzardi E, Alfieri O. Very long-term results (up to 17 years) with the double-orifice mitral valve repair combined with ring annuloplasty for degenerative mitral regurgitation. J Thorac Cardiovasc Surg. 2012;144(5):1019–24.
77. Tommaso CL, Fullerton DA, Feldman T, Dean LS, Hijazi ZM, Horlick E, Weiner BH, Zahn E, Cigarroa JE, Ruiz CE, Bavaria J, Mack MJ, Cameron DE, Bolman RM 3rd, Miller DC, Moon MR, Mukherjee D, Trento A, Aldea GS, Bacha EA. SCAI/AATS/ACC/STS operator and institutional requirements for transcatheter valve repair and replacement. Part II. Mitral valve. J Thorac Cardiovasc Surg. 2014;148(2):387–400.
78. O'Gara PT, Calhoon JH, Moon MR, Tommaso CL. Transcatheter therapies for mitral regurgitation: a professional society overview from the American College of Cardiology, The American Association for Thoracic Surgery, Society for Cardiovascular Angiography and Interventions Foundation, and The Society of Thoracic Surgeons. J Thorac Cardiovasc Surg. 2014;147(3):837–49.
79. Moon MR, DeAnda A Jr, Daughters GT 2nd, Ingels NB Jr, Miller DC. Experimental evaluation of different chordal preservation methods during mitral valve replacement. Ann Thorac Surg. 1994;58(4):931–43; discussion 943–4.
80. Moon MR, DeAnda A Jr, Daughters GT 2nd, Ingels NB Jr, Miller DC. Effects of mitral valve replacement on regional left ventricular systolic strain. Ann Thorac Surg. 1999;68(3):894–902.
81. Moon MR, DeAnda A Jr, Daughters GT 2nd, Ingels NB, Miller DC. Effects of chordal disruption on regional left ventricular torsional deformation. Circulation. 1996;94(9 Suppl):II143–51.
82. Lillehei CW, Levy MJ, Bonnabeau RC Jr. Mitral valve replacement with preservation of papillary muscles and chordae tendineae. J Thorac Cardiovasc Surg. 1964;47:532–43.
83. Reardon MJ, David TE. Mitral valve replacement with preservation of the subvalvular apparatus. Curr Opin Cardiol. 1999;14(2):104–10.
84. Cox JL, Schuessler RB, D'Agostino HJ Jr, Stone CM, Chang BC, Cain ME, Corr PB, Boineau JP. The surgical treatment of atrial fibrillation. III. Development of a definitive surgical procedure. J Thorac Cardiovasc Surg. 1991;101(4):569–83.
85. Melby SJ, Zierer A, Bailey MS, Cox JL, Lawton JS, Munfakh N, Crabtree TD, Moazami N, Huddleston CB, Moon MR, Damiano RJ Jr. A new era in the surgical treatment of atrial fibrillation: the impact of ablation technology and lesion set on procedural efficacy. Ann Surg. 2006;244(4):583–92.
86. Robertson JO, Lawrance CP, Maniar HS, Damiano RJ Jr. Surgical techniques used for the treatment of atrial fibrillation. Circ J. 2013;77(8):1941–51.
87. Ibrahim M, Rao C, Ashrafian H, Chaudhry U, Darzi A, Athanasiou T. Modern management of systolic anterior motion of the mitral valve. Eur J Cardiothorac Surg. 2012;41(6):1260–70.

7 Secondary Mitral Regurgitation

Michael J. Mack and James T. Willerson

Introduction

Mitral regurgitation (MR) is among the most common valvular heart disorders, having an estimated prevalence in the United States of 1.7% and increasing with age to 9.3% in those >75 years of age [1, 2]. MR is classified as primary when it is due to a structural or degenerative abnormality of the mitral valve (MV), chordae tendineae, papillary muscles, or mitral annulus. In contrast, secondary or functional MR occurs in the absence of organic MV disease, usually resulting from left ventricular (LV) dysfunction. Secondary MR is more common than primary MR [1, 3] and is associated with a worse prognosis, which is primarily related to the severity of the associated underlying LV dysfunction [1].

Secondary MR

Figure 7.1 shows the MV leaflets and valve. Papillary muscles, anteromedial and posterolateral, arise from the LV myocardium. Chordae tendineae support the leaflets. LV dilation due to ischemic or nonischemic cardiomyopathy can impair leaflet coaptation in a structurally normal MV, causing secondary MR. LV dysfunction and remodeling lead to apical and lateral papillary muscle displacement. These changes are dependent on loading conditions; thus, secondary MR is dynamic [1].

Papillary muscle displacement results from global LV enlargement or focal myocardial or valve scarring and can affect one or both papillary muscles, causing posteriorly directed or central MR (Fig. 7.2) [4]. Insufficient leaflet remodeling and increased mitral leaflet area sometimes cause severe MR [5, 6].

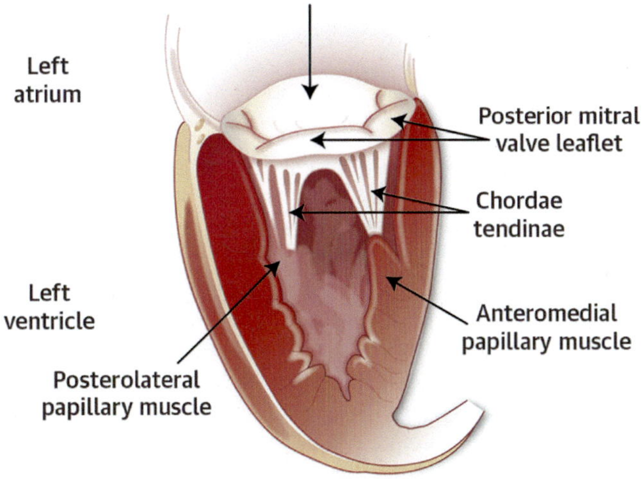

Fig. 7.1 Mitral valve anatomy. This diagram illustrates the valve and supporting structures. From Asgar et al. [1]. Reprinted with permission from Elsevier

The normal annulus is important for maintaining normal leaflet stress [1, 3, 7]. Annular deformation and flattening due to LV remodeling result in increased leaflet stress. These mitral valve changes lead to failure of leaflet coaptation, decreased valvular closing forces due to LV dysfunction, and MR.

MR is characterized as ischemic or nonischemic. Ischemic MR is more frequent. LV remodeling after myocardial infarction results in papillary muscle displacement, thereby causing systolic tenting of the MV. Regional wall motion abnormalities can result in sufficient MV tethering to cause severe MR [1, 8].

Nonischemic MR is usually caused by hypertension or idiopathic dilated cardiomyopathy. Chronic MR due to atrial flutter, atrial fibrillation, or marked left atrial (LA) enlargement can result in a dilated mitral annulus and reduced leaflet coaptation. In patients with atrial fibrillation or flutter, restoring sinus rhythm sometimes reduces MR severity [9].

M. J. Mack
Cardiovascular Service Line, Baylor Scott & White Health, Dallas, TX, USA

Department of Cardiovascular Surgery, The Heart Hospital, Baylor Plano, Plano, TX, USA

J. T. Willerson (✉)
Department of Cardiology, Texas Heart Institute, Houston, TX, USA
e-mail: jwillerson@texasheart.org

B. A. Carabello (ed.), *Valvular Heart Disease*, Cardiovascular Medicine, https://doi.org/10.1007/978-1-4471-2840-3_7

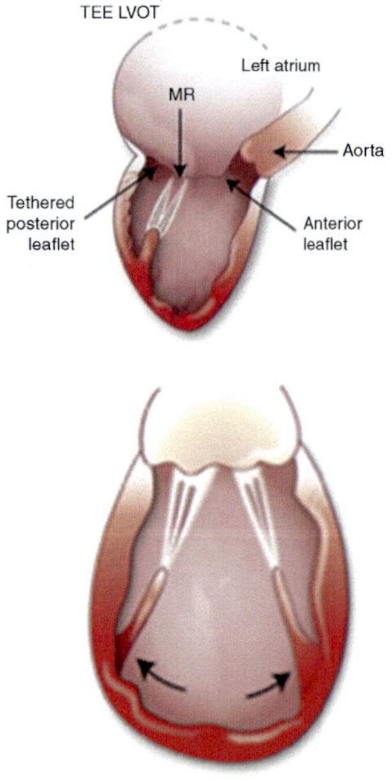

Fig. 7.2 Secondary MR due to left ventricular dilation. A diagram of ischemic MR, with posteriorly directed jet. *LVOT* left ventricular outflow tract, *MR* mitral regurgitation, *TEE* transesophageal echocardiography. From Asgar et al. [1]. Reprinted with permission from Elsevier

Secondary MR severity is associated with all-cause mortality and heart failure (HF) hospitalization [10–12]. Among 303 patients with a completed Q-wave myocardial infarction, ischemic MR was detected by echocardiography in 194 patients and was an independent predictor of mortality (relative risk: 1.88 [95% confidence interval: 1.23–2.86], $p = 0.003$) [11]. In a study from the Duke Cardiovascular Databank, qualitatively assessed 3+ to 4+ MR on left ventriculography was present in 29.8% of 2057 HF patients with an LVEF <40% and was an independent predictor of 5-year mortality (adjusted hazard ratio: 1.23 [95% confidence interval: 1.13–1.34]) [12]. Secondary MR is a predictor of death even in patients with less severe HF [13]. However, whether reducing secondary MR improves patient outcomes is uncertain.

Evaluation of Secondary MR

Secondary MR can be divided into four clinical groups that help define clinical prognosis and can assist in guiding therapy: (1) At risk of secondary MR; (2) Progressive secondary MR; (3) Asymptomatic severe secondary MR; and (4) Symptomatic severe secondary MR [14]. Diagnostic evaluation of MR is performed by echocardiography (both transesophageal and transthoracic), magnetic resonance imaging (MRI), or LV angiography. Transesophageal echocardiography and MRI most often accurately identify the underlying cause and mechanism of MR. All 3 methods allow estimation of LV volume, function, and sphericity; pulmonary artery pressure; right ventricular function; and tricuspid regurgitation.

The echocardiographic or angiographic severity of MR is classified as mild, moderate, or severe [15]. Qualitative findings include MV morphology and the color-flow and continuous-wave signals of the MR jet. Semiquantitative measures are the effective regurgitant orifice area (EROA), regurgitant volume, and regurgitant fraction [1]. Enlarged LA and LV chamber size and increased pulmonary artery pressure support the diagnosis of severe MR.

Conventional 2-dimensional (2D) assessment for MR quantification relies on measuring the MR jet core at its vena contracta. Therefore, MR severity can be significantly underestimated when the orifice is elliptical (which is common in secondary MR) [4], a problem that is compounded if multiple jets are present. Three-dimensional (3D) echocardiography overcomes this limitation by permitting direct planimetry of the vena contracta, regardless of orifice shape or the number of jets [16]. Conversely, both 2D and 3D color flow Doppler tend to overestimate the orifice area because they cannot resolve the high velocity jet core because of aliasing and blooming artifacts. Secondary MR severity also varies during the cardiac cycle and can peak in early or late systole. This further complicates the evaluation, which is traditionally done in midsystole. No single variable is sufficient to quantify the degree of MR, so multimodality assessment with both 2D and 3D echocardiography is optimal [17].

Severe primary MR is usually defined as an EROA of $\geq 40\ mm^2$ and a regurgitant volume of ≥60 mL. Enriquez-Sarano et al. [11] proposed, and the most recent U.S. and European valve guidelines have accepted, that an EROA $\geq 20\ mm^2$ and a regurgitant volume ≥30 mL are consistent with severe secondary MR (Table 7.1) [14, 18]. However, the amount of MR (assessed by either EROA or regurgitant volume) resulting in loss of >50% of total stroke volume (i.e., the regurgitant volume) is influenced by LV end-diastolic volume and LVEF [19].

Exercise echocardiography is sometimes useful when symptoms appear disproportionate to resting MR severity [20]. Exercise results in greater preload and afterload, a more spherical ventricle, increased coaptation distance, and systolic expansion of the mitral annulus. Such changes can occur in the absence of ischemia [21] and increase the patient's risk of acute pulmonary edema [22]. Patients with exercise-induced severe MR may be at heightened risk for death or HF hospitalization [23]. Quantitatively, an exercise-induced EROA increase of $\geq 13\ mm^2$ is associated with elevated morbidity and mortality rates. Exercise echocardiography can also reveal increased pulmonary artery pressure and reduced LVEF, both of which are associated with LV dysfunction and poor prognosis after MV surgery [24, 25]. Exercise can also induce greater LV dyssynchrony with

Table 7.1 Quantitative echocardiographic criteria for severe MR in primary and secondary disease of the mitral valve

	Primary (organic) MR	Secondary (functional) MR
EROA	≥0.4 cm^2	≥0.2 $cm^{2,a}$
Regurgitant volume	≥60 mL	≥30 mL
Regurgitant fraction	≥50%	≥50%
Vena contracta	≥0.7 cm	–
Jet area	Central jet >40% LA or holosystolic eccentric jet	–

In cases of secondary MR, measuring the proximal isovelocity surface area with two-dimensional transthoracic echocardiography underestimates the true EROA because of the crescent shape of the proximal convergence

EROA effective regurgitant orifice area, *LA* left atrium, *MR* mitral regurgitation

From Asgar et al. [1]. Reprinted with permission from Elsevier

[a]Measurement of the proximal isovelocity surface area by two-dimensional transthoracic echocardiography in secondary MR underestimates the true EROA because of the crescent shape of the proximal convergence

increased MR. However, the predictive value of exercise echocardiography is imperfect, given the technical issues of measuring key variables either during or immediately after exercise.

Echocardiography is also useful for determining the likelihood of successful MV repair by either surgical or transcatheter procedures (e.g., MitraClip placement) [26]. In a group of 300 patients with severe MR who underwent MitraClip implantation (68% of whom had secondary MR), the procedure failed to reduce MR to ≤2+ in 31 patients (10.3%). By multivariable analysis, predictors of failed MitraClip placement included greater EROA (odds ratio [OR]: 1.21 per 10 mm^2 increase, $p = 0.005$) and a baseline transmitral pressure gradient ≥4 mm^2 (OR: 1.26, $p = 0.03$). Success rates were similar in patients with primary and secondary MR [27].

Cardiac magnetic resonance (CMR) imaging and multidetector row computed tomography (MDCT) can provide complementary information to echocardiography in patients with MR. CMR can accurately quantify the degree of MR [28]. Given its high spatial resolution, MDCT can accurately depict MV morphology [29]. Both techniques can be used to make volumetric measurements of chamber dimensions, evaluate ventricular function, and assess myocardial fibrosis.

Therapy for Secondary MR

The goals of therapy for secondary MR are to relieve symptoms, improve quality of life, reduce HF hospitalizations, and potentially improve patient survival. Often, therapy is directed at the underlying LV dysfunction; these treatments include guideline-directed medical therapy for HF and biventricular cardiac resynchronization therapy (CRT) when appropriate. Coronary revascularization may also help patients with extensive ischemia and preserved myocardial viability, although it rarely markedly reduces or eliminates secondary MR. Regarding surgical and transcatheter MV repair, it is unclear how well these interventions interrupt the progressive cycle of LV volume overload → LV dilation → secondary MR → increasing LV volume overload and dilation → increasing MR.

Carvedilol or metoprolol, combined with angiotensin-converting enzyme inhibitors (ACEIs) or angiotensin receptor blockers, is sometimes helpful for patients with LV dysfunction and secondary MR. By reducing LV remodeling, maximal guideline-directed medical therapy sometimes reduces MR in severe cases. However, few studies have examined the effect of medical therapies on secondary MR. In a randomized trial that involved 59 patients with HF and severe dilated cardiomyopathy, treatment with carvedilol versus placebo resulted in reduced LV mass sphericity and improved systolic function. The severity of MR, assessed by the ratio of MR jet area/LA area, increased during follow-up in the placebo group but decreased in the carvedilol group ($p = 0.04$) [30]. In the largest randomized trial, among 138 patients with dilated cardiomyopathy who were taking stable doses of digoxin, diuretic agents, and ACEI, metoprolol (titrated to 50 mg, 3 times a day) produced greater 6-month reductions in LV end-diastolic and end-systolic volumes and secondary MR than did placebo [31]. However, MR improved in only ~42% of metoprolol-treated patients (vs. 20% of control-group patients), and there were no significant differences in symptoms or in rates of cardiac readmission or death during follow-up.

There is limited information about whether ACEIs and other agents reduce secondary MR. In a small study of 19 patients with severe dilated cardiomyopathy (mean LVEF ~20%) and 3+/4+ MR who were taking stable doses of digoxin and diuretic agents, the mean lisinopril dose was up-titrated from 16 to 55 mg/day, and isosorbide from 30 to 286 mg/day. At 12-month follow-up, MR had decreased to grade 0/1+ in 8 patients (42%) and remained 3+/4+ in the other 11. LVEF improved in both groups but to a greater degree in the MR responders, and the LV end-diastolic dimensions decreased in the responders but increased in the non-responders [32].

CRT

CRT is a recommended treatment for selected HF patients with LV dyssynchrony. CRT is a Class I recommendation for patients in sinus rhythm with New York Heart Association (NYHA) functional class II to IV symptoms, LVEF ≤35%, left bundle branch block (LBBB), and QRS duration ≥150 ms despite receiving guideline-directed medical therapy. CRT may also be useful in patients with LVEF ≤35%, sinus rhythm, non-LBBB pattern, and QRS duration ≥150 ms, and in those with LBBB and QRS duration 120–149 ms (Class IIa indications) [33, 34]. Randomized trials of CRT with or without a defibrillator have shown that it improves both survival and HF rehospitalization rates [35], reduces LV end-diastolic and end-systolic dimensions, and increases LVEF.

The effect of CRT on secondary MR is inconsistent, although most studies show that overall MR severity decreases with restoration of synchronous ventricular contraction and LV remodeling. In the sham-controlled MIRACLE (Multicenter InSync Randomized Clinical Evaluation) trial involving 450 NYHA functional class III/IV HF patients with LVEF ≤35% and QRS duration ≥130 ms, CRT resulted in reductions in LV end-diastolic and end-systolic volumes, improved LVEF, and sustained reductions in MR (assessed by the relative size of the mitral jet area in the LA) [36]. In a study of 63 patients with HF and moderate to severe MR, MR improved by ≥1 grade in 43% of patients, and an additional 20% had late improvement at 6 months [34]. Improvement of severe secondary MR is associated with better prognosis, but this improvement occurs in no more than one-half of patients after CRT [33].

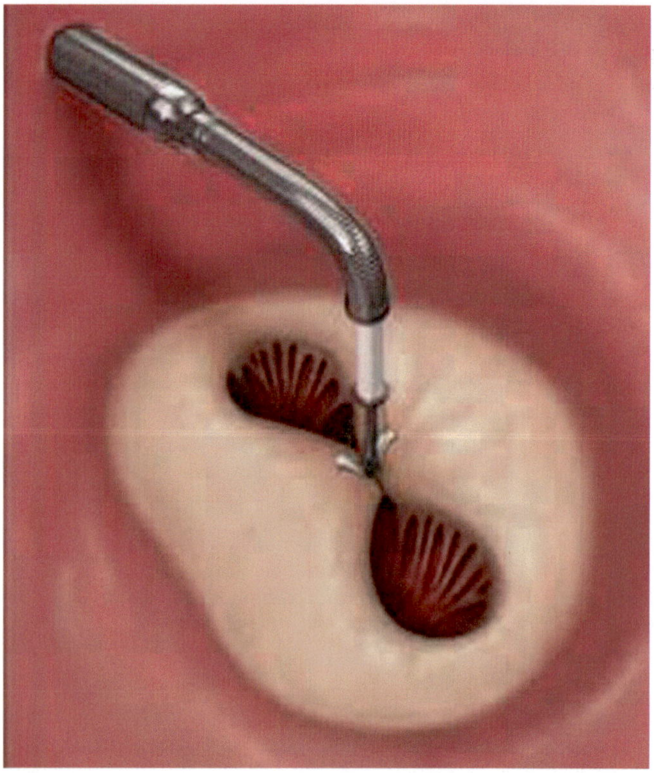

Fig. 7.3 The MitraClip is shown clipping the 2 leaflets of the mitral valve together

Mechanical Therapy

Surgical Options

As noted, secondary MR is so named because it is secondary to disease of the LV not of the valve itself. Heart failure associated with secondary MR has a worse prognosis than heart failure without MR [37, 38]. However it was unclear whether the presence of MR was merely a marker of LV dysfunction or was itself contributing to the pathology of heart failure and thus a target for therapy. Indeed surgical approaches to secondary MR have failed to demonstrate improved survival over medical therapy although some reported improved symptoms [39–43]. Recently 2 large randomized trials of the MitraClip (Fig. 7.3) have helped clarify the issue. MitraClip is a percutaneously inserted device that clips the mitral leaflets together at their midbellies, creating a figure of 8 orifice, reducing MR. In the Mitra-FR trial [44] patients with moderate to severe MR and severe LV dilitaiton were randomized to standard therapy versus standard therapy + the MitraClip. The MitraClip caused no reduction in repeated hospitlalizations or mortality. In the COAPT trial [45] patients with severe MR and modest LV dilitation who were still symptomatic after very aggressive medical therapy were randomized to receive aggressive medical therapy versus agressive medical therapy + the MitaClip. The results were virtually opposite to those of Mitra FR. The clip reduced both rehospitalizations and mortality. Only 3 patients needed to be treated to avoid 1 rehoapitalization and only 6 needed to be treated to avoid 1 death. The results of the 2 trials are in fact complementary. They indicate that patients with very severe MR and only modest LV dilitaiton who are symptomatic despite aggressive medical therapy benefit from the clip whereas patients with less severe MR yet more LV dysfucntion fail to benefit. Thus in this group of patients MR is not only a marker of LV dysfucntion but also contibutes to the pathology of the disease and thus is a target for therapy. In patients with less severe MR, the MR is not a target. On this basis there is now FDA approval for the use of MitraClip for the treatment of severe symptomatic secondary MR.

Summary

The development of secondary MR is associated with a poorer prognosis in patients with HF, regardless of its cause. Assessing MR severity accurately is helpful in making treatment decisions. Guideline-directed medical therapy for HF is sometimes effective in patients with moderate or severe secondary MR, as is coronary revascularization in patients with concomitant coronary artery disease. These measures, when applied effectively, sometimes reduce secondary MR and improve patient prognosis. The appropriate role of surgical and transcatheter interventions in treating persistent severe secondary MR is less clear.

Acknowledgement Adapted in part from de Marchena E, Badiye A, Robalino G, et al. Respective prevalence of the different Carpentier classes of mitral regurgitation: a stepping stone for future therapeutic research and development. J Card Surg 2011;26:385–392.

References

1. Asgar AW, Mack MJ, Stone GW. Secondary mitral regurgitation in heart failure: pathophysiology, prognosis, and therapeutic considerations. J Am Coll Cardiol. 2015;65:1231–48.
2. Nkomo VT, Gardin JM, Skelton TN, Gottdiener JS, Scott CG, Enriquez-Sarano M. Burden of valvular heart diseases: a population-based study. Lancet. 2006;368:1005–11.
3. de Marchena E, Badiye A, Robalino G, et al. Respective prevalence of the different Carpentier classes of mitral regurgitation: a stepping stone for future therapeutic research and development. J Card Surg. 2011;26:385–92.
4. Ray S. The echocardiographic assessment of functional mitral regurgitation. Eur J Echocardiogr. 2010;11:i11–7.
5. Chaput M, Handschumacher MD, Tournoux F, et al. Mitral leaflet adaptation to ventricular remodeling: occurrence and adequacy in patients with functional mitral regurgitation. Circulation. 2008;118:845–52.
6. Saito K, Okura H, Watanabe N, et al. Influence of chronic tethering of the mitral valve on mitral leaflet size and coaptation in functional mitral regurgitation. JACC Cardiovasc Imaging. 2012;5:337–45.
7. Dal-Bianco JP, Levine RA. Anatomy of the mitral valve apparatus: role of 2D and 3D echocardiography. Cardiol Clin. 2013;31:151–64.
8. Kumanohoso T, Otsuji Y, Yoshifuku S, et al. Mechanism of higher incidence of ischemic mitral regurgitation in patients with inferior myocardial infarction: quantitative analysis of left ventricular and mitral valve geometry in 103 patients with prior myocardial infarction. J Thorac Cardiovasc Surg. 2003;125:135–43.
9. Gertz ZM, Raina A, Saghy L, et al. Evidence of atrial functional mitral regurgitation due to atrial fibrillation: reversal with arrhythmia control. J Am Coll Cardiol. 2011;58:1474–81.
10. Chinitz JS, Chen D, Goyal P, et al. Mitral apparatus assessment by delayed enhancement CMR: relative impact of infarct distribution on mitral regurgitation. JACC Cardiovasc Imaging. 2013;6:220–34.
11. Grigioni F, Enriquez-Sarano M, Zehr KJ, Bailey KR, Tajik AJ. Ischemic mitral regurgitation: long-term outcome and prognostic implications with quantitative Doppler assessment. Circulation. 2001;103:1759–64.
12. Trichon BH, Felker GM, Shaw LK, Cabell CH, O'Connor CM. Relation of frequency and severity of mitral regurgitation to survival among patients with left ventricular systolic dysfunction and heart failure. Am J Cardiol. 2003;91:538–43.
13. Bursi F, Barbieri A, Grigioni F, et al. Prognostic implications of functional mitral regurgitation according to the severity of the underlying chronic heart failure: a long-term outcome study. Eur J Heart Fail. 2010;12:382–8.
14. Nishimura RA, Otto CM, Bonow RO, et al. 2014 AHA/ACC guideline for the management of patients with valvular heart disease: a report of the American College of Cardiology/American Heart Association Task Force on Practice Guidelines. J Am Coll Cardiol. 2014;63:e57–185.
15. Lancellotti P, Moura L, Pierard LA, et al. European Association of Echocardiography recommendations for the assessment of valvular regurgitation. Part 2: mitral and tricuspid regurgitation (native valve disease). Eur J Echocardiogr. 2010;11:307–32.
16. Thavendiranathan P, Liu S, Datta S, et al. Quantification of chronic functional mitral regurgitation by automated 3-dimensional peak and integrated proximal isovelocity surface area and stroke volume techniques using real-time 3-dimensional volume color Doppler echocardiography: in vitro and clinical validation. Circ Cardiovasc Imaging. 2013;6:125–33.
17. Grayburn PA, Carabello B, Hung J, et al. Defining "severe" secondary mitral regurgitation: emphasizing an integrated approach. J Am Coll Cardiol. 2014;64:2792–801.
18. Vahanian A, Alfieri O, Andreotti F, et al. Guidelines on the management of valvular heart disease (version 2012): the Joint Task Force on the Management of Valvular Heart Disease of the European Society of Cardiology (ESC) and the European Association for Cardio-Thoracic Surgery (EACTS). Eur J Cardiothorac Surg. 2012;42:S1–44.
19. Grayburn PA, Weissman NJ, Zamorano JL. Quantitation of mitral regurgitation. Circulation. 2012;126:2005–17.
20. Lee R, Marwick TH. Assessment of subclinical left ventricular dysfunction in asymptomatic mitral regurgitation. Eur J Echocardiogr. 2007;8:175–84.
21. Lancellotti P, Magne J. Stress testing for the evaluation of patients with mitral regurgitation. Curr Opin Cardiol. 2012;27:492–8.
22. Pierard LA, Lancellotti P. The role of ischemic mitral regurgitation in the pathogenesis of acute pulmonary edema. N Engl J Med. 2004;351:1627–34.
23. Picano E, Pibarot P, Lancellotti P, Monin JL, Bonow RO. The emerging role of exercise testing and stress echocardiography in valvular heart disease. J Am Coll Cardiol. 2009;54:2251–60.
24. Leung DY, Griffin BP, Stewart WJ, Cosgrove DM 3rd, Thomas JD, Marwick TH. Left ventricular function after valve repair for chronic mitral regurgitation: predictive value of preoperative assessment of contractile reserve by exercise echocardiography. J Am Coll Cardiol. 1996;28:1198–205.
25. Pai RG, Bansal RC, Shah PM. Doppler-derived rate of left ventricular pressure rise. Its correlation with the postoperative left ventricular function in mitral regurgitation. Circulation. 1990;82:514–20.
26. Lancellotti P, Tribouilloy C, Hagendorff A, et al. Recommendations for the echocardiographic assessment of native valvular regurgitation: an executive summary from the European Association of Cardiovascular Imaging. Eur Heart J Cardiovasc Imaging. 2013;14:611–44.
27. Lubos E, Schluter M, Vettorazzi E, et al. MitraClip therapy in surgical high-risk patients: identification of echocardiographic variables affecting acute procedural outcome. JACC Cardiovasc Interv. 2014;7:394–402.
28. Thavendiranathan P, Phelan D, Thomas JD, Flamm SD, Marwick TH. Quantitative assessment of mitral regurgitation: validation of new methods. J Am Coll Cardiol. 2012;60:1470–83.
29. Delgado V, Tops LF, Schuijf JD, et al. Assessment of mitral valve anatomy and geometry with multislice computed tomography. JACC Cardiovasc Imaging. 2009;2:556–65.
30. Lowes BD, Gill EA, Abraham WT, et al. Effects of carvedilol on left ventricular mass, chamber geometry, and mitral regurgitation in chronic heart failure. Am J Cardiol. 1999;83:1201–5.
31. Waagstein F, Stromblad O, Andersson B, et al. Increased exercise ejection fraction and reversed remodeling after long-term treatment with metoprolol in congestive heart failure: a randomized, stratified, double-blind, placebo-controlled trial in mild to moderate heart failure due to ischemic or idiopathic dilated cardiomyopathy. Eur J Heart Fail. 2003;5:679–91.
32. Levine AB, Muller C, Levine TB. Effects of high-dose lisinopril-isosorbide dinitrate on severe mitral regurgitation and heart failure remodeling. Am J Cardiol. 1998;82:1299–301, A1210.

33. van Bommel RJ, Marsan NA, Delgado V, et al. Cardiac resynchronization therapy as a therapeutic option in patients with moderate-severe functional mitral regurgitation and high operative risk. Circulation. 2011;124:912–9.
34. Ypenburg C, Lancellotti P, Tops LF, et al. Acute effects of initiation and withdrawal of cardiac resynchronization therapy on papillary muscle dyssynchrony and mitral regurgitation. J Am Coll Cardiol. 2007;50:2071–7.
35. Cleland JG, Daubert JC, Erdmann E, et al. The effect of cardiac resynchronization on morbidity and mortality in heart failure. N Engl J Med. 2005;352:1539–49.
36. St John Sutton MG, Plappert T, Abraham WT, et al. Effect of cardiac resynchronization therapy on left ventricular size and function in chronic heart failure. Circulation. 2003;107:1985–90.
37. Trichon BH, et al. Relation of frequency and severity of mitral regurgitation to survival among patients with left ventricular systolic dysfunction and heart failure. Am J Cardiol. 2003;91(5):538–43.
38. Rossi, A. et al. Independent prognostic value of functional mitral regurgitation in patients with heart failure. A quantitative analysis of 1256 patients with ischaemic and non-ischaemic dilated cardiomyopathy. Heart. 2011;97(20):1675–80.
39. Wu AH, et al. Impact of mitral valve annuloplasty on mortality risk in patients with mitral regurgitation and left ventricular systolic dysfunction. J Am Coll Cardiol. 2005;45(3):381–7.
40. Lancellotti P, Gerard PL, Pierard LA. Long-term outcome of patients with heart failure and dynamic functional mitral regurgitation. Eur. Heart J, 2005;26(15):1528–32.
41. Fattouch K, et al. POINT: Efficacy of adding mitral valve restrictive annuloplasty to coronary artery bypass grafting in patients with moderate ischemic mitral valve regurgitation: a randomized trial. J Thorac Cardiovasc Surg. 2009;138(2):278–85.
42. Mihaljevic T, et al. Impact of mitral valve annuloplasty combined with revascularization in patients with functional ischemic mitral regurgitation. J Am Coll Cardiol. 2007;49(22):2191–201.
43. Benedetto U, et al. Does combined mitral valve surgery improve survival when compared to revascularization alone in patients with ischemic mitral regurgitation? A meta-analysis on 2479 patients. J Cardiovasc Med.(Hagerstown). 2009;10(2):109–14.
44. Obadia JF, Messika-Zeitoun D, Leurent G, et al. Percutaneous repair or medical treatment for secondary mitral regurgitation. N Engl J Med. 2018;379(24):2297–306.
45. Stone GW, Lindenfeld J, Abraham WT, et al. Transcatheter mitral-valve repair in patients with heart failure. N Engl J Med. 2018;379(24):2307–318.

Innovative Approaches to Mitral Valve Repair and Replacement

8

Joseph Lamelas, Corinne M. Aberle, and Swaminadhan Gnanashanmugam

Introduction

Minimally invasive valve surgery in its most comprehensive definition involves any procedure to replace or repair a heart valve without a full sternotomy. It is not a single approach but more of a constellation of different techniques and technologies that are specific to this type of procedure. They include various enhanced visualization or exposure devices and instrumentation, as well as modified perfusion techniques, used with the ultimate goal of minimizing surgical trauma by limiting the surgical incision. Types of access typically used include partial upper or lower sternotomy with a T or J transection of the sternum, and mini-thoracotomy approaches using videoscopic or robotic assistance or direct vision.

Reported advantages of these procedures over their open surgical analogues include shorter hospital and intensive care unit stays, less postoperative pain, a more cosmetically acceptable incision, lower thoracic wound infection rates, less use of blood products, better postoperative respiratory function, a more rapid return to baseline functional status, greater patient satisfaction, and lower hospital costs [1–4]. These advantages mimic those observed with minimally invasive techniques used in other fields. Concerns remain, however, that there is a tradeoff of limited exposure against safety, operative length—including cardiopulmonary bypass time and duration of cross-clamping (if used)—ability to adequately evacuate air from the heart, quality of valve repair, potential vascular and cerebrovascular complications, and a long learning curve.

J. Lamelas (✉)
Division of Cardiac Surgery, CHI St. Luke's Health—Baylor St. Luke's Medical Center, Houston, TX, USA

Department of Cardiovascular Surgery, Texas Heart Institute, Houston, TX, USA

C. M. Aberle · S. Gnanashanmugam
Cardiothoracic Surgery, Texas Heart Institute—Baylor College of Medicine, Houston, TX, USA

The recent development and implementation of transcatheter mitral valve (MV) replacement and repair technologies, while representing the pinnacle of minimally invasive ideals, will for the near future remain limited in scope because of the heterogeneity of the MV, technical challenges, and lack of long-term data regarding durability and results. Nonetheless, transvenous/transseptal access to the MV for deployment of a mitral clip has benefited a subset of patients. Newer technologies have been developed to access and repair the MV via a transapical approach. These transcatheter/transapical approaches have been named "micro" invasive procedures to differentiate them from techniques that require cardiopulmonary bypass (CPB). Less-invasive approaches, whether surgical or transcatheter, will continue to evolve and play a major role in cardiovascular therapies.

Evolution

Minimally invasive MV surgery has undergone an evolution of different techniques and philosophies. In this chapter, we review the evolution of the procedure, including the development of CPB techniques, surgical incisions, and approaches that have led the way to its current state. In addition, we review different techniques for replacing and repairing the MV in different disease states.

The first successful use of CPB by John Gibbon in 1953 paved the way to allowing correction of complex cardiac anomalies in a bloodless field [5]. The first documented minimally invasive approach to both aortic and mitral valve disease through a right parasternal incision is attributed to Cosgrove and colleagues in 1996 [6]. Concurrently, improvements were made to minimize the circulating blood volume through a bypass circuit, with the objective of diminishing the inflammatory reaction caused by CPB. Cannulas became smaller and longer and were manufactured with non-kinking materials to maximize flow dynamics. Application of carbon dioxide to displace the oxygen in the operative field has reduced the risk of air embolism. In addition, the advent and routine use of intraoperative transesophageal echocardiography (TEE) has

B. A. Carabello (ed.), *Valvular Heart Disease*, Cardiovascular Medicine, https://doi.org/10.1007/978-1-4471-2840-3_8

aided in both confirming cannula placement and ensuring proper removal of air [7].

One of the most significant advances in the evolution of minimally invasive valve surgery is the development of alternative methods of establishing CPB. Because these procedures do not fully expose the heart, alternative techniques involving central aortic or peripheral cannulation via the femoral, subclavian/axillary, and/or jugular vessels were required. Additionally, many minimally invasive operations employ hybrid cannulation strategies involving both central and peripheral cannulation. These strategies can be used on an arrested, fibrillating, or even beating heart [8].

Several disadvantages of peripheral arterial cannulation have been documented, including elevated incidences of vascular complications and stroke [9–11]. However, results from several studies of large patient cohorts contradict these findings [12, 13]. In fact, outcomes have been similar whether central arterial or peripheral cannulation was used. Numerous variations of venous cannulation have been tried, as well. The application of vacuum-assisted drainage with a hard-shell reservoir has had a dramatic impact on venous drainage, augmenting the decompression of the right atrium and ventricle. Such drainage is performed directly via the right atrium or percutaneously from the femoral or internal jugular veins [14].

In a similar manner, cardioplegia solution can be administered either antegrade directly into the aorta or retrograde via the coronary sinus with either transjugular access or direct right atrial insertion. Additionally, extended-effect cardioplegia solutions have allowed surgeons to protect the heart for longer periods of time while performing complex valvular reconstructions.

In the beginning, minimally invasive MV operations were performed through a right parasternal incision. This required resecting the third and fourth costal cartilages, which led to significant chest-wall deformities and paradoxical chest-wall motion [15]. Thereafter, for many surgeons, ministernotomy with a T or L transection of the sternum in the fourth or fifth intercostal space became the incision of choice for minimally invasive mitral-valve repairs [16, 17]. This allows central cannulation and facilitates conversion to median sternotomy if necessary. Other incisions have included a right thoracotomy, right infra-axillary thoracotomy [18], transsternal approach [19], inverted T-sternotomy [20], and "V"-incision [1]. Today, a right mini-thoracotomy in the fourth or fifth intercostal space is the most widely used approach.

In addition, innovative technologies have been developed to facilitate minimally invasive cardiac surgery. The port-access, keyhole, or "Heart Port" method was one of the first to use aortic occlusion with an endoaortic balloon inserted through a peripheral artery, along with a retrograde cardioplegia catheter inserted through the right internal jugular vein [21]. An alternative method that is commonly used today is direct aortic clamping either via a separate port or directly through the incision [22].

In 1996, Carpentier described the use of 2-D video thoracoscopic assistance to improve visualization of the MV [23]. Shortly thereafter, a 3D version was developed to improve depth perception. In an attempt to further facilitate the procedure, a voice-activated robotic arm was attached to the scope (AESOP 3000, Computer Motion, Inc., CA, USA), allowing mitral surgery to be performed by a single surgeon [24].

In 1998, Carpentier also became the first surgeon to perform a MV operation using a robotic system, the Da Vinci® Surgical System (Intuitive Surgical, Inc., Sunnyvale, CA, USA) [25]. This telemanipulator allowed the surgeon to sit at a console and remotely control surgical instruments in the operative field with 360 degrees of motion. Robotic surgical systems were met with great enthusiasm initially but were not widely adopted because they involved an extremely steep learning curve. In addition, operative times and costs are often greater for robotic surgery than for traditional sternotomy approaches, except at a few expert centers. Nonetheless, newer generations of the Da Vinci Surgical System have been developed, and other corporations—including Google, which has teamed up with Johnson & Johnson (Verb Surgical), Medtronic, and Cambridge Medical Robotics (Versius)—are now introducing their own versions of the robotic system.

Minimally Invasive Surgical Approaches for the Mitral Valve

The most common surgical approach to the MV is through a median sternotomy with central aortic and right atrial cannulation. The MV is exposed through the intra-atrial groove or the right atrium with either a transseptal exposure or a superior approach through the dome of the left atrium.

Less-invasive approaches to the MV have also been devised. The most common include a right mini-thoracotomy with direct visualization, video thoracoscopic visualization, and robotic surgical assistance. The most important considerations are that the patient's safety not be compromised and that the mitral repair be effective and durable.

Comorbidities and Anatomic Considerations

A complete history and physical exam to identify all comorbidities should be routine before any cardiac operation. In addition, computed tomography (CT) imaging can help to determine whether a patient is a good candidate for a minimally invasive approach. When such an approach is planned, careful screening is necessary for several pertinent comorbidities. Significant lung disease is of particular concern in minimally invasive surgery because this approach may require single-lung ventilation. Furthermore, lung dysfunction places the patient at risk for postoperative respiratory failure. Any patient with symptoms of obstructive lung disease or with a heavy smoking history should be considered for pulmonary function testing.

Any history of chest trauma, chest tube placement, empyema, or chest surgery should be elucidated, because existing adhesions or scarring can complicate efforts to obtain the necessary exposure of the heart. These pulmonary adhesions may require extensive dissection, potentially leading to lung injury. Interestingly enough, imaging cannot detect intraoperative adhesions that would potentially preclude a right mini thoracotomy approach.

If a chest radiograph shows the right border of the heart adjacent to the right border of the vertebral column, the heart might be displaced toward the left side of the chest. In addition, the surgeon should know if the patient has breast implants, as these can complicate placement of the atrial retraction system. Significant obesity or extensive chest-wall musculature can place the MV further away from the surgeon, also potentially compromising exposure.

Physical examination and a CT scan help identify congenital and traumatic chest-wall and skeletal deformities that can compromise exposure during minimally invasive mitral surgery. In these specific cases, preoperative screening can potentially prevent conversion by identifying aberrant or challenging anatomy.

Although the aforementioned barriers can potentially complicate minimally invasive right thoracotomy surgery, none of them definitively contraindicate it.

Peripheral vascular disease, aortic aneurysmal disease, and aortic calcification are also of particular concern. Minimally invasive surgery often involves cannulating the femoral vessels for retrograde arterial perfusion, as well as aortic occlusion with a cross-clamp or endoaortic balloon. Existing peripheral vascular disease may preclude safe aortic cross-clamping or peripheral cannulation, thereby placing the patient at risk for perioperative limb ischemia. A complete physical examination should be made of the femoral and peripheral pulses. Any abnormalities on examination or a history of prior vascular disease warrants additional testing. Noninvasive vascular screening can be a useful adjunct to the physical exam. A more detailed assessment is obtained with CT angiography of the chest, abdomen, and pelvis, including the femoral vessels. This scan can reveal vascular dissection, thrombus, aneurysmal dilation, and occlusive disease, all of which contraindicate minimally invasive surgery. Patients with an aortic diameter >4 cm may not be suitable candidates for endoaortic balloon occlusion. A calcified aorta does not contraindicate mitral surgery, but identifying it preoperatively enables the surgeon to be prepared to perform the procedure on a fibrillating heart if necessary. In addition, evaluating the venous phase on CT can help identify barriers to successful peripheral venous cannulation, especially for patients with a history of iliofemoral deep vein thrombosis or an inferior vena cava filter. Having such a filter does not definitively contraindicate femoral venous cannulation, but cannulation should be attempted with fluoroscopic guidance.

In addition, obesity and overlying pannus can interfere with femoral cannulation and place the patient at risk for infection. Evidence of fungal infection in the groin should prompt consideration of alternate cannulation sites.

Coronary artery disease, coexisting valvular disease, reduced left ventricular ejection fraction (LVEF), right ventricular dysfunction, and severe pulmonary hypertension are additional comorbidities that should be screened for. Echocardiography should be completed on all patients preoperatively and can identify many of these comorbidities. Left heart catheterization identifies coronary disease, potentially allowing hybrid approaches with percutaneous coronary intervention and, thereafter, valve surgery in selected patients. The American Heart Association (AHA) guidelines recommend left heart catheterization for male patients over 40 and postmenopausal women undergoing valvular surgery [26]. The need for concomitant coronary revascularization may be considered a relative contraindication to minimally invasive MV replacement unless the revascularization can be performed percutaneously. Concomitant tricuspid valve and even aortic valve surgery is not a contraindication. A minimally invasive approach through the right chest can incur longer ischemic times, which places patients with severely decreased LVEF, depressed right ventricular function, and severe pulmonary hypertension at high risk if the surgeons are inexperienced. In addition, topical cooling of the heart may not be possible with a minimally invasive approach.

The only definitive contraindication to a less-invasive approach is the inability to cannulate the patient safely. Although challenging to address, anatomical variants and associated comorbidities are not definitive contraindications to minimally invasive MV surgery.

Additional Considerations

Other important factors may influence patient selection for minimally invasive mitral surgery. For example, for most reoperative MV procedures, a minimally invasive approach should be considered. Performing the procedure through the right chest and avoiding a redo sternotomy limits the associated risk of iatrogenic injuries. In the majority of cases, a right chest approach provides a field with fewer adhesions. In addition, some patients with prior stroke, limited mobility, or increased frailty may benefit from the avoidance of a sternotomy. Furthermore, many of the relative contraindications to minimally invasive surgery can be overcome with surgeon experience and modified operative techniques. Inserting transjugular retrograde coronary perfusion cannulas and pulmonary artery vents can augment cardiac protection and heart decompression in patients with existing coronary disease or aortic insufficiency. Retrograde cannulas can also be inserted directly into the right atrium from the operating port. Cold fibrillatory arrest may be an option for patients with extensive pericardial adhesions, aortic disease precluding cross-clamp or endoaortic balloon placement, or prior coronary artery bypass grafting. Hybrid approaches with percutaneous coronary intervention can further increase candidacy for these procedures. Mitral annular calcification adds significant complexity and thus can be considered a relative contraindication. The feared complication of atrioventricular disruption associated with mitral annular calcification is sometimes difficult to repair for even the most experienced limited-access surgeons. These features can be identified on both preoperative echocardiography and CT angiography. Not only should the pathology of the MV be considered, but any additional valve disease must be considered, as well. Aortic regurgitation is of particular interest, as it may complicate cardiac protection, arrest, and effective decompression and venting. As surgeon experience increases, more complex repairs, as well as concomitant procedures, can be completed with a minimally invasive platform.

Robotic Mitral Valve Surgery

Robotic mitral surgery is more technically challenging and takes longer to learn than other approaches. Patient setup in the operating room is largely the same as in other minimally invasive approaches. The trachea is intubated with either a double-lumen tube or a bronchial blocker. In some cases, a pulmonary EndoVent and transjugular retrograde cardioplegia cannula (Edwards Lifesciences, Irvine, CA, USA) are inserted. The patient is positioned with the right chest elevated by a scapula roll. The right arm hangs off the table with the elbow slightly flexed. Defibrillator pads are placed on the posterior and lateral thorax.

Robotic mitral operations usually require peripheral cannulation, usually via the femoral artery and vein, although in some cases, an additional venous cannula is inserted into the superior vena cava (SVC) through the right internal jugular vein. An endoscope port is placed in the fourth intercostal space (ICS), 2–3 cm lateral to the nipple. The right minithoracotomy working port (1.5-cm retractor) is placed in the fourth ICS as well, approximately 4 cm lateral to the camera. The left robotic arm enters through a port in the second ICS, halfway between the endoscope port and shoulder. The right robotic arm is placed in the sixth ICS in the region of the anterior axillary line. An atrial lift retractor is inserted through an additional port in the fourth ICS medial to the camera port. Aortic occlusion is performed with an endoaortic balloon catheter. In these cases, bilateral radial arterial lines are placed, and care is taken to avoid dampening of the pressures, which signals migration of the balloon and occlusion of the great vessels. If an endoaortic balloon is not used, a sixth incision or port is created in the second ICS, 10 cm posterior to the left robotic arm, for insertion of a transthoracic cross-clamp. Cardioplegia solution is delivered through the endoaortic balloon or, if the aorta is clamped externally, directly into the aortic root with a small cannula. Mitral repair techniques are similar for all minimally invasive approaches. Robotic assisted MV replacement is more challenging and should be reserved for the most experienced robotic surgeons. Suture management is challenging, and the working port needs to be large enough to permit passage of the prosthetic valve. Autoknotting devices may facilitate tying in these cases [27].

Endoscopic Mitral Valve Surgery

The intraoperative setup and patient positioning are essentially similar to those used in a robotic operation. A 4-cm working incision or port is made at the level of the fourth or fifth ICS, starting at the anterior axillary line, and thereafter a soft tissue retractor is placed. Rib spreading with an intercostal rib retractor is avoided in these procedures. Another incision is made at the level of the seventh ICS midaxillary line. Through this incision, a sump suction is tunneled and is subsequently inserted through the left atriotomy and into the left inferior pulmonary vein to help drain the pulmonary venous return. Carbon dioxide is infused into the operative field at 2–3 L/min. This facilitates evacuation of air from the heart. Peripheral cannulation is usually used with video endoscopic procedures. Aortic occlusion can be performed with an endoaortic balloon or direct external aortic clamping through a separate incision. Cardioplegia solution is administered through the endoballoon or a cardioplegia cannula inserted directly into the aortic root.

Once electromechanical arrest of the heart is established, a left atriotomy is performed. Cross-clamping, cardioplegia delivery, pericardiotomy, atriotomy, and closure can be performed with videoscopic assistance or direct vision. A 5-mm trocar is placed 1 intercostal space above and lateral to the working port. A 0° or 30° thoracoscope is inserted through the trocar to directly visualize the MV. After the left atriotomy, an atrial lift retractor is inserted through the working port and connected to a post inserted through a separate stab wound medial to the incision. Long-shafted, manually controlled instruments are inserted through the working port to perform the mitral repair or replacement. Video endoscopic operations can be challenging and take time to learn [28].

Direct Vision Right Mini-Thoracotomy Mitral Valve Surgery

A single-lumen endotracheal tube is inserted, and double-lung ventilation is used throughout the operation. If visualization of the heart is impaired by the lungs, the lungs are temporarily deflated, or CPB can be instituted early.

Single-lung ventilation with a double-lumen endotracheal tube or bronchial blocker is not commonly performed unless significant pleural adhesions limit visualization and dissection. There are reported cases of unilateral re-expansion pulmonary edema secondary to single-lung ventilation [29, 30].

Transesophageal Echocardiography

Every patient should have a thorough intraoperative 2-D and 3-D TEE assessment. The size of the mitral annulus and anterior leaflet are measured. Left ventricular function is assessed. The MV is further interrogated. Atherosclerotic disease is assessed in the ascending and descending aorta; evidence of grade 4 or 5 free-floating atheroma in the descending aorta should preclude femoral cannulation and retrograde arterial perfusion. The venous cannula is positioned in the SVC under TEE guidance, using a bicaval mid-esophageal view at 80–100°. In patients with mild-to-moderate aortic insufficiency, TEE is used to obtain a midesophageal four-chamber view at 0° to guide placement of a retrograde cardioplegia cannula.

Intraoperative fluoroscopy can also be used to aid placement of the venous guide wire and cannula when the wire cannot be visualized by TEE. Intraoperative iliac and abdominal aortic angiograms with fluoroscopy are performed when there is uncertainty after insertion of the femoral arterial cannula, or when calcified plaques are encountered during cannulation.

Cannulation and Perfusion

A femoral platform is the access site of choice. Left femoral artery and vein cannulation are preferred because most patients undergo a cardiac catheterization via the right femoral artery. If the surgeon is not yet experienced with this technique, CT angiography should be performed routinely, especially if severe peripheral vascular disease is suspected.

Before cannulation, the patient is fully heparinized (3.3 mg/kg). A 2–3-cm longitudinal skin incision is made above the inguinal crease. In our practice, using this approach, along with limited dissection of the anterior aspect of the vessels, has decreased the incidence of seroma formation. Careful attention is paid to assessing the quality of the artery. The presence of a posterior horseshoe calcified plaque does not contraindicate cannulation, but circumferential calcification does. A purse string suture is placed on the anterior aspect of each vessel. A modified Seldinger technique is used for cannulation. A guide wire is advanced through the femoral artery and subsequently into the proximal descending aorta, and its position is verified by TEE. The wire should pass through without resistance. Thereafter, a cannula is inserted into the artery. The choice of cannula size depends on the patient's body surface area.

If there is any resistance when the cannula is advanced, an alternative access site should be chosen. Additionally, if there are any concerns, an intraoperative angiogram can be performed. If an alternative cannulation site is required, the right axillary artery is the next access point of choice. During axillary cannulation, intraoperative fluoroscopy and angiography are always performed. Because all female patients are positioned with the arm placed over the head, if peripheral vascular disease is present, the axillary artery is cannulated through the axilla. Central cannulation can also be performed, although this is more challenging because of the distance from the incision.

Venous Cannulation

Femoral venous cannulation is performed by using a Seldinger technique. A wire is passed through the femoral vein and into the SVC under TEE guidance. A 0° bicaval view is obtained for placement [31].

Thereafter, a 25 Fr venous cannula is advanced deep into the SVC. To obtain adequate venous drainage, the cannula should be in the SVC, and vacuum drainage should be applied. Vacuum assistance with 35 mmHg of negative suction is applied and increased to 65 mmHg if necessary. The application of negative pressure increases the formation of gaseous microemboli, although this has not been proven to be harmful [32]. Evidence suggests that surpassing 60 mmHg of negative pressure does not increase the incidence of neurological events [33].

There are also instances in which additional venous drainage is required because of right-sided distention or dislodgement of the venous cannula into the right atrium. It is crucial to have adequate decompression of the right side of the heart, because this can lead to postoperative heart failure.

Patient Selection

When compared with standard sternotomy MV surgery, minimally invasive MV surgery appears to benefit higher-risk patients. These include patients more than 75 years old [2], obese patients (body mass index >30 kg/m^2) [4], patients with chronic obstructive pulmonary disease (COPD) [3], and patients with a low LVEF (<35%) [4].

Several series have demonstrated lower morbidity and mortality with minimally invasive MV procedures in these subsets of patients. Concomitant tricuspid and aortic valve surgery can also be performed. Unlike in minimally invasive AVR surgery, a saphenous vein bypass to the right coronary artery cannot be performed. On the other hand, reoperative MV surgery is feasible in patients with prior valve surgery or coronary revascularization via a right mini-thoracotomy approach [34]. Patients with CAD amendable to PCI can be offered a hybrid approach. A percutaneous intervention can be performed at any time before the minimally invasive valve procedure; in a select few patients, it can be performed afterward. Furthermore, a mini-thoracotomy approach can be offered to patients receiving dual antiplatelet therapy [35].

Surgical Technique

All male patients are positioned with the arm hanging slightly off of the operating table with a scapula roll allowing elevation of the right chest. Female patients are positioned with the scapula roll as well, although the right arm is positioned over the head and the breast is displaced medially to provide additional exposure. A 5–6-cm incision is made at the level of the fourth or fifth intercostal space. A soft-tissue retractor and a rib spreader provide additional exposure. Cardiopulmonary bypass is instituted, and the pericardium is opened and retracted with stay sutures. The aorta is clamped directly through the incision, and cardioplegia solution is administered into the aortic root. If there is mild-to-moderate aortic insufficiency, a retrograde cardioplegia cannula is inserted. Thereafter, an atrial lift retractor is inserted, and the MV is further exposed. If a concomitant ablation or ligation of the atrial appendage is required, it is performed before the MV operation begins. Carbon dioxide is infused into the operative field at a rate of 2 L/min. Infusing a greater volume of CO_2 will raise the patients' CO_2 level during CPB, and sweeping it off will be an arduous task for the perfusionist.

The MV repair or replacement proceeds in the usual fashion, although long-shafted surgical instruments are required. On completion, the left atriotomy is closed and pacing wires are placed on the inferior wall of the right ventricle. The cross-clamp is removed, and deairing is performed with an aortic root vent. Once TEE images confirm adequate air removal, valve function, and valve competency, the patient is weaned from CPB. After protamine is administered, the femoral arterial and venous cannulas are removed. A drain is placed in the pericardium and the right pleural cavity. An intercostal nerve block is performed, and the chest is closed in the usual fashion.

Mitral Valve: Introduction

Mitral valve disease represents the most common valvular disorder worldwide. Although mitral stenosis (MS) is on the decline because of earlier treatment of rheumatic fever, mitral regurgitation (MR) remains a more common valvular disease, especially in developed nations. In the United States, MR is the most frequent valvular disease; nearly 10% of MR patients aged 75 years or older have moderate-to-severe MR [36]. This equates to 4 million affected persons, with an estimated incidence of 250,000 new cases of severe MR per year [36, 37]. Medical therapy has a limited role in these patients' treatment; surgical repair and replacement are the mainstays of therapy [26].

However, a large discrepancy exists between patients who have MV disease and patients who undergo surgical therapy; 2009 data show that only 2% of this potential patient population was treated surgically [38–40]. The reasons for this disparity are multifold. Nearly 50% of symptomatic patients with severe MR are never referred for correction because they are deemed too high risk for surgery. Of the patients referred for surgery, only a fraction actually undergo it; the rest are not treated surgically because of age, comorbidities, or severe LV dysfunction [39]. Mitral regurgitation also has a variable natural history: some patients have stable, mild, or moderate MR for many years, while others' MR progresses over a variable time course.

Etiology and Classification of Mitral Regurgitation

The etiology of MR is multifaceted, with surgical therapy offering different results for MR of different causes. Mitral regurgitation can be classified as either primary (organic) or secondary (functional), depending on the abnormality that leads to the regurgitation, although its pathophysiology varies widely within each category. Differentiating between these two entities is crucial to choosing a therapeutic strategy and predicting its outcome. In addition, it is important to recognize that a single patient's MR can have multiple causes.

Primary or organic MR is an intrinsic valvular abnormality affecting components of the mitral apparatus (i.e., leaflets, annulus, chordae, or papillary muscles). Dysfunction of any of the structures of the MV leads to regurgitation of blood into the atrium during systole. The most common causes of primary MR are degenerative diseases: a variety of conditions that cause abnormalities of the connective tissue, leading to structural changes of the mitral apparatus. Myxomatous degeneration of the MV in its most extensive form is called Barlow disease. The mitral leaflets become thickened and redundant and commonly develop multisegmental prolapse due to a myxoid infiltration. The valves are typically large, with diffuse chordal elongation and rupture. Carpentier described a "forme fruste" of Barlow disease, understanding that many valves have some but not all of the disease's pathologic features, thus recognizing the spectrum of lesions [41, 42].

Another cause of degenerative MR is fibroelastic disease, in which there is a deficiency of connective tissue. This leads to a deficiency of collagen, elastins, and proteoglycans, causing a thinning of the leaflets. The majority of patients present with a normal-appearing annulus and valve segments with thin and elongated or ruptured chordae. Some patients present with isolated prolapsing segments of the leaflets, which can become thickened from myxoid deposition, but the mechanism of MR is usually rupture of thin chordae tendineae.

Additional causes of primary MR include other connective tissue disorders (Marfan syndrome, Ehlers-Danlos syndrome), osteogenesis imperfecta, pseudoxanthoma elasticum, endocarditis, rheumatic disease, and radiation- or drug-induced valvulopathy. Rheumatic disease is the most prevalent cause of primary MR in developing countries.

Secondary or functional MR is caused by ventricular dysfunction due to dilation, diffuse hypokinesis, or segmental damage secondary to ischemic disease or dilated cardiomyopathy. These changes in the sphericity of the ventricle displace the papillary muscles in an outward and/or apical direction and cause tethering of the leaflets, thus restricting closure during systole. Another, less common cause of functional MR occurs only with left atrial remodeling from atrial fibrillation. In these cases, annular enlargement leads to MR with preserved LV function. In both types of secondary MR, the mitral leaflets are usually structurally normal or nearly normal.

Furthermore, as disease progresses, causes can become mixed; for instance, severe untreated primary MR may lead to ventricular remodeling and associated secondary MR. Multiple causes can also arise concurrently (e.g., ischemic MR with combined degenerative MR), further complicating matters. Although surgical therapy has had good results in primary MR, results in secondary MR have been varied.

Mitral Valve Apparatus Structure and Function

A thorough understanding of MV apparatus structure and function is necessary to understand surgical and percutaneous approaches to MV repair and replacement and their potential advantages and disadvantages. One can conceive of the MV apparatus as being formed by four components: the annulus, leaflets, chordae tendineae, and papillary muscles [43, 44].

The annulus is an ellipsoid, asymmetrical structure that forms the outer perimeter of the MV apparatus. The anterior portion makes up approximately one-third of the annular circumference and consists of a fibrous portion that is in continuity with the aortic annulus [44]. The posterior portion makes up the remaining two-thirds of the annular circumference and is a dynamic structure. The apparatus contains an asymmetric bileaflet valve consisting of an anterior leaflet and a posterior leaflet. The anterior leaflet has greater leaflet length but has a narrower base than the posterior leaflet. The leaflets are demarcated by an anterolateral and posteromedial commissure [44]. The MV leaflets are attached to the papillary muscles via chordae tendineae or chords. Primary chords attach to the free edge of the leaflets, whereas secondary chords attach to the body of the leaflets. Chords to the anterior leaflet attach to the anterolateral papillary muscles, whereas posterior chords attach to the posterolateral papillary muscles. All of the papillary muscles are affixed to the LV wall.

Functionally, pre-closure of the MV leaflets begins after atrial contraction to approximate the anterior and posterior leaflets. Closure of the MV components relies on the position of the anterior leaflet and coaptation of the leaflets. During systole, when in proper position, the anterior leaflet forms a veil parallel to systolic flow in the LV outflow tract. Then, during coaptation of the leaflets, coaptation over the rough zones on the atrial surfaces of either leaflet creates high friction and resistance, producing strong shear forces. Posterior annular contraction increases this coaptation to facilitate competent closure. Improper valve coaptation or loss thereof due to disruption of any of these anatomic elements of the MV apparatus can result in MR.

Assessing the Mitral Valve

Classification of Mitral Valve Dysfunction

Carpentier's classification of leaflet dysfunction has allowed surgeons and cardiologists to describe valve disease in universal terms [45]. The classification is based on leaflet motion.

- Type I: normal leaflet motion (annular dilatation, leaflet perforation, cleft valve)
- Type II: excessive leaflet motion (prolapse, chordal elongation or rupture, papillary muscle elongation or rupture)
- Type III: restricted leaflet motion
- Type IIIa: leaflet thickening and/or retraction, chordal thickening and/or retraction, commissural fusion (during systole and diastole)
- Type IIIb: papillary muscle displacement and/or leaflet tethering (during systole only)

Table 8.1 further details this complex interplay of etiology, lesions, and function. In any given patient, multiple causes, lesions, and mechanisms of dysfunction may be present, which in turn may necessitate the use of multiple techniques and technologies for valve repair.

Table 8.1 Mitral regurgitation: causes, example lesions, and type of dysfunction

Mechanism of MR and type of dysfunction	Cause of mitral regurgitation (e.g., of lesion)	
	Ischemic	Nonischemic
Organic/primary		
Type I		• Infectious/endocarditis (perforation)
		• Degenerative (annular calcification)
		• Congenital (cleft leaflet)
Type II	Ruptured papillary muscle	• Infectious/endocarditis (ruptured chord)
		• Traumatic (ruptured chord)
		• Rheumatic (elongated chords)
		• Degenerative (billowing/flail leaflets)
Type IIIa		• Rheumatic (e.g., fibrotic chords)
		• Iatrogenic (radiation/drug)
		• Inflammatory (lupus, anticardiolipin, eosinophilic, fibrosis, endocardial diseases)
Functional/secondary		
Type I and Type IIIb	Functional ischemic MR	• Cardiomyopathy, myocarditis
		• LV dysfunction (any cause)

LV left ventricular, *MR* mitral valve regurgitation

Grading the degree of MR has its limitations, so a comprehensive process to obtain multiple measurements by transthoracic echocardiography (TTE), TEE, and Doppler color flow imaging is essential. A more comprehensive assessment should be made—with cardiac magnetic resonance imaging, if necessary—to further quantify the degree of MR and resolve any discrepancies in the echocardiographic findings.

In most cases, TTE can identify the mitral valve pathology. When additional information is required, TEE provides a more precise and detailed assessment of the MV. It has better spatial resolution, allowing more accurate MR quantification, especially with regard to jet color characteristics. In addition, 3-D visualization of the valve provides further confirmatory evidence of the mitral leaflet abnormality and delineates its exact location [46].

Identifying the cause of the MR is essential for the patient's preoperative and postoperative management, as well as for planning the operative strategy. Obtaining an echocardiogram while the patient is not under anesthesia is important because the loading conditions of the heart are not altered; the degree of regurgitation can be significantly reduced and therefore underestimated when the patient is under anesthesia. Assessing not only leaflet pathology but also the direction of the single or multiple regurgitant jets is also important in planning the operative strategy.

The quantitative assessment of the MV by echocardiography classifies the degree of regurgitation into four grades (I–IV). The degree of severity can be graded further by calculating the effective regurgitant orifice area (EROA), regurgitant volume, and regurgitant fraction. It is important to understand that the quantitative parameters used to assess of the severity of MR are different with degenerative and functional MV disease.

With MR, anatomic malcoaptation of the mitral leaflets occurs during systole, and this results in an effective regurgitant orifice (ERO) that allows abnormal flow from the LV into the left atrium (LA) during systole. The ERO is influenced by the pressure gradient between the LV and the LA and may be dynamic, depending on the cause of the MR [47]. Increased afterload or ventricular volume can increase ERO, whereas decreased afterload and improved contractility can reduce ERO [48]. The sum of the regurgitant flow through the ERO during systole is the regurgitant volume (RVol) accumulated in the LA. This RVol reenters the LV during the subsequent diastole, resulting in volume overload of the LA and LV and ensuing manifestations and consequences of disease. In acute MR, the LA is small and has low compliance; as a result, any amount of RVol increases LA pressure. For this reason, acute MR is often not well tolerated and results in significant symptoms and hemodynamic changes.

The hemodynamic responses of the heart to chronic, slowly progressive MR are different from those associated with acute MR. These responses to the excessive chronic volume overload caused by MR initially result in a chronic compensated stage of volume overload, which, if uncorrected, can progress to a decompensated stage with irreversible LV dysfunction. In chronic MR, the LA remodels to accommodate the RVol so that the LA pressure is maintained; for this reason, even severe MR may be tolerated hemodynamically and symptomatically for a long period, even years [49]. Thus, in the chronic compensated state, the LV is initially unloaded by the low-resistance runoff into the LA, which is then countered by an increase in LV size to maintain wall stress at normal levels [50, 51]. In the chronic compensated stage, LV enlargement is the chief compensatory mechanism, allowing a greater LV volume as a result of the MR while maintaining normal diastolic pressures. The chronic overload from this RVol eventually leads to LV hypertrophy and dilatation [52]. The LV end-diastolic volume, end-systolic volume, and wall stress all increase, causing the LV to become more spherical [53, 54].

In the chronic compensated state, adequate forward cardiac output and normal filling pressures are maintained. Sequelae of this pathophysiology, such as atrial fibrillation due to continued left atrial enlargement, and pulmonary hypertension due to continued pressure overload, are the presenting clinical phenomena for some patients. Diastolic dysfunction may also be present but is often difficult to diagnose and quantify; it may account for symptomaticity and reduced functional capacity in patients with normal systolic function [55, 56].

Many patients remain asymptomatic in this state, and normalized preload and wall stress sometimes help the LV maintain normal contractility. Patients can remain in a chronic compensated stage for years to decades after the onset of MR.

However, eventually, the consequence of these changes is progressive LV enlargement beyond the compensated stage; the ensuing ventricular dysfunction can be severe [56]. Progressive LV enlargement may be due to increased severity of MR, continued compensatory chamber enlargement, or both. The LV enlargement can exacerbate MR because of ventricular-valvular interdependence, resulting in a vicious cycle of worsening MR and LV dysfunction. Preload and afterload changes can make the degree of this LV dysfunction difficult to characterize [57]. Nevertheless, these cumulative effects can result in irreversible LV dysfunction, leading to decompensated MR, with an ensuing poor prognosis.

In *primary MR*, mild MR is defined as a mitral RVol <30 mL, a regurgitant fraction (RF) <30%, and an EROA <0.2 cm^2, whereas severe MR is defined as a RVol ≥60 mL with an RF ≥50% and an EROA ≥0.4 cm^2. Other indicators of severe MR include a vena contracta width ≥0.7 cm with a large central regurgitant jet occupying >40% of the LA area or with a wall-impinging jet of any size, as well as blunting of the systolic component with systolic flow reversal in the pulmonary veins. Additional supportive signs include a very dense, early-peaking triangular jet on a continuous-wave Doppler echocardiogram and a peak mitral inflow velocity >120 cm/s [58].

The 2014 AHA/American College of Cardiology (ACC) guidelines now classify primary MR into four grades: grade A, at risk of MR; grade B, progressive MR; grade C, asymptomatic severe MR; and grade D, symptomatic severe MR (Table 8.2). Patients at risk of MR are identified on echocardiography with mild valvular prolapse but normal coaptation, or mild valvular thickening and leaflet restriction. They have either no MR jet or a jet area <20% of the LA, with a vena contracta <0.3 cm. Mitral valve surgery is not indicated for patients at risk of MR [26].

Progressive, or grade B, MR is characterized by severe mitral prolapse with normal coaptation, rheumatic changes with leaflet restriction, and loss of coaptation, or by prior infective endocarditis. The central jet measures 20–40% of the LA or may be a late systolic eccentric jet. The vena contracta measures <0.7 cm and has a regurgitant volume of <60 mL, an RF <50%, and an EROA <0.4 cm^2. Concomitant MV repair is now a class IIa recommendation for patients with grade B MR undergoing cardiac surgery for other indications [26].

Asymptomatic severe MR, or grade C, can be characterized similarly to grade B, in that echocardiographic findings are consistent with rheumatic changes or prior infective endocarditis. Grade C severity is often distinguished from Grade B by prolapse with the loss of leaflet coaptation or a flail leaflet, or by thickening of the leaflets associated with radiation heart disease. Defining echocardiographic measurements are a central jet >40% of the LA, a holosystolic eccentric jet, vena contracta >0.7 cm, regurgitant volume >60 mL, RF >50%, and an EROA >0.4 cm^2. Class Ia indications for surgery for asymptomatic severe MR include LV dysfunction (defined by an LVEF of 30–60% or a LV end-systolic diameter >40 mm) and cardiac surgery for other indications, during which the MV can be repaired concomitantly. Current guidelines make a class IIa recommendation for repair for asymptomatic severe MR in patients with preserved LV function, for whom the likelihood of a successful and durable repair is >95%, with an expected mortality <1% when performed at a Heart Valve Center of Excellence [26].

Symptomatic severe MR, or grade D, is identified by the same anatomic findings and echocardiographic measurements used to identify asymptomatic MR. Symptoms of severe MR include decreased exercise tolerance and exertional dyspnea. Mitral valve surgery is a class I recommendation for patients with an LVEF >30% and symptomatic severe MR. In addition, considering MV surgery in patients with an LVEF <30% now carries a class IIb recommendation [26].

In *secondary MR*, the thresholds of 0.4 cm^2 or 60 mL/beat may still be considered severe on the basis of several arguments. A lower RVol might still represent significant overload for a compromised LV. Because the total cardiac output of the ventricle is generally lower than in primary MR with preserved LV function, the 60-mL threshold may not be reached despite a >50% RF. In addition, with secondary MR, the orifice is usually crescentic along the commissural line and may underestimate the orifice area when one uses the 2D PISA method (in contrast to 3D), which inherently assumes a hemispheric flow convergence [59].

The most recent (2017) guideline the ERO delineating "severe" MR was changed from 0.2 cm^2 to 0.4 cm^2 recognizing that LV volume interacted with orifice area in delineating severity. In the typically dilated LV in patients with MR, an ERO of 0.4 cm^2 is usually associated with a regurgitant fraction of 50% while in smaller LVs the ERO may be less than 0.4 and still be consistant with severe MR. Most importantly, no single parameter should ever be used to assess MR severity in either primary or secondary MR. Rather all parameters including physical examination should be integrated to arrive at an estimation.

Cardiac magnetic resonance (CMR) can be used not only to assess the cause but also, more importantly, to quantify the severity of MR. Use of CMR is indicated when echocardiographic and clinical findings do not agree. It is extremely useful for quantifying multiple or eccentric MR jets that are difficult to evaluate by echocardiography. In addition, CMR can assess cardiac size and function and LV scar burden, along with their interaction, in patients with secondary MR [60]. Most comparisons of CMR and TTE show concordance

Table 8.2 Stages of primary MR

Grade	Definition	Valve anatomy	Valve hemodynamics[a]	Hemodynamic consequences	Symptoms
A	At risk of MR	• Mild mitral valve prolapse with normal coaptation • Mild valve thickening and leaflet restriction	• No MR jet or small central jet area <20% LA on Doppler • Small vena contracta <0.3 cm	• None	• None
B	Progressive MR	• Severe mitral valve prolapse with normal coaptation • Rheumatic valve changes with leaflet restriction and loss of central coaptation • Prior IE	• Central jet MR 20–40% • LA or late systolic eccentric jet MR • Vena contracta <0.7 cm • Regurgitant volume <60 mL • Regurgitant fraction <50% • ERO <0.40 cm^2 • Angiographic grade 1–2+	• Mild LA enlargement • No LV enlargement • Normal pulmonary pressure	• None
C	Asymptomatic severe MR	• Severe mitral valve prolapse with loss of coaptation or flail leaflet • Rheumatic valve changes with leaflet restriction and loss of central coaptation • Prior IE • Thickening of leaflets with radiation heart disease	• Central jet MR >40% LA or holosystolic eccentric jet MR • Vena contracta ≥0.7 cm • Regurgitant volume ≥ 60 mL • Regurgitant fraction ≥50% • ERO ≥0.40 cm^2 • Angiographic grade 3–4+	• Moderate or severe LA enlargement • LV enlargement • Pulmonary hypertension may be present at rest or with exercise • C1: LVEF >60% and LVESD <40 mm • C2: LVEF ≤60% and LVESD ≥40 mm	• None
D	Symptomatic severe MR	• Severe mitral valve prolapse with loss of coaptation or flail leaflet • Rheumatic valve changes with leaflet restriction and loss of central coaptation • Prior IE • Thickening of leaflets with radiation heart disease	• Central jet MR >40% LA or holosystolic eccentric jet MR • Vena contracta ≥0.7 cm • Regurgitant volume ≥ 60 mL • Regurgitant fraction ≥50% • ERO ≥0.40 cm^2 • Angiographic grade 3–4+	• Moderate or severe LA enlargement • LV enlargement • Pulmonary hypertension present	• Decreased exercise tolerance • Exertional dyspnea

ERO effective regurgitant orifice, *IE* infective endocarditis, *LA* left atrium/atrial, *LV* left ventricular, *LVEF* left ventricular ejection fraction, *LVESD* left ventricular end-systolic dimension, *MR* mitral regurgitation

From Nishimura RA, Otto CM, Bonow RO, Carabello BA, Erwin JP, 3rd, Guyton RA, et al. 2014 AHA/ACC guideline for the management of patients with valvular heart disease: a report of the American College of Cardiology/American Heart Association Task Force on Practice Guidelines. J Thorac Cardiovasc Surg. 2014;148:e1–e132. Reprinted with permission

[a]Several valve hemodynamic criteria are provided for assessment of MR severity, but not all criteria for each category will be present in each patient. Categorization of MR severity as mild, moderate, or severe depends on data quality and integration of these parameters in conjunction with other clinical evidence

in evaluating the degree of primary MR, although not secondary MR [61, 62].

The 2017 AHA/ACC guidelines classify secondary MR into the same 4 classes as primary MR: grade A, at risk of MR; grade B, progressive MR; grade C, asymptomatic severe MR; and grade D, symptomatic severe MR. Patients at risk of secondary MR have normal valve leaflets, chords, and annular structure, with associated coronary disease or cardiomyopathy. Echocardiography reveals no MR jet or a jet <20% of the LA, and a vena contracta <0.3 cm. No intervention is recommended for patients at risk of secondary MR [26].

The most recent 2017 ACC/AHA guidelines used to describe secondary/functional MR are shown in Table 8.3.

Secondary progressive MR is identified by wall motion abnormalities on echocardiography, with mild tethering of the mitral leaflet or with annular dilation and loss of central coaptation of the leaflets. The EROA is <0.4 cm^2, regurgitant volume is <60 mL, and the RF is <50%. Mitral valve repair (not replacement) may be considered for secondary progressive MR in patients undergoing cardiac surgery for other indications (class IIb recommendation) [26].

Asymptomatic and symptomatic severe secondary MR are associated with regional wall motion abnormalities, LV dilatation with severe tethering of a mitral leaflet, or annular dilation with severe loss of mitral leaflet coaptation. The EROA is >0.4 cm^2, with a regurgitant volume >60 mL or an RF >50%. Asymptomatic patients may have symptoms due to coronary ischemia or heart failure, but these symptoms respond to revascularization and medical therapy. In contrast, patients considered symptomatic have heart failure symptoms that

Table 8.3 Stages of secondary MR

Grade	Definition	Valve anatomy	Valve hemodynamics[a]	Associated cardiac findings	Symptoms
A	At risk of MR	• Normal valve leaflets, chords, and annulus in a patient with coronary disease or cardiomyopathy	• No MR jet or small central jet area <20% LA on Doppler • Small vena contracta <0.30 cm	• Normal or mildly dilated LV size with fixed (infarction) or inducible (ischemia) regional wall motion abnormalities • Primary myocardial disease with LV dilation and systolic dysfunction	• Symptoms due to coronary ischemia or HF may be present that respond to revascularization and appropriate medical therapy
B	Progressive MR	• Regional wall motion abnormalities with mild tethering of mitral leaflet • Annular dilation with mild loss of central coaptation of the mitral leaflets	• ERO <0.40 cm[2,b] • Regurgitant volume <60 mL • Regurgitant fraction <50%	• Regional wall motion abnormalities with reduced LV systolic function • LV dilation and systolic dysfunction due to primary myocardial disease	• Symptoms due to coronary ischemia or HF may be present that respond to revascularization and appropriate medical therapy
C	Asymptomatic severe MR	• Regional wall motion abnormalities and/or LV dilation with severe tethering of mitral leaflet • Annular dilation with severe loss of central coaptation of the mitral leaflets	• ERO ≥0.40 cm[2,b] • Regurgitant volume ≥60 mL • Regurgitant fraction ≥50%	• Regional wall motion abnormalities with reduced LV systolic function • LV dilation and systolic dysfunction due to primary myocardial disease	• Symptoms due to coronary ischemia or HF may be present that respond to revascularization and appropriate medical therapy
D	Symptomatic severe MR	• Regional wall motion abnormalities and/or LV dilation with severe tethering of mitral leaflet • Annular dilation with severe loss of central coaptation of the mitral leaflets	• ERO ≥0.40 cm[2,b] • Regurgitant volume ≥60 mL • Regurgitant fraction ≥50%	• Regional wall motion abnormalities with reduced LV systolic function • LV dilation and systolic dysfunction due to primary myocardial disease	• HF symptoms due to MR persist even after revascularization and optimization of medical therapy • Decreased exercise tolerance • Exertional dyspnea

2D 2-dimensional, *ERO* effective regurgitant orifice, *HF* heart failure, *LA* left atrium, *LV* left ventricular, *MR* mitral regurgitation, *TTE* transthoracic echocardiogram

From Nishimura RA, Otto CM, Bonow RO, Carabello BA, Erwin JP, 3rd, Guyton RA, et al. 2017 Focused Update of the 2014 AHA/ACC guideline for the management of patients with valvular heart disease: a report of the American College of Cardiology/American Heart Association Task Force on Practice Guidelines. JACC 2017 70:252–289. Reprinted with permission

[a]Several valve hemodynamic criteria are provided for assessment of MR severity, but not all criteria for each category will be present in each patient. Categorization of MR severity as mild, moderate, or severe depends on data quality and integration of these parameters in conjunction with other clinical evidence

[b]The measurement of the proximal isovelocity surface area by 2D TTE in patients with secondary MR underestimates the true ERO due to the crescentic shape of the proximal convergence

persist after revascularization and do not respond to optimized medical therapy. These symptoms may include decreased exercise tolerance and exertional dyspnea. Mitral valve surgery is recommended for both asymptomatic and symptomatic severe secondary MR in patients undergoing coronary artery bypass grafting or AVR (class IIa). Mitral valve repair or replacement may be considered for symptomatic patients undergoing other cardiac operations (class IIb) [26].

Nonischemic functional MR is most often due to severe chronic LV volume overload with unknown or idiopathic causes. Other advanced valvular heart disease is the second most common cause. Functional MR can be found in 40% of patients with heart failure due to dilated cardiomyopathy [63]. Functional, ischemic MR is increasingly prevalent as the population ages and as more patients survive myocardial infarction and live with severe ischemic heart disease. Ischemic MR can result in changes in mitral annular geometry and regional and global LV geometry and function, abnormal leaflet motion, increased distance between papillary muscles, misalignment of papillary muscles, and apical tethering of the leaflets with restricted systolic leaflet motion and a typical Carpentier type IIIb pattern of dysfunction [64, 65]. Thus, ventricular dysfunction, whether the cause is ischemic or nonischemic, can cause or contribute substantially to the development of MR. Technologies aimed at ameliorating ventricular dysfunction may therefore be important in treating MR in such patients.

Mitral Valve Stenosis

Mitral valve stenosis is classified into stages similar to the grades used to classify MR: stage A, at risk of MS; stage B, progressive MS; stage C, asymptomatic severe MS; and stage D, symptomatic severe MS. Patients at risk of MS may have MV doming identified by echocardiography, but with normal transmitral velocities. No intervention is recommended at this stage [26].

Patients with progressive MS may have rheumatic changes with associated commissural fusion and diastolic doming. The planimetered valve area is <1.5 cm^2, transmitral flow velocities are increased, and the diastolic pressure half-time is <150 ms. In contrast, both asymptomatic and symptomatic severe MS are associated with similar anatomy on echocardiography but with a planimetered valve area <1.5 cm^2, a diastolic pressure half-time >150 ms, and elevated (>30 mmHg) pulmonary artery systolic pressures. Very severe MS is further characterized by MV areas <1 cm^2 and diastolic pressure half-times >220 ms. Symptoms associated with MS can include decreased exercise tolerance and exertional dyspnea [26].

For patients with mitral stenosis, percutaneous balloon commissurotomy is often the first-line therapy when anatomically feasible. Candidates for balloon commissurotomy must be free of moderate or severe MR and must have no left atrial thrombus. The AHA/ACC guidelines currently make a class I recommendation for percutaneous balloon commissurotomy in symptomatic patients with severe MS and favorable valve morphology. Furthermore, patients with asymptomatic severe or very severe MS may be considered for balloon commissurotomy. However, for patients with severe symptomatic MS who are not candidates for balloon commissurotomy or for whom it has failed, MV surgery is recommended. Additionally, concomitant MV surgery is recommended for patients with moderate or severe MS undergoing cardiac surgery for other indications. Lastly, MV surgery with ligation of the left atrial appendage can be considered for patients with severe MS who have recurrent embolic events while on anticoagulation [26].

The Current Treatment Paradigm—Natural History of MR and Timing of Surgical Therapy

Medical therapy offers little for the treatment of severe MR, so the current treatment paradigm relies primarily on surgical repair or replacement of the MV. To understand the role and timing of surgical intervention in this current treatment paradigm, one must first consider the risks and benefits of surgical intervention and understand the natural history of MR, and how the interplay of these factors determines the current surgical paradigm for MR.

Surgery for Mitral Regurgitation

Surgical therapy for MR can be broadly grouped into two categories: MV repair and MV replacement. These procedures pose a risk of morbidity and mortality that increases with worsening MR and LV dysfunction [66]. As a result, at later stages of MR, the risks associated with surgery may be prohibitively high, precluding safe surgical intervention. Therefore, one of the major goals in the current treatment paradigm is to identify cases of MR and intervene surgically before the patients become too sick to tolerate surgery and have a low likelihood of surviving the operation.

At the other end of the spectrum, with regard to patients with MR and healthy ventricles, surgery is offered only to patients for whom the potential benefits of surgical correction of MR outweigh the risks. In this regard, some patients with MR can be considered "too healthy" for surgery and are monitored for progression of the disease until they fall within the appropriate therapeutic window.

Further complexity arises when the choice is made between MV replacement and repair. Mitral valve replacement involves placing a prosthetic valve in the heart, incurring a lifelong risk of infection. One must also consider the durability of the prosthetic valve. Replacement valves can be broadly categorized into mechanical valves and bioprosthetic tissue valves. Mechanical valves are extremely durable and may last for the patient's lifetime, but they pose certain risks. These include valve thrombosis and resultant embolization, which can result in stroke or other embolic phenomena, as well as the risk of bleeding incurred by lifelong anticoagulation with warfarin to prevent such thrombosis. Mechanical valves can also fail by developing infra-annular pannus, which impairs leaflet function and reduces the effective orifice area.

Bioprosthetic valves do not necessitate systemic anticoagulation with warfarin and therefore do not pose the attendant risks. However, bioprosthetic valves have limited durability; their life span averages 10–20 years and is lower in younger patients. Significant bioprosthetic valve deterioration then results in the need for reintervention and redo valve replacement, which usually carries a higher risk of morbidity and morbidity than primary valve replacement.

In contrast, MV repair does not incur the device-related risks of anticoagulation and bioprosthetic valve deterioration, because the native valve remains in place [67, 68]. Furthermore, with contemporary valve repair, the chordal apparatus is maintained; studies show preservation of LV geometry and systolic function and also lower rates of late complications than with prosthetic MV replacement [69]. However, not all valves can be repaired, even at the best referral centers. In addition, the risks, benefits, durability, and complications of surgery must be balanced against the natural history of MR, to further elucidate the best timing for surgery and to better identify patients for whom surgical intervention is appropriate.

Natural History of MR

The natural history of MR varies substantially with severity, cause, and symptomatology. When treatment options are considered for patients with MR, it is important to distinguish between patients with symptomatic versus asymptomatic disease, and among patients with mild-to-moderate, moderate-to-severe, and severe MR.

As much as 20% of the population has trivial or mild-to-moderate MR; however, most of these individuals are asymptomatic, and for many, their MR never becomes significant enough to warrant surgical intervention [70, 71]. Furthermore, MR can remain mild or mild-to-moderate for many years without any significant worsening, either hemodynamically or in terms of symptoms. Affected patients are monitored for the development of significant hemodynamic changes or symptoms.

Although the development of symptoms is an indication for surgical intervention, it is an unpredictable and unreliable indicator of progression to moderate-to-severe or severe MR, of a chronic compensated state of MR, or of transition to a decompensated state. For example, by the time significant dyspnea arises, there may already be significant irreversible ventricular dysfunction. Thus, most patients with MR will be monitored for the development of significant anatomic, echocardiographic, or hemodynamic changes that indicate worsening MR. However; even patients with significantly worsening MR can remain asymptomatic.

The natural history of asymptomatic, moderately severe MR is controversial. Initial studies suggested a benign prognosis, without death or deterioration of LV function for up to 5 years of follow-up, but a 10% average annual risk of symptom development leading to surgical correction was noted [72]. Subsequent studies have shown a 5-year combined incidence of 42% for the onset of atrial fibrillation, heart failure, or cardiovascular death [73].

As MR progresses to the severe stage, if left untreated, its natural history involves worsening clinical deterioration, morbidity, and substantial mortality risk. This holds true in both symptomatic and asymptomatic patients. Thus, it is clear that such patients should be considered for surgery; however, as described previously, these patients are at risk for significant LV dysfunction, which can be difficult to detect and which substantially increases the likelihood of morbidity and mortality with operative intervention. Thus, patients who have developed severe LV dysfunction may be too sick for surgery and may thus fall out of the therapeutic window.

The end result of these considerations is summarized in Fig. 8.1, adapted from the 2017 ACC/AHA guidelines, describing recommendations for the timing of surgical intervention for MR.

Comorbidities

In addition to the risks and benefits of surgery and the natural history of MR itself, one must also consider comorbid conditions and the increased risks of morbidity, mortality, and complications they may pose. Two of the strongest risk factors for early mortality are age and NYHA functional class [66]. Continued heart failure is the main cause of death after surgical correction of MR [66]. Important predictors of late mortality after operation include advanced age, elevated serum creatinine level, elevated systolic blood pressure, coronary artery disease, advanced functional class heart failure, and echocardiographic evidence of reduced LVEF and worsening end-systolic dimension [66, 68, 74]. Renal failure or dysfunction, liver failure or dysfunction, a hostile chest due to prior sternotomy or radiation, COPD, prior stroke, endocarditis, and poor nutritional status are other factors and comorbidities that increase the risks associated with surgery and that may portend poorer outcomes. Thus, appropriate candidates for surgery are those patients who fall within the therapeutic window, and for whom the risks posed by comorbid conditions are low enough so as to not preclude surgical intervention.

Understanding this paradigm is important, as it lays the framework for understanding how emerging technologies for endovascular treatments—MV repair, MV replacement, and interventions to alleviate ventricular dysfunction—can alter the therapeutic window. This paradigm also informs what threshold levels of risk can be tolerated, and what threshold levels of benefit need to be exceeded, to ensure successful adoption of any given technique or technology.

Mitral Valve Repair

Despite the lack of randomized trials comparing MV repair and replacement in degenerative valve disease, comparative studies have demonstrated a survival advantage with MV repair [75–77]. In addition, repair preserves ventricular function and provides greater freedom from thromboembolic and anticoagulation-related events, as well as endocarditis.

The basic principles of any mitral repair include (1) reestablishing normal leaflet motion, (2) obtaining an adequate surface of leaflet coaptation, and (3) annular stabilization with a ring or band while maintaining an adequate mitral orifice size. To perform the most durable repair, the surgeon needs to be familiar with both the normal functional anatomy and the pathological anatomy as it relates to the lesions of the leaflets, leaflet motion, and annulus.

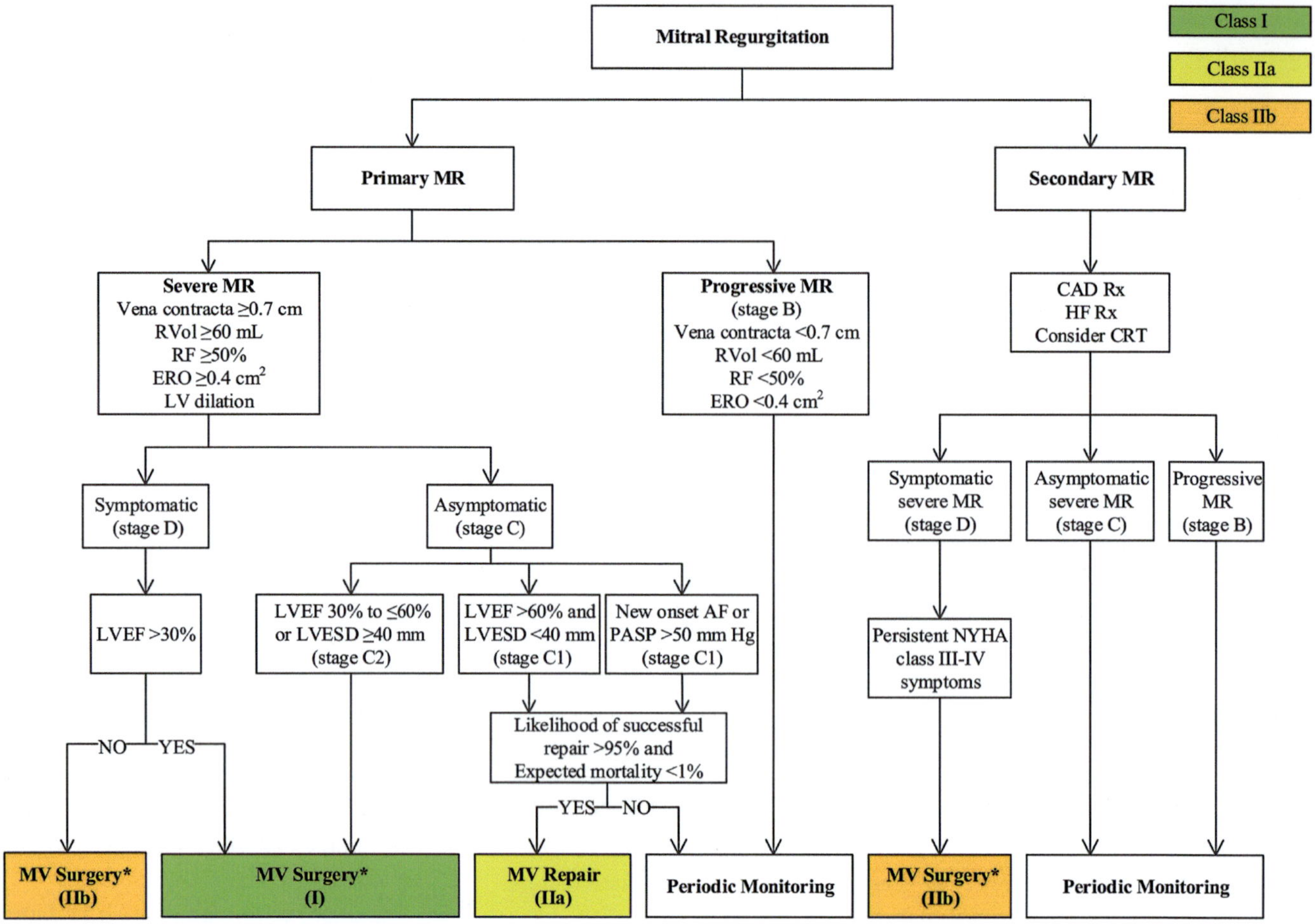

Fig. 8.1 Indications for surgery for mitral regurgitation. *AF* atrial fibrillation, *CAD* coronary artery disease, *CRT* cardiac resynchronization therapy, *ERO* effective regurgitant orifice, *HF* heart failure, *LV* left ventricular, *LVEF* left ventricular ejection fraction, *LVESD* left ventricular end-systolic dimension, *MR* mitral regurgitation, *MV* mitral valve, *MVR* mitral valve replacement, *NYHA* New York Heart Association, *PASP* pulmonary artery systolic pressure, *RF* regurgitant fraction, *RVol* regurgitant volume, *Rx* therapy. *Mitral valve repair is preferred over MVR when possible. From Nishimura et al. [26]

Repair techniques have evolved into three basic concepts. The first involves resectional techniques, which were popularized by Carpentier. This entails resecting abnormal leaflet tissue and later reconstruction. The second involves a "respect all, rather than resect" technique. With this approach, the free edges of the prolapsing leaflet segments are resuspended with artificial Gore-Tex neochords. Multiple variations of this approach have been described. The third concept combines the first 2: resecting all abnormal leaflet tissue, then using Gore-Tex neochords to address any remaining redundant leaflet tissue.

The edge-to-edge technique, which was popularized by Alfieri, has been used as both a primary repair strategy and a "bailout" technique. This technique provides a functional, as opposed to an anatomical, repair of the valve.

Carefully evaluating the valvular deformity by both preoperative and intraoperative echocardiography is essential. Thereafter, the surgeon must correlate these findings with the intraoperative valve analysis. Each of the leaflet segments, including commissures, chordae, and the subvalvular apparatus, as well as the annulus, must be carefully inspected. Many surgeons use P1 as a reference point to assess the degree of prolapse of the adjacent scallops because, in the majority of cases, P1 is free of disease. Others reject this concept and instead take a targeted approach to the valve by addressing the most significant lesion first and repairing additional defects thereafter. The surgeon must take into consideration the amount of leaflet tissue involved (volume) in relation to adjacent normal leaflet, the height of the affected leaflet, and the amount of support (chordae) that is lacking or in excess. Leaving the posterior leaflet too long (i.e., >1.5 cm) can lead to systolic anterior motion of the MV.

Today, more than 90% of cases of degenerative MV disease can be repaired at referral or expert centers. Furthermore, after surgeons obtain sufficient experience in minimally invasive surgery, essentially every repair technique can be applied. Minimally invasive approaches to mitral surgery provide unimpeded, direct, and truly anatomic visualization of the MV. One must keep in mind that these approaches do not help surgeons to improve their competency with mitral repair techniques. Proficiency with a wide variety of mitral repair techniques is acquired with experience and repetition. A significant learning curve is associated with both mitral repair and minimally invasive access. Considering that among surgeons performing MV surgery, the median number of MV repairs per surgeon is 5 per year, proficiency in repair may be difficult to obtain. In addition, among all surgeons performing mitral surgery, the median MV repair rate is 41% [78]. Therefore, the concept of centers of excellence has been proposed in order to obtain the highest possible rate of durable repairs [79].

Furthermore, in 2008, 26% of Society of Thoracic Surgeons Adult Cardiac Surgery Database centers were performing a median of 3 less-invasive procedures per year [80]. Therefore, the necessary skillsets to perform complex MV repairs via a minimally invasive approach may be obtainable only at minimally invasive MV repair referral centers.

Mitral Valve Repair Techniques

Posterior Leaflet Prolapse or Flail

A P2 prolapse is the most common dysfunction seen in degenerative MV disease. A small segment of flailed or prolapsed leaflet can be managed with a limited triangular resection. In contrast, a broad scallop with a large area of prolapse or flailed segment can be addressed with a quadrangular resection. This can be performed along with a sliding or folding plasty. With larger resections, annular compression sutures can be considered, as well. An alternative approach is a butterfly resection of a broad P2 segment. In certain cases in which a limited triangular resection is performed and there is excess height in P2, a Gore-Tex chord can be added to avoid potential systolic anterior motion (SAM) of the MV. With excessive leaflet tissue, a larger quadrangular resection of P2 will help avoid SAM, as well.

Prolapse of P1 and P3 can be addressed with limited resection, depending on the thickness and amount of tissue on the affected scallop. Alternatively, a complete "respect rather than resect" approach can be taken by placing polytetrafluoroethylene (PTFE) artificial neochords. Several methods can be used. These include placing individual chords in the papillary muscles supported with or without pledgets, running one Gore-Tex suture through the papillary muscle and then into the leaflet and back multiple times, placing one small Gore-Tex loop in the papillary muscle and then passing multiple individual Gore-Tex sutures through the loop and into the leaflets as necessary, and using the multi-loop technique. This approach displaces the leaflets into the ventricle and establishes a new line of coaptation to simulate a Roman arch.

Anterior Leaflet Prolapse or Flail

Mild anterior leaflet prolapse usually does not need to be addressed and resolves once the annuloplasty is placed. For moderate or greater anterior prolapse or flail, placing artificial neochords is the most commonly used technique. Various methods have been described. Single or multiple Gore-Tex neochords can be placed from the papillary muscle to the free edge of the leaflet. It is important that the neochords cross neither the midline nor each other. The length of the leaflet can be determined by measuring the height of an adjacent normal native chordae or with the saline test after annuloplasty implantation. Another method involves using premeasured Gore-Tex loops. The length of these loops can be determined by measuring adjacent normal chordae intraoperatively or by measuring normal chordae with intraoperative TEE. These chordal loops for the anterior leaflet usually measure between 22 and 26 mm. Aggressively shortening the anterior leaflet can lead to residual MR and even SAM. Another reference point that can be considered for determining the chordal length is the annular plane; the free edge of the leaflet should reach the level of the annulus. Even with these methods, measuring an exact length can be challenging.

In addition, anterior leaflet secondary chords (which are usually the appropriate length) can be transferred to the free edge. These chords can serve as a guide to the proper length of an artificial neochord if one is needed for additional support.

Other, infrequently used alternative techniques include chordal transposition, which is effective but can potentially damage a normal posterior leaflet; this technique involves transposing a segment of normal posterior leaflet with native chordae of normal length to the affected segment of prolapsing anterior leaflet. Papillary muscle repositioning involves anchoring the fibrous head of the anterior papillary muscle to the posterior papillary muscle. Resecting the anterior leaflet is reserved for significant localized abnormalities of the leaflet, and resection is limited to no more than 10% of the leaflet.

Bileaflet Prolapse

Bileaflet prolapse can be treated with a combination of the previously described techniques. These are the most challenging of all repairs, as well as the least durable. Bileaflet prolapse presenting with only a central jet identified by preoperative TEE can occasionally be addressed with only an annuloplasty ring that is sized to the annulus. Another approach to bileaflet prolapse is an Alfieri stitch (edge-to-edge repair) with the addition of an annuloplasty ring.

Commissural Prolapse

Limited commissural prolapse can be treated with a limited resection or folding plasty. With more extensive commissural prolapse secondary to leaflet destruction and chordal rupture, a quadrangular resection with annular plication can be performed. This procedure can be completed with a "magic stitch" to restore coaptation. In cases with more extensive involvement of the commissure, both A3 and P3 can be detached from the annulus after a quadrangular resection is performed. Annular plication and leaflet advancement are performed thereafter.

Patients with intact leaflets and elongated chordae can be treated with papillary muscle shortening or a papillary muscle sliding plasty. Another option is using artificial neochordae to reduce the height of the commissure.

Mitral Annular Calcification

Annular decalcification may be required to establish an adequate surface of leaflet coaptation in patients undergoing repair. The leaflet is detached from the annulus, and an attempt is made to resect the calcium bar en bloc. If this is not possible, fractional debridement with a rongeur can be performed, after which the leaflet is reattached. An ultrasonic debridement device can also facilitate the decalcification. Some cases may require patch repair of the atrioventricular groove to avoid a disruption. In cases of diffuse calcification, an alternative is to place annular sutures around the calcium and to modify the annuloplasty ring or band if necessary. Mitral annular calcification can pose a challenge, and the feasibility of repair may be limited.

Rheumatic Valvular Disease

In developing countries, attempts to repair a rheumatic valve in the earlier stages of the disease are complicated by the need for reoperation due to progressive distortion and fibrosis of the leaflets secondary to progression or recurrence of the rheumatic process. Replacement attempts are also plagued by several complications, as well as the risks associated with multiple operations, especially in young patients.

In developed countries, the disease process is different, and the leaflets undergo more of an advanced, end-stage histologic process that is unlikely to progress except for the development of calcium deposition. Annular dilatation is the cause of regurgitation in more than half of cases. Mitral repair is technically more feasible and yields better results in this group.

Repair for rheumatic mitral disease includes several techniques, ranging from commissurotomy, subvalvular chordal, and papillary muscle splitting to leaflet peeling and leaflet extension [81]. The initial step is to free the fused commissures and subvalvular apparatus by splitting the fused chords and papillary muscles. Shortened secondary chords are cut to free the leaflets even further. In some cases, even thickened restricted primary chords are transected and replaced with artificial Gore-Tex chords. The leaflets can be made more pliable by peeling off the inflammatory fibrotic layer and decalcification. When the leaflet and subvalvular mobilization are not enough to compensate for tissue retraction, performing leaflet augmentation techniques can increase the surface area of the leaflet, providing greater mobility and surface area for leaflet coaptation. Leaflet augmentation can be performed with autologous pericardium, bovine pericardium, or a collagen matrix, and on the anterior or posterior leaflet, or both leaflets. The leaflet extension technique also allows the insertion of a larger annuloplasty ring or band [81].

Annular Stabilization

Annular stabilization with a full ring or band is essential to the long-term durability of the repair. The choice between a full ring and a band is a topic of ongoing debate. The size of the annuloplasty is usually determined by the height of the anterior leaflet, although in cases of extreme myxomatous degeneration with voluminous leaflets and a very dilated annulus, a "true sized" annuloplasty is recommended. The annuloplasty restores the normal 4:3 ratio of the MV, increases the line of coaptation of the leaflets, and prevents annular dilatation. Some reports state that after a band is placed, the annulus between the trigones may continue to dilate and contribute to recurrent MR. On the other hand, others believe that a full ring can lead to mitral stenosis.

Edge-to-Edge

This technique, originally described by Alfieri [82], has been applied to degenerative disease with bileaflet prolapse, flail leaflet, and calcified annulus. The middle portion of each leaflet is identified by assessing the subvalvular apparatus with nerve hooks. Wide clefts are usually closed. The repair is completed by taking large bites through the rough zone of the leaflet tissue and suturing the free edge of A2 and P2 with a running 4 or 5-0 Prolene suture. The running length is variable but commonly covers the whole length of the mid scallop. With flail segments other than A2 or P2, the location of the suture will correspond to the center of the flailed segment. An annuloplasty is performed at the end of the procedure [83].

The minimum ring or band size should be 32 mm. Failure to use annular stabilization will increase the failure rate. Mitral annular calcification also contributes to long-term failure.

Mitral Valve Replacement

Mitral valve replacement is reserved for patients with end-stage Barlow disease, previous failed attempts to repair the MV, a heavily calcified mitral annulus, or certain forms of rheumatic disease. The replacement procedure should spare the chords to maintain annular papillary continuity. The different options include preserving the posterior leaflet and chords and resecting the entire anterior leaflet; preserving the posterior leaflet and chords, then detaching the entire anterior leaflet from the annulus and incorporating it into the posterior suture line; preserving the posterior leaflet and chords and resecting only A1 and a portion of P2, leaving P3 intact; and resecting all leaflets and chords and resuspending the papillary muscles with Gore-Tex neochords, which are passed through the annulus and onto the sewing cuff of the valve (typically placed at 4 and 8 o'clock). In patients with mitral annular calcification, if sutures can be passed through the calcium, decalcification may be avoidable. If a large segment of calcium is present and precludes suture placement, the segment will need to be resected.

Some patients have valves that are not amenable to repair, so replacement is indicated. These include patients with irreparable complex valve disease, as well as elderly patients with multiple comorbidities, for whom the benefit of repair is outweighed by the risks. A good MV replacement is better than a bad MV repair.

Surgical Treatment of Functional Mitral Regurgitation

Annular Techniques

Secondary MR, also known as functional MR, is most often caused by ischemic or dilated cardiomyopathy. The MR is caused by changes in the LV that distort the valvular apparatus. Specifically, dilation of the LV results in inferior and lateral papillary muscle displacement, which ultimately leads to tethering of the valve leaflets and loss of central coaptation.

Left ventricular end-systolic volume index (LVESVI) can be used as a surrogate for LV dilation and remodeling associated with ischemic myocardial disease and is a predictor of poor prognosis in these patients. The principles of mitral valve surgery are to restore valve competence, reduce the LVESVI, and induce reverse remodeling of the LV, which may be associated with better outcomes [84]. For patients with secondary MR, the most commonly used technique is implanting a downsized annuloplasty ring [84–91].

However, the high recurrence rate of MR associated with repair, as compared to mitral valve replacement, has prompted further examination of the two approaches to secondary MR. Recently, the Cardiothoracic Surgical Trials Network conducted a randomized controlled trial of MV repair versus replacement for patients with severe ischemic MR. Unlike many of the previous studies, this trial showed no difference in overall LV remodeling or survival for patients who underwent repair versus replacement [92]. Furthermore, the rate of recurrence of moderate or severe MR was much higher with repair than with replacement (32.6% vs. 2.3%). On the other hand, patients who underwent repair but did not have recurrent MR had significant reverse LV remodeling. In addition, the absence of MR recurrence was associated with better quality of life. This finding prompted a search for predictors of recurrent MR in order to improve patient selection for MV repair.

A subgroup analysis by Kron and colleagues [93] identified only basal aneurysm as an independent risk factor for MR recurrence. This finding suggests that leaflet tethering plays a significant role in the recurrence of MR after repair. Other possible predictors include specific echocardiographic measurements, including leaflet tethering height, tenting area, coaptation distance, LVESVI, and ventricular sphericity index [89, 94–100]. Recently, follow-up studies have suggested that 3D echocardiography may be superior to 2D echocardiography at predicting MR recurrence [101]. In addition, a 3D echocardiography study identified a P3 tethering angle of 29.9° or larger as an independent risk factor for MR recurrence [102].

Subvalvular Techniques of Mitral Valve Repair for Ischemic Mitral Regurgitation

Chordal Cutting

The technique of chordal cutting typically focuses on anterior mitral leaflet tethering in functional MR (FMR). This attachment can cause an abnormal bend in the anterior mitral leaflet described as a "seagull wing" by Professor Alain Carpentier [103]. In theory, second-order chordal cutting should reduce the degree of leaflet tethering and increase leaflet mobility and coaptation height, thereby limiting the

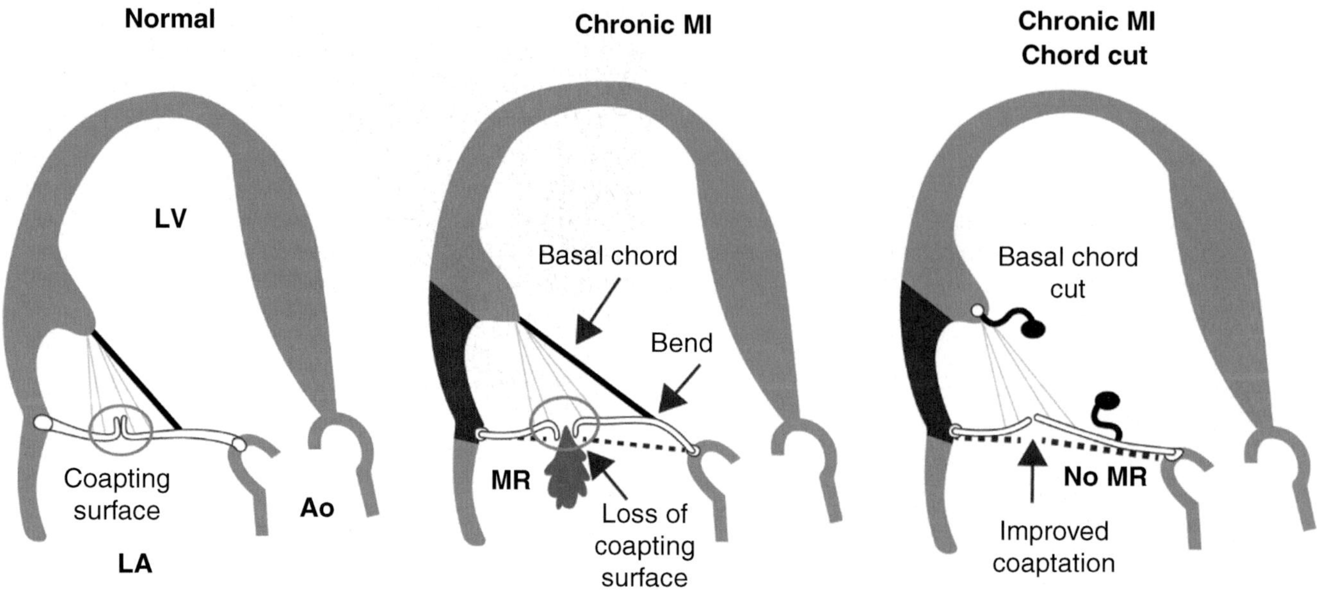

Fig. 8.2 Encircling the base of the papillary muscles with a Gore-Tex graft

degree of MR (Fig. 8.2). Chordal cutting can also be performed by dividing secondary chords to the posterior leaflet and to the commissure that arises from the papillary muscle or muscles affected by the infarcted myocardium [104]. To optimize visibility of the chords, this procedure is performed before the annuloplasty band is placed.

Compared with conventional MV repair, chordal-cutting MV repair has been associated with a reduced risk of recurrent MR because this repair produces greater reductions in tenting area and greater mobility of the anterior leaflet (as measured by a reduction in the distance between the free edge of the anterior MV leaflet and the posterior LV wall) without compromising postoperative LVEF [104].

Papillary Muscle Relocation

Papillary muscle relocation techniques for secondary MR are used to treat severe leaflet tethering and displacement of the coaptation point. One technique includes placing a 3-0 polypropylene suture through the posterior papillary muscle fibrous tip and then passing it through the adjacent mitral annulus just posterior to the right fibrous trigone [105]. After the mitral annuloplasty is performed, if the saline test reveals inadequate leaflet coaptation (typically in the P3 segment), the relocation suture is tightened, drawing the posterior papillary muscle tip closer to the annulus.

Another technique is the "ring plus string" repair [106, 107]. This technique is performed by anchoring a Teflon-pledgeted suture in the head of the posterior papillary muscle, then passing it through the fibrosa (midseptal annular saddle horn) under direct vision and exteriorizing it through the aortic wall underneath the commissure between the non-coronary and left coronary aortic cusps. The suture is then tied under echocardiographic guidance in the loaded, beating heart to reposition the displaced posterior papillary muscle toward the fibrosa. This technique has been refined to allow further reduction of the septal-lateral diameter after the loaded, beating heart is implanted with a DYANA nitinol-based dynamic annuloplasty device that can be deformed by activation with radiofrequency [108].

Papillary muscle relocation with a suture plus nonrestrictive mitral annuloplasty promotes a significant reversal of LV remodeling, a decrease in tenting area and coaptation depth, and less recurrent MR [109]. What remains to be seen is whether restrictive mitral valve annuloplasty produces better results than nonrestrictive annuloplasty. This raises the question of whether the annuloplasty technique or the subvalvular repair contributes more to the success of MV repair for FMR.

Papillary Muscle Approximation

Papillary muscle approximation (PMA) with a papillary muscle sling technique was first introduced to treat patients with ischemic LV dysfunction and FMR [110]. By restoring a more normal alignment between the mitral annulus and the laterally displaced papillary muscles, this technique could relieve the excess tethering on the mitral leaflets and significantly restore leaflet mobility. This method is performed by placing a 4-mm PTFE tube graft around the base of all the papillary muscles (Figs. 8.3 and 8.4). The graft is then progressively tightened until there is no gap between the bases of the two papillary muscles (Fig. 8.5). An annuloplasty ring that is "true sized" to the anterior leaflet is then placed (Fig. 8.6). This technique has been termed the "sling and ring" repair. It has been modified

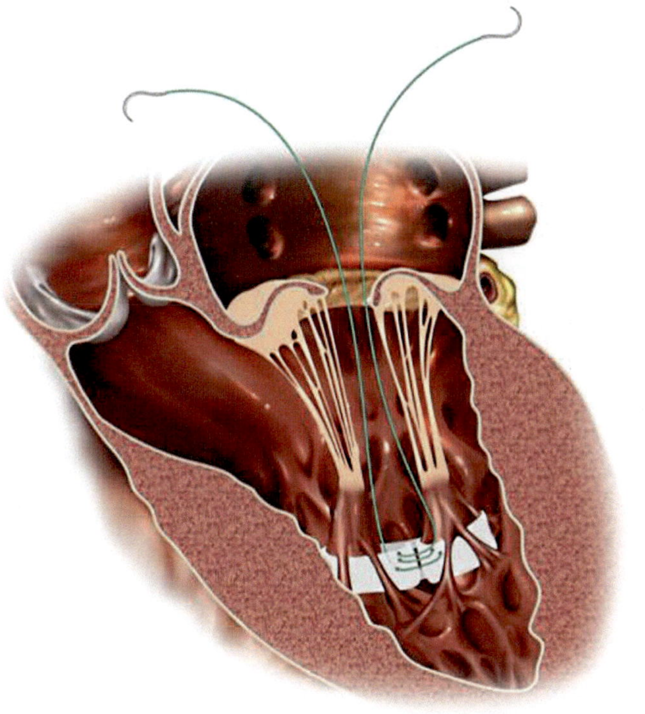

Fig. 8.3 Diagram showing sling around base of papillary muscles

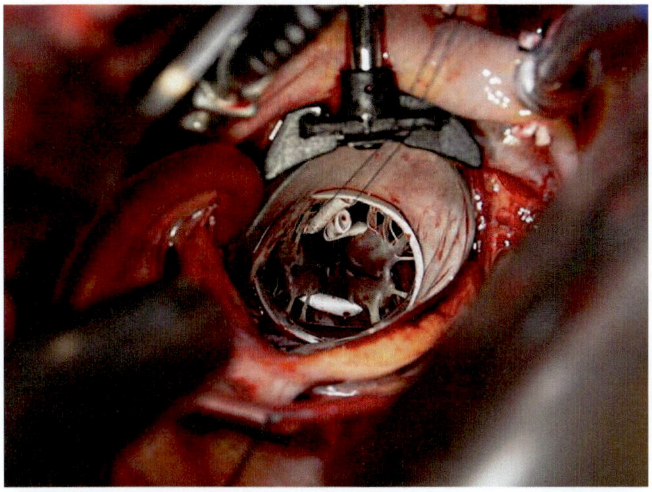

Fig. 8.4 Intraoperative photo of sling placed around the base of the papillary muscles

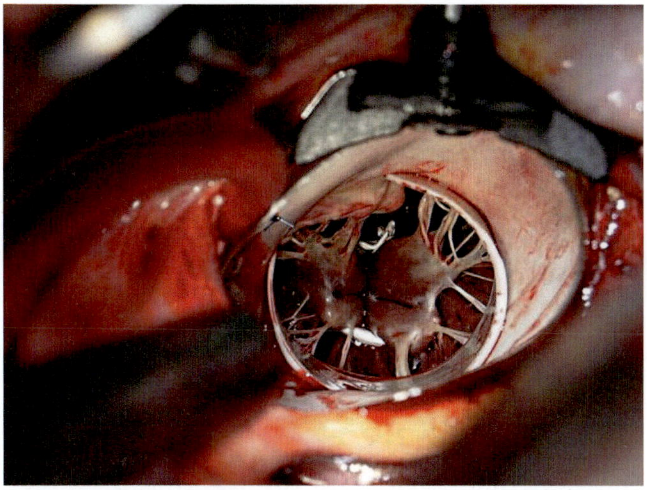

Fig. 8.5 Photo of PTFE graft tightly approximating the base of the papillary muscles

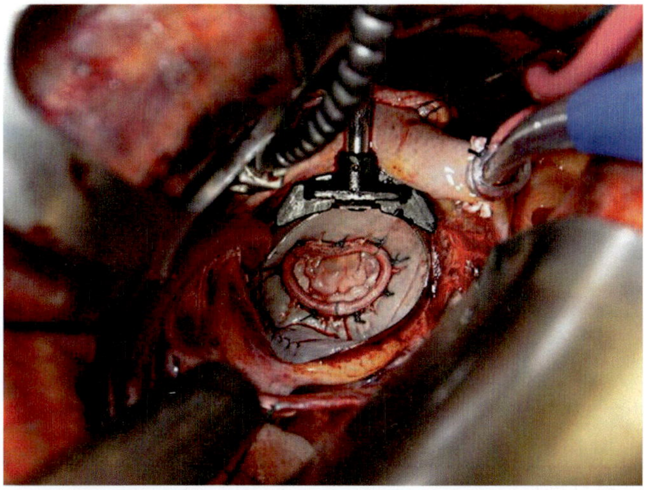

Fig. 8.6 Rigid annuloplasty ring, true sized to the anterior leaflet

and performed safely in a minimally invasive fashion via a mini-right thoracotomy [111, 112].

The "sling and ring" repair has shown promise with regard to promoting LV remodeling and leaflet mobility by limiting the tethering secondary to displacement of the papillary muscles [110]. This anatomical correction can lead to improvements in ventricular diameter, LVEF, volume, and sphericity index.

A similar subvalvular approach to PMA consists of placing a single U-shaped stitch, reinforcing it with two patches of autologous pericardium, and passing it through the posterior and anterior papillary muscles [113]. This method of PMA lowers the rate of recurrent MR [113] and is believed to promote significant ventricular remodeling, reducing mean LVEDD and increasing mean LVEF [113]. This is consistent with the Cardiothoracic Surgery Network trial that showed that patients with more complex tethering may benefit from additional subvalvular procedures [92].

Surgical Ventricular Reconstruction

In certain populations, adding left ventriculoplasty to MV repair for FMR has been associated with more effective control of MR and further improvement of LVEF than restrictive mitral annuloplasty alone [114]. Surgical ventricular reconstruction (SVR) was first popularized for the management of heart failure with LV remodeling caused by coronary artery disease, and SVR was shown to reduce LV volume, increase LVEF, and improve ventricular function [115, 116]. In the STICH trial, despite a significantly greater reduction in LV volume with SVR than with coronary artery bypass grafting alone, this improvement did not translate into a measurable survival benefit for patients [117].

An additional study has shown that when compared with annuloplasty alone, the addition of left ventriculoplasty significantly improved LVEF in patients with an enlarged LV (LVEDD >65 mm) and severe mitral tethering. There was also a nonsignificant trend toward greater improvement in MR grade when a left ventriculoplasty was performed [118].

Endovascular Devices for the Treatment of Mitral Regurgitation

In patients with severe MR, observational studies have demonstrated that surgery to repair or replace the MV was found to improve survival more effectively than medical therapy [119]. However, surgery can pose significant risks, including a 1–5% risk of mortality and a 10–20% risk of morbidities including stroke, reoperation, renal failure, and prolonged ventilation. Elderly patients and those with LV dysfunction are at even greater risk [120]. Even in patients with moderate-to-severe MR, and in asymptomatic patients, the risks posed by surgery are not trivial, which inspired the current paradigm of monitoring patients until symptom develop, MR or LV dysfunction worsens, or sequelae of MR arise such as atrial fibrillation or pulmonary hypertension—at which point the benefits of surgery justify the risks [119, 121]. In contrast, at experienced referral centers treating patients who have a >90% chance of successful repair, the benefits of surgery justify the risks for a broader range of indications, such that guidelines recommend considering MV repair even for asymptomatic patients with normal LV function [26].

The risks posed by surgery, combined with other factors such as patient preference for less-invasive therapies, the recent successes and rapid adoption of devices for transcatheter aortic valve replacement (TAVR), and the large, unmet clinical need for therapies for patients who are outside of the therapeutic window of surgery, have stimulated an explosion in the development of endovascular technologies for treating MR. Interest is especially great in therapies for high-risk patients deemed too sick for surgery.

Whereas TAVR for the treatment of aortic stenosis has enjoyed quick adoption and widespread success due to several factors (e.g., a singular pathophysiology of valve disease; the anatomy of the aortic annulus, which allows for precise stent-valve delivery; the ability to leverage conventional imaging techniques), the advancement of transcatheter MV interventions has been relatively slow. Endovascular therapy for MR poses far more complex challenges in terms of the anatomy, structure, and function of the MV apparatus, complex pathophysiological considerations, challenges in patient selection, imaging complexities, and comparison to gold-standard surgical approaches that include both repair and replacement. Nevertheless, a plethora of device technologies exist or are in development and the devices can be broadly categorized into repair and replacement devices.

Emerging Mitral Valve Repair Devices

Just as a variety of different surgical techniques exist to address and repair various lesions and associated dysfunction of the MV, a variety of devices are in development, largely mimicking surgical repair techniques, with the aim of producing results comparable to those of surgical repair but by a transvascular approach. Emerging devices can be categorized by where they are placed and their mechanism of action within the MV apparatus, including annulus-based devices, leaflet-based devices, chordal-based devices, and papillary muscle-based devices.

Annulus-Based Devices

Several device technologies are in development to replicate one of the mainstay techniques of surgical MV repair, namely mitral annuloplasty. These devices can be subdivided into direct and indirect annuloplasty devices. Direct annuloplasty devices seek to mimic surgical annuloplasty techniques; a variety of these devices are placed directly into the mitral annulus. Existing direct annuloplasty devices include the Edwards Cardioband device, the ValCare Amend device, the MitraSpan Transapical Segmented Reduction Annuloplasty (TASRA) device, and the Millipede Medical IRIS device.

Direct Annuloplasty Devices

Edwards Cardioband

The Edwards Cardioband system (Edwards Lifesciences) is an adjustable annuloplasty system that consists of a polyester sleeve implant with radiopaque markers spaced 8 mm apart. The sleeve is fastened to the mitral annulus with multiple repositionable and retrievable 6-mm anchors. The device uses a transfemoral implant delivery system and a 25 Fr transseptal steerable sheath (Fig. 8.7) [122].

A transseptal puncture is performed under TEE guidance, and an anchor is released close to the hinge of the leaflet and the anterior commissure. The implant is advanced until a radiopaque portion reaches the adjacent marker; the implant catheter is then navigated to each subsequent anchoring point along the posterior annulus until the tip reaches the last anchoring site. Thereafter, the implant is tightened to size with the adjustment tool, and the reduction of MR is assessed by TEE until the desired effect is obtained [122].

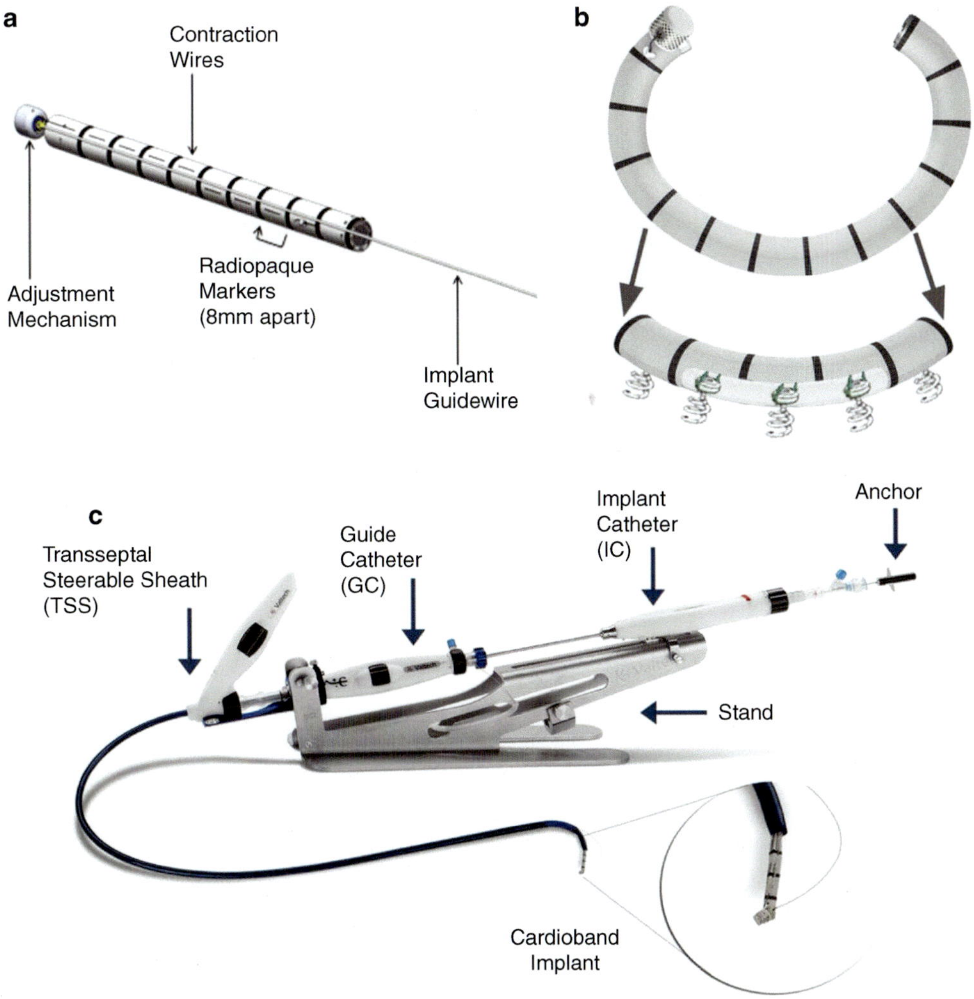

Fig. 8.7 Edwards Valtech Cardioband device, shown before (**a**) and after (**b**) implantation. (**c**) Cardioband delivery system. From Maisano et al. [122]. Reprinted with permission from Oxford University Press

Among 31 high-risk patients with symptomatic functional MR, procedural success was reported in all patients. A significant reduction in septolateral dimension was found in 29 patients, with no MR in 6 (21%), mild MR in 21 (72%), and moderate MR in 2 (7%). No procedural mortality was encountered, and in-hospital mortality was 6.5% (2/31); of note, neither death was procedure or device related. At 30 days, MR remained at 2+ or less in 22 patients (88%). Ongoing trials of the Cardioband device are described in Table 8.4 [122].

Valcare Amend Device

The Valcare Amend device is a D-shaped annuloplasty ring that is attached to the annulus with 12 independently deployed anchors positioned in 4 zones (Fig. 8.8). The posterior zones are anchored first and then pulled anteriorly to reduce the anterior-posterior dimension by 15–25%. The device is delivered by a transapical approach. The first human implantation was done in 2016 and reduced the patient's MR from severe (4+) to trace (1). Details of ongoing trials are listed in Table 8.5.

MitraSpan TASRA Device

The TASRA device (MitrasSpan Inc., Belmont, MA, USA), which is based on the concept of septal lateral annular cinching, is another direct annuloplasty device. The cinching device is delivered transapically with a low-profile (≤12-Fr) system. A suture is placed on both the anterior trigone and posterior mitral annulus, and the cinch device then compresses the annulus (Fig. 8.9).

Millipede Medical IRIS Device

Another device, the Millipede IRIS (Millipede Medical, Santa Rosa, CA, USA) seeks to replicate a semirigid, complete ring, using a zigzag-shaped nitinol frame that is placed in a supra-annular position. The delivery system uses a transseptal approach, and the device itself has anchors that attach the ring to the annulus. Collars on the peak of each zigzag contract or expand the ring when tightened or released to accomplish final sizing (Fig. 8.10) [123]. The first successful human implantation was completed in May 2017. Ongoing trial details are described in Table 8.6.

Table 8.4 Cardioband trials

Device/trial name	Trial design	Arms	Inclusion criteria	Exclusion criteria	Primary outcome measures	Secondary outcome measures	Follow-up	Est. study completion date
REPAIR (transcatheteR rEPair of mitrAl Insufficiency with caRdioband system)	Prospective, multicenter, nonrandomized trial, 50 pts	1. Experimental: Device	1. Severe secondary MR (3+ to 4+) 2. Symptomatic MR (NYHA II–IVa) despite GDMT, including CRT if indicated 3. Transfemoral/transseptal delivery feasible 4. Not offered surgery by local site heart team	1. LVEF <20% 2. LVEDD ≥7 cm 3. Heavily calcified 4. Significant CAD needing revascularization 5. Active endocarditis 6. Any endovascular or carotid intervention within 30 days, coronary within 3 months 7. Dialysis, liver disease 8. Life expectancy <12 months 9. PHtn >69 mmHg at rest 10. Right heart dysfunction 11. Bleeding or coagulation disorder 12. Prior MV repair 13. TIA or CVA within 3 months 14. Pregnancy 15. Hypersensitivity to nickel or chromium	1. Reduction in severity of MR by ≥1 on a 0–4 scale (30 days)	1. Change in 6MWD (6 months) 2. Change in MR severity (6, 12, and 24 months)	2 years	August 2019
ACTIVE—Edwards Cardioband system ACTIVE Pivotal Clinical trial	Global, multicenter RCT, 375 pts estimated	1. Experimental: Device 2. Comparator: GDMT	1. Clinically significant FMR 2. Symptomatic HF 3. Prior HF hospitalization within 12 months or elevated BNP	1. DMR 2. MAC impeding device 3. Other valve dx requiring intervention 4. Unfavorable anatomy 5. Life expectancy <12 months	1. Prevalence of MR ≤2+ 2. Time to cardiovascular death 3. Hospitalizations 4. 6MWD 5. KCCQ improvement	1. Rates of various adverse events (30 days) 2. NYHA improvement (1 year) 3. 6MWD improvement (1 year) 4. KCCQ improvement (1 year) 5. HF hospitalizations (1 year)	1 year	September 2024

6MWD 6-minute walk distance, *BNP* brain natriuretic peptide, *CAD* coronary artery disease, *CRT* cardiac resynchronization therapy, *CVA* cerebrovascular accident, *DMR* degenerative mitral regurgitation, *FMR* functional mitral regurgitation, *GDMT* goal-directed medical therapy, *HF* heart failure, *KCCQ* Kansas City Cardiomyopathy Questionnaire, *LVEDD* left ventricular end-diastolic dimension, *LVEF* left ventricular ejection fraction, *MAC* mitral annular calcification, *MAE* major adverse events, *MR* mitral regurgitation, *MV* mitral valve, *NYHA* New York Heart Association, *PHtn* pulmonary hypertension, *RCT* randomized, controlled trial, *TIA* transient ischemic attack

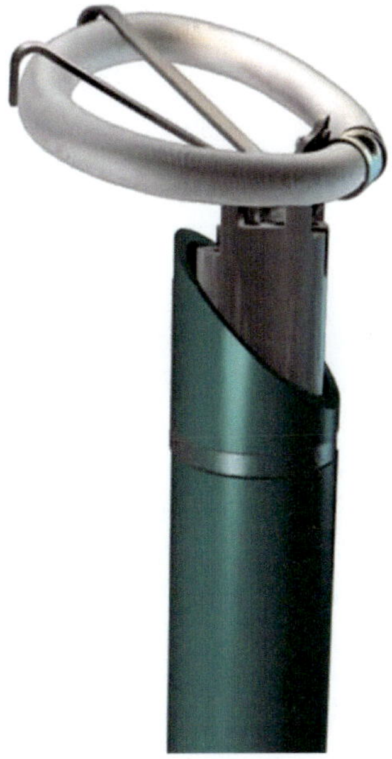

Fig. 8.8 Valcare Amend device. From https://www.medgadget.com/2016/06/amend-new-minimally-invasive-device-treating-mitral-regurgitation.html. Reprinted with permission from Valcare Medical

Indirect Annuloplasty Devices

Several device designs exist that seek to use the anatomical relationship of the coronary sinus to the mitral annulus to perform an indirect annuloplasty. The coronary sinus circumferentially tracks and surrounds the annulus along the posterior and posterolateral curvature of the heart. The devices are placed in the coronary sinus, and an attempt is made to reduce the annular size by tightening the sinus. Two such indirect annuloplasty devices, the Cardiac Dimensions Carillon system and the MVRx ARTO System, are described below.

Cardiac Dimensions Carillon System

The Carillon Mitral Contour system (Cardiac Dimensions Inc., Kirkland, WA, USA) is positioned in the coronary sinus to accomplish an indirect annuloplasty and treat functional MR. The device is a fixed-length, double-anchored nitinol structure whose distal anchor is deployed deep in the coronary sinus via a 9 Fr delivery catheter (Fig. 8.11) [124]. Traction is used to cinch the posterior periannular tissue and reduce the mitral annular circumference. When tissue plication is optimized as evidenced by a diminished degree of mitral regurgitation by TEE, the proximal anchor is deployed at the coronary sinus ostium. Angiography is performed before final release of the device, to ensure that the left circumflex coronary artery is unharmed.

The Carillon Mitral Annuloplasty Device European Union Study (AMADEUS) showed a modest (22%) reduction in MR at 6 months in 30 of the 48 patients enrolled. Similar results were shown in the Transcatheter Implantation of the Carillon Mitral Annuloplasty Device (TITAN) trial. The device was implanted successfully in 35 of 53 patients (68%), significantly reducing regurgitation and LV diastolic and systolic volumes. An additional study with the Carillon device is described in Table 8.7.

MVRx ARTO Device

Another device in development for treating FMR is the ARTO device (MVRx Inc., Belmont, CA, USA). This device employs magnet-tipped catheters positioned in the LA (through a transseptal puncture) and in the coronary sinus, which link on either side of the atrial wall behind the P2 segment of the posterior leaflet. The anchors are joined with a crossing wire to facilitate placement of a T-bar anchor in the coronary sinus. Another anchor is placed at the atrial septum at the site of transseptal puncture, and a linking suture is tensioned under TEE guidance until the anterior-posterior diameter of the mitral annulus is reduced sufficiently to reduce MR (Fig. 8.12) [125].

The first phase of the Mitral Valve Repair Clinical Trial (MAVERIC) of the ARTO device involved 11 patients with NYHA II–III symptoms and ≥2+ MR, for all of whom the risks of surgery were deemed prohibitively high by the heart team. Device implantation was successful in all 11 patients, with no procedural safety events and only 2 events at 30-day follow-up (1 pericardial effusion requiring drainage, and 1 asymptomatic device dislodgement). At 6 months, improvements were seen in MR grade, LV volumes, MR severity, regurgitant volumes, annular diameter, and functional status. The Phase II trial has yet to begin recruiting.

Leaflet-Based Devices

Several devices exist or are in development to correct leaflet disease or reapproximate leaflets in the manner of the Alfieri stitch. The most well known of these devices is the Abbott MitraClip, which is described elsewhere in this textbook. The success of the Abbott MitraClip has led to the development of other devices that work by leaflet coaptation, the best known of which is the Edwards PASCAL device.

Edwards PASCAL Device

The PASCAL device (Edwards LifeSciences) is another device that accomplishes leaflet coaptation. The device has a pair of paddles, placed 180° apart, which capture the edge of the anterior and posterior leaflet. A spacer in the middle is used to reduce the regurgitant orifice area, and the device allows independent leaflet grasping, giving it the potential for use in patients with more complex anatomy (Fig. 8.13) [123].

A multicenter prospective observational first-in-human compassionate use study is underway (Table 8.8). Preliminary (6-month) data show technical success in 28 of the first 29 patients, and less than one-quarter of patients required a

Table 8.5 Valcare Amend trials

Device/trial name	Trial design	Arms	Inclusion criteria	Exclusion criteria	Primary outcome measures	Secondary outcome measures	Follow-up	Est. study completion date
AMEND™ Mitral Valve Repair System, Annuloplasty Ring Applied in a Transcatheter Method	Prospective, multicenter, single-arm, nonrandomized trial, 40 pts	1. Experimental: Device	1. Need for MV annuloplasty without need for concomitant CT surgery 2. NYHA ≥II 3. High risk for surgery	1. Major cardiac or noncardiac disease that incurs unacceptable risk 2. Life expectancy <12 months 3. Heavily calcified annulus/leaflets 4. Active infection or hx of endocarditis 5. Previous MV intervention 6. Drug/alcohol abuse	1. Freedom from MAE (30 days) 2. Technical success of implantation	1. Freedom from MAE at 6 months	6 months	December 2018

CT cardiothoracic, *hx* history, *MAE* major adverse events, *MV* mitral valve, *NYHA* New York Heart Association

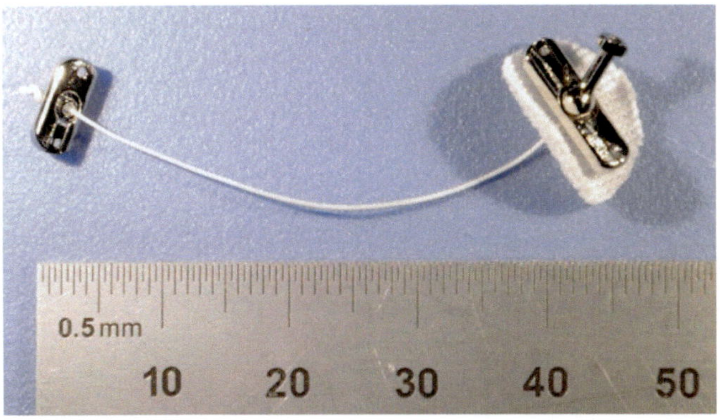

Fig. 8.9 MitraSpan Tasra device. Reprinted with permission from MitraSpan, Inc.

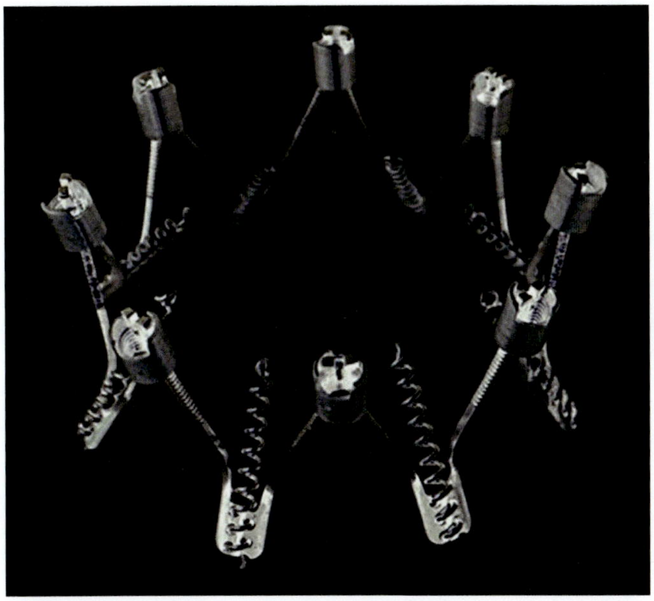

Fig. 8.10 Millipede IRIS Transcatheter Angioplasty Ring. From Sharma and Gafoor [123]. Reprinted with permission from Millipede Medical

second device implantation. Only 3 patients needed reintervention, and MR reduction and functional improvement were sustained; reverse LV remodeling was seen at 6 months, particularly in FMR patients.

Chordal Repair Devices

Numerous devices are being developed to repair chordal abnormalities. Prominent among these devices are the NEOCHORD DS1000 system, the Harpoon Medical Harpoon system, and the MISTRAL system.

NEOCHORD DS1000 System

The NEOCHORD DS1000 (NeoChord Inc., St. Louis Park, MN, USA) consists of expanded PTFE (ePTFE) sutures that are attached to the prolapsing mitral leaflet under echocardiographic guidance via an off-pump, transapical approach. Leaflets are grasped and pierced to allow fixation and retraction of the neochordae, and then are subsequently fixated at the LV apex (Fig. 8.14).

The initial Transapical Artificial Chordae Tendineae (TACT) trial involved 30 patients with severe MR due to isolated posterior leaflet prolapse. The procedure was successful in 26/30 patients, in whom at least one neochord was placed and MR was reduced from 3–4+ to ≤2+. This reduction in MR was maintained by 17/30 patients at 30 days. An ongoing trial with this device is described in Table 8.9.

Harpoon Medical Harpoon TSD-5 Device

Another device that also uses ePTFE chords, anchored to the prolapsed mitral leaflet via transapical access, is the Harpoon TSD-5 (Harpoon Medical, Baltimore, MD, USA). Under TEE guidance, the device is directed to the LV surface of the prolapsed leaflet, and the leaflet is perforated after it is stabilized and the device is actuated, perforating the leaflet with a needle that in turn is wrapped by ePTFE coils in a preformed knot. The needle is withdrawn, producing a double helix coiled knot on the atrial surface of the leaflet that secures the pair of ePTFE chords to the leaflet. Multiple devices can be deployed as needed before length is finally selected and the chords are tethered to the LV apex (Fig. 8.15). Initial data from 11 patients with severe MR for posterior leaflet prolapse show 100% procedural success, minimal postprocedural MR, and, at 1 month, mild MR and significant reductions in end-diastolic and left atrial volume. Trials have been planned for the Harpoon device.

Mitralix MISTRAL Device

Another device that reapproximates the chords is the transseptal 12-Fr MISTRAL device (Mitralix Ltd., Rehovot, Israel). This device consists of an atraumatic, spiral-shaped nitinol wire that pulls the chordae together.

Emerging Mitral Valve Replacement Devices

Although no device has yet been approved for transvascular MV replacement (TMVR), several promising devices are in development. Such TMVR devices have the potential to extend the therapeutic window into higher-risk, "too sick" patient populations, offering them relief of their MR with the potential for results comparable to those of surgical replacement with a bioprosthetic valve, but with fewer of the comorbidities associated with traditional surgery. In addition to extending the therapeutic window, TMVR devices have the potential to supplant traditional surgical valve replacement with a bioprosthetic valve for patients for whom this is the primary therapeutic option. Furthermore, TMVR devices hold an intriguing potential to treat secondary MR. Surgical

Table 8.6 Millipede IRIS trial

Device/trial name	Trial design	Arms	Inclusion criteria	Exclusion criteria	Primary outcome measures	Secondary outcome measures	Follow-up	Est. study completion date
Annular Reshaping of the Mitral Valve for MR using the Millipede IRIS System	Prospective, multicenter, single-arm, nonrandomized trial, 30 pts	1. Experimental: Device	1. Severe symptomatic MR (ERO >0.2 cm^2 for secondary MR, ERO >0.4 cm^2 for primary MR) 2. LVEF >20% and <50% 3. NYSHA II–IVa 4. Normal CK-MB 5. LVESD <6.5 cm	1. PASP >70, RV dysfunction 2. HOCM, restrictive or constrictive HD 3. Hemodynamic instability 4. CABG, PCI, or carotid intervention within 30 days 5. Need for other CT surgery 6. LVEF <20% 7. CKD, multiple others	1. Acute safety, defined as incidence of adverse events (30 days)	1. Efficacy; echo-measured reduction in MR without significant MS (48 h)	30 days	December 2019

CABG coronary artery bypass grafting, *CKD* chronic kidney disease, *CKMB* creatine kinase-muscle/brain, *CT* cardiothoracic, *ERO* effective regurgitant orifice, *HD* heart disease, *HOCM* hypertrophic obstructive cardiomyopathy, *LVEF* left ventricular ejection fraction, *LVESD* left ventricular end-systolic dimension, *MR* mitral regurgitation, *MS* mitral stenosis, *NYHA* New York Heart Association, *PASP* pulmonary artery systolic pressure, *PCI* percutaneous coronary intervention, *RV* right ventricle/ventricular results for secondary/functional MR are not as good as those for primary MR, and surgical repair with annuloplasty has been associated with a high recurrence rate of MR [92]. In such patients, a less invasive, less morbid, yet durable replacement option would be an attractive alternative.

However, the development of TMVR devices has been slow relative to the development of TAVR devices because of the complexity of the ventricular-valvular mitral apparatus, as well as the location and size of the MV. The mitral annulus is an amorphous, complex, and dynamic structure with an ellipsoid shape and variable calcification. The lack of a predominantly cylindrical structure (like the aortic valve annulus) with significant calcification has made deploying a stent-based valve prosthesis challenging in terms of anchoring and fixation, as well as properly aligning a newly placed endovascular prosthetic valve within the annulus. The pressure differential between the atrium and ventricle, which can be up to 3 times greater than that encountered in aortic valve delivery, further complicates matters. Furthermore, the large size of the mitral annulus, especially in patients with dilated ventricles, often necessitates the use of valves larger than 30 mm in diameter, making delivery of these devices challenging. This is especially true if a transfemoral/transseptal approach is used, because the size limitations of the right atrium, atrial septum, and LA would limit the maneuverability of such a device. For this reason, several valve devices are being developed to use a transapical approach. However, this approach carries an additional set of risks that have limited device development.

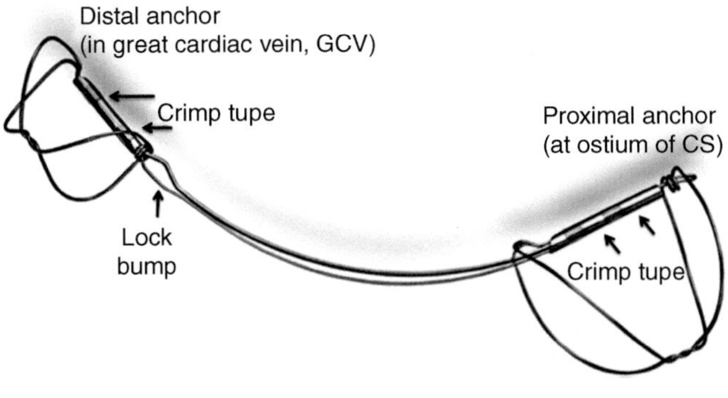

Fig. 8.11 Carillon device. The distal anchor is placed in the great cardiac vein, crimp tube, and lock bump (*left*), and the proximal anchor is placed at the ostium of the coronary sinus and the crimp tube (*right*). From Goldberg et al. [124]. Reprinted with permission from Europa Digital & Publishing

Broadly speaking, TMVR devices can be grouped according to their fixation method and their delivery approach. Delivery approaches can, in turn, be broadly categorized as transapical, transfemoral-transseptal, and transatrial. Currently, the majority of devices use a transapical approach, although future devices are being developed for a transseptal delivery approach. Fixation strategies differentiate valves into several different groups.

Wing- or Tab-Based Fixation Devices

Using wings or tabs that engage the native leaflets is the most common approach. These wings or tabs must capture healthy leaflets without becoming entangled in the chordae tendineae. This requirement may preclude or limit the use of these devices in patients with degenerative MR. These devices include the Edwards FORTIS, Neovasc Tiara, Edwards CardiAQ, and NaviGate devices.

Table 8.7 Carillon Mitral contour trial

Device/trial name	Trial design	Arms	Inclusion criteria	Exclusion criteria	Primary outcome measures	Secondary outcome measures	Follow-up	Est. study completion date
CARILLON trial: Transcatheter treatment of FMR	Prospective, multicenter, multiple-arm, double-blind RCT, 400 pts	1. Experimental: Device 2. Comparator: GDMT for HF	1. Cardiomyopathy, NYHA II, III, or IV 2. FMR >2+ and ERO >0.2 cm^2 3. 6MWD 200–450 m 4. LVEF <50% 5. LVEDD >7 cm 6. Optimized on HF medications 7. Anatomy appropriate for implant	Many criteria; refer to trial	1. Freedom from MAE (12 months) 2. Hierarchical clinical composite (12 months) 3. Change in RVol (12 months)	1. Freedom from periprocedural MAE (30 days vs. discharge) 2. Freedom from MAE (12 months) 3. 6MWD (12 months) 4. LVESV (12 months) 5. KCCQ (12 months) 6. NYHA Class (12 months)	12 months	October 2025

6MWD 6-minute walk distance, *ERO* effective regurgitant orifice, *FMR* functional mitral regurgitation, *GDMT* goal-directed medical therapy, *HF* heart failure, *KCCQ* Kansas City Cardiomyopathy Questionnaire, *LVEDD* left ventricular end-diastolic dimension, *LVEF* left ventricular ejection fraction, *LVESV* left ventricular end-systolic volume, *MAE* major adverse events, *NYHA* New York Heart Association, *RVol* regurgitant volume

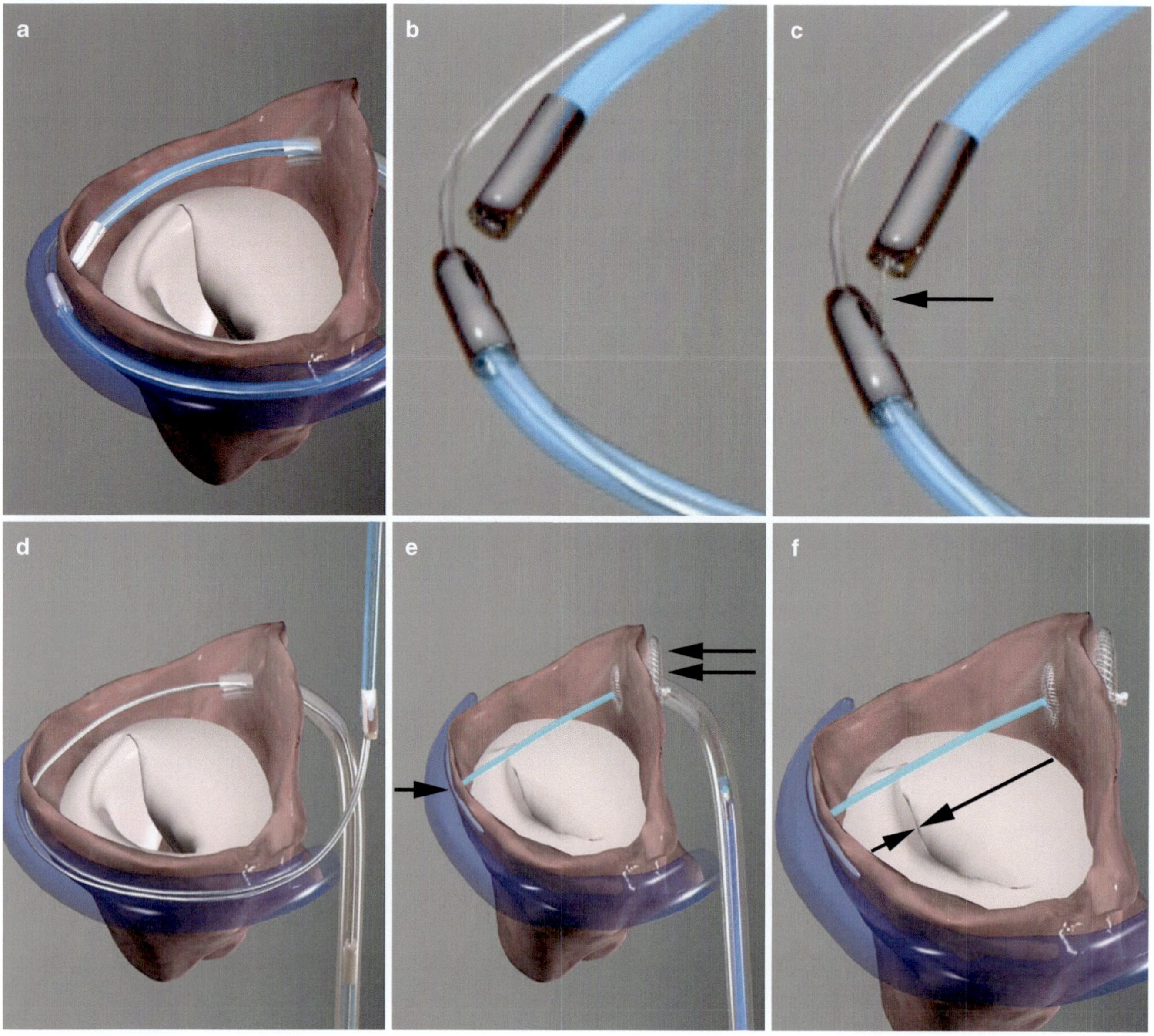

Fig. 8.12 ARTO device and implantation. (**a**) Great cardiac vein (GCV) and left atrial (LA) MagneCaths in position and magnetically linked behind the P2 segment of the posterior mitral leaflet. (**b**) Close-up of magnetically linked LA and GCV MagneCaths. Each magnetic catheter has a specific shape and lumen to direct and receive the crossing wire. (**c**) The crossing wire (*arrow*) is pushed from the GCV into the LA MagneCath. The MagneCaths are aligned to direct the wire safely from the GCV to the LA through the atrial wall. (**d**) After using an exchange catheter, the loop guidewire is placed across the left atrium. This guidewire directs the placement of the GCV anchor (T-bar, *single arrow*) and septal anchor (*double arrow*). (**e**) The Arto MVRx System in place before tensioning. (**f**) Tensioning of the bridge results in precise shortening of the mitral annulus anteroposterior diameter (*arrows*) and elimination of functional mitral regurgitation; once the final position is attained, the suture is cut and secured with a suture lock. From Erglis et al. [125]. Reprinted with permission from Europa Digital & Publishing

Edwards FORTIS Device

The Edwards Fortis TMVR device (Edwards LifeSciences) has a central cylindrical valve body composed of three pericardial leaflets sutured within a 29-mm diameter nitinol stent. It uses two paddles located in the outflow of the central valve body, allowing capture of the mitral leaflets to anchor the device. An additional atrial flange at the inflow point, made from nitinol struts covered with cloth, rests on the base of the LA and allows tissue endothelialization. The Fortis device is delivered through a 42 Fr transapical delivery system (Fig. 8.16) [126].

Twenty patients who were either inoperable or at high risk from conventional MV surgery and unsuitable for other transcatheter alternatives have received the FORTIS implant;

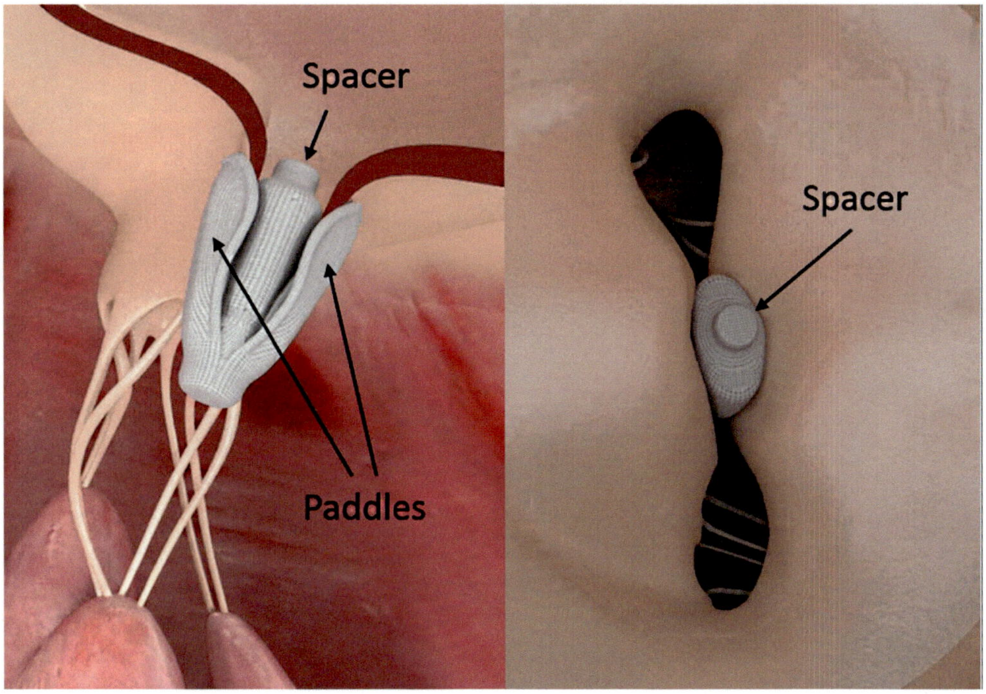

Fig. 8.13 Pascal device. The renderings show the device grasping leaflets in a cross-sectional view (*left*) and an atrial view (*right*). From Sharma et al. [123]. Reprinted with permission from Edwards Lifesciences

Table 8.8 CLASP study of the PASCAL device

Device/trial name	Trial design	Arms	Inclusion criteria	Exclusion criteria	Primary outcome measures	Secondary outcome measures	Follow-up	Est. study completion date
CLASP Edwards PASCAL Transcatheter Mitral Valve Repair System Study	Prospective, multicenter, single-arm, open-label trial, 120 pts	1. Experimental: Device	1. NYHA II–IVa despite optimal medical therapy 2. Clinically significant MR 3. Candidacy for SMVR determined by heart team 4. Non-commissural primary regurgitant jet 5. MVA >4 cm^2	1. TEE failed or not possible 2. Unsuitable anatomy 3. MVA <4 cm^2 4. RV dysfunction or failure 5. Life expectancy <12 months	1. Composite of MAE (CV mortality, stroke, MI, new need for RRT, severe bleeding, reintervention for device complications) (30 days)	1. MR reduction (30 days–1 year) 2. All-cause mortality (30 days–1 year) 3. Recurrent HF hospitalization (30 days–1 year) 4. Change in 6MWD (6 months, 1 year)	1 year	August 2021

6MWD 6-minute walk distance, *CV* cardiovascular, *HF* heart failure, *MAE* major adverse events, *MI* myocardial infarction, *MR* mitral regurgitation, *MVA* mitral valve area, *NYHA* New York Heart Association, *RRT* renal replacement therapy, *RV* right ventricle/ventricular, *SMVR* surgical mitral valve repair, *TEE* transesophageal echocardiography

13 of these patients' results have been made available [127]. The procedure was successful in 10 patients. Two patients were converted to surgery, one because of device malposition and one because the balloon system became entangled in the chords before implantation. Incomplete posterior leaflet capture resulted in partial device migration and death for 1 patient on day 4. Four patients died in the hospital, and eight survived beyond 30 days. All FORTIS implants under all protocols have been voluntarily put on hold because of evidence of thrombosis.

Neovasc Tiara Device

The Neovasc Tiara (Neovasc Inc., Richmond, BC, Canada) consists of a D-shaped, self-expanding nitinol frame with a trileaflet bovine pericardial valve. It has a full atrial skirt and three ventricular anchors, one anterior and two posterior, that

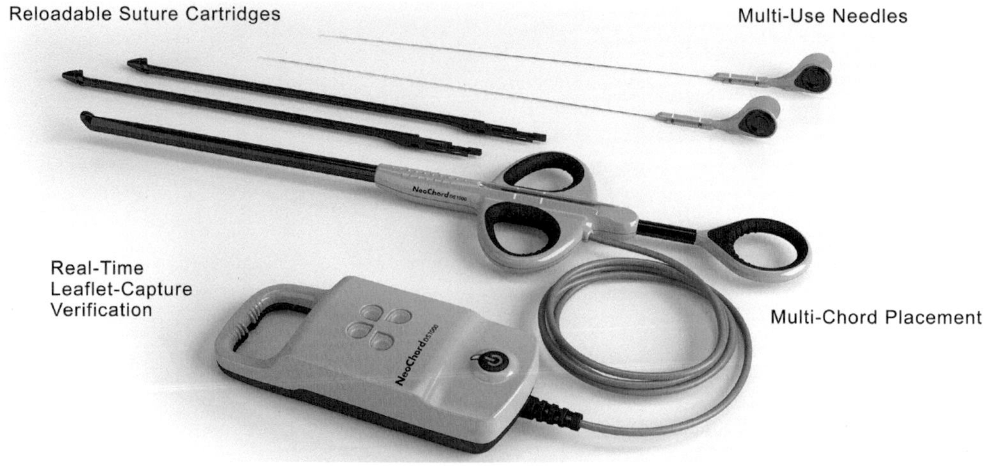

Fig. 8.14 NeoChord DS100 device with suture cartridges, multi-use needles, delivery instrument, and leaflet capture verification monitor. Reprinted with permission from NeoChord, Inc.

affix the valve to the fibrous trigone and the posterior annulus [128]. The valve currently is manufactured in two sizes, 35 and 40 mm, and the transapical delivery system is 32 Fr and 36 Fr, respectively (Fig. 8.17) [129]. The current status of ongoing trials involving the Tiara device is listed in Table 8.10.

Edwards CardiAQ Device

Another device system that uses fixation to the native valve leaflets via wings or tabs is the Edwards CardiAQ system (Edwards Lifesciences). The device is a self-expanding, nitinol frame with a trileaflet bovine pericardial valve. The frame has opposing anchors that secure the device in the annulus, and it possesses foam-covered ventricular anchors that engage the subvalvular apparatus. A polyester fabric skirt helps minimize paravalvular regurgitation. The device uses supra-annular positioning to reduce the risk of LV outflow tract obstruction, and it does not require rotational alignment [129, 130] (Fig. 8.18).

It uses a 33 Fr delivery system and can be deployed via a transapical or a transfemoral-transseptal approach. Two trials have been withdrawn and one trial was terminated to allow further design validation and testing of the valve; one trial remains ongoing and is described in Table 8.11.

"Valve and Dock" Fixation Devices

In the valve and dock approach to device fixation, a docking device is fixated to the mitral position; subsequently, a valve is docked inside this device. The Caisson TMVR and MValve devices both use this system.

Caisson TMVR Device

The Caisson TMVR device (Caisson Interventional LLC, Maple Grove, MN, USA) uses a valve and dock fixation method and is fully retrievable. The device has two components: a D-shaped, self-expanding nitinol anchor, and a self-expanding, nitinol-framed, trileaflet porcine pericardial valve. The device can be delivered through a transfemoral-transseptal approach with a 31 Fr delivery system (Fig. 8.19) [129]. The design of the Percutaneous Mitral Valve Replacement EvaLuation Utilizing IDE Early Feasibility Study (PRELUDE) of this device is summarized in Table 8.12.

MValve Device

Another novel device that uses this valve and dock approach is the MValve transcatheter mitral replacement system (MValve Technologies Ltd., Herzliyya, Israel). The device is deployed in two steps: A proprietary valve support/dock is deployed in and around the native mitral annulus, and a commercial transcatheter valve is deployed within the dock to replace the MV (Fig. 8.20) [129]. The device is designed to replicate existing valve-in-valve approaches by creating an annular dock inside the existing mitral annulus, within which any commercial valve can be placed.

Left Ventricular Tethering

Tethering to the LV is an approach wherein fixation of the valve relies on an additional anchor on the LV wall, near the apex. One concern posed by this approach is that it places an abnormal compressive load on the LV in patients who already have a compromised LV. The Abbott Tendyne valve uses this approach.

Abbott Tendyne Mitral Valve System

The Abbott Tendyne system (Abbott Vascular, Santa Clara, CA, USA) uses a transapical, fully repositionable and recapturable trileaflet porcine pericardial valve that is sewn inside two self-expanding nitinol stents. The outer stent is available in various sizes and is D-shaped to conform to the native mitral annulus. The inner circular frame has a large (>3.0 cm^2) effec-

Table 8.9 NeoChord DS1000 system trial

Device/trial name	Trial design	Arms	Inclusion criteria	Exclusion criteria	Primary outcome measures	Secondary outcome measures	Follow-up	Est. study completion date
ReChord: Randomized trial of the NeoChord DS1000 system vs. open surgical repair	Prospective, multicenter, multiple-arm, open-label RCT, 585 pts	1. Experimental: Device 2. Comparator: SMVR	1. Candidate for SMVR w/ CPB 2. Grade III moderate or Grade IV severe DMR 3. Isolated segmental prolapse of A2 or P2 segment 4. Anterior leaflet ≥65% of AP distance 5. Anatomic and general suitability	1. Prior MV surgery 2. Concomitant cardiac procedures 3. Other cardiac procedures within 3 months	1. Proportion of patients free of MAE as compared with control group (30 days) 2. Proportion of patients free of Grade II, III, or IV MR, MV replacement, or MV reintervention compared with control group (30 days)	None	1 year	July 2025

AP anterior-posterior, *CPB* cardiopulmonary bypass, *DMR* degenerative mitral regurgitation, *MAE* major adverse events, *MV* mitral valve, *RCT* randomized, controlled trial, *SMVR* surgical mitral valve repair

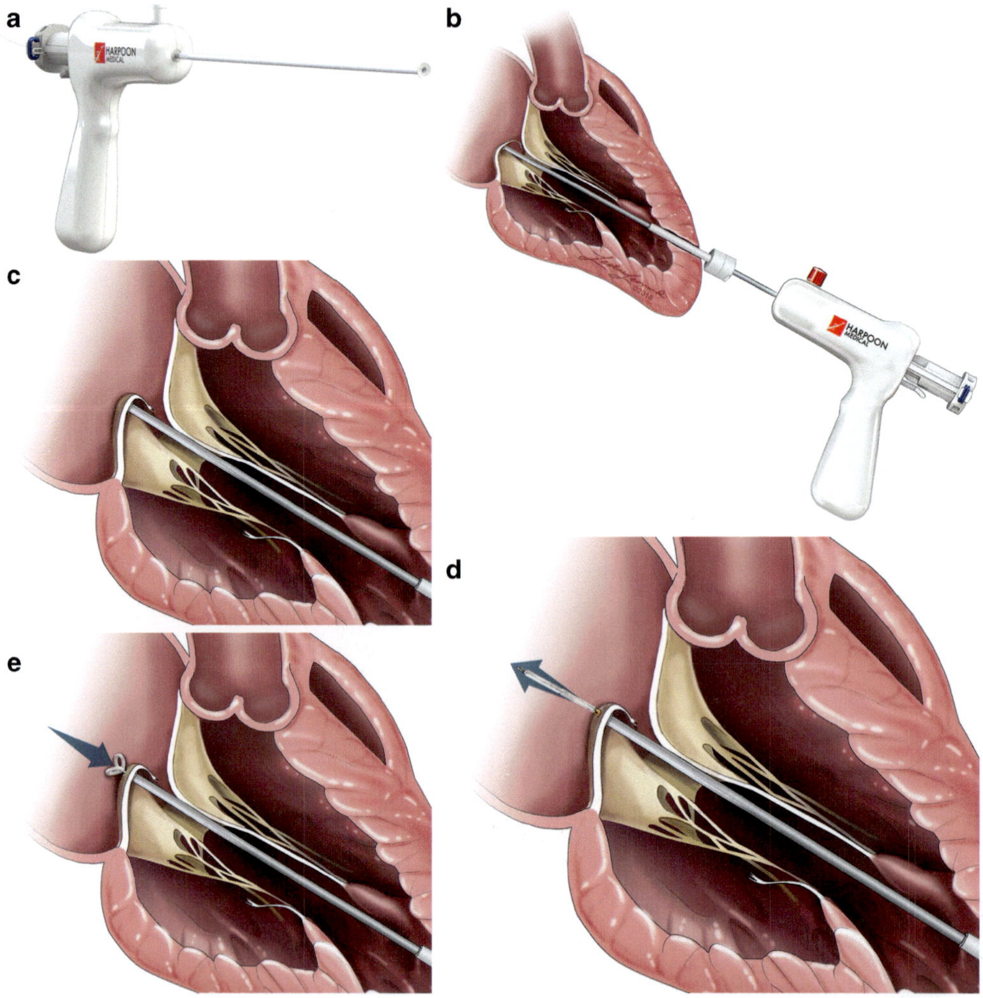

Fig. 8.15 Use of the Harpoon TSD-5 device for chordal repair in the mitral valve. (**a**) The Harpoon TSD-5. (**b**) Harpoon device inserted into left ventricle and directed toward and into contact with mitral leaflet. (**c**) Close-up view of Harpoon device in contact with mitral leaflet with ruptured chord. (**d**) Close-up view showing perforation of mitral leaflet with device needle and preformed PTFE chords. (**e**) Close-up view of deployed PTFE chords in knot configuration, secured to leaflet. Chords are then measured to appropriate length and anchored to LV apex. Images courtesy of Edwards Lifesciences LLC

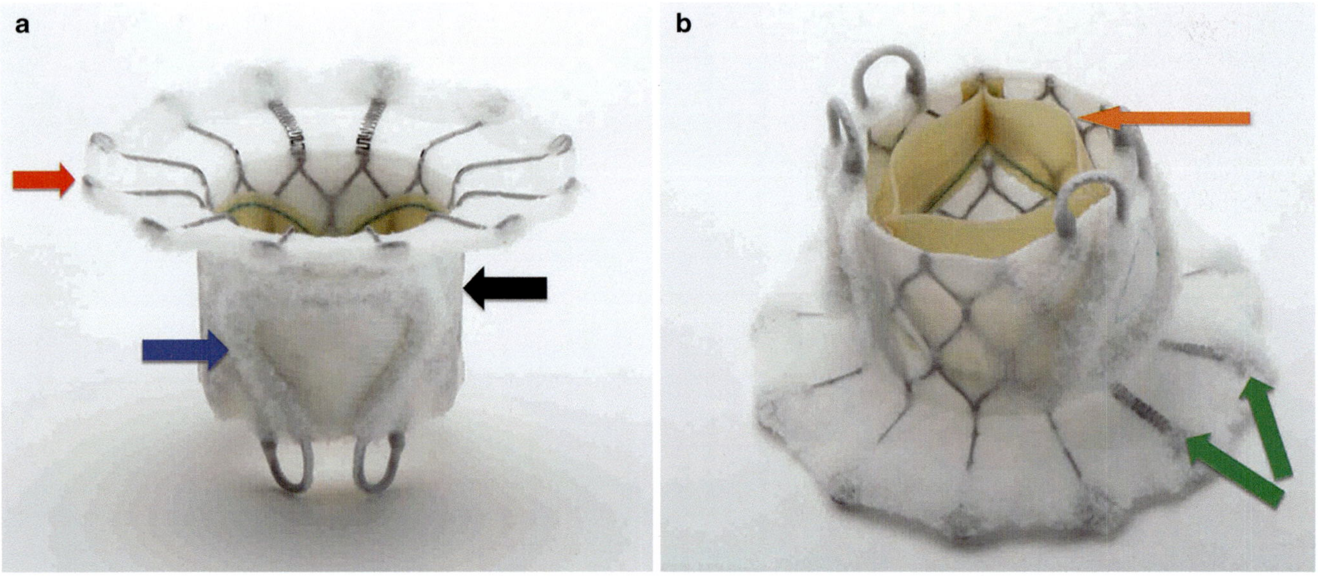

Fig. 8.16 Fortis device. (**a**) Side profile highlighting atrial flange (*red arrow*), body of valve (*black arrow*), and one of two paddles (*blue arrow*). (**b**) Side profile highlighting bovine pericardial leaflets (*orange arrow*) and flexible struts (*green arrow*), which align with the A2 segment of the mitral valve. From Bapat et al. [126]. Reprinted with permission from Europa Digital & Publishing

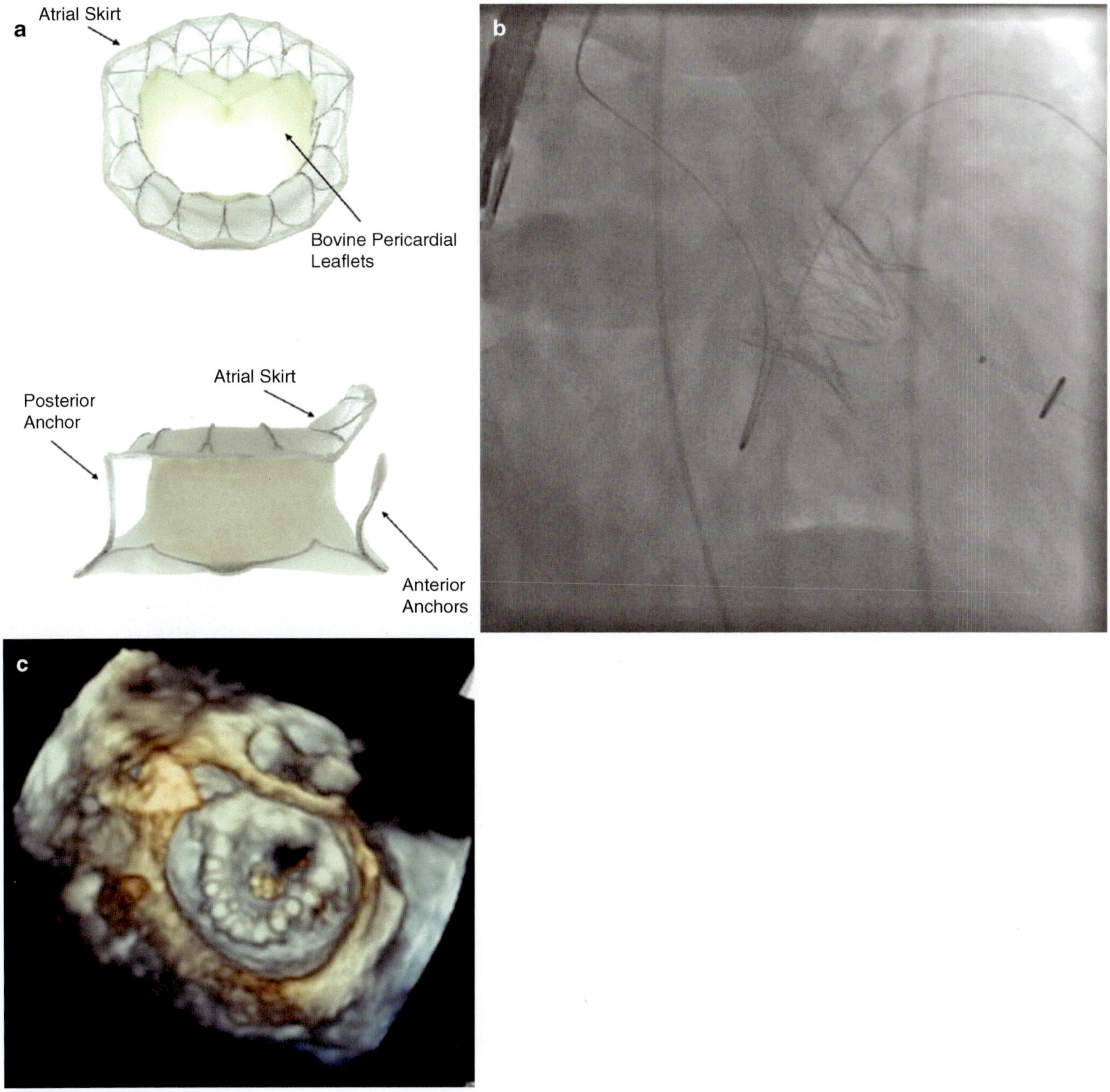

Fig. 8.17 Tiara device. (**a**) Valve prosthesis. (**b**) Valve prosthesis under fluoroscopy. (**c**) 2D TEE images of device. From Reguiero et al. [129]. Reprinted with permission from Elsevier

tive orifice area. The valve is tethered to the LV apex with an LV apical tethering system, which is designed to reduce paravalvular regurgitation and facilitate apical closure.

The device uses a 34 Fr transapical delivery sheath. The valve is positioned above the annulus, and the D-shaped outer stent is oriented such that the straight side and atrial cuff are aligned with the aortomitral continuity and the aorta. The valve is then retracted backwards into the mitral annulus with tactile guidance, and positioning is confirmed with echocardiography and fluoroscopy. Then the apical pad is positioned over the LV apical tether, and a tension gauge is used to adjust tension to keep the valve in a stable position (Fig. 8.21) [131].

An initial global feasibility study of 30 patients with grade 3/4 MR showed successful implantation in 28/30 patients, no residual MR in 26 patients, and only mild central MR (1+) in 1 patient at 30 days. At follow-up, 21 patients (75%) had NYHA Class I–II symptoms and improvement in LV end-diastolic volume index. Table 8.13 describes an ongoing trial of the Abbott Tendyne system.

Table 8.10 Neovasc Tiara trials

Device/trial name	Trial design	Arms	Inclusion criteria	Exclusion criteria	Primary outcome measures	Secondary outcome measures	Follow-up	Est. study completion date
TIARA-I	Multicenter, single-arm, prospective study, 30 pts	1. Experimental: TMVR	1. Severe symptomatic MR (Stage D) 2. High surgical risk for open MV surgery 3. Meets anatomical eligibility criteria for available sizes 4. NYHA Class III–IV	1. Operable DMR per heart team 2. Prohibitive risk, deemed too frail, or listed for transplant 3. Unsuitable cardiac structure 4. Prior stroke within 4 weeks 5. Need for coronary revascularization 6. hx of or active endocarditis 7. Renal insufficiency (Cr >2.5 mg/dL)	1. Freedom from all-cause mortality and MAE: disabling stroke, MI, renal failure necessitating dialysis, life-threatening bleeding, cardiac surgical or transcatheter reintervention (30 days or discharge, whichever is later)	1. All-cause mortality, stroke, MI, renal failure, bleeding, reintervention (30, 90, 180 days, annually to 5 years) 2. Device- and procedure-related MAE (30 days) 3. Progression of HF (1 year) 4. Procedural success (post-procedure, then annually for 5 years) 5. NYHA class, 6MWD, functional performance (up to 5 years) 6. Survival (1 year)	5 years	August 2023
TIARA-II	Global, multicenter, single-arm, prospective safety and performance study	1. Experimental: TMVR	1. Severe symptomatic MR (Stage D) 2. High surgical risk for open MV surgery 3. Meets anatomical eligibility criteria for available sizes 4. NYHA Class III–IV	1. Frailty (per objective criteria) 2. Previous CT surgery 3. Unsuitable anatomy 4. Untreated CAD 5. Chronic dialysis 6. Pregnancy 7. Bleeding or coagulation disorder 8. Active infection 9. Life expectancy <1 year	1. Freedom from all-cause mortality (30 days) 2. Freedom from major adverse events (30 days) 3. Reduction of MR to optimal or acceptable (30 days)	1. Freedom from all-cause mortality (up to 5 years) 2. Freedom from MAE (up to 5 years) 3. Technical success 4. Procedural success (30 days) 5. Device success (up to 5 years) 6. NYHA Class (up to 5 years) 7. 6MWD (up to 5 years) 8. KCCQ (up to 5 years) 9. Hemodynamic performance (up to 5 years) 10. Patient success (1 year)	Up to 5 years	January 2024

6MWD 6-minute walk distance, *CAD* coronary artery disease, *Cr* creatinine, *CT* cardiothoracic, *DMR* degenerative mitral regurgitation, *HF* heart failure, *hx* history, *KCCQ* Kansas City Cardiomyopathy Questionnaire, *MAE* major adverse events, *MI* myocardial infarction, *MR* mitral regurgitation, *MV* mitral valve, *NYHA* New York Heart Association, *TMVR* transcatheter mitral valve replacement

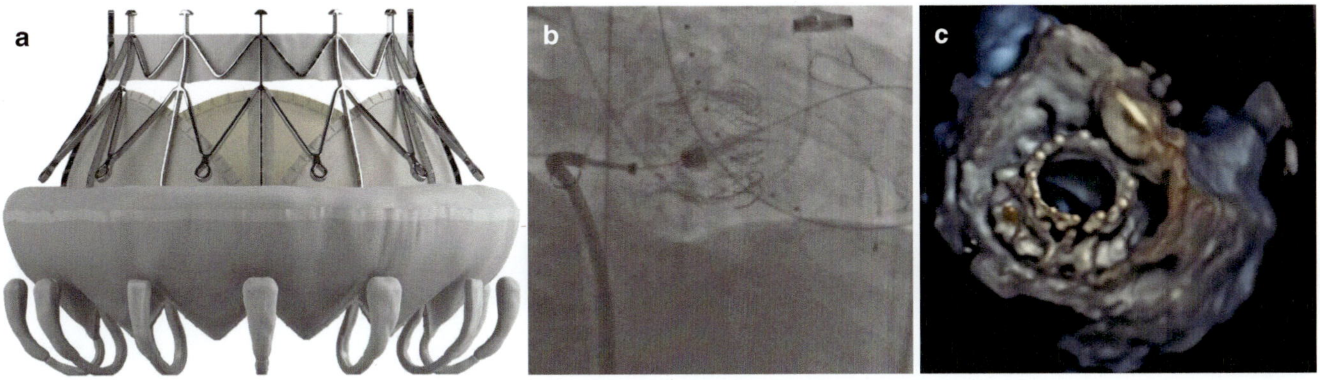

Fig. 8.18 CardiAQ device. (**a**) Valve prosthesis. (**b**) Valve prosthesis under fluoroscopy. (**c**) 2D TEE images of device. From Reguiero et al. [129]. Reprinted with permission from Elsevier

Table 8.11 Edwards CardiAQ trials

Device/trial name	Trial design	Arms	Inclusion criteria	Exclusion criteria	Primary outcome measures	Secondary outcome measures	Follow-up	Est. study completion date
CardiAQ-Edwards TMVR Early Feasibility Study	Prospective, multicenter, single-arm, nonrandomized trial, 30 pts	1. Experimental: TMVR	1. Clinically significant, symptomatic MR 2. High risk for open-heart surgery 3. Meets anatomical criteria	1. Unsuitable anatomy 2. Inoperable patient	1. Safety assessed by freedom from device or procedure-related adverse events (30 days)	1. NYHA functional class (up to 5 years) 2. 6MWD (up to 5 years) 3. Reduction in MR grade (up to 5 years)	5 years	June 2022

6MWD 6-minute walk distance, *MR* mitral regurgitation, *NYHA* New York Heart Association, *TMVR* transcatheter mitral valve replacement

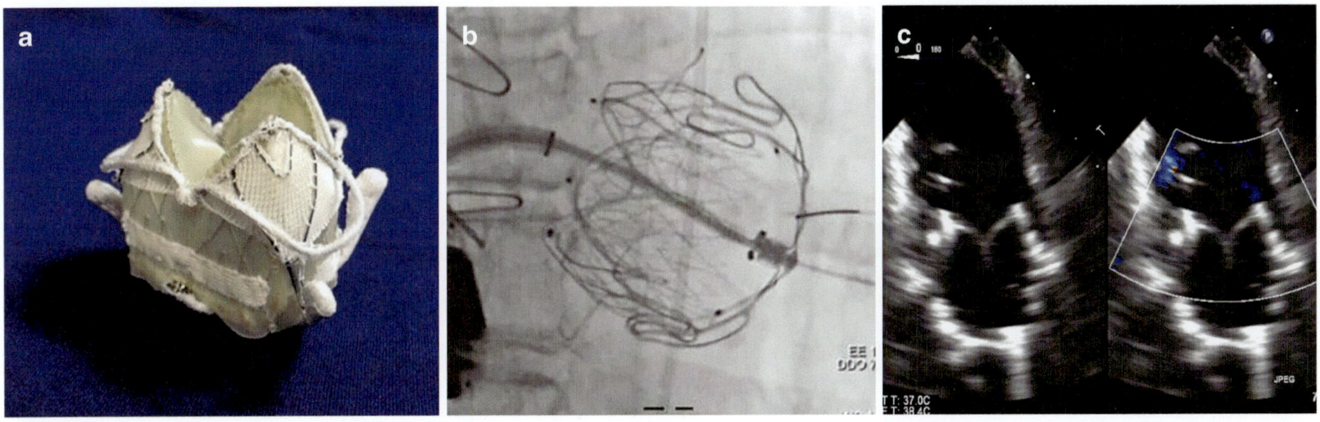

Fig. 8.19 Caisson TMVR device. (**a**). Valve prosthesis. (**b**) Valve prosthesis under fluoroscopy. (**c**) 2D TEE images of device. From Reguiero et al. [129]. Reprinted with permission from Elsevier

Clamping or Rivet Mechanisms for Annular Fixation

Yet another approach uses a clamping or rivet mechanism to surround the annulus and enable fixation. This approach may work well for certain anatomical situations, such as regurgitant MVs with an hourglass shape (i.e., a large LA and LV), but not in situations such as degenerative mitral disease in which the downstream flange of the clamp does not have a "lip" of tissue to engage. The NaviGate and HighLife valves use this approach.

Table 8.12 PRELUDE trial of Caisson TMVR

Device/trial name	Trial design	Arms	Inclusion criteria	Exclusion criteria	Primary outcome measures	Secondary outcome measures	Follow-up	Est. study completion date
Caisson TMVR system early feasibility study (PRELUDE)	Prospective, multicenter, single-arm, nonrandomized trial, 20 pts	1. Experimental: TMVR	1. Severe MR 2. High risk for open-heart surgery 3. NYSHA II–IVa or HF	1. Unsuitable anatomy 2. LVEDD >7 cm 3. LVOT obstruction 4. Severe RV dysfunction 5. Stroke within 90 days 6. TIA or MI within 30 days	1. Number of pts without MAE (30 days)	1. Number of pts with technical success (intraoperative) 2. Number of living, stroke-free pts with device success (30 days)	30 days	December 2023

LVEDD left ventricular end-diastolic dimension, *LVOT* left ventricular outflow tract, *MAE* major adverse events, *MI* myocardial infarction, *MR* mitral regurgitation, *NYHA* New York Heart Association, *RV* right ventricle/ventricular, *TIA* transient ischemic attack, *TMVR* transcatheter mitral valve replacement

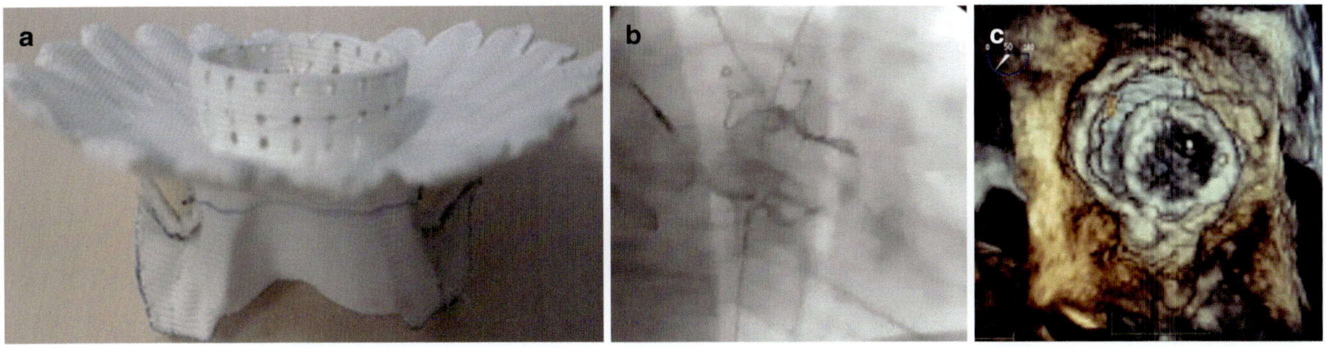

Fig. 8.20 MValve device. (**a**) Valve prosthesis. (**b**) Valve prosthesis under fluoroscopy. (**c**) 2D TEE images of device. From Reguiero et al. [129]. Reprinted with permission from Elsevier

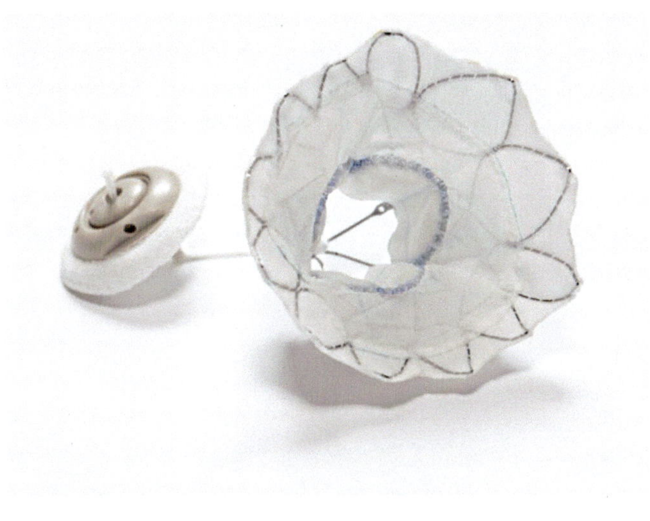

Fig. 8.21 Tendyne System. Mitral valve prosthesis (*right*) and left ventricular apical tethering device (*left*). From Perpetua and Reisman [131]. Reprinted with permission from Europa Digital & Publishing

NaviGate Cardiac Structures NaviGate Mitral Valved Stent

The NaviGate Mitral Valved Stent (NaviGate Cardiac Structures Inc., Lake Forest, CA, USA) consists of a self-expanding nitinol frame with a truncated cone. Its low profile height (21 mm) allows delivery into the heart while reducing the risk of protrusion into the atrium or ventricle. The device employs two rows of annular winglets that anchor the device to the annulus. It is available in three sizes (30/36, 30/40, and 33/44 mm) and can be delivered via transseptal, transatrial, or transapical routes with a 30 Fr system (Fig. 8.22) [132]. Early feasibility trials have been planned with this device for use in both tricuspid and mitral valve positions.

HighLife Device

With the HighLife TMVR System (HighLife SAS, Paris, France), a loop is advanced via the aortic valve, and a subannular implant is delivered via an 18 Fr femoral arterial sheath to form a loop implant in a subannular position. Transatrial or transapical delivery is then used to deliver a trileaflet bovine pericardial valve within a nitinol frame, which has a preformed annular groove to allow seating within the initially placed loop implant. The bioprosthesis expands inside the loop, and the shape of the bioprosthesis prevents migration within the ventricle (Fig. 8.23) [133]. The design of the HighLife system trial is described in Table 8.14.

Dynamic Cork Effect

The last approach uses a dynamic cork effect. In this mechanism, variable degrees of radial stiffness along the height of the structure enable the valve to compress to fit the annulus but stay larger in diameter downstream of the annulus, acting as a "cork" during systole without dilating the annulus. An advantage of this design is a high degree of adaptability to the ovoid or kidney-bean shape of the MV annulus without the need for rotational alignment. Such a design may work well in treating both degenerative and functional mitral regurgitation, but it does have some downsides. Two concen-

Table 8.13 Abbott Tendyne trial

Device/trial name	Trial design	Arms	Inclusion criteria	Exclusion criteria	Primary outcome measures	Secondary outcome measures	Follow-up	Est. study completion date
Expanded clinical study of the TENDYNE Mitral Valve System	Prospective, multicenter, single-arm, nonrandomized trial, 110 pts	1. Experimental: TMVR	1. Severe MR, primary or secondary 2. High risk/ unsuitable for open-heart surgery 3. NYSHA II–IVa	1. Severe MAC or MS 2. Chest condition precluding transapical access 3. Prior surgical or interventional treatment of mitral or aortic valves	1. Safety assessed by freedom from device- or procedure-related adverse events (30 days) 2. Performance assessed by freedom from device malfunction (30 days)	None	30 days	May 2018

MAC mitral annular calcification, *MR* mitral regurgitation, *MS* mitral stenosis, *NYHA* New York Heart Association, *TMVR* transcatheter mitral valve replacement

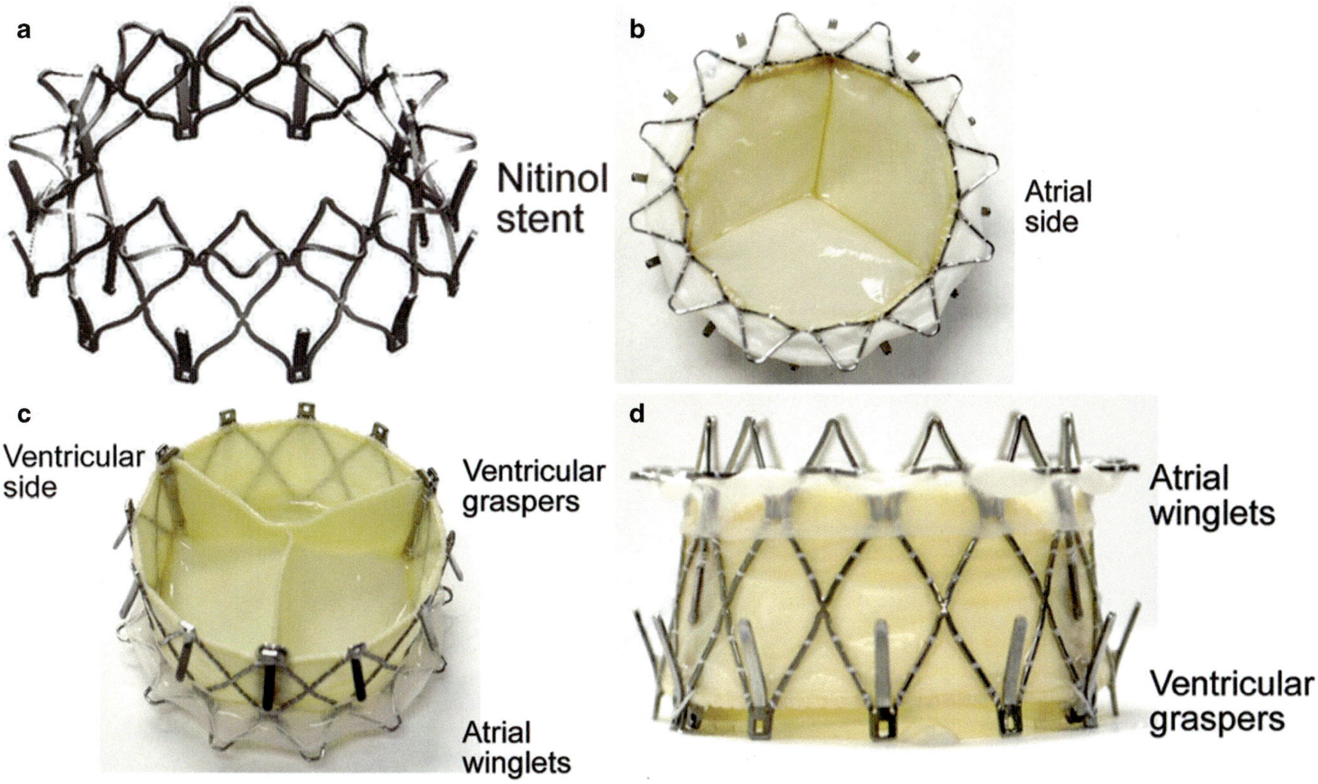

Fig. 8.22 NaviGate valved stent. (**a**) Nitinol stent frame. (**b**) Inflow (left atrial) view. (**c**) Outflow (left ventricular) view. (**d**) Side view. From Navia et al. [132]. Reprinted with permission from Europa Digital & Publishing

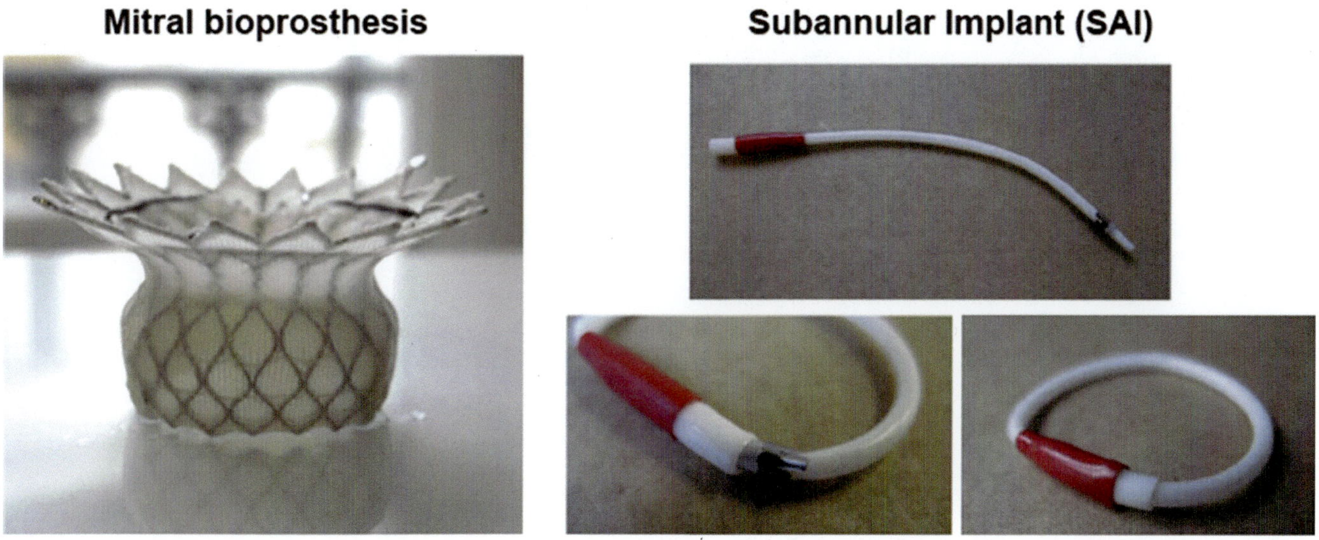

Fig. 8.23 HighLife device. Mitral bioprosthesis (*left*) and subannular implant (*right*). From Barbanti et al. [133]. Reprinted with permission from Elsevier

Table 8.14 HighLife TMVR system trial

Device/trial name	Trial design	Arms	Inclusion criteria	Exclusion criteria	Primary outcome measures	Secondary outcome measures	Follow-up	Est. study completion date
HighLife TMVR System Study	Prospective, multicenter, single-arm, nonrandomized trial, 20 pts	1. Experimental: TMVR	1. Severe MR 2. High risk/ unsuitable for open-heart surgery or other percutaneous therapy 3. NYSHA II–IVa 4. Maximally tolerated GDMT for at least 3 months 5. Meets anatomical criteria for device	1. Unsuitable anatomy 2. MS or severe MAC, or rheumatic dx 3. Prior MV intervention 4. LVEF <30% 5. LVEDD >7 cm 6. HOCM 7. Significant CAD requiring revascularization 8. Any surgery or intervention within 30 days	1. Freedom from major adverse events (30 days) 2. Continued intended performance of the valve (30 days) 3. Technical success	1. Device success (up to 12 months) 2. Procedure success (up to 12 months) 3. Patient success (up to 12 months) 4. Hemodynamic performance (up to 5 years) 5. Functional improvement (12 months) 6. Quality of life improvement (12 months)	5 years	December 2023

CAD coronary artery disease, *dx* diagnosis, *GDMT* goal-directed medical therapy, *HOCM* hypertrophic obstructive cardiomyopathy, *LVEDD* left ventricular end-diastolic dimension, *LVEF* left ventricular ejection fraction, *MAC* mitral annular calcification, *MR* mitral regurgitation, *MS* mitral stenosis, *MV* mitral valve, *NYHA* New York Heart Association, *TMVR* transcatheter mitral valve replacement

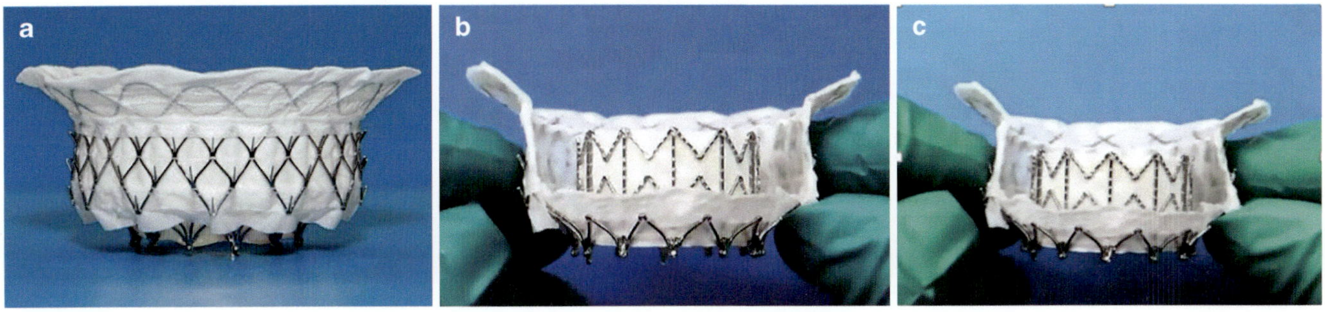

Fig. 8.24 Twelve/Intrepid valve. (**a**) The Intrepid TMVR prosthesis. Cut-outs show the device's dual-stent design (**b**) and overall flexibility (**c**), allowing the device to conform to the shape of native mitral annulus. From Meredith et al. [134]. Reprinted with permission from Europa Digital & Publishing

tric stent structures are required to make such a design work. The Medtronic/Twelve Intrepid valve is an example of such a device.

Medtronic/Twelve Intrepid Valve

The Medtronic/Twelve Intrepid system (Medtronic, Minneapolis, MN, USA) has a unique dual structure that consists of an inner self-expanding, nitinol-framed, trileaflet bovine pericardial valve that is housed concentrically within a larger, self-expanding nitinol outer fixation ring. The outer ring engages with the dynamic mitral annulus; this separates the fixation of the dynamic annulus, and movement thereof throughout the cardiac cycle, from the functioning of the inner valve. The inner stent valve has a 27-mm diameter and an effective orifice area of 2.4 cm^2, while the outer valve structure is currently available in 43-, 46-, and 50-mm outer diameter sizes. The outer ring is sized to be larger than the native MV annulus, has varying radial stiffness, and is covered by a polyester fabric skirt to prevent leaks and accommodate tissue ingrowth. The atrial portion is flexible and conforms to the native annulus, while the ventricular portion is stiffer and resists compression, thus producing a cork effect during systolic pressure to resist migration. The system need not be rotationally aligned and does not require any tethering mechanism or capture of native leaflets (Fig. 8.24) [134]. The device is housed in a transapical hydraulic delivery system that facilitates controlled expansion and deployment [134].

The intrepid valve is currently under investigation in the APOLLO trial, a multicenter, global, prospective, randomized trial comparing TMVR by the Intrepid system to conventional MV surgery. Currently active clinical trials of the Medtronic/Twelve Intrepid device are described in Table 8.15.

Table 8.15 Intrepid system trials

Device/trial name	Trial design	Arms	Inclusion criteria	Exclusion criteria	Primary outcome measures	Secondary outcome measures	Follow-up	Est. study completion date
Twelve Pilot Study	Prospective, multicenter, nonrandomized trial, 10 pts	1. Experimental: TMVR	1. Severe MR (3 to 4+) 2. Symptomatic MR (NYHA II–IV) 3. Transapical delivery feasible 4. Mitral anatomy compatible with Twelve TMVR	1. LVEF <20% 2. Intracardiac mass, thrombus, vegetation 3. Prior valve surgery or need for valve surgery 4. Prior stroke within 4 weeks 5. Need for coronary revascularization 6. hx of or active endocarditis 7. Renal insufficiency (Cr >2.5 mg/dL)	1. Adverse events (30 days)	1. Procedural success (5 years) 2. Reduction of MR (5 years)	5 years	July 2023
Intrepid/ APOLLO	Global, multicenter RCT, 1380 pts estimated	1. Experimental: Surgical candidate, TMVR 2. Comparator: Surgical candidate, SMVR 3. Experimental: Non-surgical candidate, TMVR	1. Severe, symptomatic MR 2. Candidate for MV replacement	1. Prior TMVR w/ device implant 2. Anatomic contraindications 3. Severe MAC 4. Need for emergent/urgent surgery 5. Hemodynamic instability	All-cause mortality, stroke, reoperation or reintervention, cardiovascular hospitalization (1 year)	1. All-cause mortality, stroke, AKI, prolonged ventilation, deep wound infection, reoperation/ reintervention, major bleeding (30 days or discharge) 2. Change in NYHA class (1 year) 3. Quality of life improvement per SF-12, KCCQ (30 days, 1 year) 4. Echo-degree of MR (1 year) 5. Days alive out of hospital (1 year) 6. Cardiovascular hospitalizations (1 year)	Pre- and post-procedure, discharge, 30 days, 6 months, annually through 5 years	October 2025

Cr creatinine, *hx* history, *KCCQ* Kansas City Cardiomyopathy Questionnaire, *LVEF* left ventricular ejection fraction, *MAC* mitral annular calcification, *MR* mitral regurgitation, *MV* mitral valve, *NYHA* New York Heart Association, *RCT* randomized, controlled trial, *SMVR* surgical mitral valve repair, *TMVR* transcatheter mitral valve replacement

Conclusions

One of greatest difficulties in comparing outcomes among different minimally invasive MV procedures lies in the varying techniques used. Little to no prospective data are available that compare minimally invasive MV surgery with sternotomy valve surgery, and no data are available about the relative effectiveness of the various minimally invasive methods except for retrospective reports from individual surgeons or institutions. Additionally, many of the published studies included data from institutions with a limited volume of these specialized and technically demanding procedures. Nonetheless, the data clearly demonstrate that minimally invasive valve surgery performed in the appropriate clinical setting by a high-volume institution, with a well-developed surgical method, leads to outcomes that are equivalent, if not superior, to those of valve surgery through a sternotomy.

A minimally invasive MV procedure performed via a mini-thoracotomy is a true sternal-sparing and less-invasive procedure. Benefits include shorter ventilator times and intensive care unit and hospital length of stay. In addition, patients return to their normal lifestyles sooner because of less surgical trauma and greater chest-wall stability, which allow them to regain function faster than standard sternotomy patients. Other benefits include lower transfusion and analgesic requirements and better cosmesis. A decrease has been documented in the composite complication rate in higher-risk patients (i.e., those more 75 years old, obese, COPD, and low LVEF), as has a trend toward lower surgical mortality.

Mitral valve procedures currently remain in the domain of the surgeon. Mitral valve repair techniques take time to learn and can be technically demanding. Nonetheless, surgical correction of essentially all MV abnormalities has produced excellent results and durability at experienced centers.

In addition, there exists a large, unmet clinical need for less-invasive therapies with a more favorable risk/benefit profile for the treatment of MR, and a correspondingly large potential patient population that would benefit from these therapies. The pioneering success of the MitraClip, especially in the treatment of high-risk patients, has proven the magnitude of this unmet need in clinical practice. Furthermore, the success of this device has led to a great deal of device development for transcatheter MV repair and replacement. Nonetheless, the results are still far from optimal, and for the time being, these technologies will be limited to patients not eligible for surgery.

References

1. Corbi P, Rahmati M, Donal E, et al. Prospective comparison of minimally invasive and standard techniques for aortic valve replacement: initial experience in the first hundred patients. J Card Surg. 2003;18:133–9.
2. Lamelas J, Sarria A, Santana O, Pineda AM, Lamas GA. Outcomes of minimally invasive valve surgery versus median sternotomy in patients age 75 years or greater. Ann Thorac Surg. 2011;91:79–84.
3. Santana O, Reyna J, Benjo AM, Lamas GA, Lamelas J. Outcomes of minimally invasive valve surgery in patients with chronic obstructive pulmonary disease. Eur J Cardiothorac Surg. 2012;42:648–52.
4. Santana O, Reyna J, Grana R, Buendia M, Lamas GA, Lamelas J. Outcomes of minimally invasive valve surgery versus standard sternotomy in obese patients undergoing isolated valve surgery. Ann Thorac Surg. 2011;91:406–10.
5. Cohn LH. Fifty years of open-heart surgery. Circulation. 2003;107:2168–70.
6. Cosgrove DM 3rd, Sabik JF, Navia JL. Minimally invasive valve operations. Ann Thorac Surg. 1998;65:1535–8; discussion 1538–9.
7. Chan EY, Lumbao DM, Iribarne A, et al. Evolution of cannulation techniques for minimally invasive cardiac surgery: a 10-year journey. Innovations (Phila). 2012;7:9–14.
8. Xu RB, Rahnavardi M, Nadal M, et al. Beating heart minimally invasive mitral valve surgery in patients with previous sternotomy: the operative technique and early outcomes. Open Heart. 2018;5:e000749.
9. Grossi EA, Loulmet DF, Schwartz CF, et al. Minimally invasive valve surgery with antegrade perfusion strategy is not associated with increased neurologic complications. Ann Thorac Surg. 2011;92:1346–9; discussion 1349–50.
10. Murzi M, Cerillo AG, Miceli A, et al. Antegrade and retrograde arterial perfusion strategy in minimally invasive mitral-valve surgery: a propensity score analysis on 1280 patients. Eur J Cardiothorac Surg. 2013;43:e167–72.
11. Murzi M, Glauber M. Central versus femoral cannulation during minimally invasive aortic valve replacement. Ann Cardiothorac Surg. 2015;4:59–61.
12. Lamelas J, Williams RF, Mawad M, LaPietra A. Complications associated with femoral cannulation during minimally invasive cardiac surgery. Ann Thorac Surg. 2017;103:1927–32.
13. LaPietra A, Santana O, Mihos CG, et al. Incidence of cerebrovascular accidents in patients undergoing minimally invasive valve surgery. J Thorac Cardiovasc Surg. 2014;148:156–60.
14. Iribarne A, Karpenko A, Russo MJ, et al. Eight-year experience with minimally invasive cardiothoracic surgery. World J Surg. 2010;34:611–5.
15. Navia JL, Cosgrove DM 3rd. Minimally invasive mitral valve operations. Ann Thorac Surg. 1996;62:1542–4.
16. Gillinov AM, Cosgrove DM. Minimally invasive mitral valve surgery: mini-sternotomy with extended transseptal approach. Semin Thorac Cardiovasc Surg. 1999;11:206–11.
17. Loulmet DF, Carpentier A, Cho PW, et al. Less invasive techniques for mitral valve surgery. J Thorac Cardiovasc Surg. 1998;115:772–9.
18. Wang D, Wang Q, Yang X, Wu Q, Li Q. Mitral valve replacement through a minimal right vertical infra-axillary thoracotomy versus standard median sternotomy. Ann Thorac Surg. 2009;87:704–8.

19. Cohn LH, Adams DH, Couper GS, et al. Minimally invasive cardiac valve surgery improves patient satisfaction while reducing costs of cardiac valve replacement and repair. Ann Surg. 1997;226:421–6; discussion 427–8.
20. Farhat F, Lu Z, Lefevre M, Montagna P, Mikaeloff P, Jegaden O. Prospective comparison between total sternotomy and ministernotomy for aortic valve replacement. J Card Surg. 2003;18:396–401; discussion 402–3.
21. Vanermen H, Vermeulen Y, Wellens F, De Geest R, Degrieck I, Van Praet F. Port-access mitral valve surgery. Perfusion. 1998;13:249–52.
22. Mohr FW, Falk V, Diegeler A, Walther T, van Son JA, Autschbach R. Minimally invasive port-access mitral valve surgery. J Thorac Cardiovasc Surg. 1998;115:567–74; discussion 574–6.
23. Carpentier A, Loulmet D, Carpentier A, et al. [Open heart operation under videosurgery and minithoracotomy. First case (mitral valvuloplasty) operated with success]. C R Acad Sci III. 1996;319:219–23.
24. Falk V, Walther T, Autschbach R, Diegeler A, Battellini R, Mohr FW. Robot-assisted minimally invasive solo mitral valve operation. J Thorac Cardiovasc Surg. 1998;115:470–1.
25. Carpentier A, Loulmet D, Aupecle B, et al. [Computer assisted open heart surgery. First case operated on with success]. C R Acad Sci III. 1998;321:437–42.
26. Nishimura RA, Otto CM, Bonow RO, et al. 2017 AHA/ACC Focused Update of the AHA/ACC guideline for the management of patients with valvular heart disease: a report of the American College of Cardiology/American Heart Association Task Force on Practice Guidelines. JACC. 2017;70:252–89.
27. Lehr EJ, Guy TS, Smith RL, et al. Minimally invasive mitral valve surgery III: training and robotic-assisted approaches. Innovations (Phila). 2016;11:260–7.
28. Wolfe JA, Malaisrie SC, Farivar RS, et al. Minimally invasive mitral valve surgery II: surgical technique and postoperative management. Innovations (Phila). 2016;11:251–9.
29. Irisawa Y, Hiraoka A, Totsugawa T, et al. Re-expansion pulmonary oedema after minimally invasive cardiac surgery with right minithoracotomy. Eur J Cardiothorac Surg. 2016;49:500–5.
30. Kitahara H, Okamoto K, Kudo M, et al. Successful management of severe unilateral re-expansion pulmonary edema after mitral valve repair with mini-thoracotomy using extracorporeal membrane oxygenation. Gen Thorac Cardiovasc Surg. 2017;65:164–6.
31. Wang Y, Gao CQ, Wang G, Wang JL. Transesophageal echocardiography guided cannulation for peripheral cardiopulmonary bypass during robotic cardiac surgery. Chin Med J. 2012;125:3236–9.
32. Carrier M, Cyr A, Voisine P, et al. Vacuum-assisted venous drainage does not increase the neurological risk. Heart Surg Forum. 2002;5:285–8.
33. Colangelo N, Torracca L, Lapenna E, Moriggia S, Crescenzi G, Alfieri O. Vacuum-assisted venous drainage in extrathoracic cardiopulmonary bypass management during minimally invasive cardiac surgery. Perfusion. 2006;21:361–5.
34. Mihos CG, Santana O, Lamas GA, Lamelas J. Outcomes of right minithoracotomy mitral valve surgery in patients with previous sternotomy. Ann Thorac Surg. 2011;91:1824–7.
35. Santana O, Funk M, Zamora C, Escolar E, Lamas GA, Lamelas J. Staged percutaneous coronary intervention and minimally invasive valve surgery: results of a hybrid approach to concomitant coronary and valvular disease. J Thorac Cardiovasc Surg. 2012;144:634–9.
36. Nkomo VT, Gardin JM, Skelton TN, Gottdiener JS, Scott CG, Enriquez-Sarano M. Burden of valvular heart diseases: a population-based study. Lancet. 2006;368:1005–11.
37. Doshi JV, Agrawal S, Garg J, et al. Percutaneous mitral heart valve repair—MitraClip. Cardiol Rev. 2014;22:289–96.
38. Gammie JS, Sheng S, Griffith BP, et al. Trends in mitral valve surgery in the United States: results from the Society of Thoracic Surgeons Adult Cardiac Surgery Database. Ann Thorac Surg. 2009;87:1431–7; discussion 1437–9.
39. Mirabel M, Iung B, Baron G, et al. What are the characteristics of patients with severe, symptomatic, mitral regurgitation who are denied surgery? Eur Heart J. 2007;28:1358–65.
40. Patel JB, Borgeson DD, Barnes ME, Rihal CS, Daly RC, Redfield MM. Mitral regurgitation in patients with advanced systolic heart failure. J Card Fail. 2004;10:285–91.
41. Carpentier A, Chauvaud S, Fabiani JN, et al. Reconstructive surgery of mitral valve incompetence: ten-year appraisal. J Thorac Cardiovasc Surg. 1980;79:338–48.
42. Fornes P, Heudes D, Fuzellier JF, Tixier D, Bruneval P, Carpentier A. Correlation between clinical and histologic patterns of degenerative mitral valve insufficiency: a histomorphometric study of 130 excised segments. Cardiovasc Pathol. 1999;8:81–92.
43. Lam JH, Ranganathan N, Wigle ED, Silver MD. Morphology of the human mitral valve. I. Chordae tendineae: a new classification. Circulation. 1970;41:449–58.
44. Ranganathan N, Lam JH, Wigle ED, Silver MD. Morphology of the human mitral valve. II. The value leaflets. Circulation. 1970;41:459–67.
45. Carpentier A. Cardiac valve surgery—the "French correction". J Thorac Cardiovasc Surg. 1983;86:323–37.
46. Pepi M, Tamborini G, Maltagliati A, et al. Head-to-head comparison of two- and three-dimensional transthoracic and transesophageal echocardiography in the localization of mitral valve prolapse. J Am Coll Cardiol. 2006;48:2524–30.
47. Schwammenthal E, Chen C, Benning F, Block M, Breithardt G, Levine RA. Dynamics of mitral regurgitant flow and orifice area. Physiologic application of the proximal flow convergence method: clinical data and experimental testing. Circulation. 1994;90:307–22.
48. Yoran C, Yellin EL, Becker RM, Gabbay S, Frater RW, Sonnenblick EH. Dynamic aspects of acute mitral regurgitation: effects of ventricular volume, pressure and contractility on the effective regurgitant orifice area. Circulation. 1979;60:170–6.
49. Braunwald E, Awe WC. The syndrome of severe mitral regurgitation with normal left atrial pressure. Circulation. 1963;27:29–35.
50. Carabello BA. The current therapy for mitral regurgitation. J Am Coll Cardiol. 2008;52:319–26.
51. Gaasch WH, Meyer TE. Left ventricular response to mitral regurgitation: implications for management. Circulation. 2008;118:2298–303.
52. Enriquez-Sarano M, Hannachi M, Jais JM, Acar J. [Hemodynamic and angiographic results following surgical correction of mitral insufficiency. Apropos of 51 repeated catheterizations]. Arch Mal Coeur Vaiss. 1983;76:1194–1203.
53. Starling MR, Kirsh MM, Montgomery DG, Gross MD. Impaired left ventricular contractile function in patients with long-term mitral regurgitation and normal ejection fraction. J Am Coll Cardiol. 1993;22:239–50.
54. Wisenbaugh T, Spann JF, Carabello BA. Differences in myocardial performance and load between patients with similar amounts of chronic aortic versus chronic mitral regurgitation. J Am Coll Cardiol. 1984;3:916–23.
55. Corin WJ, Murakami T, Monrad ES, Hess OM, Krayenbuehl HP. Left ventricular passive diastolic properties in chronic mitral regurgitation. Circulation. 1991;83:797–807.
56. Messika-Zeitoun D, Johnson BD, Nkomo V, et al. Cardiopulmonary exercise testing determination of functional capacity in mitral regurgitation: physiologic and outcome implications. J Am Coll Cardiol. 2006;47:2521–7.
57. Crawford MH, Souchek J, Oprian CA, et al. Determinants of survival and left ventricular performance after mitral valve replace-

ment. Department of Veterans Affairs Cooperative Study on Valvular Heart Disease. Circulation. 1990;81:1173–81.
58. Adams DH, Rosenhek R, Falk V. Degenerative mitral valve regurgitation: best practice revolution. Eur Heart J. 2010;31:1958–66.
59. El-Tallawi KC, Messika-Zeitoun D, Zoghbi WA. Assessment of the severity of native mitral valve regurgitation. Prog Cardiovasc Dis. 2017;60:322–33.
60. Chinitz JS, Chen D, Goyal P, et al. Mitral apparatus assessment by delayed enhancement CMR: relative impact of infarct distribution on mitral regurgitation. JACC Cardiovasc Imaging. 2013;6:220–34.
61. Cawley PJ, Hamilton-Craig C, Owens DS, et al. Prospective comparison of valve regurgitation quantitation by cardiac magnetic resonance imaging and transthoracic echocardiography. Circ Cardiovasc Imaging. 2013;6:48–57.
62. Lopez-Mattei JC, Ibrahim H, Shaikh KA, et al. Comparative assessment of mitral regurgitation severity by transthoracic echocardiography and cardiac magnetic resonance using an integrative and quantitative approach. Am J Cardiol. 2016;117:264–70.
63. Ngaage DL, Schaff HV. Mitral valve surgery in non-ischemic cardiomyopathy. J Cardiovasc Surg. 2004;45:477–86.
64. Dagum P, Timek TA, Green GR, et al. Coordinate-free analysis of mitral valve dynamics in normal and ischemic hearts. Circulation. 2000;102:III62–9.
65. Miller DC. Ischemic mitral regurgitation redux—to repair or to replace? J Thorac Cardiovasc Surg. 2001;122:1059–62.
66. Enriquez-Sarano M, Tajik AJ, Schaff HV, Orszulak TA, Bailey KR, Frye RL. Echocardiographic prediction of survival after surgical correction of organic mitral regurgitation. Circulation. 1994;90:830–7.
67. Ling LH, Enriquez-Sarano M, Seward JB, et al. Early surgery in patients with mitral regurgitation due to flail leaflets: a long-term outcome study. Circulation. 1997;96:1819–25.
68. Schaff HV. Asymptomatic severe mitral valve regurgitation: observation or operation? Circulation. 2009;119:768–9.
69. Magne J, Girerd N, Senechal M, et al. Mitral repair versus replacement for ischemic mitral regurgitation: comparison of short-term and long-term survival. Circulation. 2009;120:S104–11.
70. Jones EC, Devereux RB, Roman MJ, et al. Prevalence and correlates of mitral regurgitation in a population-based sample (the Strong Heart Study). Am J Cardiol. 2001;87:298–304.
71. Singh JP, Evans JC, Levy D, et al. Prevalence and clinical determinants of mitral, tricuspid, and aortic regurgitation (the Framingham Heart Study). Am J Cardiol. 1999;83:897–902.
72. Rosen SE, Borer JS, Hochreiter C, et al. Natural history of the asymptomatic/minimally symptomatic patient with severe mitral regurgitation secondary to mitral valve prolapse and normal right and left ventricular performance. Am J Cardiol. 1994;74:374–80.
73. Grigioni F, Tribouilloy C, Avierinos JF, et al. Outcomes in mitral regurgitation due to flail leaflets a multicenter European study. JACC Cardiovasc Imaging. 2008;1:133–41.
74. Tribouilloy C, Grigioni F, Avierinos JF, et al. Survival implication of left ventricular end-systolic diameter in mitral regurgitation due to flail leaflets a long-term follow-up multicenter study. J Am Coll Cardiol. 2009;54:1961–8.
75. Javadikasgari H, Gillinov AM, Idrees JJ, et al. Valve repair is superior to replacement in most patients with coexisting degenerative mitral valve and coronary artery diseases. Ann Thorac Surg. 2017;103:1833–41.
76. Mick SL, Keshavamurthy S, Gillinov AM. Mitral valve repair versus replacement. Ann Cardiothorac Surg. 2015;4:230–7.
77. Mohty D, Orszulak TA, Schaff HV, Avierinos JF, Tajik JA, Enriquez-Sarano M. Very long-term survival and durability of mitral valve repair for mitral valve prolapse. Circulation. 2001;104:I1–7.
78. Bolling SF, Li S, O'Brien SM, Brennan JM, Prager RL, Gammie JS. Predictors of mitral valve repair: clinical and surgeon factors. Ann Thorac Surg. 2010;90:1904–11; discussion 1912.
79. Bonow RO, Adams DH. The time has come to define centers of excellence in mitral valve repair. J Am Coll Cardiol. 2016;67:499–501.
80. Gammie JS, Zhao Y, Peterson ED, O'Brien SM, Rankin JS, Griffith BP. J. Maxwell Chamberlain Memorial Paper for adult cardiac surgery. Less-invasive mitral valve operations: trends and outcomes from the Society of Thoracic Surgeons Adult Cardiac Surgery Database. Ann Thorac Surg. 2010;90:1401–8, 1410.e1; discussion 1408–10.
81. Dillon J, Yakub MA, Nordin MN, Pau KK, Krishna Moorthy PS. Leaflet extension in rheumatic mitral valve reconstruction. Eur J Cardiothorac Surg. 2013;44:682–9.
82. Maisano F, Torracca L, Oppizzi M, et al. The edge-to-edge technique: a simplified method to correct mitral insufficiency. Eur J Cardiothorac Surg. 1998;13:240–5; discussion 245–6.
83. Maisano F, Schreuder JJ, Oppizzi M, Fiorani B, Fino C, Alfieri O. The double-orifice technique as a standardized approach to treat mitral regurgitation due to severe myxomatous disease: surgical technique. Eur J Cardiothorac Surg. 2000;17:201–5.
84. Milano CA, Daneshmand MA, Rankin JS, et al. Survival prognosis and surgical management of ischemic mitral regurgitation. Ann Thorac Surg. 2008;86:735–44.
85. Micovic S, Milacic P, Otasevic P, et al. Comparison of valve annuloplasty and replacement for ischemic mitral valve incompetence. Heart Surg Forum. 2008;11:E340–5.
86. Silberman S, Oren A, Klutstein MW, et al. Does mitral valve intervention have an impact on late survival in ischemic cardiomyopathy? Isr Med Assoc J. 2006;8:17–20.
87. Thourani VH, Weintraub WS, Guyton RA, et al. Outcomes and long-term survival for patients undergoing mitral valve repair versus replacement: effect of age and concomitant coronary artery bypass grafting. Circulation. 2003;108:298–304.
88. Vassileva CM, Boley T, Markwell S, Hazelrigg S. Meta-analysis of short-term and long-term survival following repair versus replacement for ischemic mitral regurgitation. Eur J Cardiothorac Surg. 2011;39:295–303.
89. Gillinov AM, Wierup PN, Blackstone EH, et al. Is repair preferable to replacement for ischemic mitral regurgitation? J Thorac Cardiovasc Surg. 2001;122:1125–41.
90. Reece TB, Tribble CG, Ellman PI, et al. Mitral repair is superior to replacement when associated with coronary artery disease. Ann Surg. 2004;239:671–5; discussion 675–7.
91. Al-Radi OO, Austin PC, Tu JV, David TE, Yau TM. Mitral repair versus replacement for ischemic mitral regurgitation. Ann Thorac Surg. 2005;79:1260–7; discussion 1260–7.
92. Acker MA, Parides MK, Perrault LP, et al. Mitral-valve repair versus replacement for severe ischemic mitral regurgitation. N Engl J Med. 2014;370:23–32.
93. Kron IL, Hung J, Overbey JR, et al. Predicting recurrent mitral regurgitation after mitral valve repair for severe ischemic mitral regurgitation. J Thorac Cardiovasc Surg. 2015;149:752–761 e751.
94. Gelsomino S, Lorusso R, De Cicco G, et al. Five-year echocardiographic results of combined undersized mitral ring annuloplasty and coronary artery bypass grafting for chronic ischaemic mitral regurgitation. Eur Heart J. 2008;29:231–40.
95. Ciarka A, Braun J, Delgado V, et al. Predictors of mitral regurgitation recurrence in patients with heart failure undergoing mitral valve annuloplasty. Am J Cardiol. 2010;106:395–401.
96. Magne J, Pibarot P, Dagenais F, Hachicha Z, Dumesnil JG, Senechal M. Preoperative posterior leaflet angle accurately predicts outcome after restrictive mitral valve annuloplasty for ischemic mitral regurgitation. Circulation. 2007;115:782–91.

97. Kongsaerepong V, Shiota M, Gillinov AM, et al. Echocardiographic predictors of successful versus unsuccessful mitral valve repair in ischemic mitral regurgitation. Am J Cardiol. 2006;98:504–8.
98. Roshanali F, Mandegar MH, Yousefnia MA, Rayatzadeh H, Alaeddini F. A prospective study of predicting factors in ischemic mitral regurgitation recurrence after ring annuloplasty. Ann Thorac Surg. 2007;84:745–9.
99. Magne J, Senechal M, Dumesnil JG, Pibarot P. Ischemic mitral regurgitation: a complex multifaceted disease. Cardiology. 2009;112:244–59.
100. De Bonis M, Lapenna E, Verzini A, et al. Recurrence of mitral regurgitation parallels the absence of left ventricular reverse remodeling after mitral repair in advanced dilated cardiomyopathy. Ann Thorac Surg. 2008;85:932–9.
101. Wijdh-den Hamer IJ, Bouma W, Lai EK, et al. The value of preoperative 3-dimensional over 2-dimensional valve analysis in predicting recurrent ischemic mitral regurgitation after mitral annuloplasty. J Thorac Cardiovasc Surg. 2016;152:847–59.
102. Bouma W, Lai EK, Levack MM, et al. Preoperative three-dimensional valve analysis predicts recurrent ischemic mitral regurgitation after mitral annuloplasty. Ann Thorac Surg. 2016;101:567–75; discussion 575.
103. Levine RA, Schwammenthal E. Ischemic mitral regurgitation on the threshold of a solution: from paradoxes to unifying concepts. Circulation. 2005;112:745–58.
104. Borger MA, Murphy PM, Alam A, et al. Initial results of the chordal-cutting operation for ischemic mitral regurgitation. J Thorac Cardiovasc Surg. 2007;133:1483–92.
105. Kron IL, Green GR, Cope JT. Surgical relocation of the posterior papillary muscle in chronic ischemic mitral regurgitation. Ann Thorac Surg. 2002;74:600–1.
106. Langer F, Rodriguez F, Ortiz S, et al. Subvalvular repair: the key to repairing ischemic mitral regurgitation? Circulation. 2005;112:I383–9.
107. Langer F, Schafers HJ. RING plus STRING: papillary muscle repositioning as an adjunctive repair technique for ischemic mitral regurgitation. J Thorac Cardiovasc Surg. 2007;133:247–9.
108. Langer F, Groesdonk HV, Kunihara T, Schafers HJ. Dynamic RING + STRING for ischemic mitral regurgitation: papillary muscle repositioning and modification of the septal-lateral diameter in the loaded beating heart under echocardiographic guidance. J Thorac Cardiovasc Surg. 2011;141:1315–6.
109. Fattouch K, Castrovinci S, Murana G, et al. Papillary muscle relocation and mitral annuloplasty in ischemic mitral valve regurgitation: midterm results. J Thorac Cardiovasc Surg. 2014;148:1947–50.
110. Hvass U, Tapia M, Baron F, Pouzet B, Shafy A. Papillary muscle sling: a new functional approach to mitral repair in patients with ischemic left ventricular dysfunction and functional mitral regurgitation. Ann Thorac Surg. 2003;75:809–11.
111. Benjo AM, Macedo FY, Santana O, Lamelas J. Papillary muscle sling placement for functional mitral regurgitation during minimally invasive valve surgery. Innovations (Phila). 2012;7:448–51.
112. Santana O, Solenkova NV, Pineda AM, Mihos CG, Lamelas J. Minimally invasive papillary muscle sling placement during mitral valve repair in patients with functional mitral regurgitation. J Thorac Cardiovasc Surg. 2014;147:496–9.
113. Nappi F, Lusini M, Spadaccio C, et al. Papillary muscle approximation versus restrictive annuloplasty alone for severe ischemic mitral regurgitation. J Am Coll Cardiol. 2016;67:2334–46.
114. Mandegar MH, Saidi B, Yousefnia MA, Alaeddini F, Roshanali F. Long-term effect of papillary muscle approximation combined with ventriculoplasty on left ventricle function in patients with ischemic cardiomyopathy and functional mitral regurgitation. Eur J Cardiothorac Surg. 2011;40:756–60.
115. Athanasuleas CL, Buckberg GD, Stanley AW, et al. Surgical ventricular restoration in the treatment of congestive heart failure due to post-infarction ventricular dilation. J Am Coll Cardiol. 2004;44:1439–45.
116. Athanasuleas CL, Stanley AW Jr, Buckberg GD. Restoration of contractile function in the enlarged left ventricle by exclusion of remodeled akinetic anterior segment: surgical strategy, myocardial protection, and angiographic results. J Card Surg. 1998;13:418–28.
117. Jones RH, Velazquez EJ, Michler RE, et al. Coronary bypass surgery with or without surgical ventricular reconstruction. N Engl J Med. 2009;360:1705–17.
118. Wakasa S, Shingu Y, Ooka T, Katoh H, Tachibana T, Matsui Y. Surgical strategy for ischemic mitral regurgitation adopting subvalvular and ventricular procedures. Ann Thorac Cardiovasc Surg. 2015;21:370–7.
119. Enriquez-Sarano M, Schaff HV, Orszulak TA, Tajik AJ, Bailey KR, Frye RL. Valve repair improves the outcome of surgery for mitral regurgitation. A multivariate analysis. Circulation. 1995;91:1022–8.
120. Gammie JS, O'Brien SM, Griffith BP, Ferguson TB, Peterson ED. Influence of hospital procedural volume on care process and mortality for patients undergoing elective surgery for mitral regurgitation. Circulation. 2007;115:881–7.
121. Bonow RO, Carabello BA, Chatterjee K, et al. 2008 focused update incorporated into the ACC/AHA 2006 guidelines for the management of patients with valvular heart disease: a report of the American College of Cardiology/American Heart Association Task Force on Practice Guidelines (Writing Committee to Revise the 1998 Guidelines for the Management of Patients With Valvular Heart Disease). J Am Coll Cardiol. 2008;52:e1–142.
122. Maisano F, Taramasso M, Nickenig G, et al. Cardioband, a transcatheter surgical-like direct mitral valve annuloplasty system: early results of the feasibility trial. Eur Heart J. 2016;37:817–25.
123. Sharma R, Gafoor S. Percutaneous mitral valve repair: the next wave. Card Interv Today. 2017;11:65–70.
124. Goldberg SL, Lipiecki J, Sievert H. The CARILLON Mitral Contour transcatheter indirect mitral valve annuloplasty system. EuroIntervention. 2015;11(Suppl W):W64–6.
125. Erglis A, Thomas M, Morice MC, et al. The Arto transcatheter mitral valve repair system. EuroIntervention. 2015;11(Suppl W):W47–8.
126. Bapat V, Buellesfeld L, Peterson MD, et al. Transcatheter mitral valve implantation (TMVI) using the Edwards FORTIS device. EuroIntervention. 2014;10(Suppl U):U120–8.
127. Bapat V, Lim ZY, Boix R, Pirone F. The Edwards Fortis transcatheter mitral valve implantation system. EuroIntervention. 2015;11(Suppl W):W73–5.
128. Verheye S, Cheung A, Leon M, Banai S. The Tiara transcatheter mitral valve implantation system. EuroIntervention. 2015;11(Suppl W):W71–2.
129. Regueiro A, Granada JF, Dagenais F, Rodes-Cabau J. Transcatheter mitral valve replacement: insights from early clinical experience and future challenges. J Am Coll Cardiol. 2017;69:2175–92.
130. Sondergaard L, Ussia GP, Dumonteil N, Quadri A. The CardiAQ transcatheter mitral valve implantation system. EuroIntervention. 2015;11(Suppl W):W76–7.
131. Perpetua EM, Reisman M. The Tendyne transcatheter mitral valve implantation system. EuroIntervention. 2015;11(Suppl W):W78–9.
132. Navia JL, Baeza C, Maluenda G, et al. Transcatheter mitral valve replacement with the NaviGate stent in a preclinical model. EuroIntervention. 2017;13:e1401–9.
133. Barbanti M, Piazza N, Mangiafico S, et al. Transcatheter mitral valve implantation using the HighLife system. JACC Cardiovasc Interv. 2017;10:1662–70.
134. Meredith I, Bapat V, Morriss J, McLean M, Prendergast B. Intrepid transcatheter mitral valve replacement system: technical and product description. EuroIntervention. 2016;12:Y78–80.

Tricuspid, Pulmonic, and Mixed Valve Disease

9

Blase A. Carabello and Rajasekhar Nekkanti

Introduction

The early part of the twenty-first century has seen a flourish of studies regarding disease of the left-sided heart valves, in part driven by newly available transcatheter treatment. However data regarding management of the right-sided valves has lagged until recently. Renewed interest has been spurred by recognition that tricuspid regurgitation persisting after successful correction of left-sided disease impacted outcome as did pulmonic regurgitation persisting into adulthood after correction of congenital heart disease. As little data that we have regarding tricuspid and pulmonary disease, we have even less regarding mixed valve disease. The foregoing will summarize the current data that we do have in these areas.

Tricuspid Valve Disease

Tricuspid Regurgitation

Etiology

Tricuspid regurgitation (TR) is classified as primary or secondary, the term "primary" indicating intrinsic valve pathology as the cause of TR while "secondary" indicates that right ventricular (RV) pressure or volume overload has caused RV dilatation in turn making a normal tricuspid valve leak. Secondary TR is far more common than primary disease. Etiologies for primary and secondary TR are listed below.

Etiology of Tricuspid Regurgitation

Primary Causes

1. Trauma
2. Ebstein's Anomaly
3. Congenital Tricuspid Hypoplasia
4. Infective Endocarditis
5. Carcinoid Syndrome
6. Serotonergic Drugs
7. Myxomatous Degeneration
8. Rheumatic Heart Disease
9. Device Leads
10. Mediastinal Irradiation

Secondary Causes

1. Left Heart Failure
2. Parenchymal Lung Disease
3. Pulmonary Vascular Disease
4. Pulmonary Embolism
5. Right Ventricular Infarction
6. Atrial Septal Defect
7. Ventricular Septal Defect
8. High Output States

Pathophysiology

The differences in function between the right and left ventricles are striking, especially because individual myocytes extracted from either ventricle are nearly identical in structure and function [1]. Volume overload appears better tolerated by the right versus left ventricle while the left ventricle better sustains a pressure overload. In the experimental animal where the tricuspid valve was removed leading to severe chronic RV volume overload and RV failure, myocytes taken from the failing RVs had normal contractile function [2]. These data suggest that it is the failing chamber rather than its contractile elements that caused RV failure in contrast to that mitral regurgitation where failure is due to myocyte dysfunction [3]. On the other hand in RV pressure overload, there is clear contractile element

B. A. Carabello (✉)
Cardiology Division, Brody School of Medicine, East Carolina University, Greenville, NC, USA

Department of Cardiovascular Sciences, Vidant Medical Center, Greenville, NC, USA
e-mail: carabellob16@ecu.edu

R. Nekkanti
Department of Cardiovascular Sciences, Vidant Medical Center, Greenville, NC, USA

B. A. Carabello (ed.), *Valvular Heart Disease*, Cardiovascular Medicine, https://doi.org/10.1007/978-1-4471-2840-3_9

dysfunction not present in compensated LV pressure overload [4, 5]. It presumably is the different geometry between the two ventricles and activation of neurohumoral systems that account for these differing responses.

When tricuspid regurgitation is primary, it imparts a volume overload on the RV, eventually leading to or exacerbating right heart failure. When TR is secondary, there is preexistent RV overload to which the TR adds an additional volume overload, perpetuating RV dilatation.

Right ventricular pressure overload. Because it is the RV that in part supplies the force that fills the left ventricle (LV), increased LV filling pressure stemming from left heart failure (requiring increased RV systolic pressure) is perhaps the most common cause of secondary TR. Mitral stenosis, pulmonary parenchymal disease, pulmonary vascular disease, pulmonary embolism, and uncorrected congenital lesions causing a left to right shunt also cause pulmonary hypertension, leading to TR.

Right ventricular volume overload. While secondary TR exacerbates RV volume overload, RV volume overload may cause TR. High output states such as pregnancy and anemia cause RV volume overload, as may intra- and extra-cardiac shunts.

Diagnosis: Assessing Etiology and Severity

Because most TR is secondary and because therapy will be aimed at treating the primary cause, a search is made for the etiology of the secondary TR. History, physical examination, and imaging studies examine for evidence of left heart failure, pulmonary embolism, intrinsic lung disease, or an intra- or extra-cardiac shunt. Or if primary TR is suspected, there should be a search for a history of trauma, rheumatic fever, congenital tricuspid valve disease, carcinoid syndrome, or the use of serotonergic drugs. A device lead crossing the tricuspid valve, causing TR, will be obvious from records, physical exam, and imaging.

Symptoms

If secondary to left heart failure or lung disease, dyspnea will already be a prominent symptom. However the onset of severe TR and attendant high right atrial pressure leads to the complaints of ascites, edema, anorexia, and if acute, right upper quadrant pain from stretch of the hepatic capsule.

Physical Examination

Unlike other valve diseases, TR may be first suspected not because of a heart murmur but rather by noting characteristic jugular venous pulsations. The neck veins are prominent with an accentuated v wave caused by systolic expansion of the right atrium due to regurgitant flow. This same hemodynamic phenomenon also causes systolic expansion of the liver (pulsatile liver) which when present is almost always due to severe TR. The murmur of TR is typically holosystolic and relatively soft, heard best along the right sternal border. While classically the murmur is said to increase with inspiration as more blood is drawn into the RV, this finding may be absent in right heart failure where the RV is already engorged and cannot receive more volume. Inspiratory augmentation of the murmur may also be blunted by the chest wall moving away from the examining stethoscope.

Imaging

Establishing Etiology. Echocardiography is the mainstay of diagnosis. Standard 2-D echocardiography gives a semiquantitative estimate of right atrial (RA) and right ventricular volumes while color flow provides an estimation of TR magnitude. Examination of the valve leaflets is made to determine if TR is due to primary valve pathology. For instance, Figs. 9.1 and 9.2 demonstrate impingement of the tricuspid

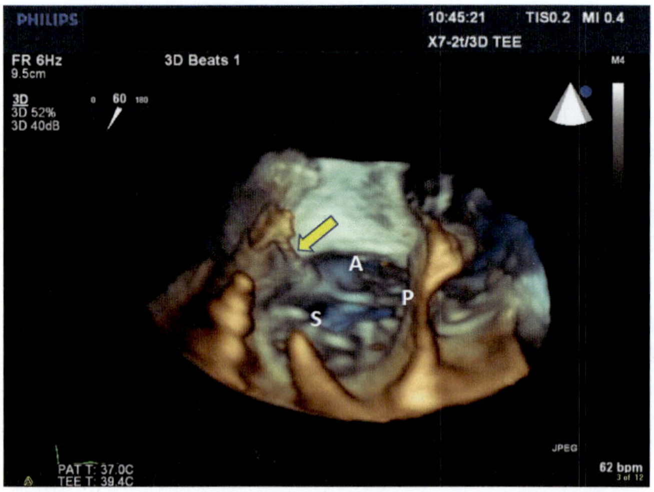

Fig. 9.1 3 D TEE of a patient demonstrating impingement of the anterior leaflet of the tricuspid valve (TV) by a defibrillator lead (arrow) as viewed from the atrial aspect (*A* anterior, *P* posterior, *S* septal)

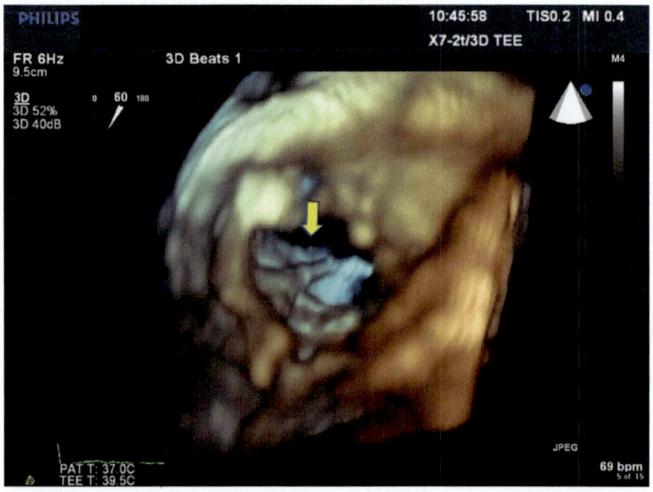

Fig. 9.2 3 D TEE of the same patient demonstrating impingement of the anterior leaflet of the TV by a defibrillator lead (arrow) as viewed from the ventricular aspect

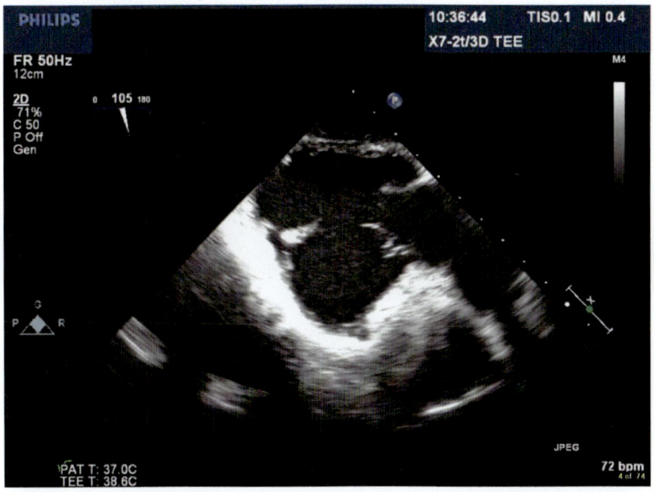

Fig. 9.3 2D TEE image of the TV from the gastric location. A case of functional tricuspid regurgitation where non-coaptation of the leaflets is noted setting the stage for very severe TR

valve by device leads. Figure 9.3 demonstrates the failure of leaflet coaptation due to RV dilatation in secondary TR.

RV Pressure Overload. The tricuspid regurgitant jet gives key information regarding RV pressure overload both as a cause of TR and also regarding general cardiac status. Central to this evaluation is an estimate of peak RV pressure in turn allowing for estimation of systolic pulmonary artery pressure (Fig. 9.4). Using the modified Bernoulli equation, the systolic trans-tricuspid pressure gradient (Δ_p) is estimated as $\Delta_p = 4V^2$, where V is the peak trans-tricuspid flow velocity. Right ventricular pressure is estimated as RVP + RAP. Thus if the peak jet velocity is 3.58 m/s and estimated RA pressure is 15 mmHg (Fig. 9.5), RVP = $4(3.58)^2 + 15 = 51 + 15$ or 66 mmHg. This determination helps establish whether pulmonary hypertension and its attendant etiologies are the cause of the patient's TR, or whether there is pure volume overload either from a primary or secondary cause. While pulmonary embolism is rarely a cause of severe TR, it often causes enough TR to estimate RV pressure. The constellation of sudden dyspnea or chest pain plus the echocardiographic findings of RV dysfunction and dilatation together with pulmonary hypertension raises the clinical suspicion of pulmonary embolus. It should

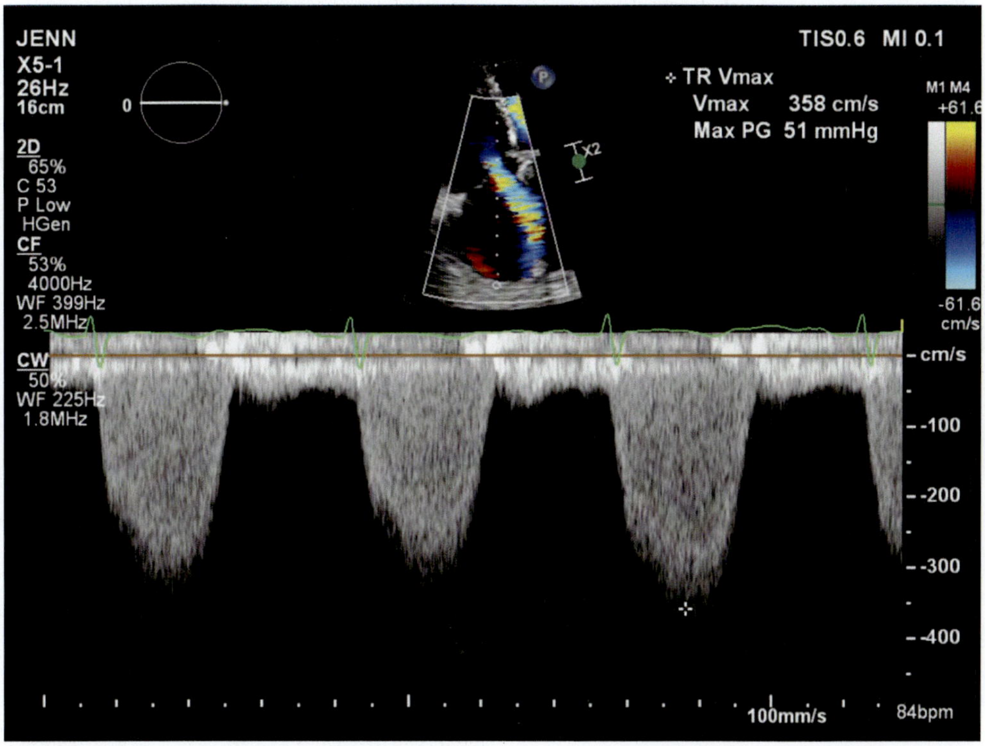

Fig. 9.4 Continuous wave Doppler of the tricuspid regurgitation jet yields a dense image which is parabolic in contour. The density of the signal is proportional to the amount of regurgitant flow into the right atrium. The right ventricular systolic pressure is estimated using TR jet velocity, employing the modified Bernoulli equation to estimate the pressure gradient between RV and RA and adding the RA pressure estimated from inferior vena cava dilatation (see Fig. 9.5). For example, as shown above the TR maximum velocity is estimated to be 3.58 m/s. Using the modified Bernoulli equation, as follows: Pressure gradient between RV and RA during systole = $4 \times (\text{TR peak velocity})^2 = 4 \times (3.58)^2 = 51$ mmHg. Assuming a RA pressure of 15 mmHg, the RVSP is estimated at 66 mmHg. Pitfalls: Density of the signal is dependent on technical factors such as "gain" settings. The intensity can be increased or decreased depending on how gain is used in the display and can therefore underestimate or overestimate the peak tricuspid regurgitation velocity, thus resulting in computation of lower or higher right ventricular systolic pressures

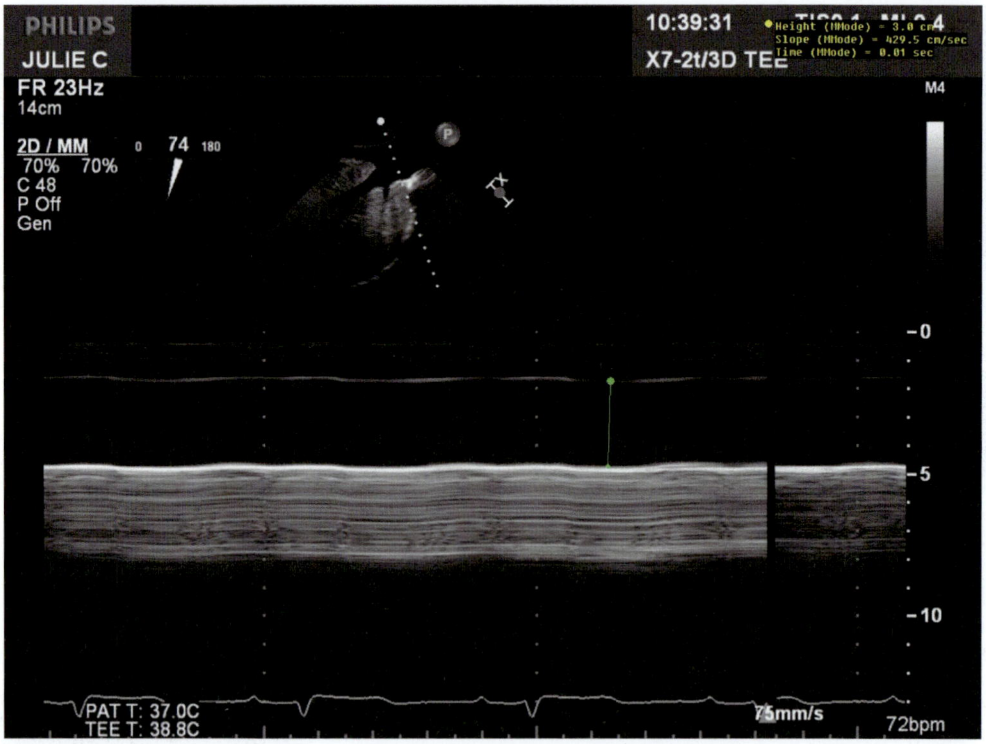

Fig. 9.5 Dilated IVC measuring at 3 cm using m-mode examination. There are respirophasic changes within the IVC. This suggests markedly elevated right atrial pressure

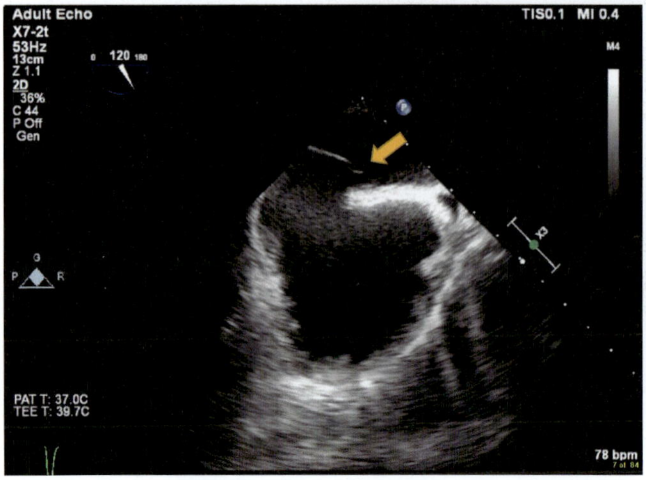

Fig. 9.6 A TEE image of a small atrial septal defect (arrow) is shown in the bicaval view

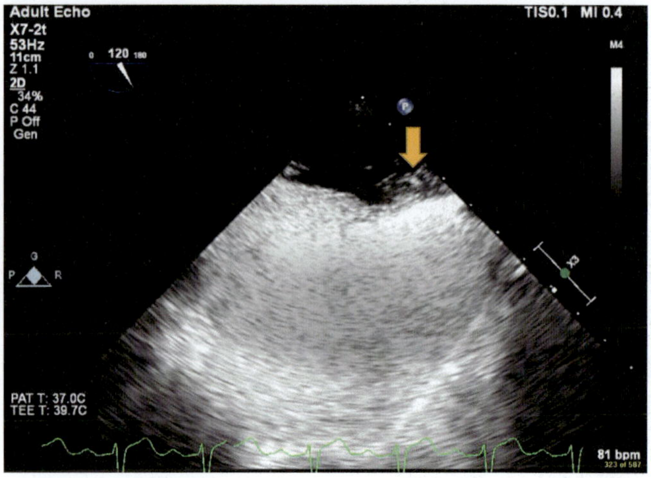

Fig. 9.7 A TEE image of agitated saline contrast bubbles crossing the shunt into the LA

be noted that the pulmonary hypertension due to an initial pulmonary embolus is not severe probably because the unhypertrophied RV is capable of generating a pressure of only about 50 mmHg [6].

If an atrial septal defect is suspected but not directly visualized, agitated saline is injected intravenously producing RA and RV contrast. A left to right shunt of un-contrasted blood produces a negative contrast at the site of the shunt (Figs. 9.6 and 9.7).

Assessment of TR severity. Assessment of TR severity is made from the size and penetration of the TR jet, the width of the vena contracta, the morphology of Doppler wave forms and reversal of flow in systemic veins. Figure 9.8 demonstrates measurement of the TR vena contracta, the size of the jet as it exits the regurgitant orifice. In general, the larger the orifice, the greater is the magnitude of TR. The morphology of the Doppler wave form provides additional information about TR severity (Fig. 9.9). In the case demonstrated a large regurgitant orifice produces severe TR despite low flow velocity. Indeed the orifice can be so wide as to produce laminar instead of turbulent flow (Fig. 9.10) and the jet velocity is low but dense in contour (Fig. 9.11).

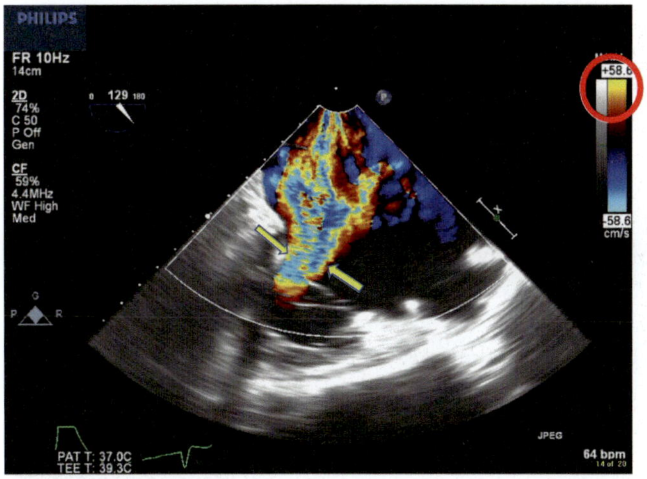

Fig. 9.8 Severe TR is demonstrated by color Doppler. The *vena contracta* measures 8 mm (arrows). Note the severely dilated right atrium. A vena contracta width greater than 7 mm signifies severe tricuspid regurgitation. The Nyquist limit (red circle) should be set between 50 and 70 cm/s. In this case the severe TR was caused by impingement of a defibrillator lead on the anterior leaflet of the tricuspid valve with severe restriction of leaflet movement. Pitfall: Strict vigilance is needed during imaging to optimize the color gain. One can increase or decrease the jet area by suboptimal color gain settings

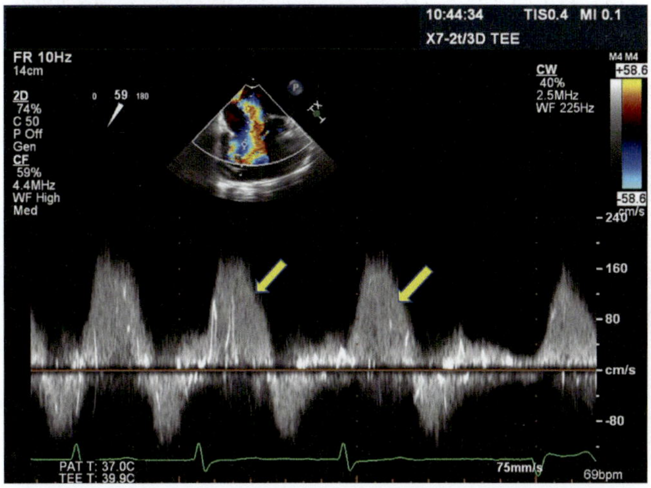

Fig. 9.9 Low velocity severe TR. Note the triangulated waveform of the TR jet (arrows) in the same patient shown in Fig. 9.8. Compare the density of the TR jet with the TV inflow which is of the same spectral density suggesting significant regurgitant flow. However, the jet velocity is low (<2 m/s). This suggests ventricularization of the RA pressure. In such instances, it is not possible to estimate RVSP. The TV inflow demonstrates an E velocity greater than 1 m/s (open arrow), which is another semiquantitative measure of severe TR

Reversal of flow into the great veins gives further evidence of severe TR (Figs. 9.12 and 9.13). While more quantitative measures such as PISA (proximal isovelocity surface area) may be employed, they have not gained the same acceptance as they have for mitral regurgitation. In accordance with the suspicion of severe TR, the RA and RV also

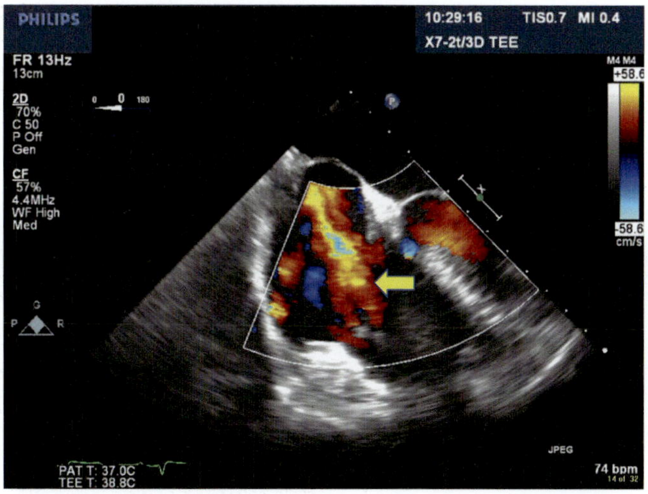

Fig. 9.10 Color Doppler examination of the tricuspid valve from an RV focused view in the mid-esophageal location. Notice the absence of any turbulent flow and that the regurgitant jet appears as laminar flow (arrow) which can sometimes be an interpreted as mild TR if a high degree of diagnostic suspicion for severe TR is not entertained

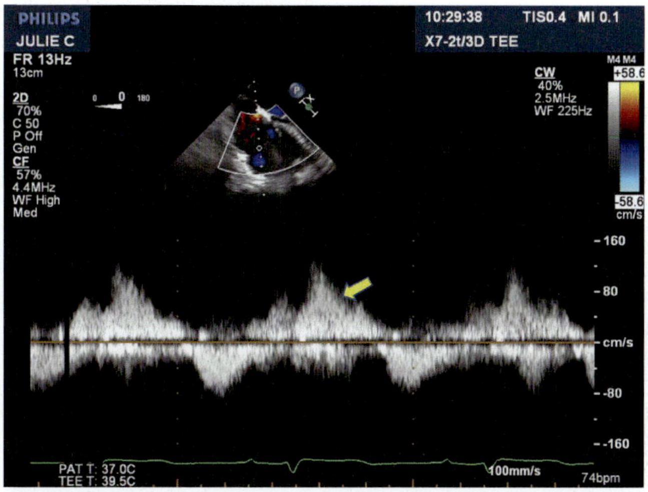

Fig. 9.11 Very low velocity but severe TR. A corresponding continuous wave Doppler examination from the patient shown in Fig. 9.10 demonstrates very low velocity but dense and triangulated envelope (arrow) consistent with very severe TR

should be enlarged. Although examination of the jugular venous pulse provides an accurate estimate of central venous pressure (CVP) in experienced hands, the pulsations may be difficult to see in some patients. In such cases echocardiographic findings of a dilated inferior vena cava indicates that CVP is elevated (Fig. 9.5).

Cardiac Catheterization

Echocardiography is clearly the main modality for diagnosing TR. However if the clinical presentation is such that catheterization is planned to resolve other clinical issues, right heart catheterization can add hemodynamic information supportive

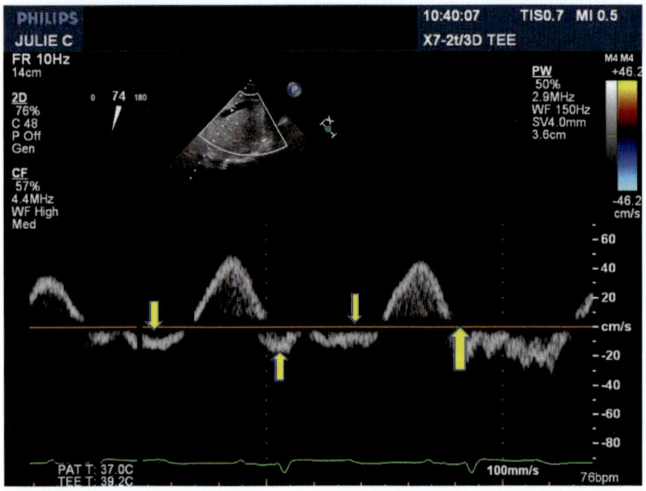

Fig. 9.12 Hepatic systolic flow reversal. In the same patient, there is systolic reversal in the hepatic veins on pulsed Doppler examination (solid downward arrows). Upward arrows indicate atrial systolic reversal which is normal. There is forward diastolic predominant flow following the reversed systolic flow

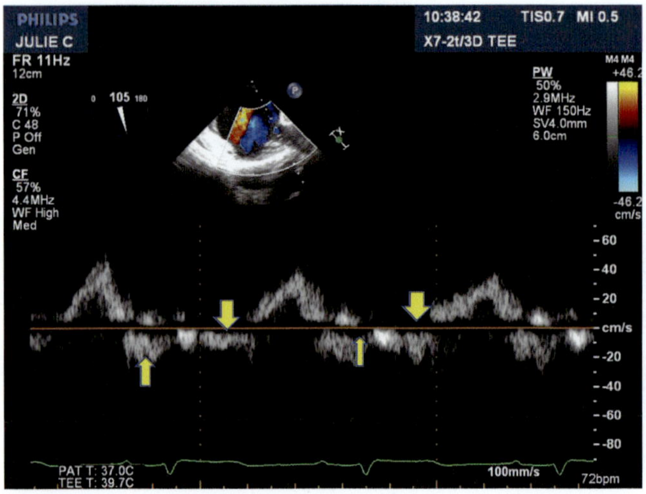

Fig. 9.13 Systolic flow reversal in the Superior Vena Cava. In the same patient, there is systolic reversal in the SVC on pulsed Doppler examination (solid downward arrows). Upward arrows indicate atrial systolic reversal which is normal. There is forward diastolic predominant flow following the reversed systolic flow

of the diagnosis of severe TR. Right atrial pressure is elevated and the tracing demonstrates a large v wave. In very severe cases, the atrial pressure becomes ventricularized, whereby the right atrial tracing appears more like an RV tracing as RA and RV nearly become one continuous chamber. It should be noted that thermodilution determination of cardiac output is unreliable in the face of severe TR.

Assessing RV Function. Unlike for mitral and aortic regurgitation, there are no well-recognized benchmarks signifying that RV dysfunction is developing that might in turn trigger therapeutic intervention. The difficult geometry of the RV further complicates estimation of RV volume and function and RV ejection fraction is not routinely reported. A common estimation of RV function is made by measuring tricuspid annular plane systolic excursion (TAPSE) [7] although its role in assessing RV function in the presence of TR is uncertain. The premise of TAPSE is that it measures RV long axis shortening and thus measures contraction in that plane. Right ventricular strain has also been employed to assess RV systolic function [8]. However both TAPSE and strain are load dependent and thus affected by TR alterations in both preload and afterload. Correction of primary severe TR is recommended when there is "progressive deterioration in RV function or progressive RV dilatation" but specific numeric cutoffs for when these conditions exist are not uniformly agreed upon. Accurate assessment of changes in RV volume and function over time is accurately made with cardiac MRI.

Therapy

For most cases of secondary TR, standard therapy is treatment of the left heart or lung disease responsible for causing the TR. Thus the treatment of left heart failure reduces LV filling pressure, in turn reducing pulmonary artery pressure, reducing RV size, and improving TR. Likewise improving lung function and oxygenation in a patient with lung disease reduces pulmonary vascular resistance, in turn reducing pulmonary artery and RV pressure, thus reducing RV size, improving secondary TR. In the case of pulmonary vascular hypertension, pulmonary vasodilators may reduce pulmonary hypertension, thereby reducing RV volume, partially restoring tricuspid competence.

Secondary TR and Left-Sided Valvular Heart Disease

An exception to the strategy for treating secondary TR by treating its primary cause is when TR is caused by the consequences of severe left-sided valvular heart disease (VHD), especially mitral regurgitation. While it is reasonable to expect that mechanical correction of left-sided VHD (valvotomy, valve repair or valve replacement) would improve secondary TR, such improvement does not always occur and is difficult to predict [9–11]. In cases where TR does not improve or even worsens following successful mitral or aortic valve surgery, the patient may then suffer from right heart failure due to TR, raising the prospect of a second heart operation to address the TR. In small reported series, such operations have led to unexpectedly-high mortality [12, 13]. While percutaneous methods are being developed to address this problem [14–16], long-term assessment of those solutions is not yet available. In most cases, **severe** TR, whether primary or secondary, will be addressed with tricuspid valve repair, usually employing a ring annuloplasty, at the time of left-sided valve surgery. More difficult is the decision to operate on **mild or moderate** secondary TR because it is uncertain whether tricuspid repair is beneficial or not.

Impact of Secondary TR on Outcome

Nath et al. have demonstrated that the presence of TR negatively affects prognosis (Figs. 9.14 and 9.15) even in patients with normal pulmonary artery pressure and normal LV ejection fraction (EF) [17], supporting TR intervention at the time of left-sided valve surgery. As noted above, it is often hoped that correction of left-sided lesions will reduce LV filling pressure, simultaneously decreasing pulmonary artery pressure, thereby relieving TR without direct TR surgery. Unfortunately existing data are confusing and lead to no definitive course of management. Yilmaz et al. found that in nearly 700 mitral repairs of primary mitral regurgitation (MR), TR untreated at the time of surgery rarely progressed and only 1 patient required re-operation at follow-up

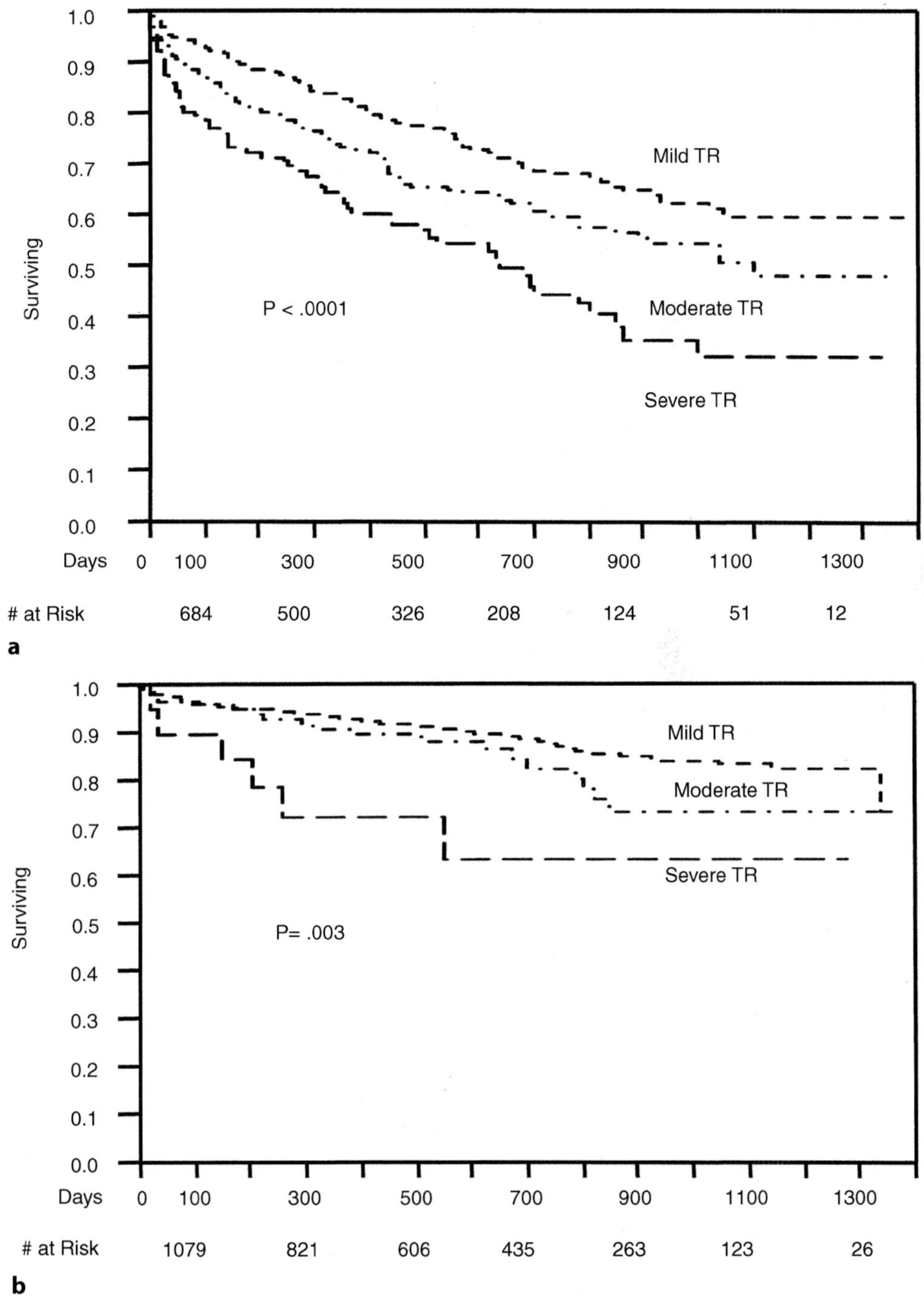

Fig. 9.14 Progressively worse TR negatively impacts prognosis both in patients with pulmonary hypertension (panel **a**) and without (panel **b**) pulmonary hypertension. From Nath J, et al. [17]. Reprinted with permission from Elsevier

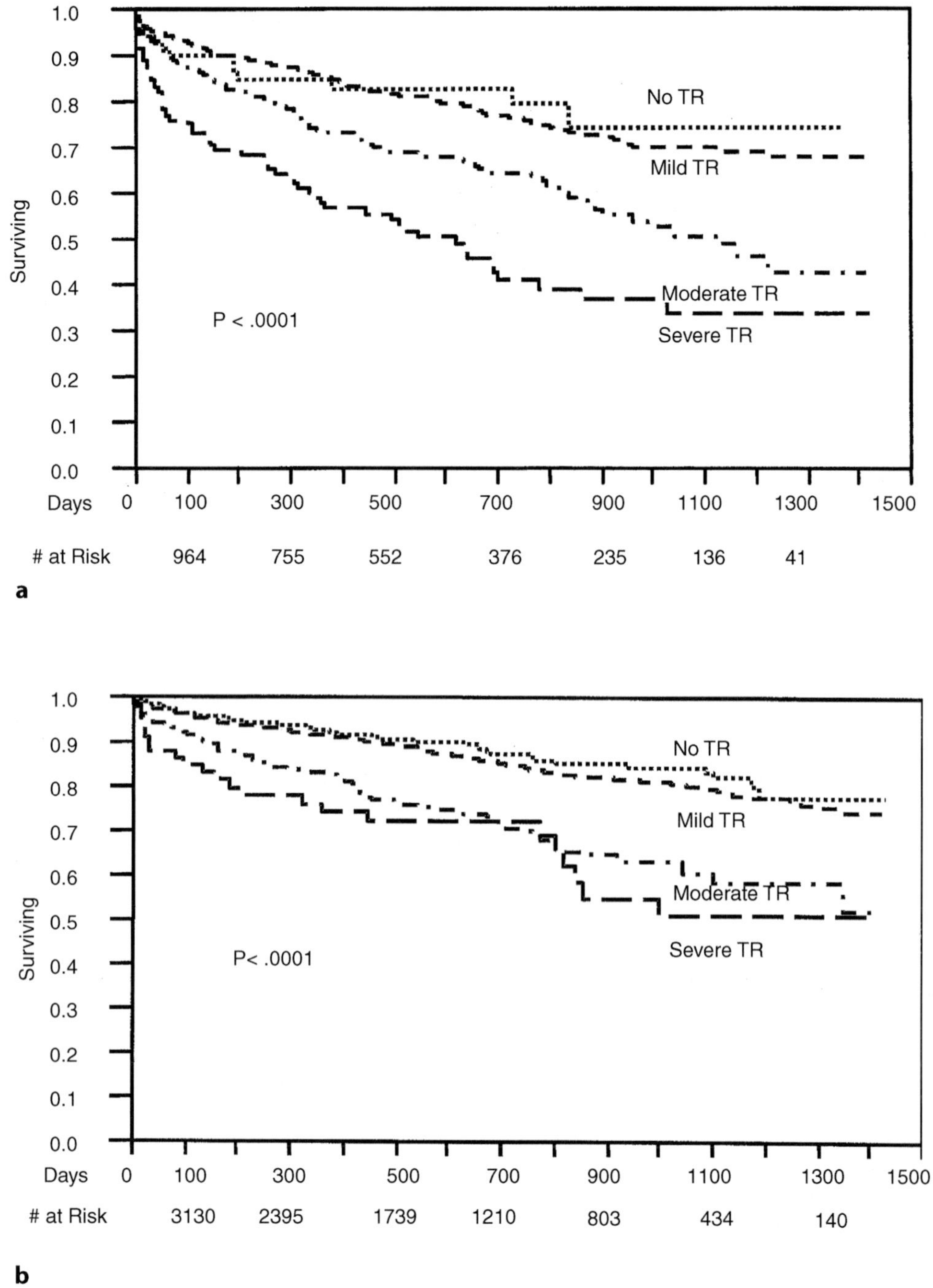

Fig. 9.15 Progressively worse TR negatively impacts prognosis both in patients with low left ventricular ejection (LVEF) (panel **a**) and with normal LVEF (panel **b**). From Nath J, et al. [17]. Reprinted with permission from Elsevier

[18]. Thus they have encouraged a conservative approach to treating TR during mitral surgery. At the other end of the spectrum, Dreyfus and colleagues have espoused tricuspid annuloplasty during mitral surgery even in the absence of TR if tricuspid annular dimension exceeded 70 mm [19] (at surgery) while Mahesh et al. have suggested the same strategy for an annular dimension >21 mm/m^2 at preoperative echocardiography [20]. This aggressive approach is supported by Kwak et al. who found that 27% of patients with no TR at the time of left-sided surgery developed moderate or severe TR within 5 years following operation, especially if atrial fibrillation occurred [10]. Several other authors also found progression or the new occurrence of TR in 14–50% of patients with untreated tricuspid valves at the time of mitral surgery [21–23].

When left unattended, existing TR often improves initially after left-sided surgery but then worsens over time (Fig. 9.16) [9]. Virtually all studies are concordant in demonstrating reduced TR when the tricuspid valve is repaired at the time of left-sided surgery [13, 24–29]. Most also found improved RV remodeling post tricuspid repair [26–29]. In addition, tricuspid surgery has reduced the incidence of

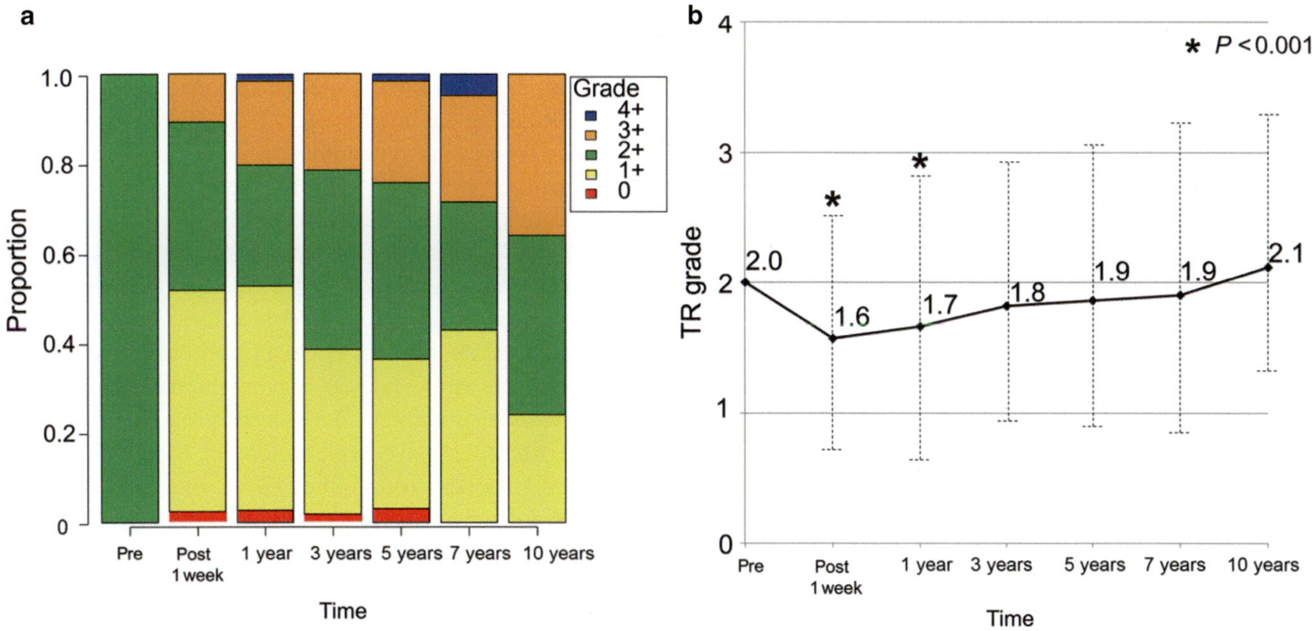

Fig. 9.16 The course of moderate TR after left-sided surgery is shown over time, color coded by grade (left) and by numerical grade (right). After initial improvement, many patients suffer gradual worsening. Kusajima K, et al. [9]. Reprinted with permission from Oxford University Press

Table 9.1 Studies of functional tricuspid regurgitation

Ref #	*N*	Background	Intervention	Result
[9]	96	MVS	None	Initial TR DEC then INC
[10]	335	MVS, AVS	None	26% with no I-TR developed 2–4+ TR in 5 years
[11]	165	MVS	None	88% vs. 46% 5 year survival 0,1+ TR vs. ≥2+ TR
[18]	699	MVS	None	Initial TR DEC then INC 1 pt needed TR Surg
[19]	311	MVS	None vs. TVR	Mortality same but NYHA better with TVR
[22]	174	MVS	None	16% with 1 = 2+ ITR became severe in 8 years
[24]	110	MVS	No TVR vs. TVR	Adjusted survival 45% no TVR vs. 75% TVR
[25]	225	MVS	No TVR vs. TVR	93% <2+ TR in TVR vs. 61% for no TVR at 4 years
[26]	645	MVS	No TVR vs. TVR	TVR predicted recovery of RV function
[27]	624	MVS	No TVR vs. TVR	TVR decreased TR and HF but not mortality
[28]	44	MVS	R_{nd} no TVR vs. TVR	2–4+ TR in 28% vs. 0% no TVR vs. TVR

AVS Aortic Valve Surgery, *DEC* Decrease, *HF* Heart Failure, *I* Initial, *INC* Increase, *MVS* Mitral Valve Surgery, R_{nd} Randomized Trial, *TR* Tricuspid Regurgitation, *TVR* Tricuspid Valve Repair

heart failure or improved functional capacity in some studies [27, 29]. No study has demonstrated that correction of mild-to-moderate TR during mitral or aortic surgery prolongs life, indeed most found no change in survival with tricuspid repair [13, 25–27] although mortality adjusted for comorbidities was improved in at least one study [24]. Most recently David et al. found that TR was relatively rare at the time of mitral surgery [30]. While TR was associated with a worse survival outcome, poor prognosis was due more to cofactors associated with TR (age, atrial fibrillation, poor LV function, etc.), than the TR itself. Probably because of these comorbidities, treatment of TR at the time of mitral surgery did not ameliorate the negative impact of preoperative TR on outcome [30].

In summary, virtually all studies demonstrate that tricuspid repair reduces the risk of TR progression following surgery. Some reports also demonstrate objective clinical improvement with less heart failure, faster return of RV function toward normal and better exercise capacity when tricuspid repair accompanied left-sided valve surgery. Whether treating TR at the time of left-sided surgery improves survival is uncertain. Because repeat heart surgery to correct residual symptomatic severe TR carries substantial risk, most surgeons prefer to address more than mild TR with tricuspid repair during left-sided valve surgery and thus surgical tricuspid interventions have increased in frequency over the past decade [31]. Several studies of TR progression are summarized in Table 9.1.

Primary Tricuspid Regurgitation

Usual causes of primary TR include deceleration injuries from motor vehicle accidents, penetrating chest wounds, interference from pacemaker leads, infective endocarditis, accidental damage during RV biopsy, and the carcinoid syndrome or use of serotonergic-like drugs (see Etiology of Tricuspid Regurgitation box above).

Diuretics form Initial therapy for primary TR in an attempt to lower right atrial pressure and relieve venous congestion but are only modestly effective in severe primary TR. The best mechanical therapy for isolated TR is uncertain and specific indications for valve repair or replacement have not been developed. As noted above, the presence of severe TR impairs prognosis so it would seem reasonable to eliminate it surgically. Using knowledge gained from left-sided VHD, it would also seem wise to operate before RV dysfunction has occurred. However unlike in left-sided VHD where data strongly indicate improved survival after timely surgery, there is no evidence that mechanical management of primary TR improves outcomes, primarily because no trials exist to assess it. Further there are no agreed-upon triggers for TR surgery (ejection fraction, RV volumes, etc.) that separate good from bad postoperative outcomes. Lack of such triggers stems from difficulties in assessing RV volumes echocardiographically. Thus in the current AHA/ACC Guidelines the only class I indication for mechanical therapy is to treat severe TR during left-sided surgery [32]. There is a class IIa indication for treating symptomatic severe TR with repair or replacement (Fig. 9.17) [32]. Valve repair is preferred over replacement by consensus with some supportive data [33] but unlike with mitral regurgitation where repair is clearly superior to replacement, the data for TR are much less robust. Of note when TR was caused by infective endocarditis in those who used intravenous drugs, in some cases the tricuspid valve was entirely excised, leaving the patient with torrential TR which was tolerated for several years but eventually required tricuspid valve replacement in a minority who developed intractable heart failure [34].

When outcomes from tricuspid valve replacement with bioprostheses were compared to those of mechanical valves in a meta-analysis, only the usual differences were noted. Structural valve deterioration was more common with bioprostheses while thromboembolic/hemorrhagic complications were more common with mechanical valves [35]. In cases of carcinoid disease, tricuspid surgery improves symptoms but outcome is primarily driven by the carcinoid tumor and not the valve disease [36].

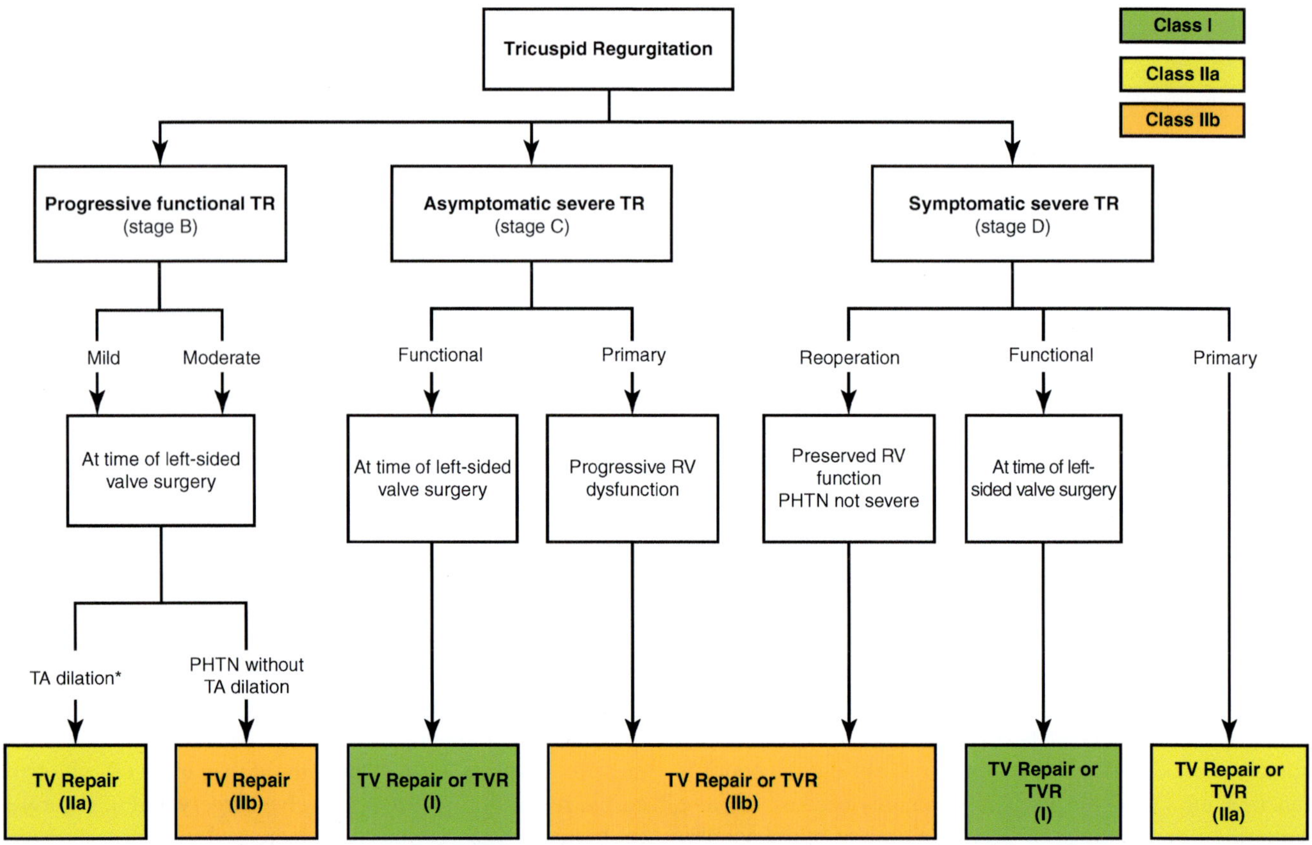

Fig. 9.17 The algorithm from ACC/AHA Guidelines for management of TR is presented. The only class 1 indication for the surgical treatment of TR is to address it at the time of left-sided surgery. From Nishimura RA, et al. [32]. Reprinted with permission from Wolters Kluwer Health, Inc.

Tricuspid Stenosis

Etiology and Symptoms
In adults worldwide the most common cause of tricuspid stenosis (TS) is rheumatic heart disease but even in rheumatic endemic areas TS is relatively rare, affecting only about 3–9% of patients. In developed countries where rheumatic heart disease is rare, TS is even rarer. In some cases TS is iatrogenic occurring when correction of TR with small valve protheses or small annuloplasty rings cause functional TS.

The symptoms of TS are primarily caused by right atrial (RA) and systemic venous hypertension; even a trans-tricuspid valve gradient of 5 mmHg results in an RA pressure of 10–12 mmHg, enough to cause right-sided congestion, ascites, and edema. Because gradient increases with the square of the cardiac output, exercise may cause very high RA pressure. Severe TS results in reduced cardiac output and fatigue.

Physical Examination
Although the typical murmur of TS is a diastolic rumble, accentuated by inspiration, the relatively low right-sided pressures reduce murmur intensity such that it may be very soft. Concomitant TR may add a systolic murmur to the exam. The neck veins are elevated with a prominent a wave and blunted y descent.

Diagnostic Imaging
As with all valve disease, imaging is the mainstay of diagnosis. However, the tricuspid valve is more difficult to image than the mitral valve and special care must be taken to obtain all views and to calculate the trans-tricuspid gradient.

Cardiac Catheterization
Because the gradient across the tricuspid valve is usually likely small, yet significant, invasive hemodynamics at rest and during exercise can be illuminating. A double lumen pigtail catheter with one lumen residing in the right atrium and the other in the RV measures the pressure difference across the valve. Obtaining cardiac output allows for valve area calculation; however there is no accepted categorization of TS severity according to valve area.

Therapy
Therapy is directed at treating symptoms. Mild symptoms are treated with diuretics. Severe TS is treated surgically at the time of left-sided valve operations because isolated TS as the most clinically important valve lesion is exceedingly rare. Valve repair, when possible, is preferred to valve replacement. While balloon valvotomy may be attempted in cases too high risk for surgery [37], most patients with TS also have a significant element of TR which may worsen following this procedure, making it less effective for treating TS than for treating mitral stenosis. However no large studies with long-term follow-up have been reported.

Pulmonic Valve Disease

Pulmonic Stenosis

Etiology and Symptoms
Most cases of pulmonic stenosis (PS) are due to congenital fusion of the valve leaflets and are addressed by balloon valvotomy in childhood. Occasionally PS patients are identified for the first time during adulthood. Most PS patients are asymptomatic. However severe PS may cause dyspnea on exertion, fatigue, and chest pain. Overt right-sided heart failure causing ascites and edema is rare. Unlike aortic stenosis where the calcific lesion progresses over time, the leaflets in PS usually remain thin and pliable and severity is typically static (once patients reach adulthood) and stenosis progression is unusual.

Physical Examination
Pulmonic stenosis is often recognized from the typical systolic ejection murmur heard in the pulmonic area, sometimes increasing with inspiration. The murmur is often preceded by an ejection click as the thin but fused leaflets dome in early systole. The click typically lessens in intensity or disappears during inspiration as inspiration alone may cause diastolic pulmonary blood flow, doming the valve before ventricular systole, reducing or obliterating the click. In severe disease the ejection click is usually lost. Severe PS is accompanied by right ventricular (RV) hypertrophy causing an RV lift. The jugular venous pulse displays a prominent a wave and neck vein distension accompanies RV failure. The second heart sound is widely split as pressure overload prolongs RV systole. S2 splitting widens with inspiration.

The severity of PS is usually gauged by peak gradient because it is on this parameter that outcomes have been correlated. Symptom-free survival worsens when the peak gradient exceeds 50 mmHg (Fig. 9.18) [38].

Imaging
Echocardiography demonstrates doming of the valve in systole (Fig. 9.19). Doppler interrogation determines jet velocity from which the transvalvular gradient is obtained (Fig. 9.20). Echocardiography may also reveal downstream pulmonary artery stenosis (Fig. 9.21) that can be further evaluated by cardiac CT and or MRI.

Management
Conservative management is indicated for less-than-severe **asymptomatic** PS. Balloon valvotomy is indicated for severe asymptomatic disease (peak gradient ≥50 mmHg) or for borderline **symptomatic** disease since prognosis worsens when gradient exceeds 50 mmHg (Fig. 9.18). Because valvotomy often damages the valve at the time of the procedure, its most serious sequela is creation of pulmonary regurgitation (PR).

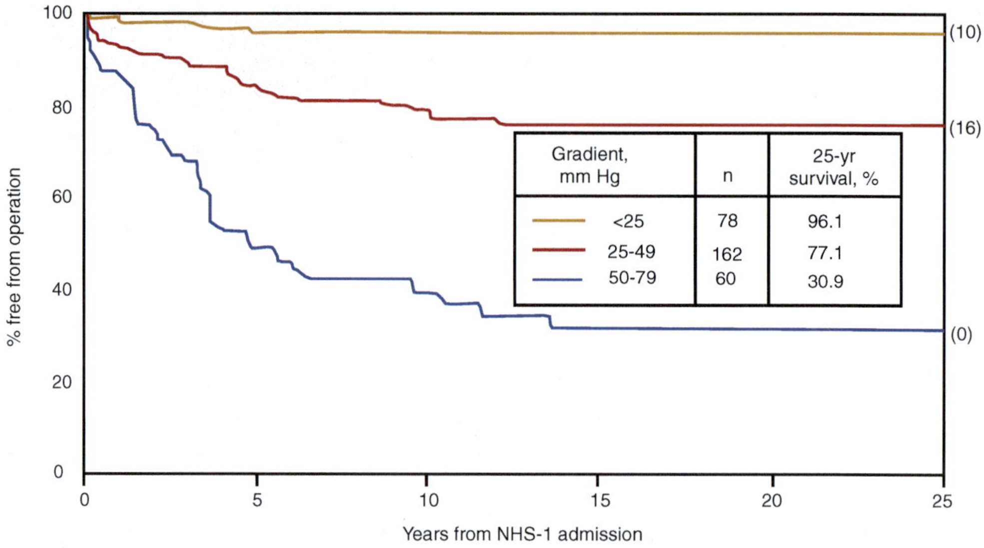

Fig. 9.18 The outcome of pulmonic stenosis patients treated medically is plotted against pulmonic valve gradient. A marked increase in mortality occurs when gradient exceeds 50 mmHg. From Hayes CJ, et al. [38]. Reprinted with permission from Wolters Kluwer Health, Inc.

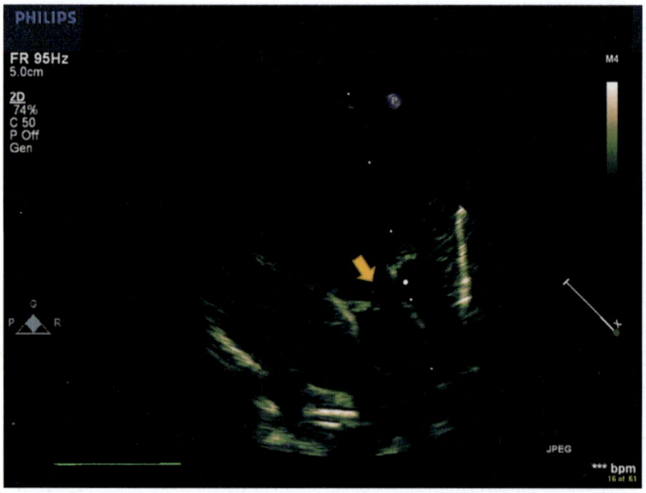

Fig. 9.19 Systolic doming (arrow) of the PV is demonstrated. *PA* pulmonary artery

In a recent study, 60% of patients had more than moderate PR 10 years following balloon pulmonary valvotomy but only 3% of patients required pulmonary valve replacement [39].

Pulmonic Regurgitation

Etiology

Trivial pulmonic regurgitation (PR) is present in most normal subjects. However most clinically important primary PR occurs secondary to previous correction of congenital heart disease, either from balloon valvotomy [39] for PS or from failure of valved conduits used to treat a variety of congenital conditions, most often tetralogy of Fallot. Occasionally primary PR is caused by carcinoid syndrome or rheumatic heart disease. In other cases, PR is secondary to severe pulmonary hypertension (PHTN). In general PR is well tolerated, owing to the low resistance of the pulmonary circuit. Blood pumped forward during systole continues on its normal path through the pulmonary bed eventually into the left heart from where it is not regurgitated back into the pulmonary circuit. Thus regurgitant fraction in severe PR is rarely >40%, whereas in severe left-sided regurgitation, regurgitant fraction usually exceeds 50%.

Symptoms and Physical Examination

Most patients with PR are asymptomatic. When symptoms develop in severe PR, they usually consist of dyspnea on exertion and fatigue and may occasionally include those of RV failure, ascites, and edema. The murmur of PR is a high pitched diastolic blowing sound heard best in the pulmonic area. In severe PR with RV enlargement an RV lift is usually palpated.

Imaging

Echocardiography is usually adequate to detect and assess the severity of PR semiquantitatively. However, echocardiography does not visualize the RV well, a deficit because progressive RV enlargement and reduction in RV ejection fraction may be indicators for pulmonic valve replacement (PVR). Currently cardiac magnetic resonance imaging is the most precise method for assessing RV volumes and function [40].

Management

Mild-to-moderate PR is well tolerated and is managed conservatively. If PR is secondary to pulmonary hypertension, the conditions causing it are addressed to reduce pulmonary pressure, in turn reducing PR. When severe PR has caused symptoms or a progressive decline in RV function or increased RV size, mechanical treatment is indicated [41–43]. While the presence of severe PR impairs prognosis (Fig. 9.22) [41], the exact triggers for intervention in terms of RV volume or ejection fraction have not been delineated.

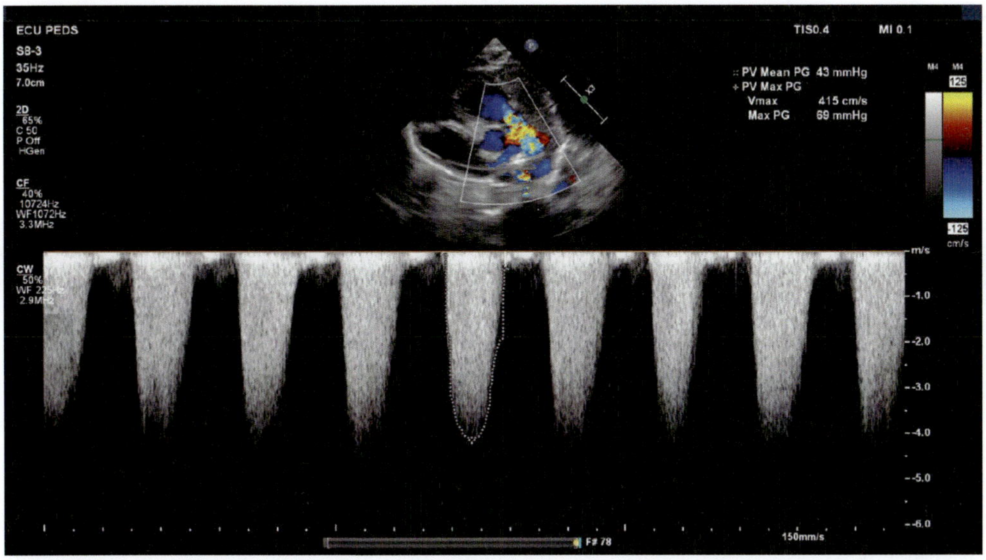

Fig. 9.20 Spectral waveforms with continuous wave Doppler demonstrating a peak flow velocity of 4.15 m/s with an estimated gradient of 60 mmHg between the right ventricle and the pulmonary artery

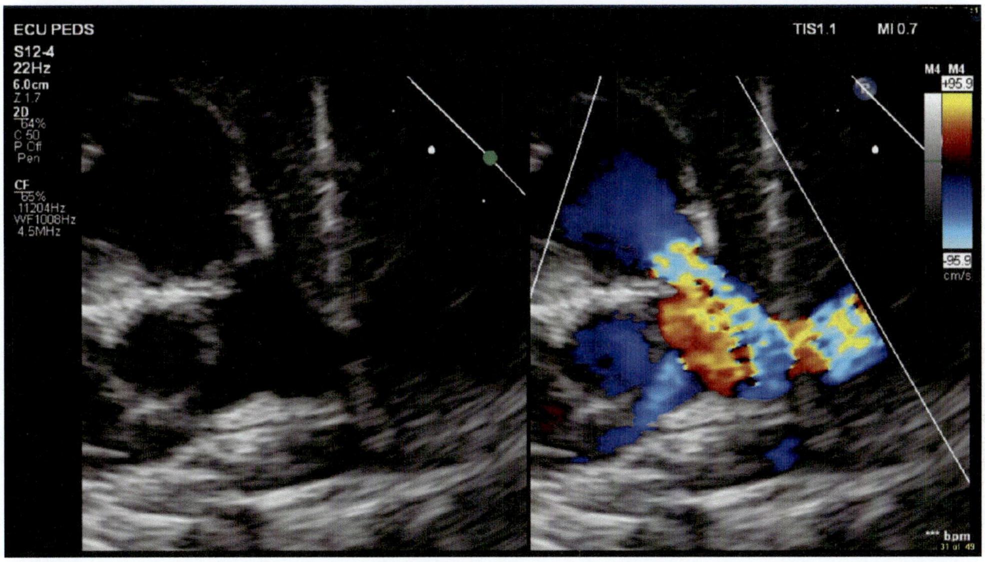

Fig. 9.21 Color Doppler flow mapping demonstrating turbulent flow across the pulmonary valve and the pulmonary artery and its branches raising the question of downstream pulmonary artery stenosis

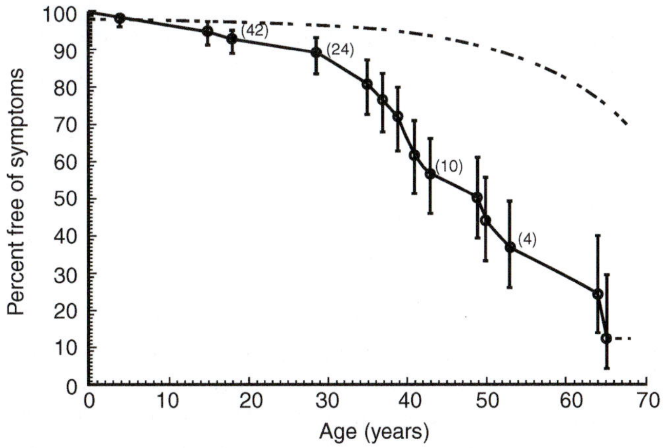

Fig. 9.22 Life expectancy for patients with severe PR (solid line) is compared to normal life expectancy. From Bouzas B, et al. [41]. Reprinted with permission from Oxford University Press

Surgical pulmonary valve replacement is the gold standard of care. If a failed pulmonary conduit is the cause of the PR it can be treated with percutaneous valve replacement with a stented tissue valve (Melody). Recently the Edwards SAPIEN valve has also been approved for this use. Off label use of larger percutaneous aortic valves has also been attempted [44].

Mixed Valve Disease

Aortic Stenosis and Mitral Regurgitation

Aortic stenosis (AS) in the developed world is usually due to calcific atherosclerotic disease and usually occurs in isolation. However it is sometimes accompanied by mitral regurgitation which is usually secondary to ventricular remodeling but is occasionally due to concomitant mitral leaflet pathology. Normally the pressure overload of AS results in concentric hypertrophy or concentric remodeling with small LV volumes and a competent mitral valve. However in far-advanced AS there may be LV dilatation and papillary muscle displacement leading to secondary MR. Therefore secondary MR represents advanced disease and not surprisingly is associated with a worse prognosis compared to isolated AS [45].

It is often hoped that relief of the pressure overload of AS by aortic valve replacement (AVR) will allow for improvement in secondary MR both because the LV may undergo reverse remodeling and because the pressure driving flow backwards across the mitral valve will be reduced. Unfortunately the fate of secondary MR following both surgical and transcatheter AVR (SAVR, TAVR) is unpredictable as is its effects on outcome. MR does often improve following AVR but sometimes it does not. Several studies have found no impact of untreated secondary MR at the time of AVR [46–48] while another found the opposite [49]. However the unpredictability of the course of untreated secondary MR following TAVR is obvious and well summarized by Nombela-Franco [48, 50–73] in Fig. 9.23. During surgical AVR the surgeon has the opportunity to address persistent MR with mitral annuloplasty and/or mitral valve repair, techniques obviously not apt for TAVR. While it is clear that primary MR often does not improve following AVR because there are intrinsic mitral anatomic lesions [48], why secondary MR fails to improve in some cases is not well understood but atrial fibrillation and low transvalvular aortic gradient are predictive of failure. Persistent atrial fibrillation may cause atrial remodeling perpetuating annular dilatation and MR. A low initial aortic gradient means less of a decrease in LV pressure driving MR after outflow obstruction is relieved. Further, low aortic gradient AS is usually due to LV dysfunction that may persist post AVR, perpetuating secondary MR. Finally relief of AS may allow for increased cardiac output, increasing the volume pumped by the LV, engendering a relative volume overload that might cause MR to persist. This conundrum is most important for patients who can undergo either SAVR or TAVR since SAVR offers a direct approach to MR that TAVR does not. On the other hand while favorable hemodynamic changes might reduce primary MR following AVR, the persisting mitral anatomic lesions are likely to worsen over time so that primary MR should be addressed surgically unless the patient is inoperable and TAVR is the only option.

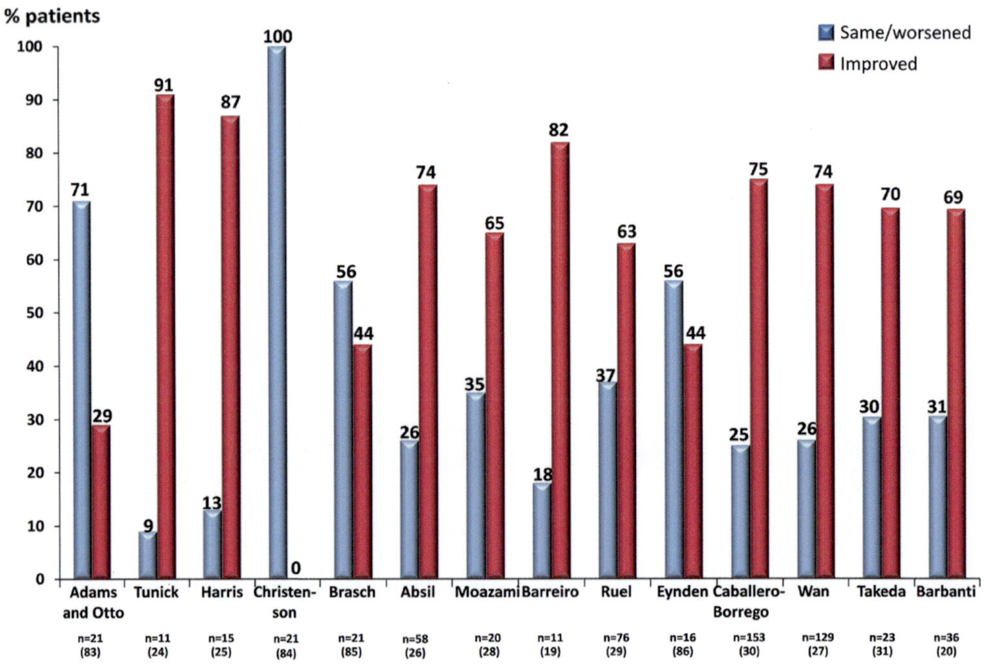

Fig. 9.23 The percentages of patients with MR whose MR improved (red bars) or remained unchanged or worsened following TAVR (blue bars). From Nombela-Franco L, et al. [50]. Reprinted with permission from Elsevier

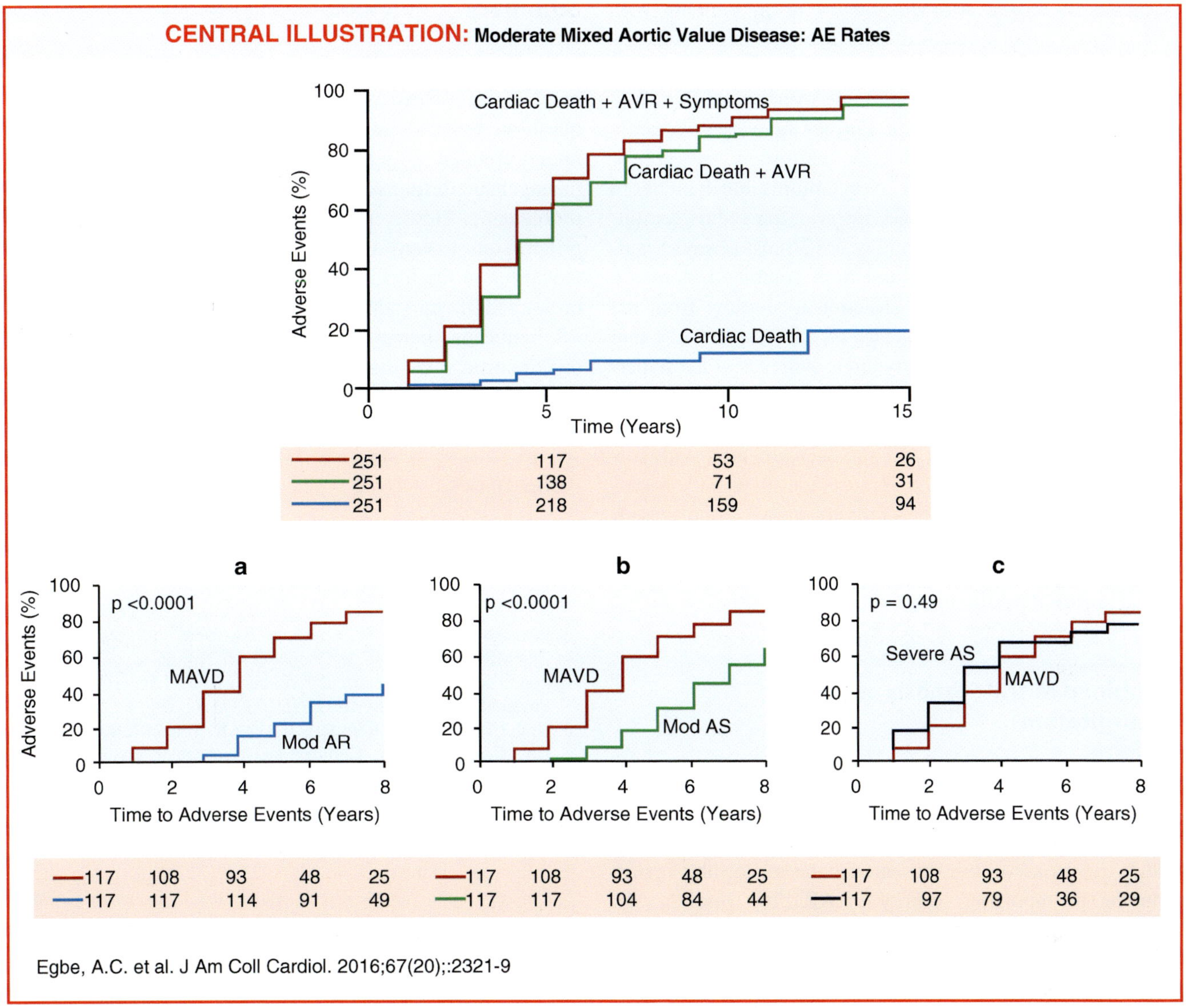

Fig. 9.24 Adverse events for patients with mixed AS/AR are shown in the upper panel. In the lower panel the natural history of mixed aortic disease follows the natural history of pure AS. *MAVD* mixed aortic valve disease, *AS* aortic stenosis, *AVR* aortic valve repalcement. From Egbe AC, et al. [75]. Reprinted with permission from Elsevier

Mixed Aortic Valve Disease

In most cases of mixed aortic valve disease, one lesion, either aortic stenosis (AS) or aortic regurgitation (AR) dominates and the patient's LV usually behaves accordingly. Thus when there is predominate AS, the LV remodels concentrically while predominate AR leads to LV dilatation and eccentric remodeling. Most perplexing to clinician is the combination of moderate AS and moderate AR, especially when the patient is symptomatic. In this case neither lesion by itself would be severe enough to warrant intervention while the combined lesion might create enough hemodynamic disturbance for the patient to benefit from valve replacement. The topic has been addressed recently and the data seem consistent. Combined AS/AR behaves primarily like isolated AS (Fig. 9.24) [74, 75]. Aortic regurgitation requires increased total stroke volume to make up for that lost by backward flow. Increased total stroke volume increases the systolic aortic pressure gradient thereby increasing the total systolic LV pressure, imposing primarily a pressure overload on the LV, mimicking pure AS. Thus the presence of symptoms and a peak transvalvular jet velocity of 4 m/s or a mean gradient of 40 mmHg should trigger AVR even if the AVA > 1.0 cm^2.

Mixed Mitral Disease

The presence of mixed mitral stenosis (MS) and MR occurs almost always in patients with rheumatic valve disease.

Occasionally mixed MS/MR can occur in patients with severe mitral annular calcification. Asymptomatic mixed disease rarely requires therapy since the copresence of MS protects the LV from the severe volume overload of pure MR that can lead to LV dysfunction. Further there are no specific objective findings in mixed disease that form a "trigger" for valve intervention. However if symptoms attributable to mixed mitral disease do occur, intervention seems reasonable. When symptoms occur, they are almost always resultant from increased LA pressure from combined increased LA inflow from MR and obstruction to outflow from the LA. Echocardiographic evidence of an enlarged LA and invasive or noninvasive hemodynamic evidence of LA hypertension either at rest or, if necessary, during exercise suggests a valvular basis for the patient's symptoms. Because the presence of significant MR precludes therapy with balloon valvotomy, mitral valve replacement is usually necessary if therapy with diuretics fails to relieve symptoms. It should be noted that neither guidelines for the management of mitral stenosis or mitral regurgitation are necessarily helpful in combined disease.

Combined Mitral Stenosis and Aortic Regurgitation

Combined MS and AR result from rheumatic heart disease. When they occur concomitantly, MS is usually the more severe lesion. However because MS limits LV filling, it may reduce the stroke volume presented to the aortic valve in turn reducing the apparent severity of AR [76]. Further, MS reduces LV cavity size for any degree of AR causing further potential underestimating of AR severity. It is in this regard that contrast aortography that visualizes AR flow instead of the echocardiographic visualization of AR velocity of flow may be helpful as is precise assessment of AR regurgitant fraction.

Mechanical intervention is indicated for symptomatic disease not easily controlled by diuretics. If mitral anatomy is favorable, balloon valvotomy should be employed to treat the MS followed by SAVR or TAVR, in this way avoiding the increased mortality of double valve replacement [77].

Aortic and Mitral Stenosis

Almost always the product of rheumatic heart disease, this combination can be very confusing to the clinician. When either lesion is severe, it may limit cardiac output, resulting in reduced flow to the other valve, reducing transvalvular gradient, leading to underestimation of lesion severity.

Summary

Key advances are emerging in the understanding and treatment of right-sided and mixed valvular lesions yet many questions remain unanswered. Persistent or worsening TR after left-sided surgery reduces quality of life but proper management during surgery for less-than-severe TR remains problematic. However in the surgical community there is progression toward treating TR at the time of surgery. Advances in the treatment of congenital heart disease have prolonged life into adulthood but often leave the patient with PR, requiring therapy later in life. Finally it appears that mixed aortic valve disease behaves and should be treated as severe AS.

References

1. Urabe Y, Hamada Y, Spinale FG, Carabello BA, Kent RL, Cooper G 4th, Mann DL. Cardiocyte contractile performance in experimental biventricular volume-overload hypertrophy. Am J Phys. 1993;264(5 Pt 2):H1615–23.
2. Ishibashi Y, Rembert JC, Carabello BA, Nemoto S, Hamawaki M, Zile MR, Greenfield JC Jr, Cooper G 4th. Normal myocardial function in severe right ventricular volume overload hypertrophy. Am J Physiol Heart Circ Physiol. 2001;280(1):H11–6.
3. Urabe Y, Mann DL, Kent RL, Nakano K, Tomanek RJ, Carabello BA, Cooper G 4th. Cellular and ventricular contractile dysfunction in experimental canine mitral regurgitation. Circ Res. 1992;70(1):131–47.
4. Cooper G 4th, Puga FJ, Zujko KJ, Harrison CE, Coleman HN 3rd. Normal myocardial function and energetics in volume-overload hypertrophy in the cat. Circ Res. 1973;32(2):140–8.
5. Cooper G 4th, Satava RM Jr, Harrison CE, Coleman HN 3rd. Mechanisms for the abnormal energetics of pressure-induced hypertrophy of cat myocardium. Circ Res. 1973;33(2):213–23.
6. Jardin F, Dubourg O, Guéret P, Delorme G, Bourdarias JP. Quantitative two-dimensional echocardiography in massive pulmonary embolism: emphasis on ventricular interdependence and leftward septal displacement. J Am Coll Cardiol. 1987;10(6):1201–6.
7. Ueti OM, Camargo EE, Ueti Ade A, de Lima-Filho EC, Nogueira EA. Assessment of right ventricular function with Doppler echocardiographic indices derived from tricuspid annular motion: comparison with radionuclide angiography. Heart. 2002;88(3):244–8.
8. Cameli M, Righini FM, Lisi M, Mondillo S. Right ventricular strain as a novel approach to analyze right ventricular performance in patients with heart failure. Heart Fail Rev. 2014;19(5):603–10.
9. Kusajima K, Fujita T, Hata H, Shimahara Y, Miura S, Kobayashi J. Long-term echocardiographic follow-up of untreated 2+ functional tricuspid regurgitation in patients undergoing mitral valve surgery. Interact Cardiovasc Thorac Surg. 2016;23(1):96–103.
10. Kwak JJ, Kim YJ, Kim MK, et al. Development of tricuspid regurgitation late after left-sided valve surgery: a single-center experience with long-term echocardiographic examinations. Am Heart J. 2008;155:732–7.
11. Di Mauro M, Bivona A, Iaco AL, et al. Mitral valve surgery for functional mitral regurgitation: prognostic role of tricuspid regurgitation. Eur J Cardiothorac Surg. 2009;35:635–9.

12. King RM, Schaff HV, Danielson GK, et al. Surgery for tricuspid regurgitation late after mitral valve replacement. Circulation. 1984;70:1193–7.
13. Kwon DA, Park JS, Chang HJ, et al. Prediction of outcome in patients undergoing surgery for severe tricuspid regurgitation following mitral valve surgery and role of tricuspid annular systolic velocity. Am J Cardiol. 2006;98:659–61.
14. Vismara R, Gelpi G, Prabhu S, et al. Transcatheter edge-to-edge treatment of functional tricuspid regurgitation in an ex vivo pulsatile heart model. J Am Coll Cardiol. 2016;68(10):1024–33.
15. Asmarats L, Puri R, Latib A, Navia JL, Rodés-Cabau J. Transcatheter tricuspid valve interventions: landscape, challenges, and future directions. J Am Coll Cardiol. 2018;71(25):2935–56.
16. Nickenig G, Kowalski M, Hausleiter J, et al. Transcatheter treatment of severe tricuspid regurgitation with the edge-to-edge MitraClip technique. Circulation. 2017;135(19):1802–14.
17. Nath J, Foster E, Heidenreich PA. Impact of tricuspid regurgitation on long-term survival. J Am Coll Cardiol. 2004;43(3):405–9.
18. Yilmaz O, Suri RM, Dearani JA, et al. Functional tricuspid regurgitation at the time of mitral valve repair for degenerative leaflet prolapse: the case for a selective approach. J Thorac Cardiovasc Surg. 2011;142(3):608–13.
19. Dreyfus GD, Corbi PJ, Chan KM, Bahrami T. Secondary tricuspid regurgitation or dilatation: which should be the criteria for surgical repair? Ann Thorac Surg. 2005;79:127–32.
20. Mahesh B, Wells F, Nashef S, Nair S. Role of concomitant tricuspid surgery in moderate functional tricuspid regurgitation in patients undergoing left heart valve surgery. Eur J Cardiothorac Surg. 2013;43(1):2–8.
21. Matsunaga A, Duran CM. Progression of tricuspid regurgitation after repaired functional ischemic mitral regurgitation. Circulation. 2005;112:1453–7.
22. Matsuyama K, Matsumoto M, Sugita T, Nishizawa J, Tokuda Y, Matsuo T. Predictors of residual tricuspid regurgitation after mitral valve surgery. Ann Thorac Surg. 2003;75:1826–8.
23. Izumi C, Iga K, Konishi T. Progression of isolated tricuspid regurgitation late after mitral valve surgery for rheumatic mitral valve disease. J Heart Valve Dis. 2002;11:353–6.
24. Calafiore AM, Gallina S, Iac AL, et al. Mitral valve surgery for functional mitral regurgitation: should moderate-or-more tricuspid regurgitation be treated? A propensity score analysis. Ann Thorac Surg. 2009;87(3):698–703.
25. Kim JB, Yoo DG, Kim GS, et al. Mild-to-moderate functional tricuspid regurgitation in patients undergoing valve replacement for rheumatic mitral disease: the influence of tricuspid valve repair on clinical echocardiographic outcomes. Heart. 2012;98(1):24–30.
26. Chikwe J, Itagaki S, Anyanwu A, Adams D. Impact of concomitant tricuspid annuloplasty on tricuspid regurgitation, right ventricular function, and pulmonary artery hypertension after repair of mitral valve prolapse. J Am Coll Cardiol. 2015;65(18):1931–8.
27. Chan V, Burwash IG, Lam BK, et al. Clinical and echocardiographic impact of functional tricuspid regurgitation repair at the time of mitral valve replacement. Ann Thorac Surg. 2009;88(4):1209–15.
28. Benedetto U, Melina G, Angeloni E, et al. Prophylactic tricuspid annuloplasty in patients with dilated tricuspid annulus undergoing mitral valve surgery. J Thorac Cardiovasc Surg. 2012;143(3):632–8.
29. Navia JL, Brozzi NA, Klein AL, et al. Moderate tricuspid regurgitation with left-sided degenerative heart valve disease: to repair or not to repair? Ann Thorac Surg. 2012;93:59–69.
30. David TE, David CM, Fan CS, Manlhiot C. Tricuspid regurgitation is uncommon after mitral valve repair for degenerative diseases. J Thorac Cardiovasc Surg. 2017;154(1):110–22.
31. Vassileva CM, Shabosky J, Boley T, Markwell S, Hazelrigg S. Tricuspid valve surgery: the past 10 years from the Nationwide Inpatient Sample (NIS) database. J Thorac Cardiovasc Surg. 2012;143(5):1043–9.
32. Nishimura RA, Otto CM, Carabello BA, et al. AHA/ACC guideline for the management of patients with valvular heart disease: executive summary: a report of the American College of Cardiology/American Heart Association Task Force on Practice Guidelines. J Am Coll Cardiol. 2014;63(22):2438–88.
33. Singh SK, Tang GH, Maganti MD, et al. Midterm outcomes of tricuspid valve repair versus replacement for organic tricuspid disease. Ann Thorac Surg. 2006;82(5):1735–41.
34. Arbulu A, Holmes RJ, Asfaw I. Tricuspid valvulectomy without replacement. Twenty years' experience. J Thorac Cardiovasc Surg. 1991;102(6):917–22.
35. Kunadian B, Vijayalakshmi K, Balasubramanian S, Dunning J. Should the tricuspid valve be replaced with a mechanical or biological valve? Interact Cardiovasc Thorac Surg. 2007;6(4):551–7.
36. Manoly I, McAnelly SL, Sriskandarajah S, McLaughlin KE. Prognosis of patients with carcinoid heart disease after valvular surgery. Interact Cardiovasc Thorac Surg. 2014;19(2):302–5.
37. Ribeiro PA, Al Zaibag M, Idris MT. Percutaneous double balloon tricuspid valvotomy for severe tricuspid stenosis: 3-year follow-up study. Eur Heart J. 1990;11(12):1109–12.
38. Hayes CJ, Gersony WM, Driscoll DJ, et al. Second natural history study of congenital heart defects. Results of treatment of patients with pulmonary valvar stenosis. Circulation. 1993;87(2 Suppl):I28–37.
39. Devanagondi R, Peck D, Sagi J, et al. Long-term outcomes of balloon Valvuloplasty for isolated pulmonary valve stenosis. Pediatr Cardiol. 2017;38(2):247–54.
40. Geva T, Sandweiss BM, Gauvreau K, et al. Factors associated with impaired clinical status in long-term survivors of tetralogy of Fallot repair evaluated by magnetic resonance imaging. J Am Coll Cardiol. 2004;43:1068–74.
41. Bouzas B, Kilner PJ, Gatzoulis MA. Pulmonary regurgitation: not a benign lesion. Eur Heart J. 2005;26(5):433–9.
42. Fathallah M, Krasuski RA. Pulmonic valve disease: review of pathology and current treatment options. Curr Cardiol Rep. 2017;19(11):108.
43. Gatzoulis MA, Balaji S, Webber SA, et al. Risk factors for arrhythmia and sudden cardiac death late after repair of tetralogy of Fallot: a multicentre study. Lancet. 2000;356(9234):975–81.
44. Ruiz CE, Kliger C, Perk G, et al. Transcatheter therapies for the treatment of valvular and paravalvular regurgitation in acquired and congenital valvular heart disease. J Am Coll Cardiol. 2015;66(2):169–83.
45. Jeong DS, Park PW, Sung K, Kim WS, Yang JH, Jun TG, Lee YT. Long-term clinical impact of functional mitral regurgitation after aortic valve replacement. Ann Thorac Surg. 2011;92(4):1339–45.
46. Absil B, Dagenais F, Mathieu P, et al. Does moderate mitral regurgitation impact early mid-term clinical outcome in patients undergoing isolated aortic valve replacement for aortic stenosis? Eur J Cardiothorac Surg. 2003;24:217–22.
47. Wan CK, Suri RM, Li Z, et al. Management of moderate functional mitral regurgitation at the time of aortic valve replacement: is concomitant mitral valve repair necessary? J Thorac Cardiovasc Surg. 2009;137:635–40.
48. Takeda K, Matsumiya G, Sakaguchi T, et al. Impact of untreated mild-to-moderate mitral regurgitation at the time of isolated aortic valve replacement on late adverse outcomes. Eur J Cardiothorac Surg. 2010;37:1033–8.
49. Coutinho GF, Correia PM, Pancas R, Antunes MJ. Management of moderate secondary mitral regurgitation at the time of aortic valve surgery. Eur J Cardiothorac Surg. 2013;44:32–40.
50. Nombela-Franco L, Ribeiro HB, Urena M, et al. Significant mitral regurgitation left untreated at the time of aortic valve replacement. J Am Coll Cardiol. 2014;63(24):2643–58.
51. Tzikas A, Piazza N, van Dalen BM, et al. Changes in mitral regurgitation after transcatheter aortic valve implantation. Catheter Cardiovasc Interv. 2010;75:43–9.

52. Gotzmann M, Lindstaedt M, Bojara W, Mügge A, Germing A. Hemodynamic results and changes in myocardial function after transcatheter aortic valve implantation. Am Heart J. 2010;159:926–32.
53. Masson JB, Lee M, Boone RH, et al. Impact of coronary artery disease on outcomes after transcatheter aortic valve implantation. Catheter Cardiovasc Interv. 2010;76:165–73.
54. Durst R, Avelar E, McCarty D, et al. Outcome and improvement predictors of mitral regurgitation after transcatheter aortic valve implantation. J Heart Valve Dis. 2011;20:272–81.
55. De Chiara B, Moreo A, De Marco F, et al. Influence of CoreValve revalving system implantation on mitral valve function: an echocardiographic study in selected patients. Catheter Cardiovasc Interv. 2011;78:638–44.
56. Samim M, Stella PR, Agostoni P, et al. Transcatheter aortic implantation of the Edwards-SAPIEN bioprosthesis: insights on early benefit of TAVR on mitral regurgitation. Int J Cardiol. 2011;152:124–6.
57. Hekimian G, Detaint D, Messika-Zeitoun D, et al. Mitral regurgitation in patients referred for transcatheter aortic valve implantation using the Edwards Sapien prosthesis: mechanisms and early post procedural changes. J Am Soc Echocardiogr. 2012;25:160–5.
58. Toggweiler S, Boone RH, Rodés-Cabau J, et al. Transcatheter aortic valve replacement: outcomes of patients with moderate or severe mitral regurgitation. J Am Coll Cardiol. 2012;59:2068–74.
59. D'Onofrio A, Gasparetto V, Napodano M, et al. Impact of preoperative mitral valve regurgitation on outcomes after transcatheter aortic valve implantation. Eur J Cardiothorac Surg. 2012;41:1271–6.
60. Hutter A, Bleiziffer S, Richter V, et al. Transcatheter aortic valve implantation in patients with concomitant mitral and tricuspid regurgitation. Ann Thorac Surg. 2013;95:77–84.
61. Giordana F, Capriolo M, Frea S, et al. Impact of TAVR on mitral regurgitation: a prospective echocardiographic study. Echocardiography. 2013;30:250–7.
62. Barbanti M, Webb J, Hahn RT, et al. Impact of preoperative moderate/severe mitral regurgitation on 2-year outcome after transcatheter and surgical aortic valve replacement: insight from the PARTNER (Placement of AoRTic TraNscathetER Valve) Trial Cohort A. Circulation. 2013;128:2776–84.
63. Bedogni F, Latib A, Brambilla N, et al. Interplay between mitral regurgitation and transcatheter aortic valve replacement with the CoreValve revalving system: a multicenter registry. Circulation. 2013;128:2145–53.
64. Barreiro CJ, Patel ND, Fitton TP, et al. Aortic valve replacement and concomitant mitral valve regurgitation in the elderly: impact on survival and functional outcome. Circulation. 2005;112:I443–7.
65. Tunick PA, Gindea A, Kronzon I. Effect of aortic valve replacement for aortic stenosis on severity of mitral regurgitation. Am J Cardiol. 1990;65:1219–21.
66. Caballero-Borrego J, Gómez-Doblas JJ, Cabrera-Bueno F, et al. Incidence, associated factors and evolution of non-severe functional mitral regurgitation in patients with severe aortic stenosis undergoing aortic valve replacement. Eur J Cardiothorac Surg. 2008;34:62–6.
67. Harris KM, Malenka DJ, Haney MF, et al. Improvement in mitral regurgitation after aortic valve replacement. Am J Cardiol. 1997;80:741–5.
68. Moazami N, Diodato MD, Moon MR, et al. Does functional mitral regurgitation improve with isolated aortic valve replacement? J Card Surg. 2004;19:444–8.
69. Adams PB, Ott CM. Lack of improvement in coexisting mitral regurgitation after relief of valvular aortic stenosis. Am J Cardiol. 1990;66:105–7.
70. Christenson JT, Jordan B, Bloch A, et al. Should a regurgitant mitral valve be replaced simultaneously with a stenotic aortic valve? Texas Heart Inst J. 2000;27:350–5.
71. Brasch AV, Khan SS, DeRobertis MA, et al. Change in mitral regurgitation severity after aortic valve replacement for aortic stenosis. Am J Cardiol. 2000;85:1271–4.
72. Vanden Eyden F, Bouchard D, El-Hamamsy I, et al. Effect of aortic valve replacement for aortic stenosis on severity of mitral regurgitation. Ann Thorac Surg. 2007;83:1279–84.
73. Ruel M, Kapila V, Price J, Kulik A, Burwash IG, Mesana TG. Natural history and predictors of outcome in patients with concomitant functional mitral regurgitation at the time of aortic valve replacement. Circulation. 2006;114:I541–6.
74. Zilberszac R, Gabriel H, Schemper M, et al. Outcome of combined stenotic and regurgitant aortic valve disease. J Am Coll Cardiol. 2013;61(14):1489–9.
75. Egbe AC, Luis SA, Padang R, Warnes CA. Outcomes in moderate mixed aortic valve disease: is it time for a paradigm shift? J Am Coll Cardiol. 2016;67(20):2321–9.
76. Gash AK, Carabello BA, Kent RL, Frazier JA, Spann JF. Left ventricular performance in patients with coexistent mitral stenosis and aortic insufficiency. J Am Coll Cardiol. 1984;3(3):703–11.
77. Gillinov AM, Blackstone EH, Cosgrove DM 3rd, et al. Mitral valve repair with aortic valve replacement is superior to double valve replacement. J Thorac Cardiovasc Surg. 2003;125(6):1372–8.

Transcatheter Aortic Valve Replacement

10

Sukhdeep Singh Basra, Hani Jneid, and Biswajit Kar

Introduction

Calcific aortic stenosis (AS) remains the most frequently encountered valvular heart disease in the Western world and represents a major health-care burden. The disease process has a slow, progressive asymptomatic phase [1] followed by a poor prognosis once symptoms develop with a 5-year survival rate of only 15–50% when managed without valve replacement [2]. The prevalence of aortic stenosis increases with age and its burden has been increasing with the aging world population. The Euro Heart Survey of patients with valvular heart disease in 92 centers across 25 countries showed that aortic stenosis was the most common left-sided native valvular heart disease and was present in 43.1% of patients with valvular heart disease [3]. Similarly, the National Heart, Lung and Blood Institute population-based study of 11,911 adults who underwent systematic echocardiography showed an age-dependent increase in prevalence of aortic stenosis from 0.02% in patients aged 18–44 years to 2.8% in those aged more than 75 years [4]. Until recently, surgical aortic valve replacement (SAVR) was the only effective treatment option for patients with aortic stenosis and has been shown to prolong life even in patients over 80 years of age [5]. However, a relatively large percentage (33% of patients with severe AS above age 75 years) is not a candidate for SAVR due to a high burden of comorbidities [6]. Transcatheter aortic valve replacement (TAVR) has emerged as a viable treatment option in AS patients who are at intermediate surgical risk, high surgical risk, or who are inoperable due to advanced age and associated comorbidities.

The first-in-man reported TAVR was performed by Dr. Alan Cribier in 2002 and since then more than 1,00,000 such procedures have been done all over the world. At this time there are two major valve platforms approved for use in the USA and include the Edwards SAPIEN Balloon-Expandable Valve (BEV) and the Medtronic CoreValve Self-Expanding Valve (SEV). These have been extensively studied and FDA approved through several multicenter registries as well as randomized trials including the PARTNER trial for Edwards SAPIEN BEV and the US Pivotal Trials for CoreValve SEV in inoperable, high-risk, and intermediate-risk patients. Results of recent trials found TAVR to be non-inferior or superior to SAVR for low risk patients and TAVR is likely to recieve FDA apporival in this group. Additionally, there are several other valve platforms being developed with several undergoing clinical trials at this time.

Indications/Contraindications

The current approved indications for TAVR include patients with severe symptomatic aortic stenosis who are likely to gain improvement in quality of life and have a life expectancy of more than 1 year but are either "inoperable" candidates for SAVR as assessed by a "heart team" or have a high or intermediate surgical risk and are offered TAVR as an alternative. The indications/contraindications for TAVR are listed below.

S. S. Basra (✉)
UT Center for Advanced Heart Failure, Interventional Cardiology, Section of Cardiology, University of Texas McGovern Medical School Houston, Houston, TX, USA
e-mail: sukhdeep.s.basra@uth.tmc.edu

H. Jneid
Department of Medicine, Baylor College of Medicine, Interventional Cardiology, Houston, TX, USA

Interventional Cardiology, Michael E. DeBakey VA Medical Center, Houston, TX, USA

B. Kar
UT Center for Advanced Heart Failure, Interventional Cardiology, Section of Cardiology, University of Texas McGovern Medical School Houston, Houston, TX, USA

Department of Medicine, Baylor College of Medicine, Interventional Cardiology, Houston, TX, USA

Interventional Cardiology, Michael E. DeBakey VA Medical Center, Houston, TX, USA

B. A. Carabello (ed.), *Valvular Heart Disease*, Cardiovascular Medicine, https://doi.org/10.1007/978-1-4471-2840-3_10

Absolute and relative contraindications for transcatheter aortic valve replacement
Absolute contraindications
Absence of a "heart team" and no cardiac surgery on the site
Appropriateness of TAVI as an alternative to AVR, not confirmed by a "heart team"
Clinical
Estimated life expectancy less than 1 year
Improvement of quality of life by TAVI unlikely because of comorbidities
Severe primary associated disease of other valve with major contribution to the patient's symptoms that can be treated only by surgery
Anatomic
Inadequate annulus size (<18 mm, >29 mm[a])
Thrombus in the left ventricle
Active endocarditis
Elevated risk of coronary ostium obstruction (asymmetric valve calcification, short distance between annulus and coronary ostium, small aortic sinuses)
Plaques with mobile thrombi in the ascending aorta or arch
For transfemoral/subclavian approach: inadequate vascular access (vessel size, calcification, tortuosity)
Relative contraindications
Bicuspid or noncalcified valves
Untreated coronary artery disease requiring revascularization
Hemodynamic instability
LVEF less than 20%
For the transapical approach: severe pulmonary disease, LV apex not accessible

Abbreviations: AVR aortic valve replacement, *LV* left ventricle, *LVEF* left ventricular ejection fraction, *TAVI* transcatheter aortic valve implementation

Data from: Joint Task Force on the Management of Valvular Heart Disease of the European Society of Cardiology (ESC)1; European Association for Cardio-Thoracic Surgery (EACTS), Vahanian A, Alfieri O, et al. Guidelines on the management of valvular heart disease (version 2012). Eur Heart J. 2012 Oct;33(19):2451–96

[a]Contraindication when using the current devices

The current recommendations for use of TAVR as laid out by the American College of Cardiology/American Heart Association guidelines and the European Society of Cardiology/European Association of Cardio-Thoracic Surgery are listed in Fig. 10.1 [7, 8]. However it is likely that guidelines for TAVR use will move progressively to lower risk patients.

Risk Stratification

Patients being evaluated for TAVR must be evaluated by a "heart team" which includes cardiologists, cardiac surgeons, anesthesiologists, and other specialists as needed to develop a comprehensive understanding of each patient's risk and guide them towards appropriate therapies. Patients must be evaluated with a goal to separate patients who are severely ill **with** aortic stenosis from those who are severely ill **due** to severe aortic stenosis.

Risk stratification is key in the TAVR evaluation because appropriateness of use is in part determined by level of risk. The current accepted method for risk stratification includes calculation of either the Society of Thoracic Surgeons (STS) projected risk of mortality (PROM) score [9] or the Logistic European Score for Cardiac Operative Risk Evaluation (LES Euroscore) [10]. Both these scoring systems have been used in several TAVR registries as well as randomized clinical trials to risk stratify patients for TAVR. Overall, the LES Euroscore overestimates mortality in high-risk patients undergoing SAVR and was not appropriately calibrated to estimate mortality after TAVR. The STS score is probably more realistic in estimating mortality and morbidity after SAVR. An STS mortality score cutoff of >4% is used to certify intermediate or surgical high risk, the current criteria for TAVR use.

Newer scoring systems including the EuroSCORE II [11], ACEF (Age, creatinine, ejection fraction) score, TVT TAVR In Hospital Mortality Score, and the Aortenklappenregister score [12] have been developed to better predict patient outcomes after TAVR. Although the STS and EuroSCORE II score are well established in predicting surgical risk, neither was specifically developed for TAVR patients. Newer models that incorporate frailty, prohibitive anatomy including porcelain aorta and severe aortic calcification, oxygen dependency, pulmonary hypertension, RV dysfunction, cirrhosis, dementia, physical deconditioning and malnutrition, and access options are greatly needed and are being developed to better stratify patients for whom TAVR is a better option than SAVR. Such a model should accurately predict both early and late mortality as well as improvement in quality of life metrics. Hopefully, with the combined analyses of the PARTNER trials, CoreValve trials, and the US Transcatheter valve Therapeutics (TVT) National Database, a TAVR specific risk algorithm could be developed and validated [13].

Patient Screening

Appropriate patient screening is the cornerstone for the success of any TAVR program. Optimal screening includes a comprehensive evaluation by the heart team followed by a thorough review of patient's anatomical, functional, and imaging data to delineate the appropriate treatment strategy, procedural details, as well as post procedure care. Figure 10.2 is a representation of the

Fig. 10.1 Recommendations for choice of mechanical biological aortic valve prosthesis. Class I indicated recommended; class IIa indicates should be considered; and class IIb indicates may be considered. *Abbreviations: AHA* American Heart Association guidelines, *ESC* European Society of Cardiology guidelines. From Otto CM, Baumgartner H. Updated 2017 European and American guidelines for prosthesis type and implantation mode in severe aortic stenosis. Heart. 2018 May;104(9):710–713. Reprinted with permission from BMJ Publishing Group Ltd.

Recommendations for choice of mechanical versus biological aortic valve prosthesis		
Class	**Source**	
Shared decision making and informed patient		
I	AHA	Valve choice should be based on a shared decision process considering: • patient values, preferences, and desires • indications for and risks of long term anticoagulation • potential need for and risk associated with re-intervention.
I	ESC	A mechanical or bioprosthetic valve is recommended • according to informed patient desires if there are no contraindications to long-term anticoagulation
Anticoagulation and bleeding risk considerations		
I	AHA & ESC	Bioprosthetic valve recommended or should be considered: • if anticoagulant therapy is contraindicated, cannot be managed appropriately, or is not desired.
I	ESC	• for reoperation for mechanical valve thrombosis despite good long-term anticoagulation control.
IIa	ESC	• in young women contemplating pregnancy.
IIa	ESC	Mechanical prosthesis should or may be considered if: • already on anti-coagulation for another mechanical prosthesis
IIb	ESC	• already on long-term anticoagulation due to a high risk for thromboembolism
IIb	AHA	A pulmonary autograft (the Ross procedure) may be considered for: • young patients if anticoagulation is contraindicated or undesirable), when performed by an experienced surgeon
Risk of structural valve deterioration and redo surgery		
I	ESC	A mechanical prosthesis is recommended or should be considered in patients: • at risk of accelerated structural valve deterioration
IIa	ESC	• with a reasonable life expectancy if future redo valve surgery would be high risk
IIa	ESC	A bioprosthesis should be considered for patients with a: • low likelihood and/or a low operative risk of future redo valve surgery.
Expected patient longevity		
IIa	AHA	A mechanical valve is reasonable/should be considered for patients: • < 50 years of age if no contraindication to anticoagulation
IIa	ESC	• < 60 years of age in aortic position
IIa	AHA	Either a mechanical or bioprosthetic valve prosthesis is reasonable for patients: • between 50 and 70 years of age, based on individual patient factors and preferences.
IIa	ESC	A bioprosthetic valve should be considered/is reasonable for patients: • > 65 years of age in aortic and in those with a life expectancy lower than expected valve durability
IIa	AHA	• > 70 years of age

workflow associated with optimal patient screening by the heart team.

Imaging

Imaging is key in the workup of a patient for TAVR and is typically done using several modalities including transthoracic echocardiography (TTE), multi-slice detector computed tomography (MDCT), angiography, transesophageal echocardiography (TEE) including 3D TEE as well as MRI (Table 10.1). A comprehensive preprocedural echocardiogram is performed to evaluate the aortic valve morphology, calcification, hemodynamics, concomitant mitral valve disease, left ventricular dimensions and function, right heart function, and pulmonary hypertension. One of the most important aspects of imaging includes evaluation of the ilio-femoral access for size, tortuosity, and calcification for transfemoral approach. This is typically accomplished using MDCT, although some centers

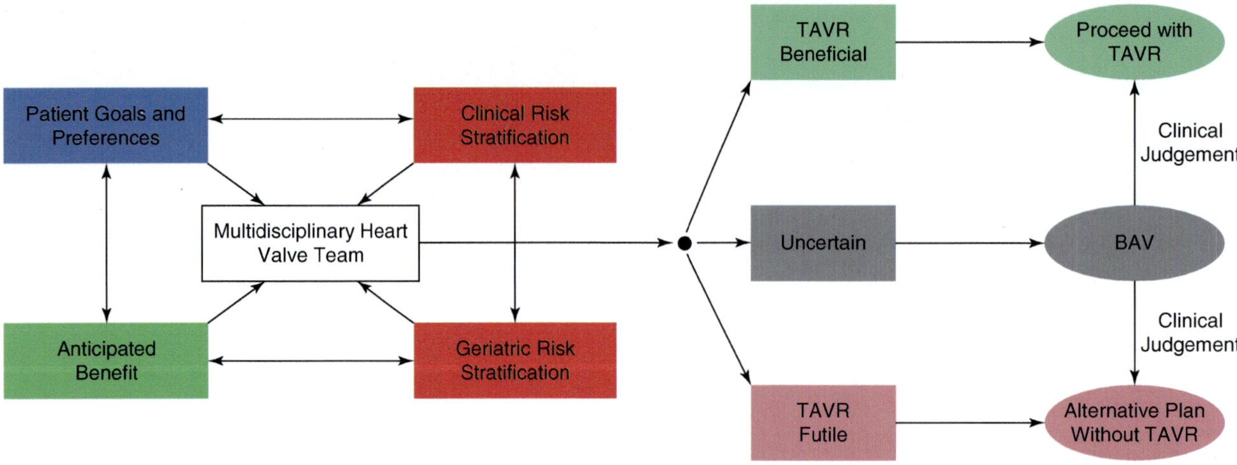

Fig. 10.2 Decision-making by the multidisciplinary heart team on patients referred for transcatheter aortic valve replacement (TAVR). The multidisciplinary team considers and weighs the various risk factors shown and makes a decision regarding whether TAVR would be beneficial or futile. *BAV indicates balloon aortic valvuloplasty.* From Agarwal S, Tuzcu EM, Kapadia SR. Choice and Selection of Treatment Modalities for Cardiac Patients: An Interventional Cardiology Perspective. J Am Heart Assoc. 2015 Oct;4(10):e002353. Published online 2015 Oct 20. https://dx.doi.org/10.1161%2FJAHA.115.002353. Copyright © 2015 The Authors. Published on behalf of the American Heart Association, Inc., by Wiley Blackwell. Open Access

Table 10.1 Preprocedural transthoracic assessment

Pre-procedural echocardiographic imaging
• Aortic valve and root – Aortic valve morphology Bicuspid versus tricuspid Degree and location of calcium – Annular dimensions Minimum and maximum diameters Perimeter Area – Aortic valve hemodynamics Aortic valve gradients and area Stroke volume Impedance – Left ventricular outflow tract Extent and distribution of calcium Presence of sigmoid septum – Aortic root dimensions and calcification Sinus of Valsalva diameter Sinotubular junction diameter and calcification Location of coronary ostia and risk of obstruction
• Mitral valve – Severity of mitral regurgitation – Presence of mitral stenosis – Severity of ectopic calcification Anterior leaflet calcification
• Left ventricular size and function – Wall motion assessment Exclude intracardiac thrombus – Left ventricular mass Hypertrophy and septal morphology – Assessments of function Ejection fraction Strain and torsion Diastolic function
• Right heart – Right ventricular size and function – Tricuspid valve morphology and function – Estimate of pulmonary artery pressures

From: Hahn RT, et al. Recommendations for comprehensive intraprocedural echocardiographic imaging during TAVR. JACC Cardiovasc Imaging. 2015 Mar;8(3):261–87. Reprinted with permission from Elsevier

use angiography for the same purpose. Assessment of aortic annulus size is crucial to determine the appropriate size of the prosthesis and is accomplished using 3D TEE and MDCT (Figs. 10.3 and 10.4).

Specific Comorbidities and Their Roles in Patient Selection

Comorbidities play an important role in evaluating patients for TAVR. Certain conditions pose a prohibitive surgical risk from a technical standpoint and may lead to TAVR being the preferred treatment option in patients with severe symptomatic AS. However, these conditions also increase the risk associated with TAVR implantation and must be carefully considered during patient screening. They include radiation heart disease, heavily calcified ascending aorta (porcelain aorta), multiple prior chest surgeries, prior sternal wound infection, and bypass graft anatomy including left internal mammary artery adherent anteriorly to the posterior wall of the sternum. Similarly severe LV dysfunction, small (<18 mm) or large (>27 mm) aortic annulus, left main coronary ostia within 10 mm of the annulus, intracardiac mass/thrombus/vegetation as well as severe pulmonary hypertension are relative contraindications for the implantation of TAVR. Other specific comorbidities including chronic kidney disease, concomitant mitral valve disease, underlying coronary artery disease, chronic lung disease, and systolic left ventricular dysfunction are associated with worse outcomes in patients undergoing TAVR and must be considered in detail during the preprocedural assessment (Table 10.2).

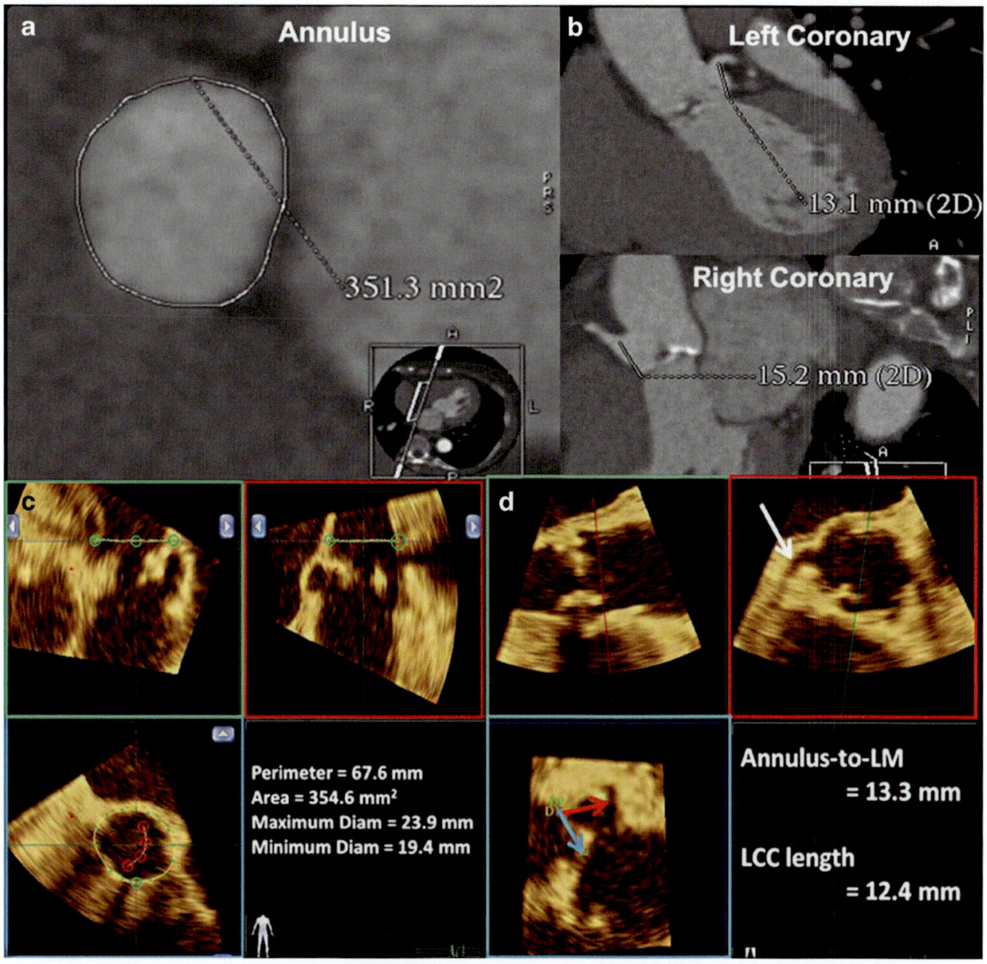

Fig. 10.3 Annular measurements by three-dimensional (3D) imaging. Panels A and B are MSCT images with annular area measurement of 351 mm^2 and left main coronary height of 13.1 mm. Panels C and D are 3D TEE images with annular area of 354 mm^2 and left main coronary height of 13.3 mm. From Hahn RT. Guidance of transcatheter aortic valve replacement by echocardiography. Curr Cardiol Rep. 2014 Jan;16(1):442. Reprinted with permission from Springer

Chronic Kidney Disease (CKD)

Patients with severe CKD and those on dialysis have been excluded from TAVR randomized trials and the long-term benefits of the procedure in these patients are unknown. Additionally, patients with CKD have a higher risk of prosthesis degeneration possibly due to abnormal calcium metabolism.

Preoperative renal function is an important predictor of mortality and morbidity in patients undergoing surgery for valvular heart disease [14]. Underlying CKD is a risk factor for acute kidney injury postoperatively. In patients with CKD, TAVR is associated with a lesser risk of acute kidney injury than SAVR and may even result in improved renal function post intervention [15–17]. Despite this, underlying CKD is still associated with worse outcomes and a higher chance of AKI post TAVR [18]. Patients who develop AKI post procedure have a higher mortality and increased cost and length of hospitalization. Preprocedural creatinine more than 1.58 mg/dL was associated with a sixfold increased risk of death in one study [19]. A meta-analysis of over 40,000 patients found worse in-hospital morbidity and mortality for CKD patients and an even worse prognosis for patients with end-stage renal disease compared to patients with normal renal function [20]. Special emphasis must be given to limit the amount of contrast and space contrast studies to prevent contrast-induced nephropathy in these patients.

Coronary Artery Disease

Significant coronary artery disease is common in up to 40–75% of patients with severe AS being evaluated for TAVR [21]. Patients with severe CAD usually have worse vascular disease and may have a higher likelihood of needing the transapical approach for valve deployment. Although a commonly encountered comorbidity, the overall impact of the presence of concomitant CAD on outcomes in patients undergoing TAVR is not well understood and needs further exploration. In a recent study, CAD increased 2 year TAVR mortality by twofold [22]. Additionally, the optimum the timing of revascularization and stent type need to be further investigated in trials. Revascularization before TAVR may be pursued due to a simpler access to the coronaries and lower risk of ischemia and hemodynamic instability during rapid pacing and valve deployment. The ischemic burden, complexity of procedure, and anticipated contrast load should be taken into account while planning revascularization prior to TAVR. Revascularization with percutaneous coronary

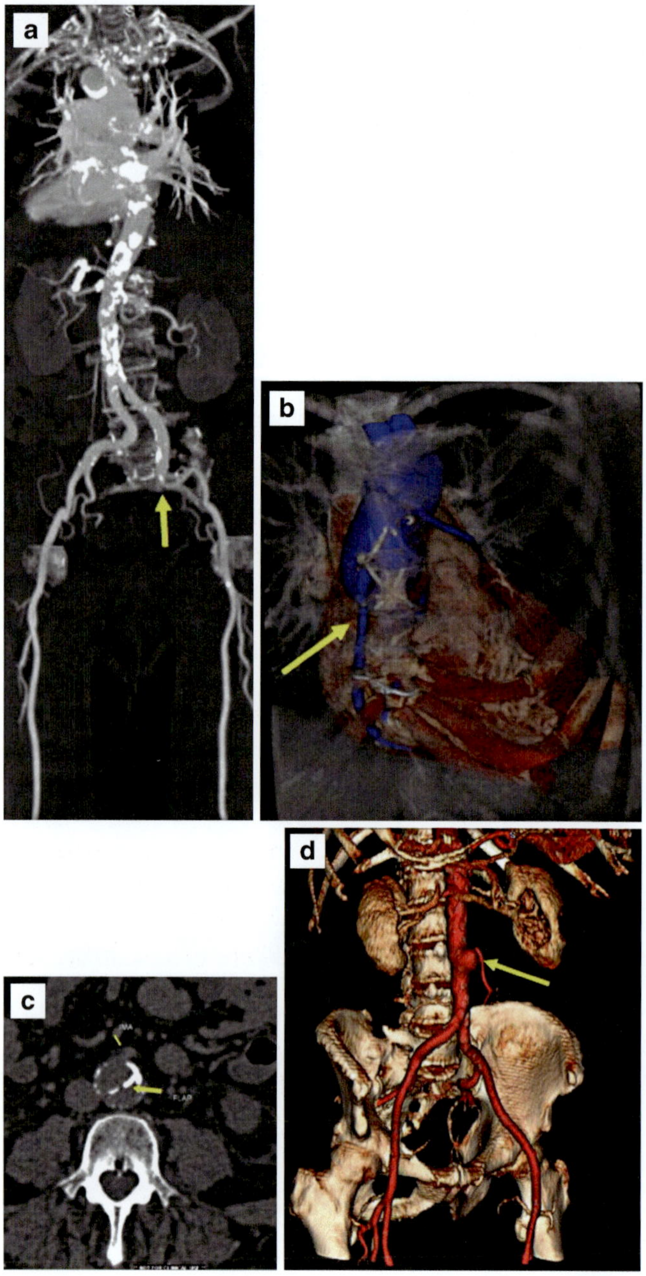

Fig. 10.4 MDCT should be used to assess safety and ideal access approach for TAVR. Identification of patients with severe iliofemoral tortuosity and calcification (**a**), previous bypass grafts and their relationship to the sternum to plan transaortic procedures (**b**) and aortic disease such as dissection (**c**) and aneurysm (**d**) is critical to evaluate prior to TAVR. From Sintek M, Zajarias A. Patient evaluation and selection for transcatheter aortic valve replacement: the heart team approach. Prog Cardiovasc Dis. 2014 May–Jun;56(6):572–82. Reprinted with permission from Elsevier

intervention should be pursued for severely stenotic lesions, which subtend a large area of myocardium at risk with several centers reporting successful staged and concomitant PCI with 1 year survival of more than 80% [23–25]. Whether revascularization should be done before TAVR vs. as a com-

Table 10.2 Specific comorbidities influencing patient selection for TAVR

Comorbidity	Relevance to selection for TAVR
CKD	Presence of CKD predicts worse outcome after TAVR. Preprocedural creatinine >1.58 mg/dL is associated with six fold increased risk of mortality
Coronary artery disease	Presence indicates more extensive vascular disease. Need for staged or concomitant revascularization needs to be assessed. The ongoing ACTIVATION trial is evaluating the role of PCI in TAVR patients
Mitral valve disease	Up to one-third of patients evaluated for TAVR have severe MVD. Presence indicates more extensive CVD limiting TAVR effectiveness
Systolic dysfunction	TAVR is generally safe and efficacious. More adverse events but similar overall mortality. Marked improvements in LVEF have been reported after TAVR at 30 days
CLD	Present in 20–30% of TAVR patients. Improved survival and functional capacity compared with medical therapy. Frail patients may not benefit from TAVR in presence of CLD

From: Sarkar K, Sarkar M, Ussia GP. Current status of transcatheter aortic valve replacement. Med Clin North Am. 2015 Jul;99(4):805–33. Reprinted with permission from Elsevier. *CKD* chronic liver disease; *CLD* chronic lung disease.

bined procedure is an important question and the currently enrolling ACTIVATION trial will help in clarifying this conundrum [26, 27].

Mitral Valve Disease

Concomitant mitral regurgitation (MR) may be present in up to one-third of patients being evaluated for TAVR [28]. Patients with severe mitral valve disease who undergo TAVR usually have a higher incidence of atrial fibrillation, pulmonary arterial hypertension, and RV dysfunction. Although it is expected that severe MR will improve after TAVR, it is not clear which patients will improve the most and in some cases MR worsens instead of improves [29]. In general patients with organic mitral disease and lower transaortic gradients are most likely to have persistent MR post TAVR. A recent multivariate analysis suggests that mitral regurgitation is not associated with worsening survival after TAVR [30], although the presence of concomitant mitral valve disease is a marker of more advanced disease and may limit the effectiveness of TAVR. Patients with significant mitral regurgitation and severe aortic stenosis may be considered for percutaneous treatment of both lesions with the recent approval of the MitraClip device [31].

Systolic Dysfunction

Patients with LVEF <20% were excluded from the PARTNER trial and most patients had LVEF >45% [21]. A single-center retrospective study by Ewe et al. showed that patients undergoing TAVR implantation with EF < 50% had higher adverse events but similar procedural and total mortality compared to those with LVEF >50% [32]. Another study showed that in patients with EF <35% implanted with a Medtronic Corevalve device, the 30-day mortality was similar to those with LVEF >35% and that a greater proportion of TAVR low EF patients showed improvement in LVEF when compared to matched SAVR controls [33, 34]. Indeed, most patients with systolic dysfunction show an improvement in LVEF after TAVR. RV function often worsens after SAVR, but usually remains stable post TAVR [35, 36].

Low-gradient severe AS (LG-AS) is associated with a worse prognosis in patients undergoing SAVR [37], with mortality as high as 35% in patients with no contractile reserve [38]. In patients with LG-AS who survive SAVR, there is improvement in outcomes suggesting a role for TAVR in these patients. Mortality is higher in patients with LG-AS who undergo TAVR as compared to those with normal gradients and may approach 33% at 6 months [39]. This is due in part to underlying LV dysfunction and also to a higher prevalence of pulmonary arterial hypertension, severe mitral regurgitation, CAD, and PAD in these patients, all of which affect outcomes in patients undergoing TAVR [40]. Nonetheless survival is improved in LG-AS patients compared to "medical" therapy [41] and patients with LG-AS who survive TAVR have an improvement in functional capacity, six-minute walk distance as well as larger improvement in LVEF compared to matched SAVR patients [34, 39, 40]. Low-dose dobutamine stress echocardiography has been used successfully to assess for contractile reserve and SAVR outcome in patients with LG-AS [38]. This technique has also been used to separate patients with true from pseudo aortic stenosis undergoing TAVR. Patients with low-flow, low-gradient, low-EF AS have the worst prognosis while high-gradient patients have the best prognosis [42]. The former patients have low EF because of severe LV dysfunction while the latter have low EF based upon high afterload that is immediately corrected by TAVR.

Chronic Lung Disease (CLD)

About 20–30% patients in TAVR and SAVR registries have chronic lung disease [43–45]. Presence of severe chronic lung disease is associated with an increased 1 year mortality in patients who undergo SAVR as well as TAVR [45]. Patients with severe chronic lung disease who undergo TAVR have an improvement in their 1 year outcomes as compared to patients treated with medical management [46]. However, oxygen-dependent chronic lung disease is associated with worse outcomes, especially 1 year all-cause mortality [46]. Severe CLD when associated with a poor 6-minute walk test is associated with a fivefold increased risk of non-CV mortality [46]. All patients undergoing evaluation for TAVR should have lung function assessed and the presence of chronic lung disease, especially in frail patients, should be carefully evaluated as these patients may not benefit as much from TAVR [47].

Frailty vs. Futility

Frailty is described as a state of decreased physiological reserve predisposing to poor outcomes, but not necessitating poor outcomes. It is affected by physical disability and medical comorbidities and is an impairment in medical systems that leads to a decline in resiliency and homeostatic reserve. Commonly accepted key domains of frailty include weakness, slowness, exhaustion, low activity, weight loss, and poor nutrition. Frailty is defined by a composite of several other factors including gait speed, grip strength, 6-min walk test, serum albumin, Katz activities of daily living, weakness, cognitive dysfunction, and several others [48]. Although it is not completely captured in the current risk stratification models, frailty is noted in about 50% of the patients referred for TAVR and has been associated with worse outcomes in patients undergoing TAVR [49–51].

Gait speed is a simple test that has been shown to be predictive of frailty in TAVR and overall mortality [52–54]. Patients who ambulate slower than 0.5 m/s or who ambulate less than 128.5 m during a 6-min walk test have similar procedural mortality but have increased long-term mortality [55]. Frailty in the PARTNER clinical trials was assessed by walk speed, grip strength, serum albumin, and the Katz activity of daily living dependency questionnaire; to be considered inoperable on the basis of frailty, three of those four domains must have been abnormal [50]. Further assessment of frailty using the Multi-Dimensional Geriatric assessment (MGA) showed that adding MGA-based information to risk models improved prediction of 30 day and 1 year mortality and MACCE [49]. Green et al. developed a frailty score for TAVR patients and noted that impaired gait speed, grip strength, reduced serum albumin, and diminished Katz activities of daily living were associated with increased 1 year mortality as well as longer post TAVR hospital stay [55]. In the recent multicenter FRAILTY-AVR study which compared outcomes in elderly patients undergoing TAVR and SAVR, the Essential Frailty Toolset that employed lower extremity weakness, cognitive impairment, anemia, and hypoalbuminemia was superior to other frailty indexes and was prognostic of 30-day mortality and worsening disability at 1 year [56].

A comprehensive frailty assessment also helps differentiate patients with "futility" rather than "high-risk" or "inoperability" as these patients have both poor survival

Table 10.3 Frailty assessment for patients being evaluated for transcatheter aortic valve replacement

Frailty test	Description
Gait speed	>7 s to walk 5 m abnormal
Grip strength	Dynamometer; <30 kg in nonobese man and <18 kg in nonobese woman is abnormal
6-min walk test	<128.5 m during 6-min walk test
Comprehensive Assessment of Frailty (CAF)	Grip strength, gait speed, instrumental activities of daily living questionnaire, standing balance test, serum albumin, brain natriuretic peptide, and creatinine. Proprietary scoring algorithm used to measure frailty
Multidimensional Geriatric Assessment (MGA)	Mini-mental state examination, timed get up and go test, basic and instrumental activities of daily living questionnaires. Frailty index score generated and score ≥3 indicated frailty

From: Sarkar K, Sarkar M, Ussia GP. Current status of transcatheter aortic valve replacement. Med Clin North Am. 2015;99(4):805–33. Reprinted with permission from Elsevier

(less than 1 year) and poor quality of life despite successful TAVR. Common clinical characteristics associated with these patients include a high STS score (STS > 15), extreme frailty usually with dependent social status, severe pulmonary and liver disease, severe dementia, chronic kidney disease (dialysis dependent), and hemodynamic instability (especially requiring pressors). Further research is needed to help better identify patients unlikely to benefit from TAVR during the screening phase based on frailty metrics and risk stratification models (Table 10.3).

Access Screening

The first TAVR by Dr. Cribier was performed using the antegrade trans-septal approach. However, most TAVRs currently use the transfemoral (TF) approach, the default route for valve implantation in patients with suitable ilio-femoral anatomy. Access screening is an important part of the procedure preparation and includes assessment of ileo-femoral size, tortuosity and calcification using MDCT or angiography so as to establish feasibility of TF approach. In patients with unsuitable ilio-femoral anatomy, alternative access sites include transapical (TA), transaortic (TAo), trans-axillary, transcarotid, and trans-caval access. The most common alternative access route for the Edwards valve is the TA route, wherein the valve prosthesis is delivered in an antegrade fashion through the LV apex, while a trans-axillary access route is used for CoreValve implantation for patients with unsuitable ilio-femoral anatomy. Newer generation devices have a lower profile with sheath size as small as 14 Fr for the 23 and 26 mm TF Edward Sapien 3 valve. As a result, most patients being evaluated

Table 10.4 Transfemoral (TF) transcatheter aortic valve replacement (TAVR): procedural steps

• Access. A 6-F to 7-F introducer is used to access femoral artery that is upsized to an 18-F to 22-F introducer sheath
• The native stenotic aortic valve is crossed with a diagnostic Amplatz Left (AL-1) catheter and straight tip wire
• A Super Stiff Amplatz (SSA-1 wire) with a hand-shaped pigtail loop at the end is placed in the LV apex in stable position using the right anterior oblique projection
• A preimplantation balloon aortic valvuloplasty is routinely performed under rapid right-ventricular pacing with an undersized balloon (1–2 mm smaller than the measured aortic annulus diameter) for preparing the native annulus in all cases except pure aortic regurgitation or degenerated aortic bioprosthesis
• A pigtail catheter is positioned in the noncoronary cusp as a marker for the annular plane and for contrast injections during the valve deployment. The image intensifier is positioned at the implant angle defined as the optimal left anterior oblique (LAO) projection for aligning the nadir of all three coronary cusps in a straight line. The valve is positioned across the aortic annulus and deployed under rapid pacing (Edwards)
• For self-expandable core valve (CRS) deployment, the delivery catheter system (DCS) is positioned such that the horizontal markers of the device are positioned (4–6 mm) below the level of the pigtail catheter (CRS)
• The DCS is maintained as perpendicular to the annular plane as possible and the release is initiated under fluoroscopic and angiographic guidance with repeated small contrast injections (10 mL to 10 mL/s at 900 psi) through the pigtail catheter

From: Sarkar K, Sarkar M, Ussia GP. Current status of transcatheter aortic valve replacement. Med Clin North Am. 2015 Jul;99(4):805–33. Reprinted with permission from Elsevier

for TAVR will likely be candidates for a TF approach. In the recent PARTNER II trial 77% of patients were treated from the femoral approach while in the SURTAVI trial 93% were treated from the femoral approach [57, 58] and it is likely that this approach will become even more dominant as TAVR valves become increasingly smaller in profile. The potential advantages of the TA approach include avoiding tortuous and diseased ilio-femoral vasculature, and having a prosthesis co-axial with the aortic annulus. The disadvantages of this approach include the need for a thoracotomy, myocardial injury and left ventricular pseudo-aneurysm from apical perforation of the ventricle and bleeding complications from the surgical site. In patients who are not candidates for either TF or TA or trans-axillary approach because of poor vascular access, poor pulmonary function or chest pathology, the valve prosthesis may be delivered using a retrograde approach by direct cannulation of the ascending aorta or the carotid artery or the subclavian artery. Additionally, in a smaller subset of patients trans-caval aortic access can be performed, which involves accessing the femoral vein to facilitate entry into the abdominal aorta through puncture of the inferior vena cava followed by standard valve implantation using TF technique. The technique for TF and TAVR is described in Table 10.4.

Valve Sizing and Positioning

There are several guidelines and consensus statements regarding the essential role of multidisciplinary imaging in patient selection and procedural guidance for patients undergoing TAVR implantation [59, 60]. Imaging guidance with multi detector CT (MDCT) and TEE are both key in valve sizing and positioning. Valve sizing is established using protocols specific for the valve type employed and implantation is optimized by concurrent TEE and fluoroscopy after determination of the appropriate co-planar implantation view and appropriate height and implantation depth of the prosthesis. A three-dimensional understanding of the complex anatomy of the aorta, LVOT and the aorto-mitral continuity is essential to appropriate valve deployment and functioning. Appropriate sizing and placement of the device will lead to excellent hemodynamics, minimal paravalvular leak, low pacemaker implantation rate and prevention of coronary obstruction and injury to the annulus.

Current Transcatheter Valve Replacement Platforms

The Edwards-Sapien Valve

The Edwards Sapien Valve (Edwards Lifesciences, Irvine, CA) was an improved version of the first balloon-expandable valve (BEV) implanted by Cribier et al. in 2002 (Fig. 10.5). The original Edwards Sapien valve consisted of a tubular slotted stainless steel frame and leaflets made of bovine pericardium, which were pretreated to decrease valve calcification. Additionally the fabric skirt, made of polyethylene terephthalate, was extended further to improve sealing and potentially reduce paravalvular regurgitation. This valve was available in two sizes (23 and 26 mm) requiring 22 F and 24 F delivery catheters for TF approach implantation, respectively.

The Sapien XT valve (Edwards Lifesciences, Irvine, CA) is a third generation of balloon-expandable Edwards valves, consisting of a trileaflet pericardial bovine valve, mounted in a cobalt chromium stent frame. The Sapien XT valve is available in 20-, 23-, 26-, and 29-mm sizes, and is implanted through the transfemoral approach using the NovaFlex delivery system implanted through 16 F (20-, 23-mm valves), 18 F (26-mm valve), or 20 F (29-mm valve) expandable sheaths (e-sheath, Edwards Lifesciences, Irvine, CA).

The Sapien 3 THV (Edwards Lifesciences, Irvine, CA) is the latest iteration of the balloon-expandable valves, and also consists of a trileaflet pericardial bovine valve that is mounted in a cobalt chromium stent. It too incorporates an additional outer skirt to further reduce the risk of paravalvular leak. The expanded length (20 mm) is slightly longer than the Sapien (16.1 mm) and Sapien XT (17.2 mm) THVs, which helps facilitate optimal positioning within the native aortic valve and annulus. Additionally, the delivery system (Commander) has an even lower profile and has been further improved to facilitate valve alignment and proper positioning Table 10.5).

The PARTNER I trial [61] was the first prospective randomized trial of the balloon-expandable Edwards-Sapien valve and included two distinct cohorts of patients: those considered to be inoperable or cohort B (i.e., comorbidities leading to a predicted risk of 50% or more of either death within 30 days after surgery or a serious irreversible condition); and those considered to be at high surgical risk or cohort A (i.e., predicted risk of operative mortality ≥15% as determined by site surgeon and cardiologist and/or a minimum STS score

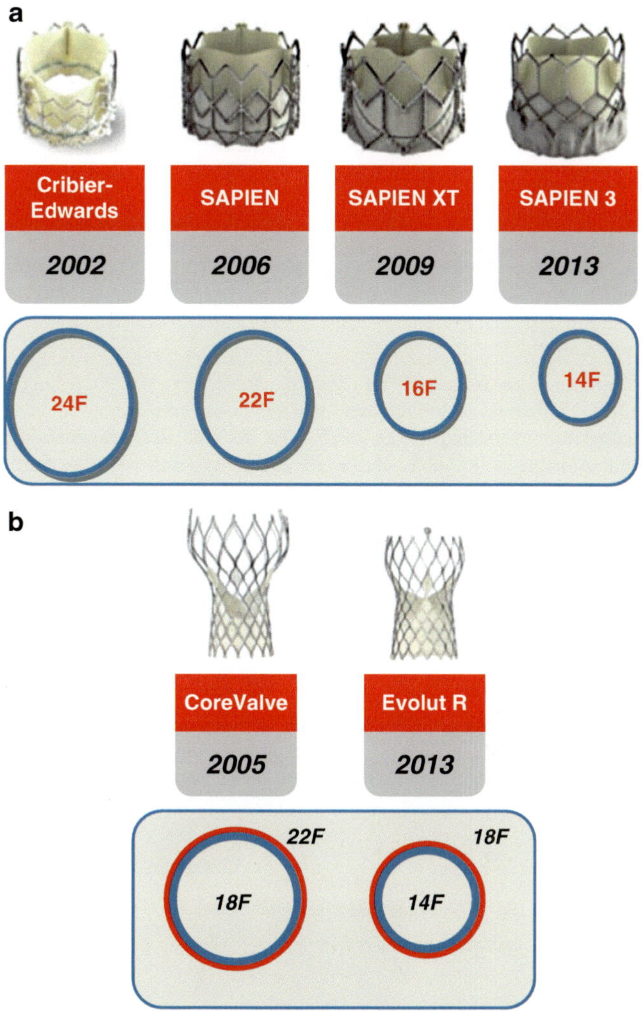

Fig. 10.5 Evolution of the Edwards balloon-expandable transcatheter valves (**a**) and Medtronic self-expandable valves (**b**) (sheath compatibility for a 23 mm valve.) From Hamm CW, Arsalan M, Mack MJ. The future of transcatheter aortic valve implantation. Eur Heart J. 2016 Mar 7;37(10):803–10. Reprinted with permission from Oxford University Press

Table 10.5 Proposed sizing algorithm using annular area (mm²) for the second- and third-generation balloon-expandable valves

	Valve size			
	20 mm	23 mm	26 mm	29 mm
Nominal area, mm²	314	415	531	661
Annular range for second-generation balloon-expandable valve, mm²	257–310	298–410	420–530	530–660
Annular range for third-generation balloon-expandable valve, mm²	273–345	338–430	430–546	540–683

The nominal areas for each balloon-expandable valve size are listed (in mm²). The ranges of annular areas that can be covered are based on an acceptable oversizing range of 5–20% for the second-generation balloon-expandable valve, and a −5–20% oversizing with the third-generation balloon-expandable valve. (Note: a negative oversizing equates to undersizing of the valve, in which the native annulus can be up to 5% larger than the nominal area of the transcatheter valve)
From: Hahn RT, et al. Recommendations for comprehensive intraprocedural echocardiographic imaging during TAVR. JACC Cardiovasc Imaging. 2015 Mar;8(3):261–87. Reprinted with permission from Elsevier

of 10) (Fig. 10.6, Tables 10.6 and 10.7). In the inoperable cohort, all-cause mortality (30.7% vs. 50.7%; $P < 0.001$), cardiovascular mortality (19.6% vs. 41.9%; $P < 0.001$), repeat hospitalization (22.3% vs. 44.1%; $P < 0.001$), and the composite endpoint of death or repeat hospitalization (42.5% vs. 71.6%; $P < 0.001$) were much lower in patients who were randomized to TAVR [61] (Figs. 10.7 and 10.8). TAVR resulted in a significant improvement in health-related quality of life as determined by the Kansas City Cardiomyopathy Questionnaire (KCCQ) [63] (Fig. 10.9). During follow-up, there was no evidence of degeneration of the valvular prosthesis or restenosis at 2 years [64]. At 5-year follow-up, the advantage of TAVR over medical therapy persisted [62]. Heart failure symptoms were less severe in patients treated with TAVR, but the TAVR patients also had a higher incidence of major vascular complications (16.2% vs. 1.1%; $P < 0.001$), major bleeding (22.3% vs. 11.2%; $P < 0.001$), and major strokes (5.0% vs. 1.1%; $P = 0.06$). Based on the results of this trial, TAVR became the new standard of care in patients with severe AS who are considered inoperable.

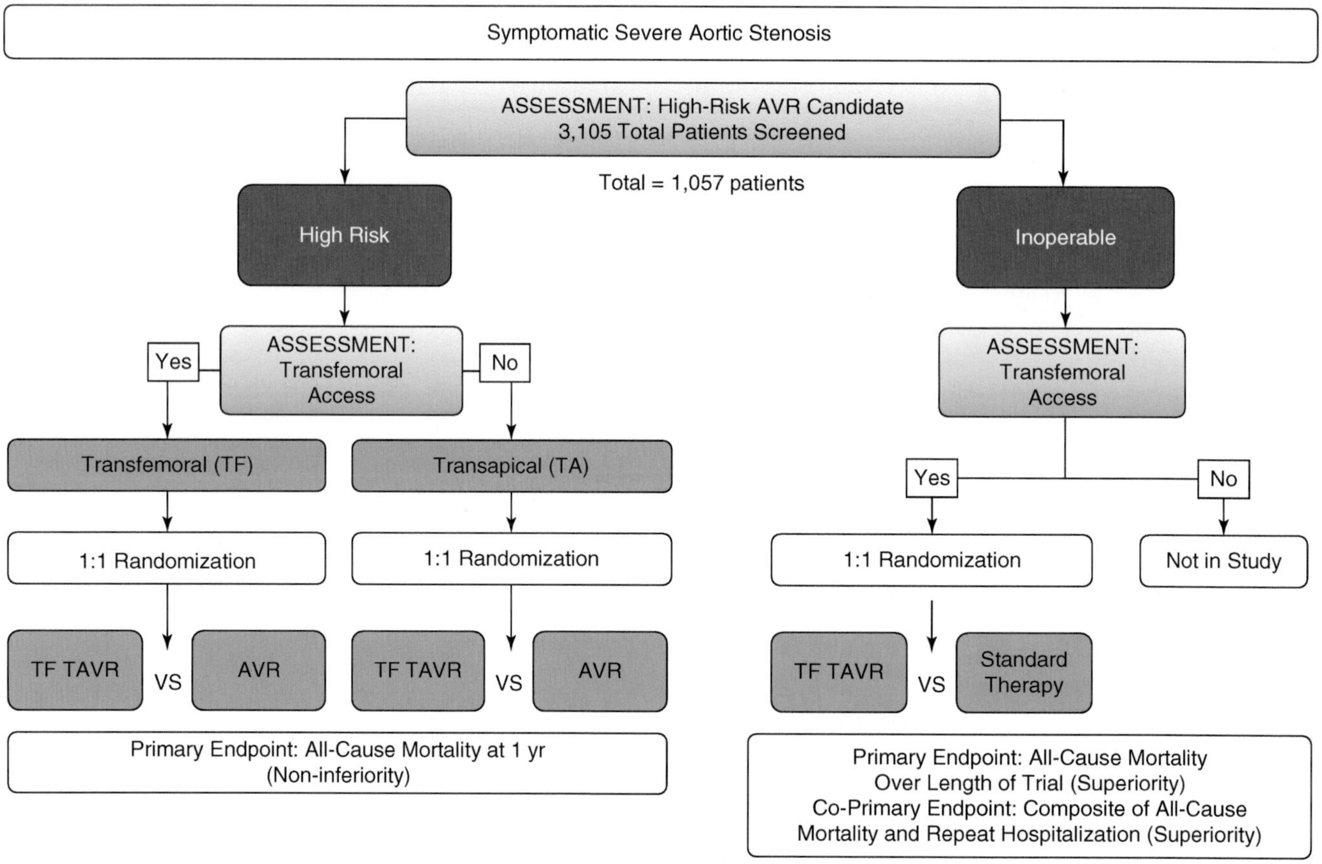

Fig. 10.6 PARTNER trial design. From Holmes DR Jr., et al. 2012 ACCF/AATS/SCAI/STS expert consensus document on transcatheter aortic valve replacement. J Am Coll Cardiol. 2012 Mar 27;59(13):1200–54. Reprinted with permission from Elsevier

Table 10.6 Major outcomes at 30 days and 1 year in Cohort B of the PARTNER trial

	30 days			1 year		
Characteristic	TAVR ($N = 179$)	Standard Rx ($N = 179$)	p value	TAVR ($N = 179$)	Standard Rx ($N = 179$)	p value
All-cause death (%)	5.0	2.8	0.41	30.7	49.7	<0.001
All-cause death or rehospitalization (%)	11.2	12.3	0.74	43.6	70.4	<0.001
Event-free MACCE (%)	90.5	94.4	NR	65.4	47.1	0.003
All stroke (%)	7.3	1.7	0.02	11.2	4.5	0.03
Major stroke (%)	5.6	1.1	0.04	8.4	3.9	0.12
All-cause death or major stroke (%)[a]	8.4	3.9	0.12	33.0	50.3	0.001
Major vascular complications (%)	16.8	1.1	<0.0001	17.3	2.2	<0.0001
Major bleeding (%)	20.6	3.9	<0.0001	28.4	14.4	<0.001
Pacemaker insertion (%)	3.4	5.0	0.60	4.5	7.8	0.27
Echocardiographic endpoints						
AV area (EOA) (cm^2)	1.5 ± 0.4	0.8 ± 0.2	<0.0001	1.6 ± 0.5	0.7 ± 0.32	<0.0001
Mean AV gradient (mmHg)	11.1 ± 6.6	33.0 ± 12.5	<0.0001	12.5 ± 10.3	44.4 ± 15.7	<0.0001

Cohort B includes only nonsurgical candidates in whom "inoperability" was formally defined as greater than 50% predicted probability of mortality or serious irreversible complication by 30 days by 1 cardiologist and 2 cardiothoracic surgeons

AV indicates aortic valve, *EOA* effective orifice area, *MACCE* major adverse cardiac and cerebrovascular events, *NR* not reported, *Rx* therapy, *TAVR* transcatheter aortic valve replacement

Data are based on Edwards Lifesciences' briefing document for the U.S. FDA Circulatory Devices Advisory Panel meeting on TAVR on July 21, 2011 (http://www.accessdata.fda.gov/cdrh_docs/pdf10/P100041b.pdf), and may show some discrepancies compared with the published manuscripts

From Holmes DR Jr., et al. 2012 ACCF/AATS/SCAI/STS expert consensus document on transcatheter aortic valve replacement. J Am Coll Cardiol. 2012 Mar 27;59(13):1200–54. Reprinted with permission from Elsevier

[a]All-cause death or major stroke was not a predefined endpoint

Table 10.7 Major outcomes at 30 days and 1 year in Cohort A of the PARTNER trial

	30 days			1 year		
Characteristic	TAVR ($N = 348$)	Surgical AVR ($N = 351$)	p value	TAVR ($N = 348$)	Surgical AVR ($N = 351$)	p value
Clinical outcomes						
All-cause death (%)	3.4	6.5	0.07	24.2	26.8	0.44
All-cause death or rehospitalization (%)	7.2	9.7	0.24	34.6	35.9	0.73
All stroke (%)	5.5	2.4	0.04	8.3	4.3	0.04
Major stroke (%)	3.8	2.1	0.20	5.1	2.4	0.07
All-cause death or major stroke (%)*	6.9	8.2	0.52	26.5	28.0	0.68
Major vascular complications (%)	17.0	3.8	<0.01	18.0	4.8	<0.01
Major bleeding (%)	9.3	19.5	<0.01	14.7	25.7	<0.01
Atrial fibrillation (%)	8.6	16.0	<0.01	12.1	17.1	0.07
Pacemaker insertion (%)	3.8	3.6	0.89	5.7	5.0	0.68
Echocardiographic endpoints						
AV area (EOA) (cm^2)	1.7 ± 0.5	1.5 ± 0.4	0.001	1.6 ± 0.5	1.4 ± 0.5	0.002
Mean AV gradient (mmHg)	9.9 ± 4.8	10.8 ± 5.0	0.16	10.2 ± 4.3	11.5 ± 5.4	0.008

Cohort A includes patients determined to be at high operative risk defined as predicted operative mortality of ≥15% and/or an STS risk score of ≥10%. The STS risk algorithm is based on the presence of coexisting illnesses in order to predict 30-day operative mortality

AV indicates aortic valve, *AVR* aortic valve replacement, *EOA* effective orifice area, *TAVR* transcatheter aortic valve replacement

From Holmes DR Jr., et al. 2012 ACCF/AATS/SCAI/STS expert consensus document on transcatheter aortic valve replacement. J Am Coll Cardiol. 2012 Mar 27;59(13):1200–54. Reprinted with permission from Elsevier

The results of the high-risk operative cohort (Cohort A) demonstrated a statistically nonsignificant difference in all-cause mortality at 30-days (TAVR vs. SAVR, 3.4% vs. 6.5%; $P = 0.07$), 1-year (24.2% vs. 26.8%), 2-year (33.9% vs. 35%), 3-year (44.2% vs. 44.8%), and 5-year (67.8% vs. 62.4%) follow-up [21, 62]. Although the rates of all neurologic events were higher after TAVR at 30 days and 1 year (5.5% vs. 2.4% and 8.3% vs. 4.3%, respectively; $P < 0.05$), there was no difference in 5 year outcome (15.9% vs. 14.7%, $p = 0.35$), and rates of major strokes were not significantly different between TAVR and SAVR at 30 days (3.8% vs. 2.1%; $P = 0.2$) or at 1 year (5.1% vs. 2.4%; $P = 0.07$) and 5 years (10.4% vs. 11.3%, $p = 0.61$). Repeat hospitalization rates were similar between the two groups at 5 years (42.3%

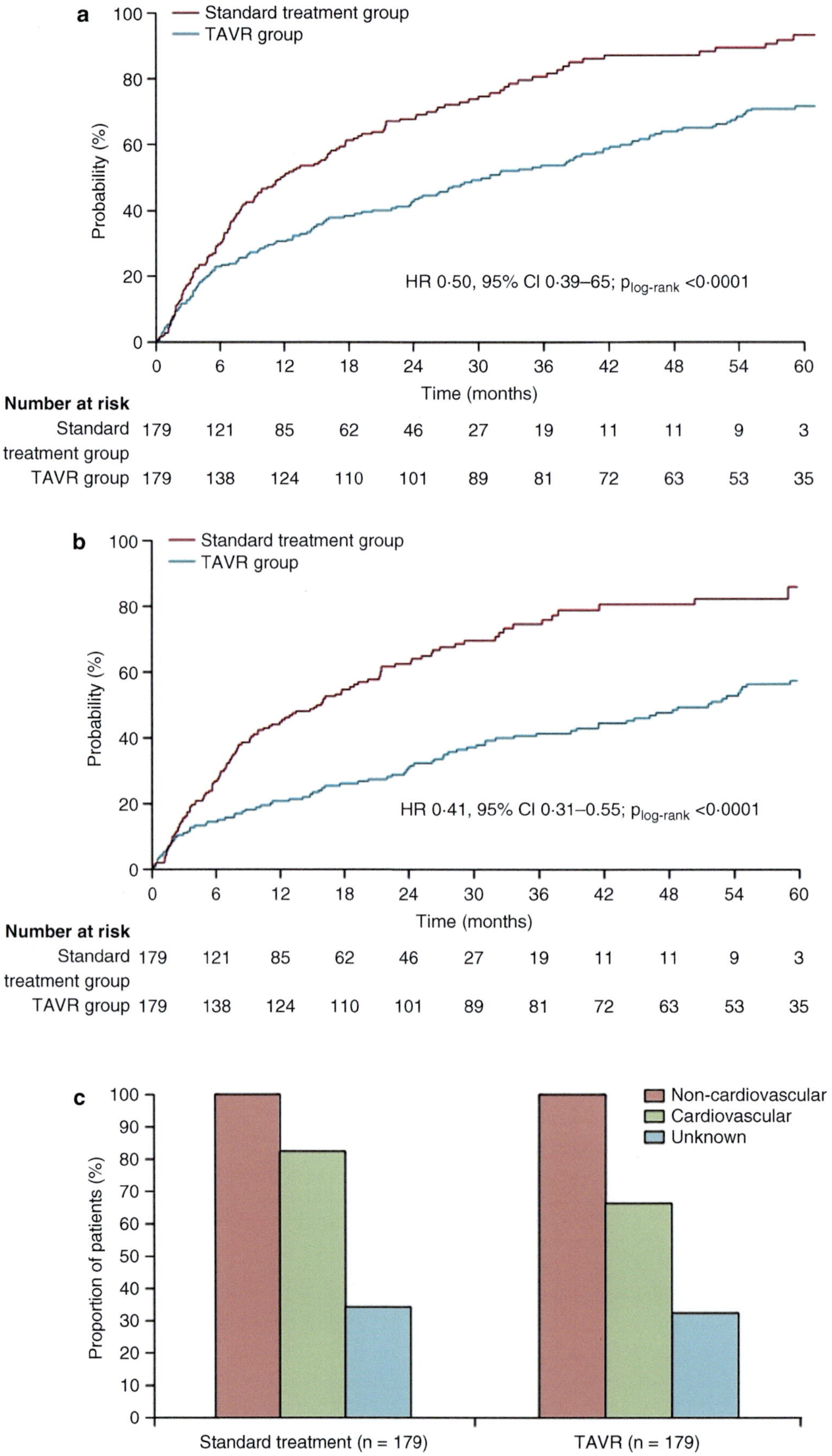

Fig. 10.7 (**a**) Kaplan-Meier analysis of all-cause mortality for the intention-to-treat population. (**b**) Cardiovascular mortality and causes of death (**c**) *TAVR* transcatheter aortic valve replacement, *HR* hazard ratio. From Kapadia SR, et al. [62]. Reprinted with permission from Elsevier

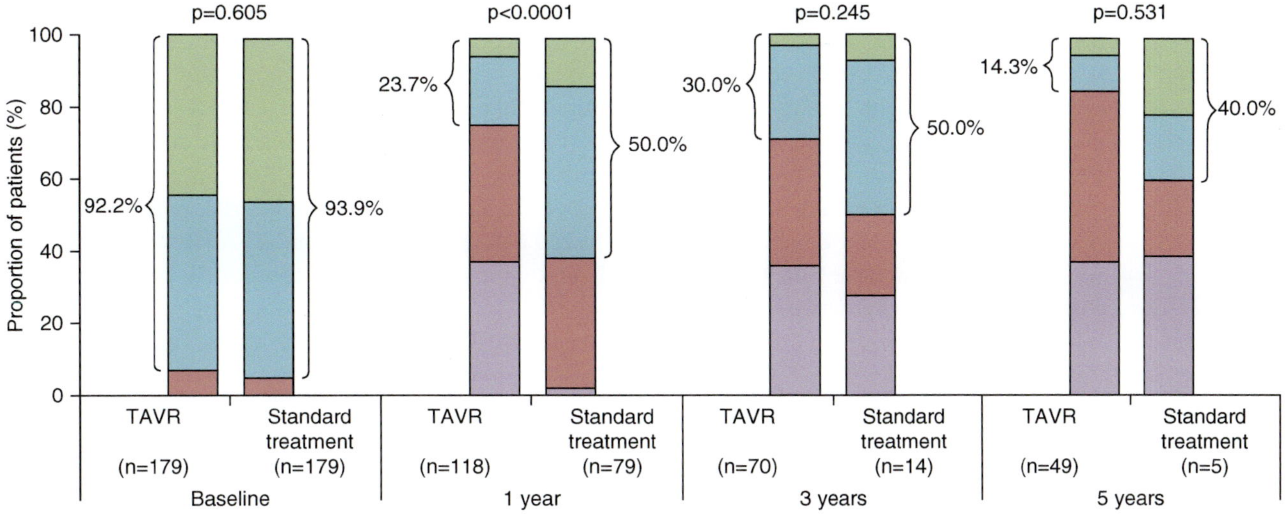

Fig. 10.8 New York Heart Association functional class of the survivors. *p* values are for TAVR versus standard treatment for the full range of functional classes. *TAVR* transcatheter aortic valve replacement (green = class IV, Aqua = class III. Brown = Class II and Lilac = Class I. From Kapadia SR, et al. [62]. Reprinted with permission from Elsevier

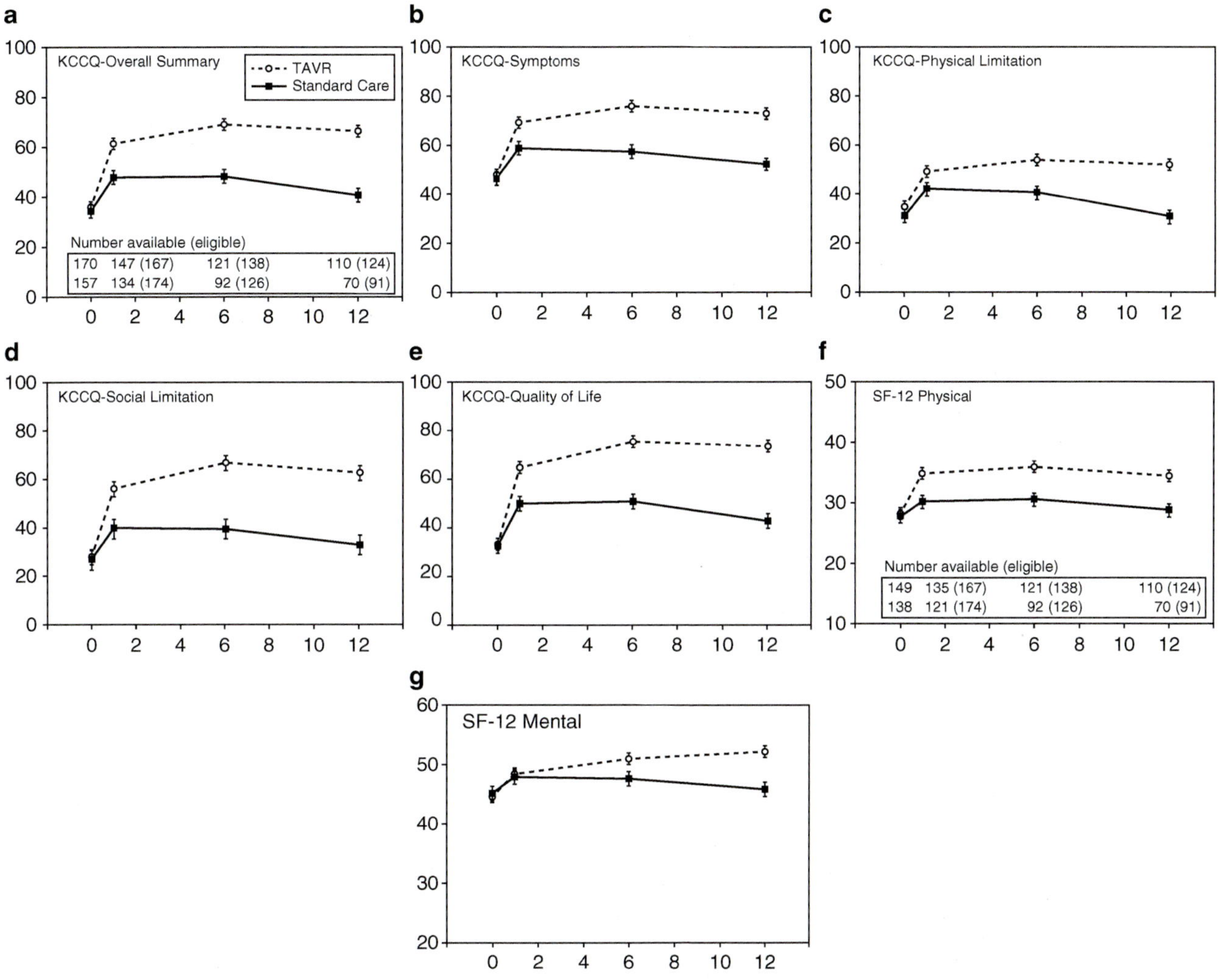

Fig. 10.9 Predicted mean values with SEs, derived from longitudinal growth curve models for the Kansas City Cardiomyopathy Questionnaire (KCCQ) overall summary scale (**a**), KCCQ Sub-Scales (**b–e**), and Short-Form 12 General Health Survey (SF-12) physical and mental health scales (**f–g**) plotted by group over time (in months). The numbers of respondents by group at each time point are shown at the bottom of panels **a** and **f**. The numbers in parentheses are the number eligible (alive and not withdrawn) for evaluation at each time point. TAVR indicates transcatheter aortic valve replacement. From Reynolds MR, et al. [63]. Reprinted with permission from Wolters Kluwer Health, Inc.

vs. 34.2%, $p = 0.17$). There were other important differences in between the two groups [65], including more major vascular complications at 30 days after TAVR (11% vs. 3.2%; $P < 0.001$) and more major bleeding with SAVR (19.5% vs. 9.3%; $P < 0.001$) and new-onset atrial fibrillation (16% vs. 8.6%; $P = 0.006$) after SAVR. Five year valve hemodynamics were similar between the two groups. The improvement of symptoms was similar after TAVR and SAVR and was sustained at 3 years in both groups. Based on the above results TAVR was considered a viable alternative to SAVR in patients classified at high risk, after a thorough evaluation by the "heart team" (Figs. 10.10 and 10.11).

The PARTNER II trial clarified the role of SAPIEN and SAPIEN XT valves in patients with severe AS with varying degrees of surgical risk (inoperable, high risk [STS score > 8%] and intermediate risk [STS score 4–8%]) [66, 67]. It had two arms: (1) an inoperable cohort, which randomized patients to SAPIEN XT versus SAPIEN via a TF approach [66]; and (2) a moderate-risk cohort, which randomized patients to SAVR versus TAVR with the SAPIEN XT and included the TA, transaortic, or TF approach (Fig. 10.12) [67]. In the first arm, there was no difference between SAPIEN and SAPIEN XT in mortality or stroke but vascular complications were fewer in the lower profile

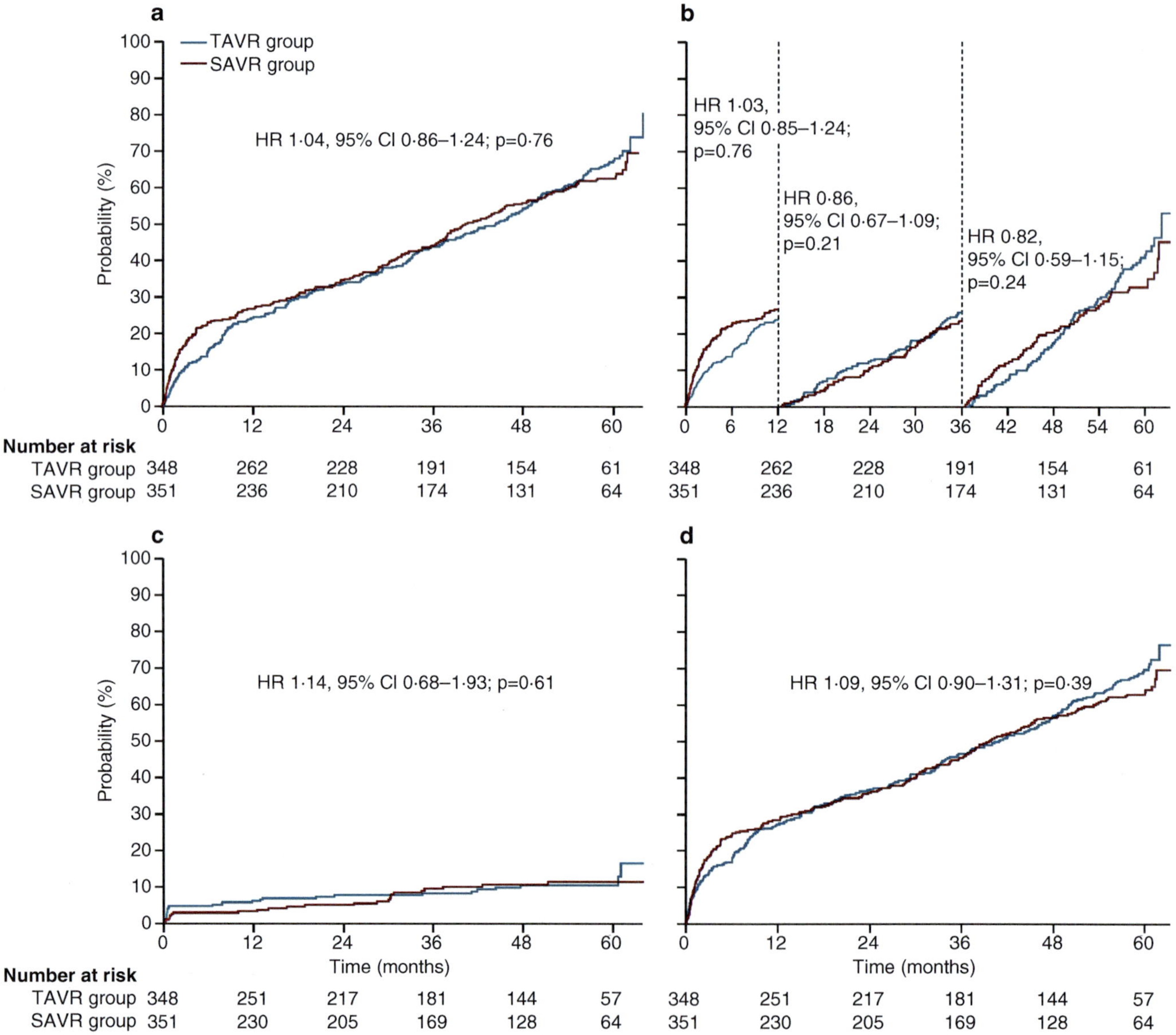

Fig. 10.10 Mortality and cardiovascular outcomes. Kaplan-Meier analysis of all-cause death in the intention-to-treat population (**a**) and by landmark analysis (**b**); stroke or transient ischemic attack (**c**); and stroke, transient ischemic attack, or death from any cause (**d**). *HR* hazard ration, *TAVR* transcatheter aortic valve replacement, *SAVR* surgical aortic valve replacement. From Mack MJ, et al. [65]. Reprinted with permission from Elsevier

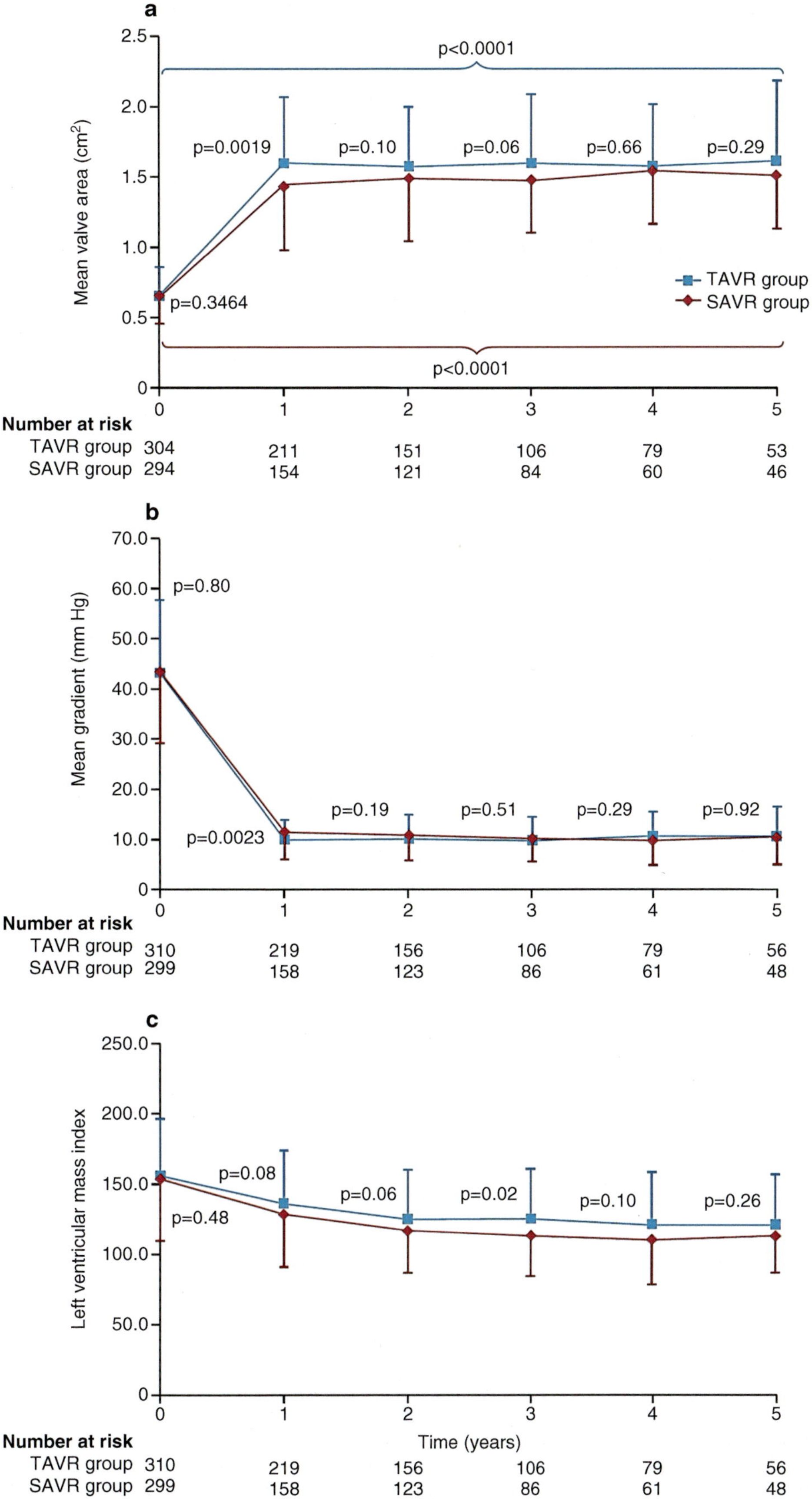

Fig. 10.11 Echocardiographic findings. Aortic valve area (**a**); mean gradient (**b**); and left ventricular mass regression (**c**). Points are means, bars are SDs. *TAVR* transcatheter aortic valve replacement, *SAVR* surgical aortic valve replacement. From Mack MJ, et al. [65]. Reprinted with permission from Elsevier

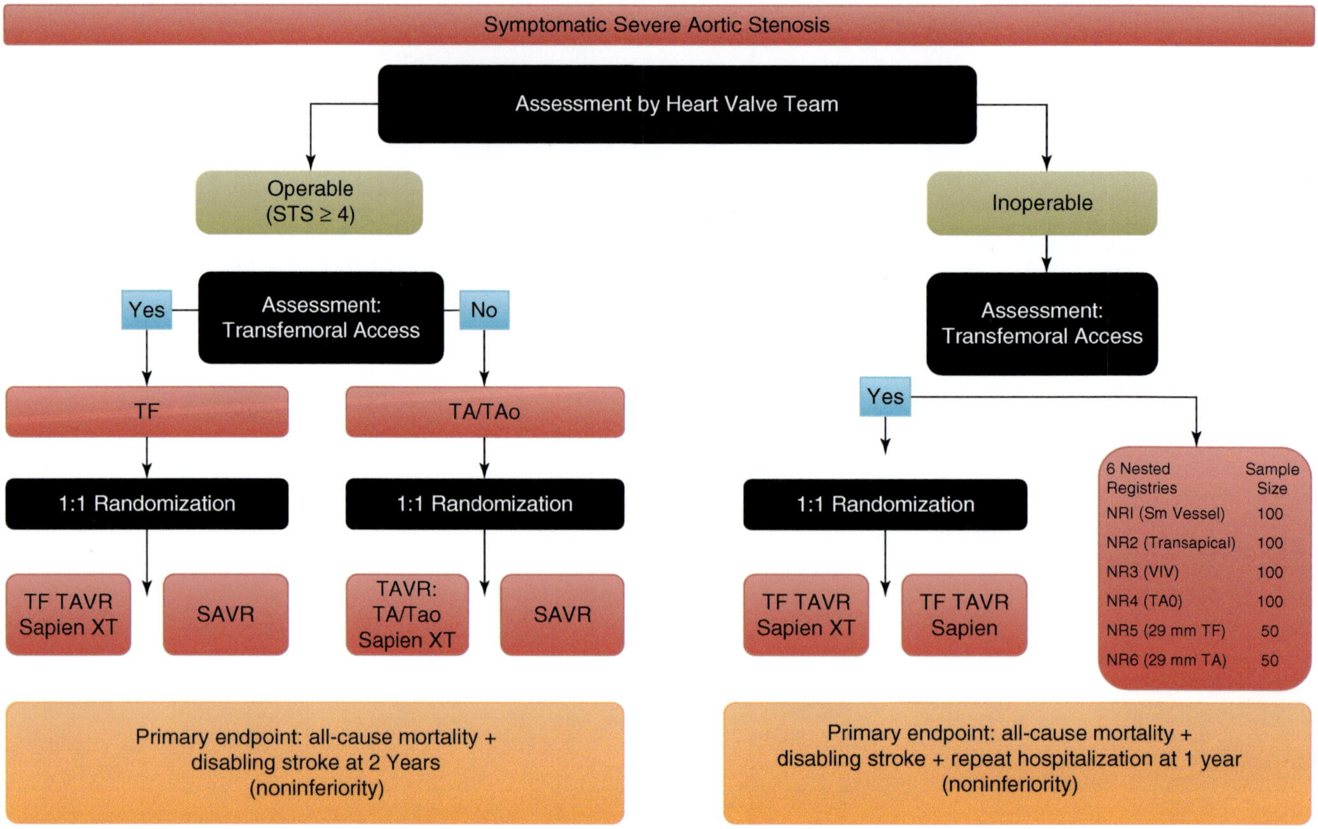

Fig. 10.12 PARTNER II study design. The PARTNER II study was designed to compare Sapien XT with the Sapien valve in surgically inoperable patients. The second arm randomized patients in the intermediate-surgical-risk category to undergo TAVR versus SAVR. *TAo* transaortic. From Rao RS et al. [68]. Reprinted with permission from Cardiac Interventions Today, Bryn Mawr Communications

SAPIEN XT TAVR. In the second arm, TAVR and SAVR were similar in mortality and stroke. However from the femoral approach (a prespecified endpoint) TAVR was superior to SAVR with respect to mortality and disabling stroke.

Moderate/severe paravalvular aortic regurgitation has been associated with adverse clinical outcomes, including higher mortality on long term in the PARTNER trial [69]. Even mild paravalvular regurgitation was associated with increased 1 year and 2-year mortality as compared to patients with no or trace paravalvular regurgitation. The Sapien 3 valve, as described above, was developed with the intent to reduce paravalvular leak as one of its main goals and early results confirm a low incidence of aortic insufficiency with the SAPIEN 3 TAVR. In a propensity-matched comparison of the SAPIEN 3 TAVR with SAVR, 98% of TAVR patients were free of more than mild aortic regurgitation [70]. SAPIEN 3 was superior to SAVR with respect to a combined endpoint of mortality, stroke and aortic regurgitation and the balloon-expandable platform has shown consistent reductions in mortality and stroke over time (Fig. 10.13).

Medtronic CoreValve Self-Expanding Valve

The CoreValve comprises a single layer, trileaflet porcine pericardial tissue valve in a nitinol frame. Nitinol is a nickel–titanium alloy with shape memory making it a desirable material for self-expanding transcatheter valves. The valve is available in four sizes (23, 26, 29, and 31 mm) (Table 10.8). The inflow segment, which is deployed within the aortic annulus, is intended to extend 4–6 mm below the annulus where the highest radial strength displaces the native aortic valve leaflets and apposes the stent against the annulus. The physical properties of the nitinol frame allow all sizes of the CoreValve prosthesis to be compressed and loaded into an 18Fr delivery system, and regain the original shape after deployment.

CoreValve was approved for commercial use in extreme risk patients in the United States in January 2013 based on the results of the CoreValve US Pivotal Extreme Risk Trial [71]. This was a non-randomized evaluation of CoreValve in 471 patients with severe symptomatic AS who were at extreme risk of SAVR (i.e., >50% chance of mortality or irreversible morbidity). The average patient age was 83 years and had high surgical risk (STS-PROM, 10.3% ± 5.6%; 92%

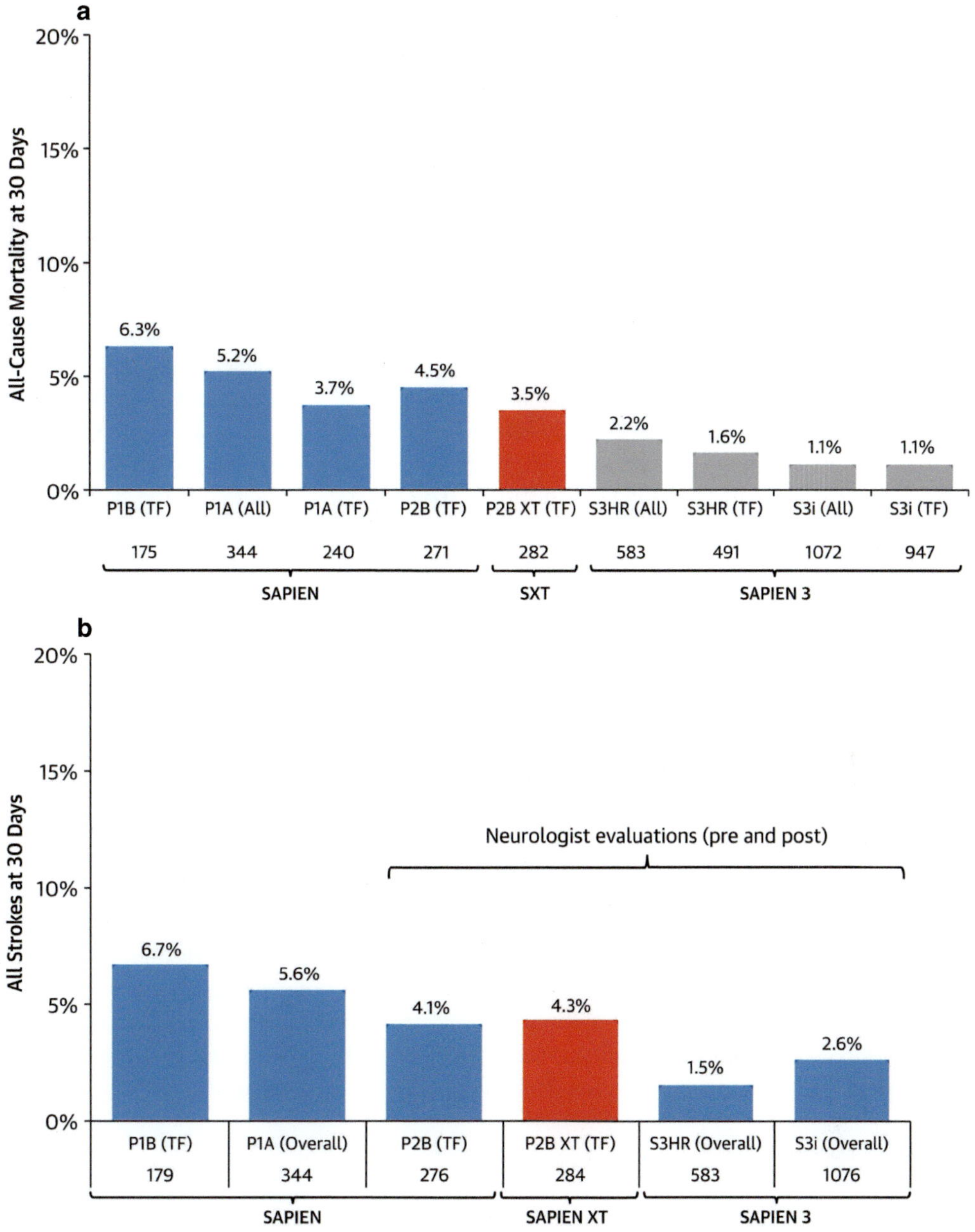

Fig. 10.13 Temporal trends in mortality and stroke after TAVR. (**a**) Reduction in all-cause mortality at 30 days with subsequent generations of Edwards Lifesciences Sapien valves (as-treated analysis) in the PARTNER I and II trials. (**b**) Reduction in strokes with different generations of Sapien valves in the PARTNER I and III trials. *P1A* PARTNER (Placement of Aortic Transcatheter Valve Trial) 1A trial, *P1B* PARTNER 1B trial, *P2B* PARTNER 2B trial, *S3HR* PARTNER 2 Sapien 3 high-risk cohort, *S3i* PAETNER 2 Sapien 3 intermediate-risk cohort, *SXT* Sapien XT valve, *TAVR* transcatheter aortic valve replacement, *TF* transfemoral. From Vahl TP, Kodali SK, Leon MB. Transcatheter Aortic Valve Replacement 2016: A Modern-Day "Through the Looking-Glass" Adventure. J Am Coll Cardiol. 2016 Mar 29;67(12):1472–1487. Reprinted with permission from Elsevier

Table 10.8 Manufacturer's recommended sizing algorithm for the self-expanding valve

Annular dimension	Valve size 23 mm	26 mm	29 mm	31 mm
Mean diameter range, mm	18–20	20–23	23–27	26–29
Perimeter range, mm	56.5–62.8	62.8–72.3	72.3–84.8	81.7–91.1
Area range, mm^2	254.5–314.2	314.2–415.5	415.5–572.6	530.9–660.5

For the self-expanding valve, the mean annular diameter and perimeter oversizing ranges from 7% to 30%. The annular area oversizing ranges from 7% to 69% according to the manufacturer

From: Hahn RT, et al. Recommendations for comprehensive intraprocedural echocardiographic imaging during TAVR. JACC Cardiovasc Imaging. 2015 Mar;8(3):261–87. Reprinted with permission from Elsevier

with NYHA class III or IV symptoms). The primary endpoint of death or major stroke in the CoreValve US Pivotal Trial occurred in 25.5%, which was lower than the lower band of the 95% confidence interval of medically treated patients with PARTNER B trial (43%). The rate of major stroke at 1 year and 2 year was 4.3 and 5.1%, respectively. Procedural events at 30 days included life-threatening/disabling bleeding (12.7%), and major vascular complications (8.2%), and need for permanent pacemaker placement (22.2%). Interestingly, moderate or severe paravalvular aortic regurgitation, which was 10.5% immediately after the procedure, decreased to 4.1% in follow-up at 1 year. There was a significant improvement in the NYHA status with 92% patients noting improvement in at least 1 functional class and 58% improvement in at least 2 functional classes by 2 years.

The randomized arm of the CoreValve US Pivotal trial (high-risk study) comparing CoreValve TAVR with SAVR showed interesting results [72]. For the first time in a large trial overall, all-cause mortality at 1 year was significantly lower in the TAVR group compared with the surgical group (14.1 vs. 18.9% at 1 year and 22.2% vs. 28.6% at 2 years, $p = 0.04$). There was no significant difference in the stroke rate between the two groups (8.7% vs. 12.5% at 1 year but was less with TAVR 10.9 vs. 16.6% at 2 years, $p = 0.05$). The rate of permanent pacemaker implantation at 1 year and 2 years was 20% and 22.5%. The rates of moderate or severe paravalvular regurgitation were higher in the TAVR group; however, most of these patients (76.2%) had mild or no regurgitation at 1 year. Patients undergoing SAVR had a significantly higher incidence of new-onset or worsening atrial fibrillation, acute kidney injury, and major bleeding. Interestingly, TAVR was shown to have better echocardiographic indices of valve stenosis with lower mean gradient and higher valve area at 1 year and 2 year as compared to SAVR.

The rate of permanent pacemaker implantations after self-expanding valves, including CoreValve, is noted to be significantly higher as compared to balloon-expandable valves. A recent meta-analysis showed 6.5% permanent pacemaker implantation rate with SAPIEN valve as compared to 25.8% with CoreValve ($p < 0.001$) [73]. On a similar note, the frequency of left bundle branch block (LBBB) after CoreValve is much higher than the SAPIEN valve. This was likely from the increased radial force applied at the annulus and LVOT by the self-expanding valves leading to edema and inflammation of the underlying conduction system. A combined analysis of all PARTNER data showed that 10.5% of all patients undergoing TAVR with normal baseline conduction developed persistent LBBB and this was associated with higher rate of pacemaker implantation and lack of improvement in the LVEF after TAVR. There was no association with increased all-cause mortality with persistent LBBB [74].

The CHOICE (Comparison of Transcatheter Heart Valves in High Risk Patients With Severe Aortic Stenosis: Medtronic CoreValve vs. Edwards SAPIEN XT) trial is the only randomized comparison of the balloon-expandable valve with the self-expanding valve [75]. The trial was an investigator-initiated, multicenter, randomized trial which evaluated procedural success (composite end point of successful vascular access and deployment of the device and retrieval of the delivery system, correct position of the device, intended performance of the heart valve without moderate or severe regurgitation, and only 1 valve implanted in the proper anatomical location) with both valve platforms in high-risk patients who were candidates for TF TAVR. Device success was noted in 77.5% of the patients in the self-expanding valve group as compared to 95.9% patients in the balloon-expandable valve group. This difference was primarily associated with increased frequency of moderate to severe paravalvular regurgitation (18.3% vs. 4.1%, $p < 0.001$) and higher rate of implant of more than 1 valve (5.8% vs. 0.8%) in the self-expanding valve group. Cardiovascular mortality, bleeding, and vascular complications were similar in both the groups. Placement of new permanent pacemaker was more common with the self-expanding valves (34.6% vs. 17.3%, $p = 0.001$) [75] (Figs. 10.14, 10.15, 10.16, 10.17, 10.18, 10.19, 10.20, and 10.21).

In the SURTAVI trial CoreValve was compared to SAVR in intermediate risk patients. The combined endpoint of mortality and disabling stroke at 2 years did not differ between TAVR(12.6%) and SAVR (14%). The TAVR group had less kidney injury and transfusion requirement but more aortic insufficiency and need for a pacemaker than the surgical group [58].

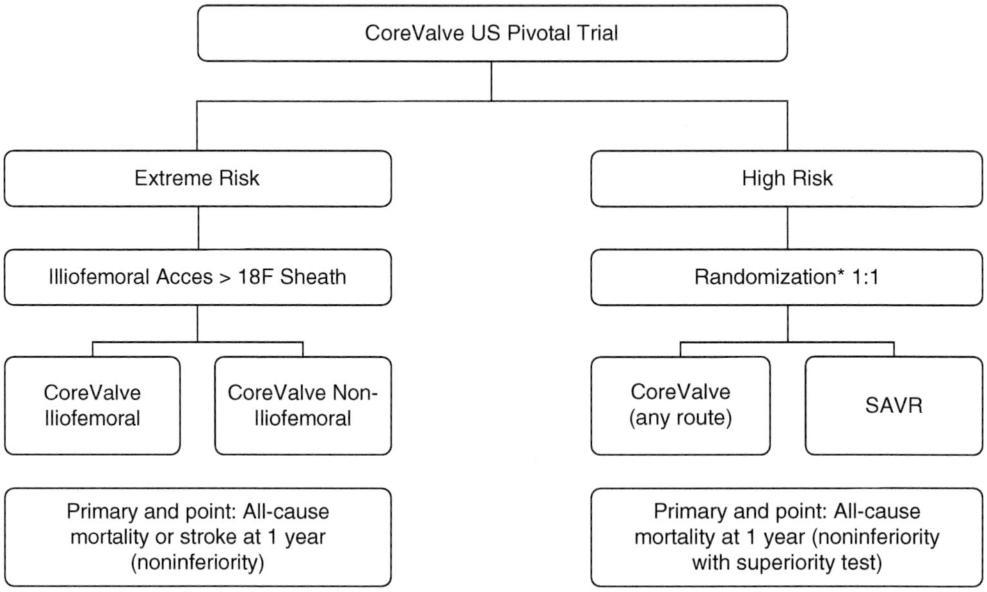

Fig. 10.14 The CoreValve US pivotal trial design. *Randomization stratified by intended access route. From Barker CM, Reardon MJ. The CoreValve US Pivotal Trial. Semin Thorac Cardiovasc Surg. 2014 Autumn;26(3):179–86. Reprinted with permission from Elsevier

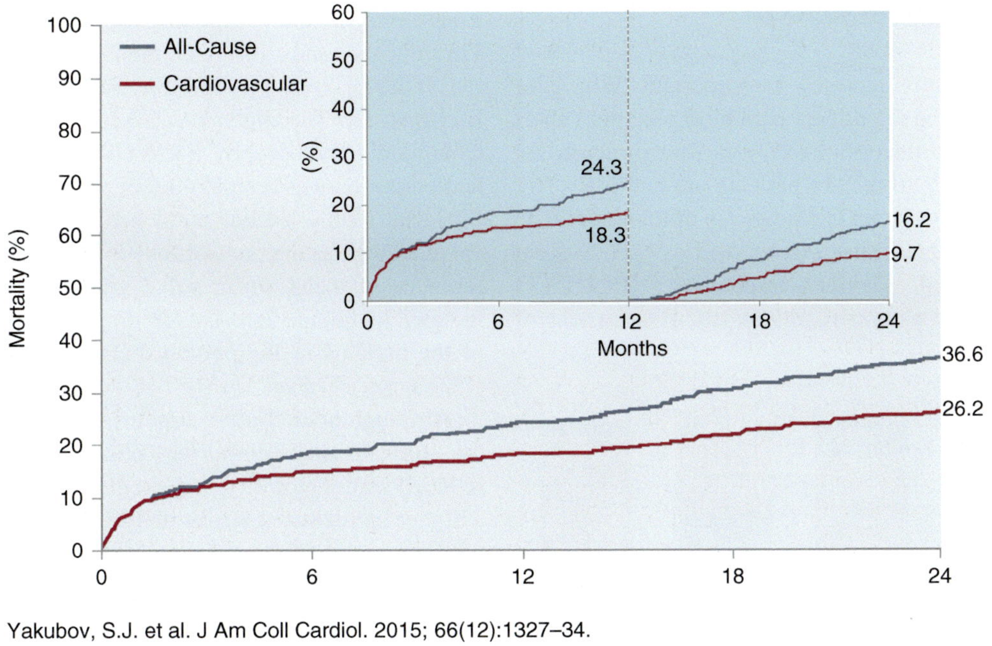

Fig. 10.15 Long-term outcomes after TAVR: Kaplan-Meier estimates of all-cause and cardiovascular mortality through 2 years. (Inset) Landmark survival analysis of all-cause and cardiovascular mortality for the 1st year after TAVR for all patients (left) and during the second year after TAVR for patients alive at 1 year (right). *TAVR* transcatheter aortic valve replacement. From Yakubov SJ, Adams DH, Watson DR, et al. 2-Year Outcomes After Iliofemoral Self-Expanding Transcatheter Aortic Valve Replacement in Patients With Severe Aortic Stenosis Deemed Extreme Risk for Surgery. J Am Coll Cardiol. 2015 Sep 22;66(12):1327–34. Reprinted with permission from Elsevier

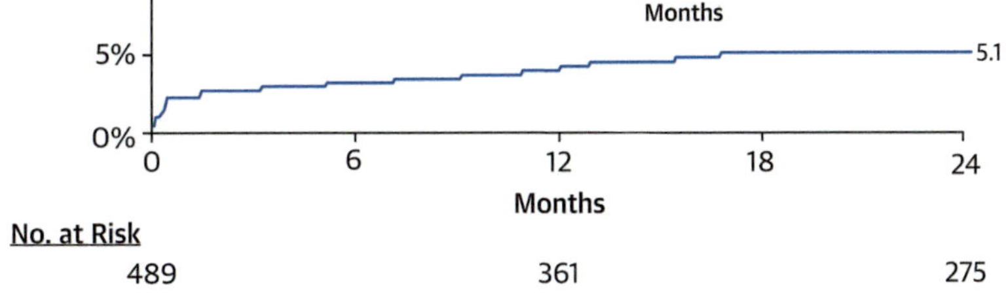

Fig. 10.16 Kaplan-Meier estimates of major stroke through 2 years. (Inset) Landmark analysis for the first year after TAVR for all patients (left) and during the second year after TAVR for patients alive at 1 year (right). *TAVR* transcatheter aortic valve replacement. From Yakubov SJ, Adams DH, Watson DR, et al. 2-Year Outcomes After Iliofemoral Self-Expanding Transcatheter Aortic Valve Replacement in Patients With Severe Aortic Stenosis Deemed Extreme Risk for Surgery. J Am Coll Cardiol. 2015 Sep 22;66(12):1327–34. Reprinted with permission from Elsevier

Subclinical Leaflet Thrombosis

Makkar et al. recently reported an important finding of reduced leaflet motion in patients with bioprosthetic valves based on analysis of data obtained from four dimensional volume-rendered CT from 187 patients after TAVR [76]. This was based on data from CT subgroup of the PORTICO (Portico Re-sheathable Transcatheter Aortic Valve System U.S. Investigational Device Exemption [PORTICO IDE]) study as well as two registries (the Assessment of Transcatheter and Surgical Aortic Bioprosthetic Valve Thrombosis and Its Treatment with Anticoagulation [RESOLVE] registry, and the Subclinical Aortic Valve Bioprosthesis Thrombosis Assessed with Four-Dimensional Computed Tomography [SAVORY] registry). Reduced leaflet motion was seen in 40% of patients in the PORTICO IDE trial with a similar incidence noted in the PORTICO valve as well as the control SAPIEN XT valve with no differences in mean aortic valve gradients in patients with reduced leaflet motion. This finding was also noted in 13% of the patients in the pooled registries as well as in 2/27 (7%) surgical valves.

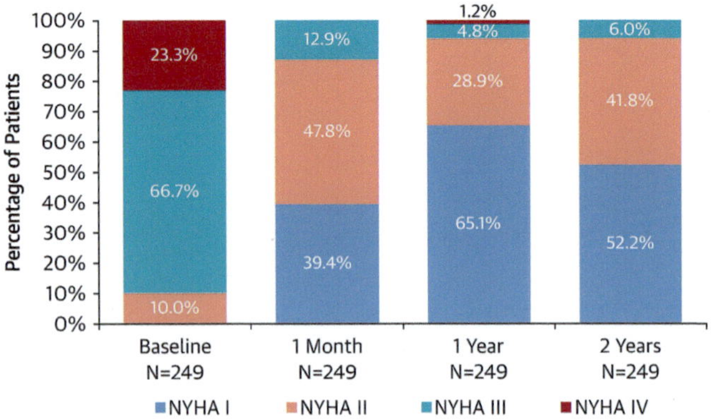

Fig. 10.17 NYHA functional classification through 2 years. Symptom status for 249 patients with matched datasets at all time points are presented. *NYHA* New York Heart Association. From Yakubov SJ, Adams DH, Watson DR, et al. 2-Year Outcomes After Iliofemoral Self-Expanding Transcatheter Aortic Valve Replacement in Patients With Severe Aortic Stenosis Deemed Extreme Risk for Surgery. J Am Coll Cardiol. 2015 Sep 22;66(12):1327–34. Reprinted with permission from Elsevier

Although no definitive conclusions could be made from the study, it made important observations. Patients with reduced leaflet mobility in the registries were noted to have a higher incidence of stroke or TIA as compared to patients with normal leaflet mobility (18% vs. 1%, $P = 0.007$). Additionally, as compared to patients on dual antiplatelet therapy, those on therapeutic anticoagulation after TAVR were noted to have a much lower risk of reduced leaflet motion on CT (21/41 patients vs. 0/8 patients, $p = 0.007$). Importantly, in follow-up CT in the PORTICO IDE, all 11 patients with reduced leaflet motion who received therapeutic anticoagulation showed full recovery of normal leaflet motion, suggesting possible subclinical leaflet thrombosis as the cause of the reduced leaflet mobility in these patients. Further studies are needed to evaluate the long-term relevance of these findings as well as to establish protocols to help prevent "possible subclinical leaflet thrombosis."

Fig. 10.18 PVAR at discharge and 1 year. The proportion of patients with varying degrees of paravalvular aortic regurgitation (PVAR) in 383 patients with paired echocardiography studies available. From Oh JK, Little SH, Abdelmoneim SS, et al. Regression of Paravalvular Aortic Regurgitation and Remodeling of Self-Expanding Transcatheter Aortic Valve: An Observation From the CoreValve U.S. Pivotal Trial. JACC Cardiovasc Imaging. 2015 Dec;8(12):1364–1375. Reprinted with permission from Elsevier

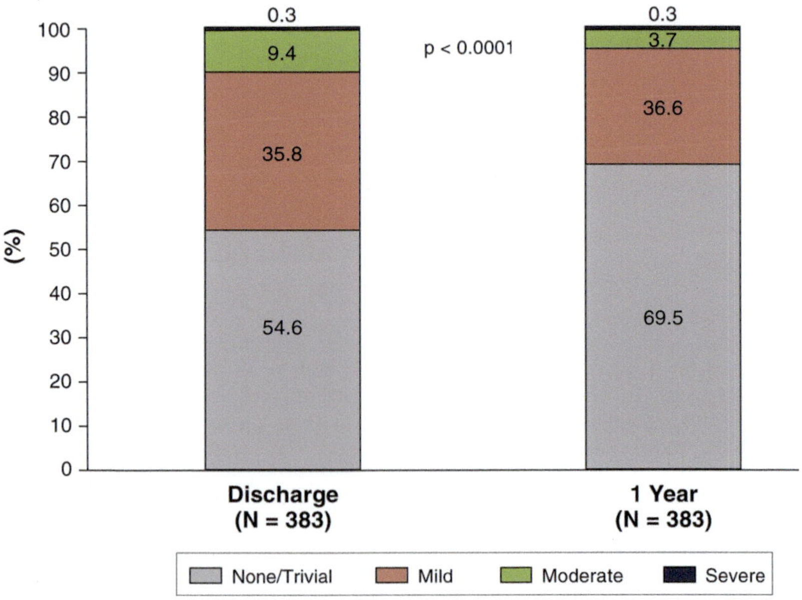

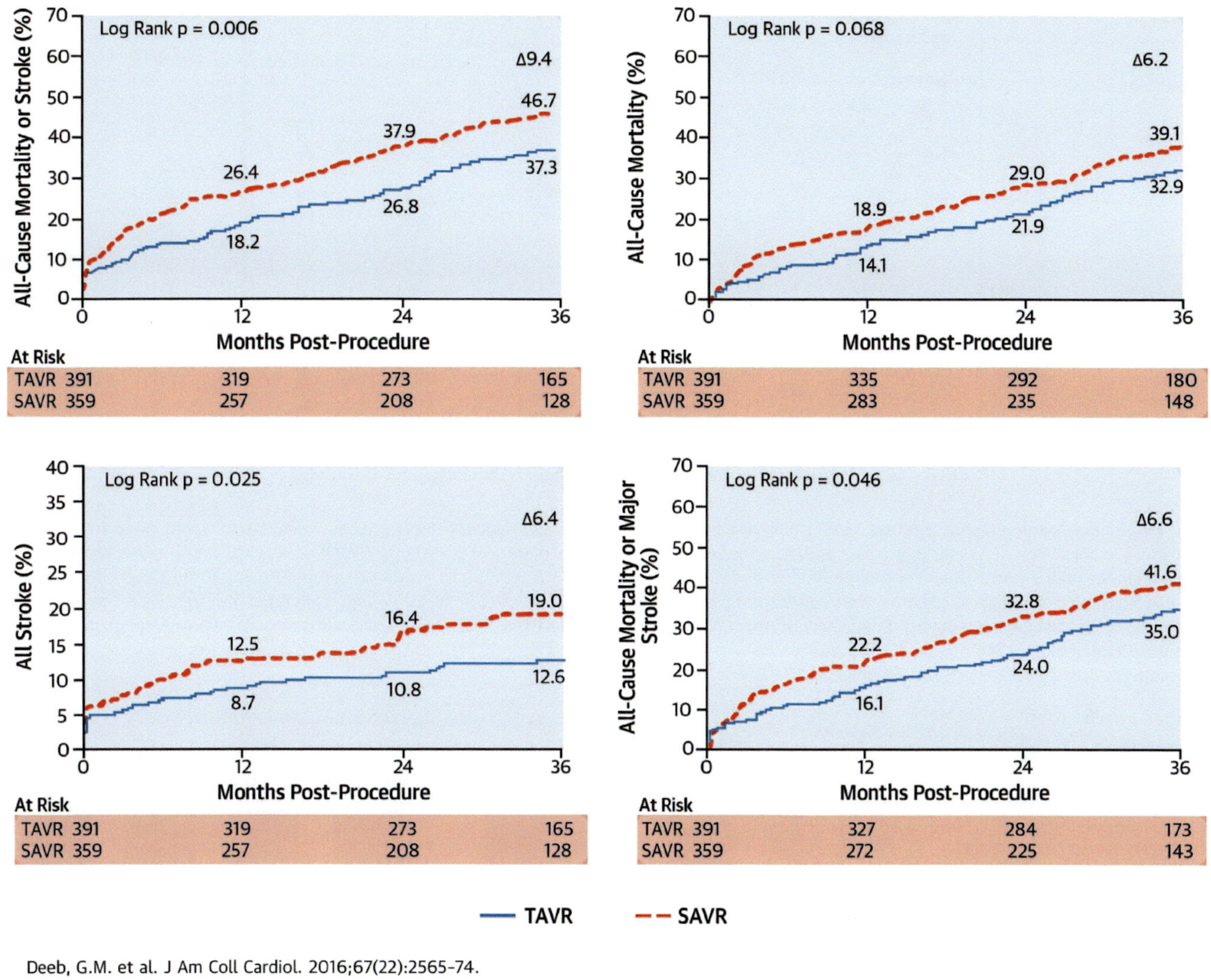

Fig. 10.19 TAVR versus SAVR: clinical outcomes at 3 years. Kaplan-Meier survival estimates for all-cause mortality or any stroke, all-cause mortality, any stroke, and all-cause mortality or major stroke. *SAVR* surgical aortic valve replacement, *TAVR* transcatheter aortic valve replacement. From Deeb GM, Reardon MJ, Chetcuti S, et al. 3-Year Outcomes in High-Risk Patients Who Underwent Surgical or Transcatheter Aortic Valve Replacement. J Am Coll Cardiol. 2016 Jun 7;67(22):2565–74

Newer Valve Systems

Although there have been promising results from the first- and second-generation TAVR platforms, they still suffer from limitations which have contributed to suboptimal outcomes. This includes large delivery sheaths contributing to vascular complications and necessitating other access routes, lack of precise positioning control of the delivery system resulting in improper valve positioning leading to coronary obstruction (too high placement) or conduction abnormalities (too low placement), as well as paravalvular regurgitation (either from under-sizing or improper placement or increased Aorta-LVOT angulation). Several newer devices are in development that aim to reduce these limitations.

New TAVR Systems Currently Undergoing Trials

The new Edwards self-expanding TAVR system, Centera, has a contoured short frame height, and is made from treated bovine pericardium attached to a nitinol frame with a polyethylene terephthalate skirt to reduce paravalvular regurgitation. It is incorporated within a 14 French motorized delivery catheter allowing the valve to be fully retrieved and redeployed before final implantation. The current version of the device was improved based on preliminary studies with a 0% pacemaker rate and a low rate of paravalvular regurgitation, which makes this device an attractive option.

The CoreValve Evolut R is a next generation self-expanding TAVR system, which is designed to be fully

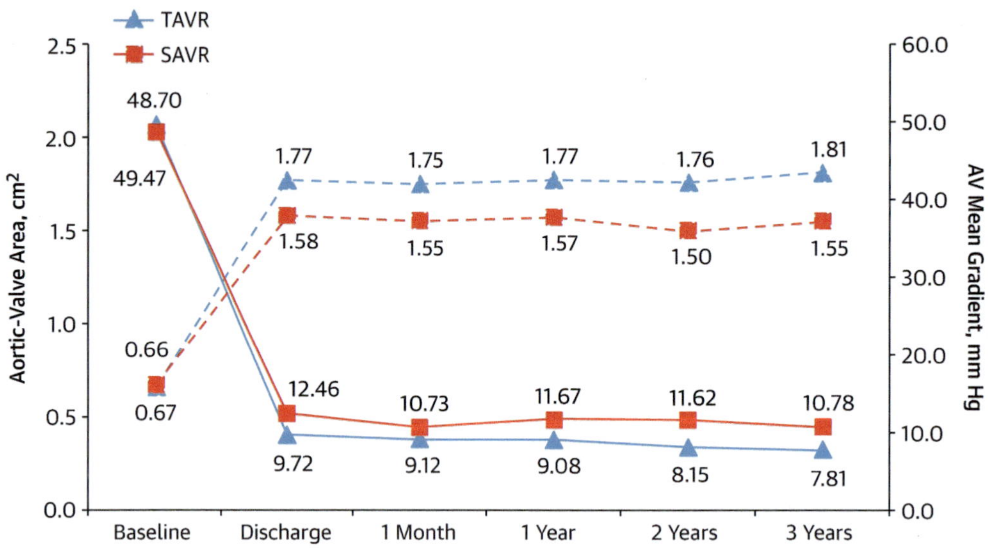

Fig. 10.20 Echocardiographic findings over time: paired analysis. Reduction in aortic valve (AV) mean gradient and increased AV area are maintained through 3 years. Data reported on the basis of site-reported echocardiographic findings in patients with echocardiographic measurements at all time points reported. Paired sets of mean AV gradient data were available for 174 TAVR and 113 SAVR patients; AV area was available for 126 TAVR and 85 SAVR patients. TAVR was associated with significantly lower gradients; and larger aortic valve areas at each time point (all $p < 0.05$). SAVR = surgical aortic valve replacement; *TAVR* transcatheter aortic valve replacement. From Deeb GM, Reardon MJ, Chetcuti S, et al. 3-Year Outcomes in High-Risk Patients Who Underwent Surgical or Transcatheter Aortic Valve Replacement. J Am Coll Cardiol. 2016 Jun 7;67(22):2565–74

Fig. 10.21 Total aortic regurgitation over time: paired analysis. Site-reported total aortic regurgitation at discharge, 1 year, 2 years, and 3 years for patients with echocardiographic measurements at each time point reported. Abbreviations as in Fig. 10.19. From Deeb GM, Reardon MJ, Chetcuti S, et al. 3-Year Outcomes in High-Risk Patients Who Underwent Surgical or Transcatheter Aortic Valve Replacement. J Am Coll Cardiol. 2016 Jun 7;67(22):2565–74

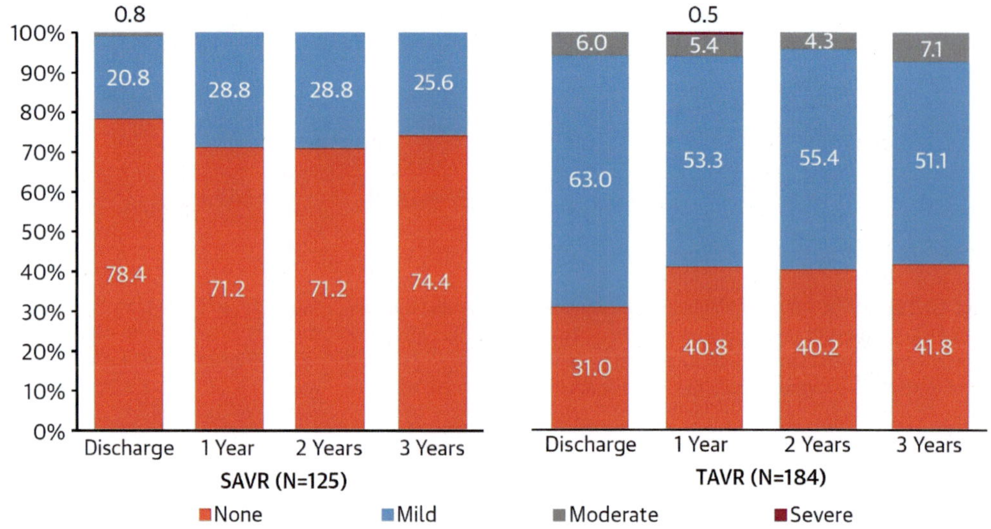

repositionable, resheathable, and recapturable through an 18F system. It retains the cell design of the first-generation CoreValve® device, with the large cell design facilitating coronary artery access and preserving conformability in order to fit noncircular and heavily calcified annuli. The overall height of the Evolut® is about 10 mm shorter than the first-generation CoreValve® in order to optimize the fit in patients with angulated aortic anatomy. However, the height of the pericardial skirt (12 mm) is preserved to provide a seal and reduce paravalvular leaks. This was tested in a valve-in-valve study with 100% procedural success and 0% pacemaker implantation rate [77]. In a series of over 1000 patients the repositioning feature was employed in 26% resulting in an overall successful implantation rate of 99.5%, a mean gradient of 8.5 mmHg and a 30 day mortality 1.9% with a rate of aortic insufficiency of <moderate of 98.1% [78].

The St. Jude Medical Portico device is similar to the CoreValve with key differentiating features including an intra-annular bovine pericardial valve with a porcine pericardial sealing cuff, larger stent cells to improve anatomic conformation and coronary access, and complete retrievability, resheathability, and repositionability of the valve. It has been evaluated in two feasibility and outcome studies (a total of 50 patients with no major strokes, no moderate or severe paravalvular leaks, and no deaths occurred within 12 months) [79].

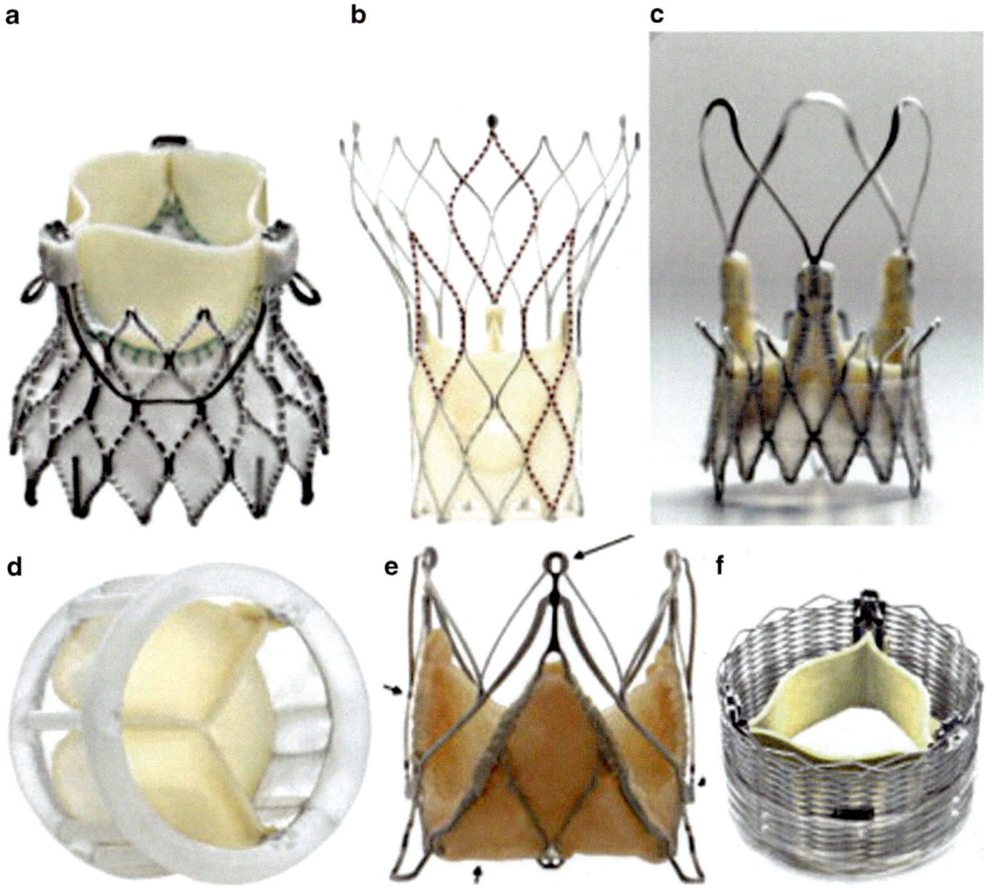

Fig. 10.22 New TAVR systems approved for clinical use in Europe (and elsewhere). (**a**) Medtronic Engager. (**b**) St. Jude Portico. (**c**) Symetis Acurate. (**d**) Direct Flow Medical. (**e**) Jena Valve. (**f**) Boston Scientific SADRA Lotus. From Leon MB, Gada H, Fontana GP. Challenges and future opportunities for transcatheter aortic valve therapy. Prog Cardiovasc Dis. 2014 May–Jun;56(6):635–45. Reprinted with permission from Elsevier

The JenaValve is a short self-expanding nitinol frame housing a valve derived from native porcine valve material, with a porcine pericardial skirt, and arms or "feelers" that are positioned behind the native valve leaflets allowing "clipping" of the valve against the lower stent, preventing embolization and eliminating radial forces on the cardiac and aortic structures. With optimal placement, there is correct commissural alignment, intra-annular position avoiding conduction defects and sparing of the coronary arteries. The device was evaluated in the Jupiter multicenter registry of 180 patients who were implanted via TA approach. The device showed excellent results with 95.5% procedural success, and no strokes and 97.6% patients with mild or lesser paravalvular regurgitation [80]. Due to the unique clip fixation mechanism of the JenaValve, the device is ideal to be anchored in patients with severe aortic insufficiency who have no aortic calcifications. This was tested in a small subset of patients with severe aortic insufficiency who were thought to be high risk for a surgical aortic valve replacement. All patients had successful device implantation with improvement in aortic regurgitation and improved exercise tolerance at 3 months [81].

The Lotus® valve system (Boston Scientific, USA) comprises an intra-annular bovine pericardial leaflets in a woven nitinol frame and a catheter-based delivery system for transfemoral introduction and delivery. The device is repositionable and has an adaptive seal surrounding the ventricular portion of the device to reduce paravalvular aortic regurgitation. The 23 and 27 mm Lotus® valves were evaluated in the REPRISE II trials. 76.1% of patients had no paravalvular regurgitation and there were no cases of moderate or severe regurgitation. Device success and performance rates were 100%. Safe valve repositioning and retrieval was performed in 16 and 4 patients, respectively. Clinical outcomes at 30 days revealed all-cause mortality in 4.2%, strokes in 5.9%, moderate or severe paravalvular regurgitation in 1%, and pacemaker implantation in 28.6% [82].

The Medtronic Engager® aortic valve bioprosthesis (Medtronic) is composed of three bovine pericardium leaflets sewn to a polyester sleeve and mounted on a compressible and self-expanding nitinol frame. The stent assembly consists of a shaped main frame and a support frame, coupled together to form the commissural posts of the valve. Two sizes are available: 23 and 26 mm for TA approach. The valve can be repositioned before final deployment. The multicenter Engager® CE pivotal trial evaluated the safety and efficacy of the device in 125 patients (mean age 82 ± 4.7 years, mean logistic EuroSCORE 18.4 ± 9%). Overall device success was 94.8%, and the prosthesis was successfully implanted in 100% of patients. Thirty day mortality was 8.1% and the stroke rate was 1.7%; life-threatening bleeding was observed in 6.5% of patients and permanent pacemaker implantation was needed in 28% of patients. The incidence of paravalvular leak was extremely low: in 95.5% of patients paravalvular leakage was absent or trivial and was mild in 4.2% of patients [83] (Fig. 10.22 and Table 10.9).

Table 10.9 The main characteristics of selected new transcatheter aortic valves

Valve type	Valve material	Stent material	Route	Delivery system (Fr)	Expansion	Repositioning
Edwards CENTERA (Edwards Lifesciences, Irvine, CA)	Bovine pericardium	Nitinol	Femoral	14	Self-expandable	Yes
Direct Flow Medical (Direct Flow Medical, Santa Rosa, CA)	Bovine pericardium	No stent (polyester fabric cuff)	Femoral and subclavian	18	Polymer expansion	Yes
JenaValve (JenaValve Technology, Munich, Germany)	Porcine native aortic valve leaflets	Nitinol	Apical	32	Self-expandable	Yes
Portico (St. Jude Medical, St. Paul, MN)	Bovine pericardium	Nitinol	Femoral	18	Self-expandable	Yes
The Lotus Valve System (Boston Scientific Corporation, Natick, MA)	Bovine pericardium	Nitinol	Femoral	18	Mechanically expanding	Yes
Symetis Acurate (Symetis, Ecublens, Switzerland)	Porcine pericardium	Nitinol	Apical and femoral	28, 18	Self-expandable	Yes
Engager (Medtronic Inc., Minneapolis, MN)	Bovine pericardium	Nitinol	Apical	29	Self-expandable	Yes
CoreValve Evolut R (Medtronic Inc., Minneapolis, MN)	Porcine pericardium	Nitinol	All except transapical	14	Self-expandable	Yes

From Abdel-Wahab M, El-Mawardy M, Richardt G. Update on transcatheter aortic valve replacement. Trends Cardiovasc Med. 2015 Feb;25(2):154–61. Reprinted with permission from Elsevier

Future Implications: Expanded TAVR Indications

Valve in Valve

Bioprosthetic surgical aortic valves have limited durability and often degenerate in 10–20 years resulting in stenosis or regurgitation. Reoperation is associated with worse morbidity and mortality due to increased complexity of the procedure as well as the increased comorbidities of aging. TAVR is an attractive option in these patients with failed bioprosthesis in which the TAVR is implanted inside the failed SAVR valve (valve-in-valve, (VIV)). Both balloon-expandable and self-expanding valve platforms have been use for the same with favorable outcomes. In a recent report of 365 VIV patients, the predicted STS mortality for reoperation was 9.1%, yet the 30 day VIV mortality was 2.7%. The mean transaortic gradient was 17.6 mmHg [84]. FDA has now approved valve-in-valve TAVR for commercial use in previously placed bioprosthetic aortic or mitral valves in patients at high risk for surgical valve replacement.

Bicuspid Aortic Valve

Patients with bicuspid aortic valve (BAV) have traditionally been excluded from TAVR clinical trials. The specific concerns with implanting transcatheter heart valves in these patients include elliptical shaped annulus with leaflet asymmetry and calcification leading to impaired valve positioning and sealing, bicuspid aortopathy with potentially a higher risk of dissection and rupture during valve delivery and implantation and high risk of residual aortic regurgitation due to disruption of commissures. In a meta-analysis of TAVR in 758 bicuspid valve patients, procedure success rate 95% with more than mild aortic insufficiency present in 12.2%, new pacemaker implantation rate of 18% with all-cause mortality of 3.7% [85].

Conclusions

TAVR now represents an established treatment modality for patients with severe aortic stenosis who are inoperable, high risk or intermediate risk for surgery. Results of the low-risk trials for TAVR are now available. Both the balloon-expandable [86] and self expandable [87] valves were either non-inferior or superior to SAVR in low risk patients making it highly likley that FDA will apporve TAVR in that group. Increasing operator experience and continuous improvements in the technology has led to improved outcomes, which has paved the way for clinical trials, which continue to seek to expand the current indications for TAVR implantations (Fig. 10.23). Long-term durability studies and data from the ongoing clinical trials will help further understand its role in lower risk

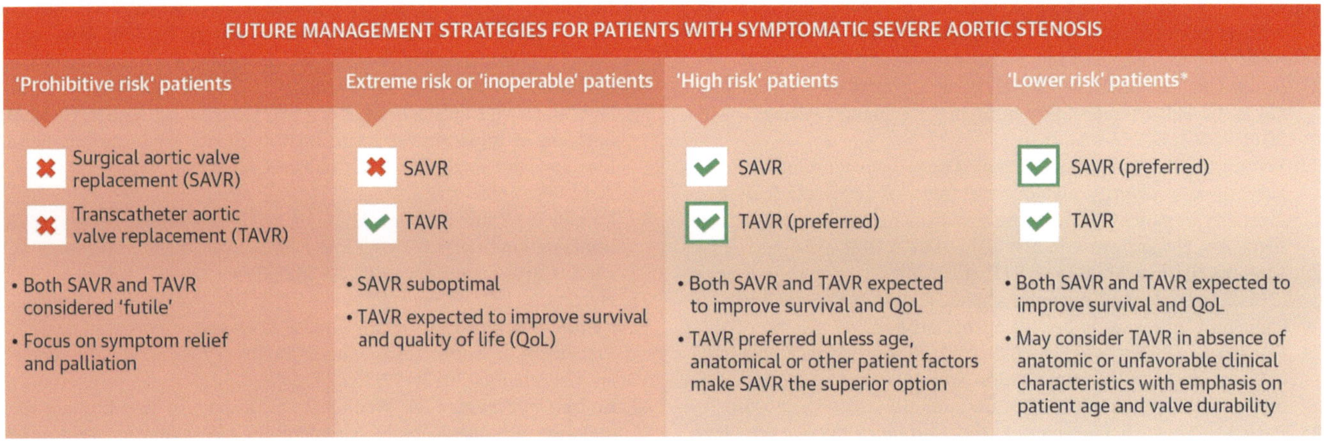

Fig. 10.23 TAVR: future expectations and barriers. Patients with severe aortic stenosis present with a spectrum of comorbidities that influence the treatment options available to them. The heart team will chose the optimal treatment strategy for individual patients based on their age, frailty, and anatomic and clinical characteristics. For patients undergoing transcatheter aortic valve replacement (TAVR), the bar for the performance standard is set by surgical aortic valve replacement (SAVR). TAVR has evolved as the preferred treatment for high-risk and inoperable patients. *Because the durability of transcatheter heart valves and outcomes in lower risk patients requires further studies, SAVR remains the treatment of choice for such patients. From Vahl TP, Kodali SK, Leon MB. Transcatheter Aortic Valve Replacement 2016: A Modern-Day "Through the Looking-Glass" Adventure. J Am Coll Cardiol. 2016 Mar 29;67(12):1472–1487. Reprinted with permission from Elsevier

patients with severe aortic stenosis and formulate appropriate treatment algorithms for optimal treatment of these patients.

References

1. Rosenhek R, Binder T, Porenta G, et al. Predictors of outcome in severe, asymptomatic aortic stenosis. N Engl J Med. 2000;343(9):611–7.
2. Carabello BA, Paulus WJ. Aortic stenosis. Lancet. 2009;373(9667):956–66.
3. Iung B, Baron G, Butchart EG, et al. A prospective survey of patients with valvular heart disease in Europe: the Euro Heart Survey on valvular heart disease. Eur Heart J. 2003;24(13):1231–43.
4. Nkomo VT, Gardin JM, Skelton TN, Gottdiener JS, Scott CG, Enriquez-Sarano M. Burden of valvular heart diseases: a population-based study. Lancet. 2006;368(9540):1005–11.
5. Varadarajan P, Kapoor N, Bansal RC, Pai RG. Survival in elderly patients with severe aortic stenosis is dramatically improved by aortic valve replacement: results from a cohort of 277 patients aged > or =80 years. Eur J Cardiothorac Surg. 2006;30(5):722–7.
6. Iung B, Cachier A, Baron G, et al. Decision-making in elderly patients with severe aortic stenosis: why are so many denied surgery? Eur Heart J. 2005;26(24):2714–20.
7. Nishimura RA, Otto CM, Bonow R, et al. 2017 AHA/ACC focused update of the 2014 AHA/ACC guideline for the management of patients with valvular heart disease: a report of the American College of Cardiology/American Heart Association Task Force on Clinical Practice Guidelines. J Am Coll Cardiol. 2017;70(2):252–89.
8. Falk V, Baumgartner H, Bax JJ, et al. ESC Scientific Document Group 2017 ESC/EACTS Guidelines for the management of valvular heart disease. Eur J Cardiothorac Surg. 2017;52(4):616–64.
9. O'Brien SM, Shahian DM, Filardo G, et al. The Society of Thoracic Surgeons 2008 cardiac surgery risk models: Part 2—isolated valve surgery. Ann Thorac Surg. 2009;88(1 Suppl):S23–42.
10. Nashef SA, Roques F, Michel P, Gauducheau E, Lemeshow S, Salamon R. European system for cardiac operative risk evaluation (EuroSCORE). Eur J Cardiothorac Surg. 1999;16(1):9–13.
11. Nashef SA, Roques F, Sharples LD, et al. EuroSCORE II. Eur J Cardiothorac Surg. 2012;41(4):734–44; discussion 744–5
12. Mohr FW, Holzhey D, Mollmann H, et al. The German Aortic Valve Registry: 1-year results from 13,680 patients with aortic valve disease. Eur J Cardiothorac Surg. 2014;46(5):808–16.
13. Mack MJ, Holmes DR, Webb J, et al. Patient selection for transcatheter aortic valve replacement. J Am Coll Cardiol. 2013;62(17 Suppl):S1–10.
14. Rosner MH, Okusa MD. Acute kidney injury associated with cardiac surgery. Clin J Am Soc Nephrol. 2006;1(1):19–32.
15. Bagur R, Webb JG, Nietlispach F, et al. Acute kidney injury following transcatheter aortic valve implantation: predictive factors, prognostic value, and comparison with surgical aortic valve replacement. Eur Heart J. 2010;31(7):865–74.
16. Aregger F, Wenaweser P, Hellige GJ, et al. Risk of acute kidney injury in patients with severe aortic valve stenosis undergoing transcatheter valve replacement. Nephrol Dial Transplant. 2009;24(7):2175–9.
17. Kong WY, Yong G, Irish A. Incidence, risk factors and prognosis of acute kidney injury after transcatheter aortic valve implantation. Nephrology. 2012;17(5):445–51.
18. Thomas M, Schymik G, Walther T, et al. One-year outcomes of cohort 1 in the Edwards SAPIEN Aortic Bioprosthesis European Outcome (SOURCE) registry: the European registry of transcatheter aortic valve implantation using the Edwards SAPIEN valve. Circulation. 2011;124(4):425–33.
19. Sinning JM, Ghanem A, Steinhauser H, et al. Renal function as predictor of mortality in patients after percutaneous transcatheter aortic valve implantation. JACC Cardiovasc Interv. 2010;3(11):1141–9.

20. Gupta T, Goel K. Kolte et al. Association of chronic kidney disease with in-hospital outcomes of transcatheter aortic valve replacement. JACC Cardiovasc Interv. 2017;10(20):2050–60.
21. Smith CR, Leon MB, Mack MJ, et al. Transcatheter versus surgical aortic-valve replacement in high-risk patients. N Engl J Med. 2011;364(23):2187–98.
22. Witberg G, Regev E, Chen S, et al. The prognostic effects of coronary disease severity and completeness of revascularization on mortality in patients undergoing transcatheter aortic valve replacement. JACC Cardiovasc Interv. 2017;10(14):1428–35.
23. Masson JB, Lee M, Boone RH, et al. Impact of coronary artery disease on outcomes after transcatheter aortic valve implantation. Catheter Cardiovasc Interv. 2010;76(2):165–73.
24. Conradi L, Seiffert M, Franzen O, et al. First experience with transcatheter aortic valve implantation and concomitant percutaneous coronary intervention. Clin Res Cardiol. 2011;100(4):311–6.
25. Pasic M, Dreysse S, Unbehaun A, et al. Combined elective percutaneous coronary intervention and transapical transcatheter aortic valve implantation. Interact Cardiovasc Thorac Surg. 2012;14(4):463–8.
26. Goel SS, Ige M, Tuzcu EM, et al. Severe aortic stenosis and coronary artery disease—implications for management in the transcatheter aortic valve replacement era: a comprehensive review. J Am Coll Cardiol. 2013;62(1):1–10.
27. Khawaja MZ, Wang D, Pocock S, Redwood SR, Thomas MR. The percutaneous coronary intervention prior to transcatheter aortic valve implantation (ACTIVATION) trial: study protocol for a randomized controlled trial. Trials. 2014;15:300.
28. Hutter A, Bleiziffer S, Richter V, et al. Transcatheter aortic valve implantation in patients with concomitant mitral and tricuspid regurgitation. Ann Thorac Surg. 2013;95(1):77–84.
29. Nombela-Franco L, Ribeiro HB, et al. Significant mitral regurgitation left untreated at the time of aortic valve replacement: a comprehensive review of a frequent entity in the transcatheter aortic valve replacement era. J Am Coll Cardiol. 2014;63(24):2643–58.
30. Hahn RT, Pibarot P, Stewart WJ, et al. Comparison of transcatheter and surgical aortic valve replacement in severe aortic stenosis: a longitudinal study of echocardiography parameters in cohort A of the PARTNER trial (placement of aortic transcatheter valves). J Am Coll Cardiol. 2013;61(25):2514–21.
31. Rudolph V, Schirmer J, Franzen O, et al. Bivalvular transcatheter treatment of high-surgical-risk patients with coexisting severe aortic stenosis and significant mitral regurgitation. Int J Cardiol. 2013;167(3):716–20.
32. Ewe SH, Ajmone Marsan N, Pepi M, et al. Impact of left ventricular systolic function on clinical and echocardiographic outcomes following transcatheter aortic valve implantation for severe aortic stenosis. Am Heart J. 2010;160(6):1113–20.
33. Clavel MA, Webb JG, Rodes-Cabau J, et al. Comparison between transcatheter and surgical prosthetic valve implantation in patients with severe aortic stenosis and reduced left ventricular ejection fraction. Circulation. 2010;122(19):1928–36.
34. van der Boon RM, Nuis RJ, Van Mieghem NM, et al. Clinical outcome following transcatheter aortic valve implantation in patients with impaired left ventricular systolic function. Catheteriz Cardiovasc Interv. 2012;79(5):702–10.
35. Zhao Y, Lindqvist P, Nilsson J, Holmgren A, Naslund U, Henein MY. Trans-catheter aortic valve implantation--early recovery of left and preservation of right ventricular function. Interact Cardiovasc Thorac Surg. 2011;12(1):35–9.
36. Forsberg LM, Tamas E, Vanky F, Nielsen NE, Engvall J, Nylander E. Left and right ventricular function in aortic stenosis patients 8 weeks post-transcatheter aortic valve implantation or surgical aortic valve replacement. Eur J Echocardiogr. 2011;12(8):603–11.
37. Carabello BA. Low-gradient, low-ejection fraction aortic stenosis: what we know and what we do not know. JACC Cardiovasc Interv. 2012;5(5):560–2.
38. Monin JL, Quéré JP, Monchi M, et al. Low-gradient aortic stenosis: operative risk stratification and predictors for long-term outcome: a multicenter study using dobutamine stress hemodynamics. Circulation. 2003;108(3):319–24.
39. Gotzmann M, Lindstaedt M, Bojara W, Ewers A, Mugge A. Clinical outcome of transcatheter aortic valve implantation in patients with low-flow, low gradient aortic stenosis. Catheteriz Cardiovasc Interv. 2012;79(5):693–701.
40. Lauten A, Zahn R, Horack M, et al. Transcatheter aortic valve implantation in patients with low-flow, low-gradient aortic stenosis. JACC Cardiovasc Interv. 2012;5(5):552–9.
41. Herrmann HC, Pibarot P, Hueter I, et al. Predictors of mortality and outcomes of therapy in low-flow severe aortic stenosis: a Placement of Aortic Transcatheter Valves (PARTNER) trial analysis. Circulation. 2013;127(23):2316–26.
42. Le Ven F, Freeman M, Webb J, et al. Impact of low flow on the outcome of high-risk patients undergoing transcatheter aortic valve replacement. J Am Coll Cardiol. 2013;62(9):782–82.
43. Gunter RL, Kilgo P, Guyton RA, et al. Impact of preoperative chronic lung disease on survival after surgical aortic valve replacement. Ann Thorac Surg. 2013;96(4):1322–8.
44. Moat NE, Ludman P, de Belder MA, et al. Long-term outcomes after transcatheter aortic valve implantation in high-risk patients with severe aortic stenosis: the U.K. TAVI (United Kingdom Transcatheter Aortic Valve Implantation) Registry. J Am Coll Cardiol. 2011;58(20):2130–8.
45. Rodes-Cabau J, Webb JG, Cheung A, et al. Long-term outcomes after transcatheter aortic valve implantation: insights on prognostic factors and valve durability from the Canadian multicenter experience. J Am Coll Cardiol. 2012;60(19):1864–75.
46. Dvir D, Waksman R, Barbash IM, et al. Outcomes of patients with chronic lung disease and severe aortic stenosis treated with transcatheter versus surgical aortic valve replacement or standard therapy: insights from the PARTNER trial (placement of AoRTic TraNscathetER Valve). J Am Coll Cardiol. 2014;63(3):269–79.
47. Arnold SV, Spertus JA, Lei Y, et al. How to define a poor outcome after transcatheter aortic valve replacement: conceptual framework and empirical observations from the placement of aortic transcatheter valve (PARTNER) trial. Circ Cardiovasc Qual Outcomes. 2013;6(5):591–7.
48. Burke GL, Arnold AM, Bild DE, et al. Factors associated with healthy aging: the cardiovascular health study. J Am Geriatr Soc. 2001;49(3):254–62.
49. Stortecky S, Schoenenberger AW, Moser A, et al. Evaluation of multidimensional geriatric assessment as a predictor of mortality and cardiovascular events after transcatheter aortic valve implantation. JACC Cardiovasc Interv. 2012;5(5):489–96.
50. Mack M. Frailty and aortic valve disease. J Thorac Cardiovasc Surg. 2013;145(3 Suppl):S7–10.51.
51. Please provide bibliographic details.
52. Green P, Woglom AE, Genereux P, et al. Gait speed and dependence in activities of daily living in older adults with severe aortic stenosis. Clin Cardiol. May 2012;35(5):307–14.
53. Studenski S, Perera S, Patel K, et al. Gait speed and survival in older adults. JAMA. 2011;305(1):50–8.
54. Green P, Arnold SV, Cohen DJ, et al. Relation of frailty to outcomes after transcatheter aortic valve replacement (from the PARTNER Trial). Am J Cardiol. 2015;116(2):264–9.
55. Green P, Cohen DJ, Genereux P, et al. Relation between six-minute walk test performance and outcomes after transcatheter aortic valve implantation (from the PARTNER trial). Am J Cardiol. 2013;112(5):700–6.
56. Afilalo J, Lauck S, Kim DH, et al. Frailty in older adults undergoing aortic valve replacement: the FRAILTY-AVR Study. J Am Coll Cardiol. 2017;70(6):689–700.
57. Leon MB, Smith CR, Mack MJ, et al. Investigators transcatheter or surgical aortic-valve replacement in intermediate-risk patients. N Engl J Med. 2016;374(17):1609–20.

58. Reardon MJ, Van Mieghem NM, Popma JJ, et al. Surgical or transcatheter aortic-valve replacement in intermediate-risk patients. N Engl J Med. 2017;376(14):1321–31.
59. Bloomfield GS, Gillam LD, Hahn RT, et al. A practical guide to multimodality imaging of transcatheter aortic valve replacement. JACC Cardiovasc Imaging. 2012;5(4):441–55.
60. Binder RK, Webb JG, Willson AB, et al. The impact of integration of a multidetector computed tomography annulus area sizing algorithm on outcomes of transcatheter aortic valve replacement: a prospective, multicenter, controlled trial. J Am Coll Cardiol. 2013;62(5):431–8.
61. Leon MB, Smith CR, Mack M, et al. Transcatheter aortic-valve implantation for aortic stenosis in patients who cannot undergo surgery. N Engl J Med. 2010;363(17):1597–607.
62. Kapadia SR, Leon MB, Makkar RR, et al. 5-Year outcomes of transcatheter aortic valve replacement compared with standard treatment for patients with inoperable aortic stenosis (PARTNER 1): a randomised controlled trial. Lancet. 2015;385(9986):2485–91.
63. Reynolds MR, Magnuson EA, Lei Y, et al. Health-related quality of life after transcatheter aortic valve replacement in inoperable patients with severe aortic stenosis. Circulation. 2011;124(18):1964–72.
64. Makkar RR, Fontana GP, Jilaihawi H, et al. Transcatheter aortic-valve replacement for inoperable severe aortic stenosis. N Engl J Med. 2012;366(18):1696–704.
65. Mack MJ, Leon MB, Smith CR, et al. 5-Year outcomes of transcatheter aortic valve replacement or surgical aortic valve replacement for high surgical risk patients with aortic stenosis (PARTNER 1): a randomised controlled trial. Lancet. 2015;385(9986):2477–84.
66. Webb JG, Doshi D, Mack MJ, et al. A randomized evaluation of the SAPIEN XT transcatheter heart valve system in patients with aortic stenosis who are not candidates for surgery. JACC Cardiovasc Interv. 2015;8(14):1797–806.
67. Leon MB, Smith CR, Mack MJ, et al. Transcatheter or surgical aortic-valve replacement in intermediate-risk patients. N Engl J Med. 2016;374(17):1609–20.
68. Rao RS, Maniar H, Zajarias A. Sapien valve: past, present, and future. Cardiac Interv Today. 2015;9:35–41.
69. Kodali SK, Williams MR, Smith CR, et al. Two-year outcomes after transcatheter or surgical aortic-valve replacement. N Engl J Med. 2012;366(18):1686–95.
70. Thourani VH, Kodali S, Makkar RR, et al. Transcatheter aortic valve replacement versus surgical valve replacement in intermediate-risk patients: a propensity score analysis. Lancet. 2016;387(10034):2218–25.
71. Popma JJ, Adams DH, Reardon MJ, et al. Transcatheter aortic valve replacement using a self-expanding bioprosthesis in patients with severe aortic stenosis at extreme risk for surgery. J Am Coll Cardiol. 2014;63(19):1972–81.
72. Reardon MJ, Adams DH, Kleiman NS, et al. 2-Year outcomes in patients undergoing surgical or self-expanding transcatheter aortic valve replacement. J Am Coll Cardiol. 2015;66(2):113–21.
73. Erkapic D, De Rosa S, Kelava A, Lehmann R, Fichtlscherer S, Hohnloser SH. Risk for permanent pacemaker after transcatheter aortic valve implantation: a comprehensive analysis of the literature. J Cardiovasc Electrophysiol. 2012;23(4):391–7.
74. Nazif TM, Williams MR, Hahn RT, et al. Clinical implications of new-onset left bundle branch block after transcatheter aortic valve replacement: analysis of the PARTNER experience. Eur Heart J. 2014;35(24):1599–607.
75. Abdel-Wahab M, Mehilli J, Frerker C, et al. Comparison of balloon-expandable vs self-expandable valves in patients undergoing transcatheter aortic valve replacement: the CHOICE randomized clinical trial. JAMA. 2014;311(15):1503–14.
76. Makkar RR, Fontana G, Jilaihawi H, et al. Possible subclinical leaflet thrombosis in bioprosthetic aortic valves. N Engl J Med. 2015;373:2015–24.
77. Diemert P, Seiffert M, Frerker C, et al. Valve-in-valve implantation of a novel and small self-expandable transcatheter heart valve in degenerated small surgical bioprostheses: the Hamburg experience. Catheteriz Cardiovasc Interv. 2014;84(3):486–93.
78. Grube E, Van Mieghem NM, Bleiziffer S, et al. Clinical outcomes with a repositionable self-expanding transcatheter aortic valve prosthesis: the International FORWARD Study. J Am Coll Cardiol. 2017;70(7):845–53.
79. Willson AB, Rodes-Cabau J, Wood DA, et al. Transcatheter aortic valve replacement with the St. Jude Medical Portico valve: first-in-human experience. J Am Coll Cardiol. 2012;60(7):581–6.
80. S E. First results of the JUPITER Registry on long-term performance and safety of the transapical JenaValve. Paper presented at EuroPCR; 2013.
81. Seiffert M, Diemert P, Koschyk D, et al. Transapical implantation of a second-generation transcatheter heart valve in patients with noncalcified aortic regurgitation. JACC Cardiovasc Interv. 2013;6(6):590–7.
82. Meredith IT, Worthley SG, Whitbourn RJ, et al. Transfemoral aortic valve replacement with the repositionable Lotus Valve System in high surgical risk patients: the REPRISE I study. EuroIntervention. 2014;9(11):1264–70.
83. Sundermann SH, Holzhey D, Bleiziffer S, Treede H, Falk V. Medtronic Engager bioprosthesis for transapical transcatheter aortic valve implantation. EuroIntervention. 2013;9(Suppl):S97–100.
84. Webb JG, Mack MJ, White JM, et al. Transcatheter aortic valve implantation within degenerated aortic surgical bioprostheses: PARTNER 2 Valve-in-Valve Registry. J Am Coll Cardiol. 2017;69(18):2253–62.
85. Reddy G, Wang Z, Nishimura RA, et al. Transcatheter aortic valve replacement for stenotic bicuspid aortic valves: systematic review and meta analyses of observational studies. Catheter Cardiovasc Interv. 2018;91(5):975–83.
86. Mack MJ, Leon MB, Thourani VH, Makkar R, et al. Transcatheter Aortic-Valve Replacement with a Balloon-Expandable Valve in Low-Risk Patients. N Engl J Med. 2019;380(18):1695–705.
87. Popma JJ, Deeb GM, Yakubov SJ, Mumtaz M, et al. Transcatheter Aortic-Valve Replacement with a Self-Expanding Valve in Low-Risk Patients. N Engl J Med. 2019;380(18):1706–15.

Valve Prosthesis

11

Corinne M. Aberle, Chrisita L. Powlett,
and Jennifer R. Cozart

Introduction

Modern valve surgery began its evolution after World War II, when Harken successfully operated on the heart to remove foreign bodies [1]. Attention was then turned toward correcting congenital defects such as valve insufficiency and stenosis. Eventually, surgery for acquired valve disease was possible in the 1950s after cardiopulmonary bypass and open heart surgery was developed. Since that time, surgical treatment for valvular heart disease has continued to advance through the development of numerous repair techniques and valve prostheses. This chapter describes the surgical approaches to valvular heart disease, indications for treatment, and decision-making criteria to ensure the optimal treatment for each patient.

Aortic Valve

A variety of pathologies develop in adults which may necessitate intervention on the aortic valve including stenosis, insufficiency and aneurysmal disease of the root and ascending aorta. While select cases may be considered for aortic valve repair, most adult aortic valvular pathologies require aortic valve replacement.

C. M. Aberle · J. R. Cozart (✉)
Division of Cardiothoracic Surgery, Baylor College of Medicine, Baylor St. Luke's Medical Center, Houston, TX, USA

Cardiovascular Surgery, Texas Heart Institute at Baylor St. Luke's Medical Center, Houston, TX, USA
e-mail: jcozart@texasheart.org

C. L. Powlett
Cardiovascular Surgery, Texas Heart Institute at Baylor St. Luke's Medical Center, Houston, TX, USA

Aortic Valve Replacement

Indications for Replacement

Aortic Stenosis

In developed countries, aortic stenosis (AS) is the most prevalent valvular heart disease in adults [2]. Common causes of AS include acquired degenerative calcific disease, bicuspid aortic valve, and rheumatic heart disease. The presence of symptoms including angina, syncope, or dyspnea on exertion is the primary indications for aortic valve surgery. The severity of AS is determined by evaluating the aortic valve area (AVA) and mean systolic gradient as shown in Table 11.1.

According to the 2014 AHA/ACC guidelines, indications for aortic valve replacement (AVR) in AS include symptomatic patients with severe AS, symptomatic patients with low flow/low gradient severe AS both with and without reduced left ventricular ejection fraction (LVEF), as well as asymptomatic patients with severe AS. In patients with moderate AS, AVR is reasonable if undergoing cardiac surgery for other reasons. Table 11.2 outlines the indications for AVR in aortic stenosis [3].

Aortic Regurgitation

Aortic regurgitation (AR) can originate either from primary leaflet disease or from disease of the aortic root, and may occur alone or in combination with aortic stenosis. Common diseases leading to leaflet malfunction include calcific degeneration, myxomatous degeneration, rheumatic disease, infective endocarditis, and bicuspid aortic valves. Dilation of the aortic root leading to regurgitation may result from aortic dissection, trauma, chronic hypertension,

Table 11.1 AHA/ACC guidelines for severity of aortic stenosis

	Mild	Moderate	Severe
Aortic valve area (cm^2)	>1.5	1.0–1.5	<1.0
Mean pressure gradient (mmHg)	<20	20–39	>40

B. A. Carabello (ed.), *Valvular Heart Disease*, Cardiovascular Medicine, https://doi.org/10.1007/978-1-4471-2840-3_11

Table 11.2 Indications for aortic valve replacement in aortic stenosis

Indication	Class of evidence
Symptomatic patients with severe high-gradient AS	I
Asymptomatic patients with severe AS and LVEF <50%	I
Severe AS undergoing other cardiac surgery	I
Symptomatic patients with low-flow/low-gradient severe AS with reduced LVEF with mean pressure gradient ≥40 mmHg or AVA ≤1.0 cm² on dobutamine stress study	IIa
Asymptomatic patients with – Very severe AS and low surgical risk – Severe AS and decreased exercise tolerance or exercise fall in BP	IIa
Moderate AS undergoing other cardiac surgery	IIa
Asymptomatic patients with severe AS, rapid disease progression and low surgical risk	IIb

AS aortic stenosis, *AVA* aortic valve area, *LVEF* left ventricular ejection fraction

Table 11.3 AHA/ACC guidelines for the severity of aortic regurgitation

	Mild	Moderate	Severe
Jet width (% LVOT diameter)	<25	25–64	≥65
Vena contracta (cm)	<0.3	0.3–0.6	>0.6
Regurgitant volume (mL/beat)	<30	30–59	≥60
Regurgitant fraction (%)	<30	30–49	≥50
Effective regurgitant orifice area (cm²)	<0.10	0.10–0.29	≥0.3

LVOT left ventricular outflow tract

Table 11.4 AHA/ACC recommendations for aortic regurgitation surgical intervention

Recommendation	COR
Symptomatically patients with severe AR regardless of LVEF	I
Asymptomatic patients with chronic severe AR and LVEF < than 50%	I
Severe AR undergoing other cardiac surgery	I
Asymptomatic patients with severe AR with LVEF >50% and severe LV dilatation	IIa
Moderate AR undergoing other cardiac surgery	IIa
Asymptomatic patients with severe AR with LVEF >50% and with progressive severe LV dilatation and low surgical risk	IIb

AR aortic regurgitation, *COR* class of recommendation, *LV* left ventricular, *LVEF* left ventricular ejection fraction

connective tissue disorders, and syphilis induced aortitis. Table 11.3 shows the criteria used to determine the severity of aortic regurgitation. Indications for aortic valve replacement for regurgitation, shown in Table 11.4, include symptomatic severe AR, asymptomatic severe AR with reduced LVEF or with left ventricular dilation, and asymptomatic moderate or severe AR undergoing cardiac surgery for other indications [3].

Patient Factors and Limitations

When considering an AVR, some patient factors and limitations may affect surgical planning and prosthesis choice. Specifically, the patient's age, ability to tolerate long-term anticoagulation, and aortic root size are important factors for consideration. Each valve replacement option has a different expected durability. A younger patient may be better suited with a valve with a longer durability, to avoid the need for reoperation. However, if the patient's life expectancy is shorter, valve durability may be less important when deciding on a valve prosthesis. In addition, some valve prostheses require life-long anticoagulation. Older patients or patients at higher risk of fall, patients at higher risk of bleeding, or patients who may desire future pregnancy may not be candidates for therapeutic anticoagulation. Alternatively, patients with an existing condition which already requires anticoagulation, such as atrial fibrillation or thrombotic disorders, may not need to consider anticoagulation when choosing a valve prosthesis. Lastly, aortic root size is an equally important determinant during aortic valve replacement. A small or heavily calcified aortic root may limit the size of the valve prosthesis which can be placed. Replacing the valve with too small a valve may place the patient at risk for an ongoing functional stenosis. Some valve prosthesis options have improved hemodynamics and flow compared to other valves of similar size, which may be important when faced with a small aortic root.

Options for Replacement

Mechanical Valve

One of the earliest valve replacement options developed was the mechanical ball and cage valve [4]. However, these initial valves required intense anticoagulation and were somewhat limited in their hemodynamic performance [5]. Mechanical valves have since evolved and are now designed as tilting discs (Fig. 11.1). Overall, mechanical valves have several advantages. The durability of these valves remains excellent, with a valve replacement rate of less than 2% over 25 years [6]. Furthermore, long-term studies comparing mechanical to biologic prosthesis have shown a greater freedom from valve-related events and from reoperation with mechanical prosthesis [7, 8]. Some studies also suggest improved survival with mechanical prosthesis, while maintaining a similar quality of life to that of a biologic prosthesis [9, 10]. In addition, mechanical valves boast excellent hemodynamics, with large effective flow orifices, which translate into functionally larger prostheses for any given tissue annulus diameter [10].

Mechanical valves have some disadvantages as well. Perhaps the most prominent disadvantage is the need for anticoagulation. Anticoagulation-related hemorrhage is the

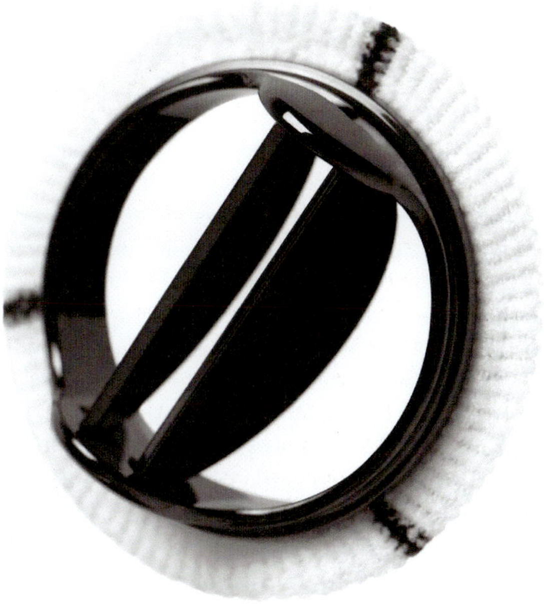

Fig. 11.1 St. Jude Medical (SJM) Regent™ mechanical heart valve. Reproduced with permission of St. Jude Medical, ©2017

most common valve-related event, and accounts for the highest mortality associated with valve-related events [7, 8, 11–15]. The target INR can vary based on patient risk factors, as well as valve choice. Thromboembolism is the second most common valve-related event, with rates ranging from 0.8% to 2.3% per patient year when anticoagulated, which is similar to that of bioprosthesis [8, 11–17]. Finally, the risk for prosthetic valve endocarditis must be considered as well. The incidence is similar between mechanical and biologic valves, with freedom from endocarditis with a mechanical valve around approximately 98% at 25 years [11, 15].

Overall, mechanical valves should be considered for younger patients, especially patients less than 60 years of age [11]. Any patients who require indefinite anticoagulation for other reasons should receive a mechanical valve [18]. Lastly, patients who would be considered high risk during any potential subsequent reoperations, such as patients with prior valve replacement or prior coronary bypass, should be considered for a mechanical valve [6, 19].

Bioprosthetic Valve

Numerous bioprosthetic valve options are available currently, which may be stented or non-stented, and are typically bovine or porcine. Figures 11.2 and 11.3 show an example of bioprosthetic aortic valve and implantation. Similar to mechanical valves, bioprosthetic valves carry their own

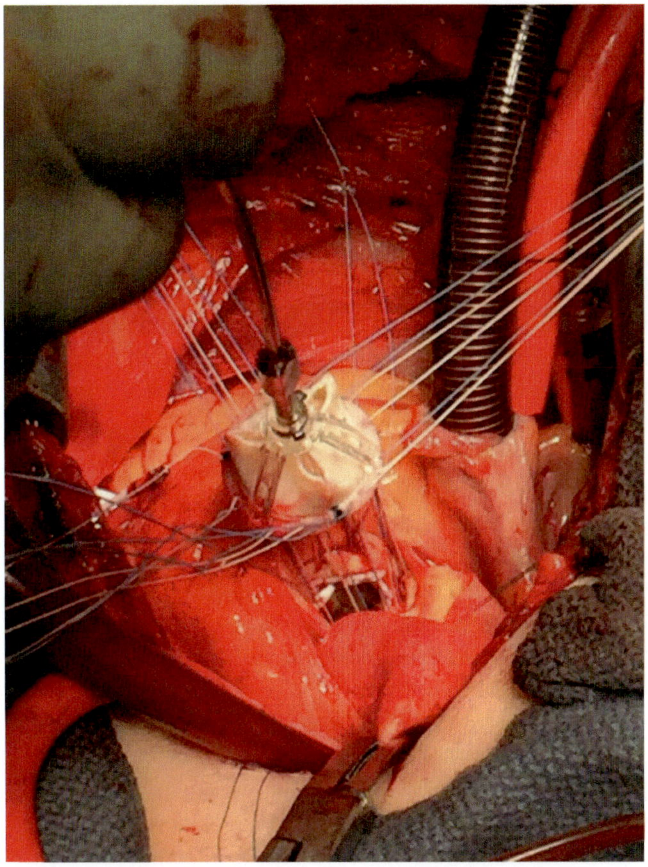

Fig. 11.2 Bioprosthetic aortic valve implantation with St. Jude Trifecta™ aortic valve

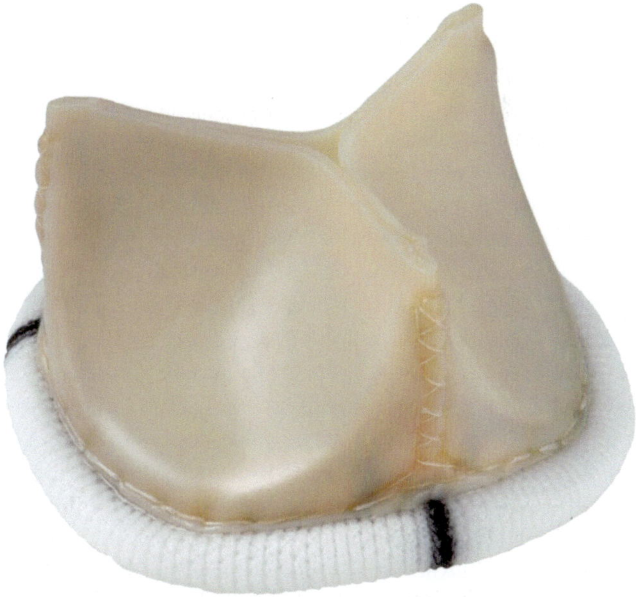

Fig. 11.3 St. Jude Medical (SJM) Trifecta™ aortic tissue valve. Reproduced with permission of St. Jude Medical, ©2017

inherent advantages and disadvantages. A major advantage with bioprosthetic valves is the freedom from therapeutic anticoagulation. The risk of thromboembolism without anticoagulation for a bioprosthetic valve is similar to the risk for a mechanical valve with anticoagulation [8, 11–17]. In addition, bioprosthetic valves also offer the potential benefit of a future transcatheter valve-in-valve implantation, which is not an option with mechanical valves.

Studies have shown higher reoperation rates in patients with bioprosthetic valves, as well as more structural valve deterioration (SVD) [20]. In most series, freedom from SVD falls rapidly after the 15 year follow-up [7, 20–22]. In addition, younger patients may be predisposed to premature bioprosthetic SVD [23, 24]. Stented bioprosthetic valves generally have lower effective orifice areas compared to that of mechanical valves, and may not be ideal in patients with small aortic roots. However, stentless biologic valves may have less residual gradients than stented valves [25]. Stentless valves are more complex to implant, requiring longer cross clamp times. Overall, bioprosthetic valves can be considered for older patients, specifically patients over 70 years old. A bioprosthesis is also a good option for patients with contraindications to anticoagulation, such as women of childbearing age who wish to become pregnant, patients with bleeding disorders, contraindication to anticoagulation, or patients who are noncompliant or refuse anticoagulation.

Homograft

Aortic root homografts (allografts) and porcine root xenografts are additional options for valve replacement. These options replace the aortic valve and the aortic root. They offer various advantages, including an excellent hemodynamic profile with low transvalvular gradients [26]. Homografts have a low risk of thromboembolism without the need for systemic anticoagulation. Furthermore, they offer potentially the lowest risk of prosthetic valve infection compared to other replacement options. However, these conduits carry the risk of structural deterioration which is inversely proportional to recipient age. In addition, older homograft donor age may contribute to higher rates of degeneration. The availability of homografts may also be limited, especially in larger sizes.

Overall, homografts and xenografts may be considered in various scenarios. The most common indication for a homograft is for the treatment of aortic valve endocarditis which has also affected the root [27, 28]. Compared to a valved conduit graft, a homograft or xenograft possesses minimal prosthetic material, which may be preferable in the setting of infection [29]. Another indication is use in a patient with a small aortic root. These conduits are stentless, which provides improved hemodynamics over other valve options. In addition, because the root is replaced, the risk of coronary obstruction by an oversized prosthesis is eliminated in these patients. Finally, because these conduits have a low risk of thromboembolism, they may be considered for patients who require valve and root replacement who cannot be anticoagulated [30].

Ross Procedure

The Ross procedure was first reported by Donald Ross in 1967 as an option for valve replacement in aortic valve disease. The procedure involves replacement of the diseased aortic valve with a pulmonary autograft and reconstruction of the right ventricular outflow tract (RVOT) with a homograft or xenograft. This procedure has proven long-term durability and the benefit of avoiding formal anticoagulation [31]. In 1987, Elkins and Stelzer began performing this operation in children leading to its adoption in the United States [32].

The main benefit of the Ross procedure is better hemodynamics across the replaced aortic valve when compared to a prosthetic valve. In the pediatric population, the Ross procedure remains a preferred choice for patients with left ventricular outflow tract (LVOT) obstruction. A significant benefit is that the valve can grow with the child, thereby avoiding multiple valve replacements. Additionally, long-term anticoagulation is not required and thrombosis occurs infrequently. The superior hemodynamics and freedom from anticoagulation makes the Ross procedure the ideal operation for active young patients with aortic valve disease.

Ideal patients for the Ross procedure are young adults with aortic valve disease and a normal-sized annulus [33]. Other patients to consider for the Ross procedure are women of childbearing age, high-level athletes, young patients with bleeding disorders or other factors preventing anticoagulation, and patients with greater than 20-year life expectancy who do not want full anticoagulation. With regard to age, some authors suggest the surgery should not be done in patients at the extremes of age. However, Schmidtke et al. reported on their experience with the Ross procedure in patients over the age of 60. They concluded that the procedure could be safely performed with excellent 7-year results in selected elderly patients up to the age of 70 [34]. After this age, the long-term benefits would be lost as the life expectancy is significantly reduced. Conversely, Willams et al. reported on their experience in infants less than 18 months of age and the results were also excellent [35]. These reports reinforce the applicability of the Ross procedure for patients regardless of age.

Contraindications to the Ross procedure include multivessel coronary artery disease, severely depressed left ventricular function, multiple valvular pathology, disease of the native pulmonary valve, connective tissue disease, and significant aortic root dilation.

One major criticism of the Ross procedure is that the operation converts a single valve pathology to a double-valve pathology (aortic and pulmonary), thereby increasing the incidence of reoperations on both the pulmonary autograft and the homograft [36, 37]. Reported incidences of reoperation range from 8 to 15% at 10 years [36]. The major indication for reoperation is dilation of the pulmonary autograft. However, revised surgical techniques at the index operation as well as better selection of surgical candidates can mitigate this complication.

The long-term outcomes of the Ross procedure are excellent. Compared to aortic valve replacement with either a mechanical or bioprosthetic valve, only patients who underwent the Ross procedure have shown survival which approached that of the general population [38]. The Ross procedure is a complex and technically demanding operation with a steep learning curve. Therefore, it should only be performed in highly specialized cardiac centers by experienced surgeons.

Valve Conduit

An additional option for AVR with aortic root or ascending aortic replacement is a valve conduit. The valve conduit typically consists of a mechanical valve which is annealed to a Dacron graft from the manufacturer. Alternatively, the surgeon may also create a valve conduit by suturing a bioprosthetic or mechanical valve to a graft. Valve conduits are considered the gold standard for aortic root replacement, but do carry the risk of prosthetic graft material and the potential for infection. Grafts are spared from degeneration and can last for a patient's lifetime.

Aortic Root Enlargement

A small aortic root can be a potential limitation to aortic valve replacement. Patient prosthesis mismatch (PPM) can occur when a valve prosthesis effective orifice area is not sufficient for the patient's body surface area, which can result in elevated gradients across the valve postoperatively. Several studies have shown that severe PPM has an adverse impact on survival. When faced with a small aortic root, a surgeon may consider aortic root enlargement in order to safely place a larger valve.

One option for aortic root enlargement involves incorporation of a bovine pericardial or Dacron patch to enlarge the diameter. There are three specific surgical techniques for aortic annular enlargement. In the Nicks procedure, the aortotomy is extended into the nadir of the non-coronary sinus and into the basal third of the anterior leaflet of the mitral valve. An autologous pericardial patch or a Dacron patch is fashioned in a teardrop shape to enlarge the annulus. The valve implantation sutures are then placed across the patch itself, as well as the remainder of the annulus. This procedure can allow the surgeon to place a valve up to two sizes larger than the native annulus [39]. Similarly, the Manougian procedure involves extending the aortotomy more posteriorly along the commissure of the non-coronary and left coronary cusps. This incision is carried through the aortic-mitral septum and onto the anterior leaflet of the mitral valve, while also opening the roof of the left atrium. A patch is then implanted along the mitral valve incision and the aortotomy, and the valve sutures may then be utilized to close the atriotomy [40]. The last and perhaps most radical option is the Konno-Rastan procedure, which involves making an enlarging incision to the left of the right coronary orifice, into the ventricular septum and along the free wall of the right ventricle [41]. A patch is utilized to repair the septum, as well as a second patch for the closure of the right ventriculotomy and annular enlargement. All root enlargement procedures may increase the operative risk with aortic valve replacement, and therefore should only be undertaken with caution.

Transcatheter Aortic Valve Replacement

Transcatheter aortic valve replacement (TAVR) is an alternative option to open surgical aortic valve replacement. Figure 11.4 shows an example of a transcatheter aortic heart valve prosthesis. Multiple approaches for TAVR have been developed including transapical, axillary, and open or percutaneous femoral. Currently, the percutaneous femoral approach is the most commonly utilized access for TAVR (Fig. 11.5).

The PARTNER and CoreValve Pivotal Trials examined the utility of TAVR in the setting of inoperable, as well as high-risk, surgical patients. Overall, TAVR was associated with improved one and two-year mortality compared with medical management [42]. When TAVR was compared to surgery for high-risk patients, both the PARTNER and the

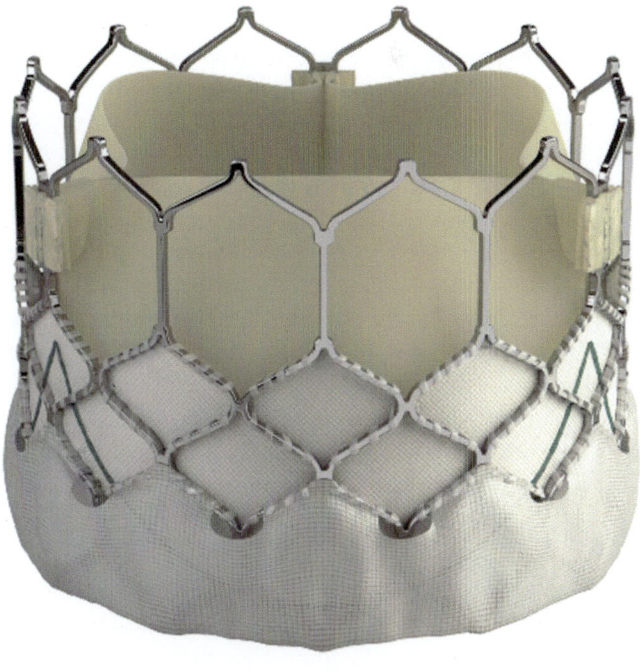

Fig. 11.4 Edwards SAPIEN 3™ transcatheter heart valve. Courtesy of Edwards Lifesciences LLC, Irvine, California

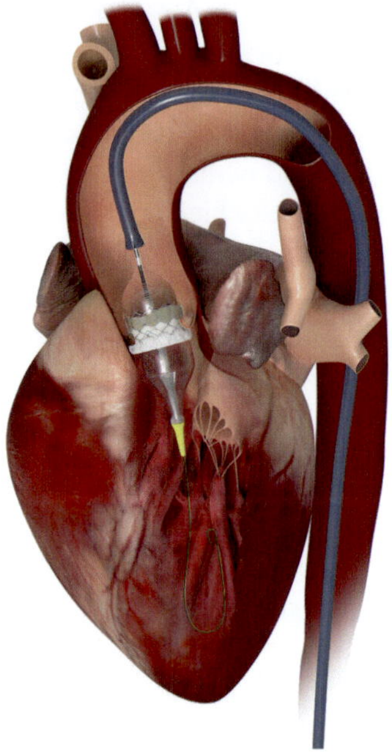

Fig. 11.5 Edwards Commander™ delivery system for TAVR. Courtesy of Edwards Lifesciences LLC, Irvine, California

CoreValve Trials found no difference in mortality at 30 days between the two groups. However, at 1 year, the CoreValve study noted a lower mortality with TAVR as compared to the surgical arm, while the PARTNER study found no difference [43, 44].

These trials have formed the basis of the current indications for TAVR. The AHA/ACC guidelines recommend surgical AVR for patients with low or intermediate surgical risk. Patients who have a prohibitive risk for surgery and a predicted post TAVR survival of greater than 12 months should be considered for TAVR. In addition, TAVR is a reasonable alternative to surgical AVR for patients who are high surgical risk [3]. It is likely that TAVR will be approved for use in low risk patients in the near future.

An additional PARTNER trial, the 2A trial, studied TAVR in intermediate-risk populations. There was no difference in disabling stroke, but the need for permanent pacemaker and the incidence of paravalvular leak was higher in the TAVR arm compared to the surgical arm. TAVR has since been approved by the US Food and Drug Administration for use in intermediate-risk populations. However, surgical AVR remains the gold standard for low- and intermediate-risk populations. For a more in depth review of TAVR, see Chap. 10.

Aortic Valve Repair

Aortic valve repair may be an option for selected patients who have aortic insufficiency or a normally functioning aortic valve associated with an aortic root or ascending aortic aneurysm. When considering a patient for aortic valve repair, the cause of the aortic insufficiency as well as the aortic cusp integrity are important determinants. Cusps with mobile and smooth-free margins may be good candidates for repair, while calcified, scarred, and fibrotic cusps may preclude an effective repair.

Overall, bicuspid aortic valve with prolapse is the most commonly performed aortic valve repair in adults [45, 46]. The prolapsing and elongated cusp can be plicated to shorten the free margin and improve coaptation. In addition, selected congenital disease and rheumatic disease may be repaired by cusp extension using autologous or bovine pericardium. Occasionally, a cusp perforation may be the sole cause of aortic insufficiency. Simple patch repair with pericardium can provide a durable repair in such circumstance. Finally, dilation of the sinotubular junction can increase the stress along the free margin of the cusps, which can ultimately lead to thinning and fenestrations. These fenestrations can be potentially repaired by running a suture along the free margin of the cusp. Careful evaluation of the valve is required for successful aortic valve repair [47].

Mitral Valve

Mitral valve disease including mitral regurgitation (MR) and mitral stenosis (MS) is caused by many different pathologies. Repair of the mitral valve is preferred to replacement in most cases of mitral regurgitation when appropriate.

Mitral Valve Repair

For patients with rheumatic, mixed, and degenerative mitral valve disease, mitral valve repair provides an improved quality of life with less morbidity and improved long-term survival when compared to mitral valve replacement [48]. Mitral repair is considered very durable, with many patients remaining free of reoperation up to 30 years from repair [49]. For this reason, repair should be performed whenever possible, specifically in the setting of mitral regurgitation (MR). However, in contrast to MR, mitral stenosis (MS) is often not amenable to repair. Furthermore, some retrospective data suggests that for patients with MS, replacement may have a better outcome than commissurotomy or valvuloplasty [50].

Indications

The indications for mitral valve repair are broadening as techniques for mitral repair have improved and overall outcomes have improved. The AHA/ACC guidelines recommend mitral valve surgery for all patients both symptomatic and asymptomatic with severe, primary MR and an LVEF

>30%. For patients with severe MR and an LVEF <30%, mitral valve repair can be considered. In addition, patients with moderate MR who are undergoing cardiac surgery for other indications can be considered for mitral valve repair.

For patients with secondary MR, mitral valve surgery is recommended if the MR is severe and the patient is undergoing coronary artery bypass or aortic valve replacement. Mitral valve repair can be considered for moderate secondary MR for patients undergoing other cardiac surgery. Lastly, mitral valve surgery can be considered for severely symptomatic patients with severe secondary MR with persistent symptoms despite optimal medical management of heart failure.

For all patients being considered for mitral valve surgery, adequate functional status before mitral valve surgery is preferred. Patients with symptoms of heart failure should be optimized as much as possible with diuresis preoperatively. Ventricular function is also important to consider when evaluating operative candidacy. For patients with severe MR, the left ventricular ejection fraction (LVEF) often decreases postoperatively, even for patients with a normal LVEF preoperatively [3].

Mitral Valve Repair Techniques

Various techniques have been developed for mitral valve repair. The choice regarding which technique to utilize is based on the pathology of valve dysfunction. In general, repair techniques are aimed at stabilizing the dilated or weakened annulus, as well as reducing the height of the prolapsing or flail leaflet to restore proper leaflet coaptation and prevent systolic anterior motion (SAM).

Annuloplasty Rings

The cornerstone of mitral valve repair is the annuloplasty. An annuloplasty should be performed with all mitral valve repairs and has been shown to improve the durability of repair significantly [51]. Various device options are available, including rigid vs. flexible rings, and partial vs. complete rings. Figure 11.6 shows an example of a mitral annuloplasty ring. Debate still exists over which type of ring should be used, but no definitive data is available. Some data suggest that a flexible ring may incur less systolic anterior motion of anterior mitral valve leaflet and a partial ring may be safer with respect to SAM [52]. However, the greatest risk for SAM occurs when a ring is undersized; therefore, oversizing is generally recommended [53, 54]. Ultimately, the choice on annuloplasty device is often based on surgeon experience and preference.

Leaflet Resections

Two types of leaflet resections are commonly used, the quadrangular resection and the triangular resection. The quadrangular resection is utilized for posterior leaflet prolapse or flail leaflet, particularly of the P2 segment [55]. In this resection, a rectangular piece of leaflet tissue is excised to the annulus. Reapproximation of the remaining posterior leaflet edges can then be accomplished by a variety of techniques often including an annular plication [56].

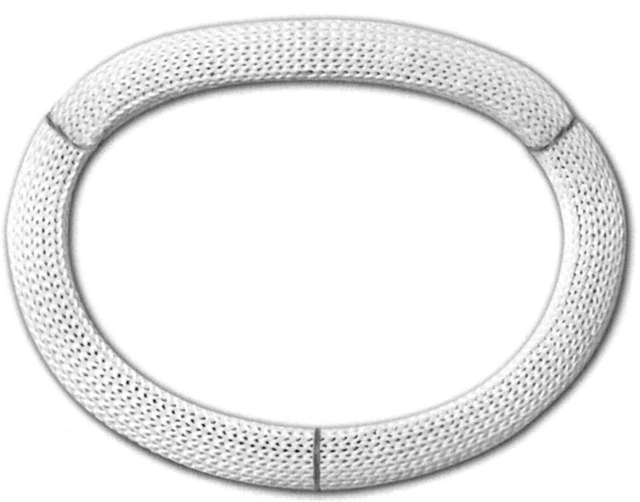

Fig. 11.6 Carpentier-Edwards Physio II mitral annuloplasty ring. Courtesy of Edwards Lifesciences LLC, Irvine, California

The triangular resection similarly resects a flail or prolapsing segment involving either leaflet, but the resection is tapered toward the annulus in a triangular fashion and does not require annular plication [57, 58]. In general, the anterior mitral leaflet should be preserved, but a triangular resection can be considered for a true flail segment. After resection, the remaining leaflet is reapproximated and the repair is completed with addition of an annuloplasty ring in most cases [57].

Artificial Chordae and Chordae Transfer

For both anterior and posterior leaflet prolapse, the creation of artificial chordae is another option for repair. Polytetrafluoroethylene (PTFE) or Gore-Tex suture is placed through the papillary muscle and then the free edge of the leaflet. These new chords can be fashioned as loops, or as figure of eight sutures, which can be adjusted while testing the valve to ensure proper leaflet height and coaptation [59, 60].

Chordal transfer is utilized for elongated or ruptured leaflet chords. In this repair, the flail segment of the affected leaflet is resected. Next, a portion of the opposite leaflet with its associated chords is resected and transferred to the affected leaflet, to replace the resected flail segment. The donor leaflet is then primarily repaired. This repair requires altering an otherwise normal leaflet, which may be considered a downside to this technique [61].

Alfieri or Edge-to-Edge Repair

The Alfieri technique, also known as the edge-to-edge repair, consists of suturing the anterior and the posterior leaflet together at the midpoint of the coaptation line [62, 63]. This creates a double-orifice valve. This technique can be useful for bi-leaflet prolapse, and helps maintain an equal height of the anterior and posterior leaflet. This technique is helpful in preventing SAM, but can place the patient at risk for mitral stenosis [54, 64]. Therefore, the suture line should not extend for more than 1 cm in length and the surgeon should ensure that each valve orifice side has at least a 2 cm opening to prevent mitral stenosis.

Transcatheter Mitral Valve Repair: MitraClip

The MitraClip device (Abbott Vascular, Menlo Park, California) is a percutaneous device used to treat patients with symptomatic chronic mitral regurgitation who are at high risk for surgery. The MitraClip was first implanted in 2003, and in 2013, it became the first device approved by the U.S. Food and Drug Administration as an alternative to open mitral valve surgery in patients with primary mitral regurgitation. It has also recently been approved for patients with severe secondary MR who remain symptomatic despite aggressive medical therapy.

The indications for MitraClip use are severe symptomatic mitral regurgitation (MR > 3+) in patients with prohibitive risk for open mitral valve surgery, favorable valve anatomy for repair, and reasonable life expectancy [3].

MitraClip is contraindicated in patients who cannot tolerate procedural anticoagulation or antiplatelet agents post-procedure. Also, patients with rheumatic mitral valve disease, active endocarditis, thrombus within the femoral vein, inferior vena cava or intracardiac thrombus, and patients with unfavorable valve anatomy (heavily calcified leaflets, cleft leaflets, large flail gap) are not candidates for this device [3].

Percutaneous mitral valve repair using the MitraClip device is based on the edge-to-edge repair as described by Alfieri. The device attaches the free edges of the middle segments (A2 and P2) of the mitral leaflets to create a double-orifice valve. This results in improved coaptation of the mitral leaflets and a reduction in the regurgitant jet. The procedure involves venous access via the femoral veins, advancement of the device into the right atrium, and a trans-septal puncture to access the mitral valve. Transesophageal echocardiographic (TEE) guidance is used to align the device with the regurgitant leaflets. The leaflets are grasped and TEE is used to evaluate the reduction in MR prior to deployment of the clip. Additional clips may be placed as necessary to reduce the regurgitant jets further. The procedure is generally performed under general anesthesia and heparin is administered to achieve an activated clotting time above 250 s [65].

The efficacy of the MitraClip was evaluated in the EVEREST II clinical trial, in which patients with severe symptomatic or asymptomatic mitral regurgitation were randomized to either percutaneous repair or surgical repair. The patients were followed for 12 months at the time of reporting. The rates of primary end-point for efficacy were 55% in the MitraClip group as compared to 73% in the surgery group. The rate of death was 6% in either group. Surgery for persistent or recurrent mitral regurgitation was 20% in the MitraClip group and 2% in the surgery group. 30-day rates of major adverse events were 15% in the MitraClip group and 48% in the surgery group. At 12 months, both groups had improved left ventricular size, New York Heart Association functional class and quality-of-life measures as compared with baseline [66].

A major disadvantage of the MitraClip procedure is that it may further damage a potentially repairable valve. For patients who fail MitraClip and then go on to an open surgical intervention, valve replacement is more likely than repair as a result of valve damage from the device. This underscores the need for proper patient selection for the MitraClip procedure, as patients with potentially repairable valves with acceptable surgical risk should be offered open surgery rather than a percutaneous repair [67].

Mitral Valve Replacement

When mitral valve repair is not feasible, mitral valve replacement (MVR) can be undertaken. Multiple prosthesis options exist for mitral replacement, and decisions regarding prosthesis type are similar to that for aortic valve replacement. Consideration for patient age, ability to anticoagulate, and patient preference are all important.

Indications

For patients with mitral regurgitation, the same criteria exist as for mitral repair. However, for patients with primary MR, replacement should only be undertaken if a successful repair cannot be achieved [3]. For patients with severe ischemic or secondary MR, the decision for repair versus replacement is less clear [68]. Some data suggests that repair has a higher recurrence rate of moderate-to-severe MR when compared with replacement, but no overall difference in mortality and left ventricular (LV) remodeling [69].

For patients with mitral stenosis (MS), percutaneous balloon commissurotomy is often the first line therapy when anatomically feasible. However, the AHA/ACC guidelines recommend mitral valve surgery for patients with symptomatic severe MS who are not candidates for or have failed balloon commissurotomy, patients with severe MS with recurrent embolic events while on anticoagulation, and for patients with moderate or severe MS undergoing cardiac surgery for other indications [3].

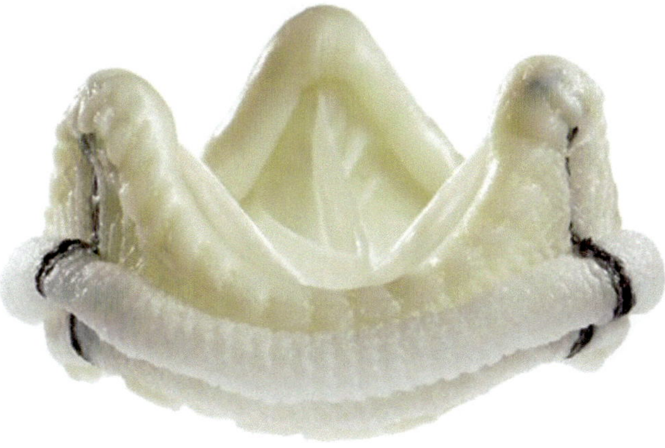

Fig. 11.7 St. Jude Epic™ stented tissue valve. Reproduced with permission of St. Jude Medical, ©2017

Choosing a Prosthesis

Similar to aortic valve replacement, multiple options for mitral valve replacements exist, which includes both mechanical and bioprosthetic valves (Fig. 11.7). In addition, mechanical and bioprosthetic mitral valves offer similar benefits and risk profiles as their counterparts for aortic valve replacement.

Mechanical valves should be considered for young patients, especially patients under 60 years of age, patients with chronic atrial fibrillation, patients already requiring long-term anticoagulation, and patients who wish to minimize the risk of reoperation [70]. Furthermore, patients with a small left ventricular size may benefit from a mechanical valve, as it offers a better hemodynamic profile compared to a bioprosthetic, while also maintaining a lower profile. However, mechanical valves may not be suitable for women of childbearing age due to the need for anticoagulation. In addition, noncompliant patients, patients with bleeding or fall risk, and patients who have other contraindications to anticoagulation should not receive a mechanical valve.

Bioprosthetic valves do not require long-term anticoagulation, which may be considered an advantage. However, they are less durable and more prone to structural valve deterioration (SVD) [71–77]. SVD is accelerated in younger patients compared to older patients. For these reasons, bioprosthetic valves should be considered for older patients, specifically patients older than 65 years old, patients with contraindications to anticoagulation, and patients of any age in sinus rhythm who wish to avoid anticoagulation.

Technique

Unlike replacement of the aortic valve, replacement of the mitral valve does not require leaflet excision. In fact, a chordal sparing technique for mitral valve replacement may help to preserve left ventricular function and is associated with improved survival [50, 78, 79]. The posterior leaflet can often be left in situ, or partially excised while preserving the chordae and subvalvular apparatus. The remaining leaflet tissue is then attached to the annulus with the sutures used for securing the prosthesis. The central portion of the anterior leaflet is often excised, while preserving the anterolateral and posteromedial aspects with the underlying chordae. The remaining anterior leaflet is similarly attached to the annulus with the valve insertion sutures [80].

Anticoagulation

In general, all valves in the mitral position are associated with a greater risk of thromboembolism than valves in the aortic position [81]. For this reason, the recommended INR for mechanical valves in the mitral position is higher than that for valves in the aortic position. The usual recommendation is a goal INR of 2.5–3.5 [3, 81]. In addition, some surgeons advocate for anticoagulation for all patients who undergo mitral valve replacement for the initial 3 months after surgery, including patients with a bioprosthesis. The atriotomy and potential stasis in the left atrial appendage, as well as the high risk of arrhythmias such as atrial fibrillation, may place patients at higher risk for thromboembolic events during this time [5, 82–86]. Patients with a bioprosthesis may then be re-evaluated at 3 months, and anticoagulation discontinued if the patient remains in sinus rhythm without other indications for anticoagulation. Aspirin should be considered for all patients with mitral replacements [87].

Future Considerations

The increasing adoption and success of TAVR has led to an increased interest in transcatheter mitral valve replacement. However, various limitations exist which has delayed the development and implementation of transcatheter mitral valve replacement (TMVR). Structurally, the mitral valve and its relationship to left ventricular function and outflow track is much more complex than that of the aortic valve. An especially important consideration is the mitral annulus. The annulus in mitral regurgitation is often not calcified and may not offer a reliable landing zone for a percutaneous device. However, some centers have achieved success with TMVR for patients with a prior bioprosthetic mitral valve or annuloplasty ring. The annuloplasty ring or stent of the implanted bioprosthesis may provide a solid landing zone for TMVR, and might provide a platform for increased implementation of valve-in-valve procedures in the mitral valve position [88–92]. Several devices for primary TMVR have been developed, but further trials are required before they may be adopted into regular use.

Tricuspid Valve

Valvular disease is infrequently isolated to the tricuspid valve (TV). Congenital lesions of the tricuspid valve occur in less than 1% of the population, and include Ebstein's anomaly, tricuspid atresia, and tricuspid stenosis. Acquired lesions of the tricuspid valve may be classified as either primary or secondary, and occur more commonly than congenital lesions. Careful evaluation is necessary to achieve the optimal individualized treatment and chance for long-term success.

Primary Lesions

Primary lesions of the tricuspid valve occur from direct involvement of the tricuspid valve by a variety of diseases. These diseases include endocarditis, rheumatic valvulitis, carcinoid disease, blunt chest trauma, and iatrogenic injuries. There has been a gradual increase in the incidence of iatrogenic injuries as a result of pacemaker/defibrillator implantation and endomyocardial biopsies, as these procedures are being performed with increasing frequency. Patients with indwelling transvalvular cardiac leads who require tricuspid surgery often have epicardial leads implanted at the time of surgery to reduce the risk of recurrence. Alternatively, the device lead may be stabilized by endocardial suture fixation at the commissure.

Secondary Lesions

The majority of tricuspid valve lesions are secondary, which occur as a result of a separate cardiac pathology. Left sided valve lesions of the mitral or aortic position are a common cause of secondary lesions. This can be observed in a variety of diseases which produce pulmonary hypertension and right ventricular dilatation which results in failure of tricuspid leaflet coaptation and "functional" regurgitation. Secondary tricuspid lesions can vary greatly and treatment requires careful evaluation.

With regard to bacterial endocarditis of the tricuspid valve, this condition occurs most frequently in patients who are intravenous drug abusers. These patients represent a unique cohort, and the optimal management of these patients remains somewhat controversial. Previously, such patients underwent valvectomy, as there has been some reluctance to implant prosthetic material in IV drug users. Once the bacteremia had been treated and the patient rehabilitated with respect to the substance abuse, they then underwent valve replacement. The process typically lasted 12–16 weeks and the tricuspid regurgitation was relatively well tolerated for that period of time. However, patients who defaulted often re-presented months to years later with severe right ventricular dysfunction. Surgery in this setting carries a high mortality. To avoid this complication, most programs offer definitive surgery at the time of presentation, acknowledging the risks of reinfection in poorly rehabilitated patients. Drug rehabilitation remains an integral part of the management of these patients, and as such, a multidisciplinary approach is undertaken.

Surgical Management

According to a recent review of the Society of Thoracic Surgery (STS) Database, between 2000 and 2010, a total of 54,375 adults underwent tricuspid valve surgery in North America [93]. Of these, 86% were performed concomitant with another major procedure. Less than 8000 cases over the 10-year period were isolated tricuspid valve surgeries. This underscores the relative rarity of this condition [94].

The 2014 AHA/ACC Guidelines recommend isolated tricuspid valve surgery only in patients with symptomatic severe tricuspid stenosis (Class I), for patients with symptomatic severe tricuspid regurgitation unresponsive to medical therapy (Class IIa), or in the setting of progressive right ventricular dysfunction (Class IIb). The only other class I indications for tricuspid valve surgery are in the setting of concomitant left sided surgery [3].

There are numerous surgical techniques for the management of tricuspid valve disease. Valve repair is preferable to replacement whenever possible. This has been reflected in the review of the STS database, where replacement rates have decreased from 15.4% in 2000 to 10.2% in 2010. The rate of permanent pacemaker implantation is lower in repairs compared to replacements (4.2% vs. 5.6%). In patients with tricuspid disease as a result of carcinoid or Ebstein's anomaly, replacement may be preferable to repair due to the extensive leaflet damage and dysplasia seen in these conditions. In addition, there are ongoing trials to evaluate the efficacy of a transcatheter system for the management of severe tricuspid regurgitation [95, 96].

The most common TV repair procedure is tricuspid annuloplasty, which may be performed using a ring or running stitch around the annulus (Fig. 11.8). Ring repair corrects

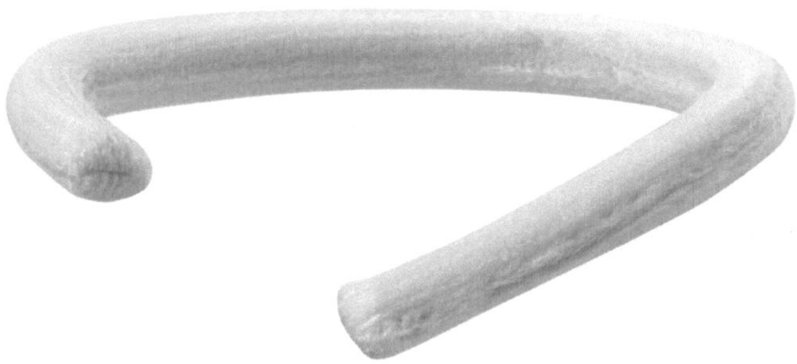

Fig. 11.8 Edwards MC3 Tricuspid™ annuloplasty ring. Courtesy of Edwards Lifesciences LLC, Irvine, California

regurgitation by reducing the annulus size and plicating the annular tissue. This improves leaflet coaptation which improves regurgitation. The atrioventricular (AV) node must be avoided to prevent arrhythmia by not placing sutures near the Triangle of Koch. Tricuspid annuloplasty rings are often incomplete for this reason.

Several factors have been shown to be predictors of poor prognosis in patients undergoing tricuspid valve surgery. These include impaired left ventricular systolic function, the presence of a permanent pacemaker, and high pulmonary artery pressures. However, a review of the STS adult cardiac surgery database found that the most important indicator of a poor outcome in this group of patients was the presence of dialysis dependent renal failure preoperatively. Overall, the operative mortality for tricuspid valve surgery has declined from 10.6% in 2000 to 8.2% in 2010 [93]. Repeat tricuspid valve surgery after a previous repair also carries a significant mortality, with rates quoted as high as 37% [97].

There is still work to be done to determine the optimal timing of surgery in patients with tricuspid valve disease, as the guidelines for asymptomatic or mildly symptomatic patients are currently based low levels of evidence. The Cardiothoracic Surgical Trials Network is currently enrolling patients in the "Evaluating the Benefit of Concurrent Tricuspid Valve Repair During Mitral Surgery" trial. The aim of this trial is to determine whether tricuspid valve repair in patients with mild to moderate tricuspid regurgitation at the time of planned mitral valve surgery is safe and efficacious [98]. It is hoped that sufficient information be gleaned from this and other trials so that the guideline recommendations can be based on strong clinical evidence.

Summary

Since the mid-twentieth century when valve repair and replacement were developed, the surgical techniques and available prostheses have continued to evolve. Valvular heart disease remains a significant challenge which accounts for a large percentage of cardiac surgical and interventional procedures today. With continued advancement, minimally invasive surgery and transcatheter valves are providing improved treatment for higher risk patients with valvular disease. Open surgical procedures for valve disease remain the gold standard for treatment for most patients.

References

1. Harken DE. Management of retained foreign bodies in the heart and great vessels, European Theater of Operations. In: Surgery in World War II. Vol. 2: Thoracic surgery. Washington, DC: Office at the Surgeon General, Department of the Army; 1965. p. 393–5.
2. Carabello BA, Paulus WJ. Aortic stenosis. Lancet. 2009;373:956–66.
3. Nishimura RA, Otto CM, Bonow RO, et al. 2014 AHA/ACC guideline for the management of patients with valvular heart disease: a report of the American College of Cardiology/American Heart Association Task Force on Practice Guidelines. J Am Coll Cardiol. 2014;63:e57.
4. Hufnagel CA, Harvey WP. The surgical correction of aortic regurgitation preliminary report. Bull Georgetown Univ Med Cent. 1953;6:60.
5. Ezekowitz MD. Anticoagulation management of valve replacement patients. J Heart Valve Dis. 2002;11(Suppl 1):S56.
6. Emery RW, Arom KV, Krogh CC, et al. Reoperative valve replacement with the St. Jude Medical valve prosthesis: long-term follow up. J Am Coll Cardiol. 2004;435:438A.
7. Oxenham H, Bloomfield P, Wheatley DJ, et al. Twenty-year comparison of a Bjork-Shiley mechanical heart valve with porcine bioprostheses. Heart. 2003;89:697.
8. Khan SS, Trento A, DeRobertis M, et al. Twenty-year comparison of tissue and mechanical valve replacement. J Thorac Cardiovasc Surg. 2001;122:257.
9. Brown ML, Schare HV, Lahr BD, et al. Aortic valve replacement in patients aged 50 to 70 years: improved outcome with mechanical versus biologic prosthesis. J Thorac Cardiovasc Surg. 2008;135:878.
10. DeVincentiis C, Kunkl AB, Trimarchi S, et al. Aortic valve replacement in octogenarians: is biologic valve the unique solution? Ann Thorac Surg. 2008;85:1296.
11. Emery RW, Krogh CC, Arom DV, et al. The St. Jude Medical cardiac valve prosthesis: a 25-year experience with single valve replacement. Ann Thorac Surg. 2005;79:776.
12. Lund O, Nielsen SL, Arildsen H, et al. Standard aortic St. Jude valve at 18 years: performance, profile and determinants of outcome. Ann Thorac Surg. 2000;69:1459.
13. Aagaard J, Tingleff J, Hansen CN, et al. Twelve years' clinical experience with the CarboMedics prosthetic heart valve. J Heart Valve Dis. 2001;10:177.
14. Butchart EG, Li H, Payne N, et al. Twenty years' experience with the Medtronic Hall valve. J Thorac Cardiovasc Surg. 2001;121:1090.
15. Ikonomidis JS, Kratz JM, Crumbley AJ, et al. Twenty-year experience with the St. Jude Medical mechanical valve prosthesis. J Thorac Cardiovasc Surg. 2003;126:200.
16. Puskas J, Gerdisch M, Nichols D, et al. Reduced anticoagulation after mechanical aortic valve replacement: interim results for the prospective randomized on-X valve anticoagulation clinic trial randomized Food and Drug Administration Investicational Device Exemption Trail. J Thorac Cardiovasc Surg. 2014;147:1202.
17. Wu YX, Burchart EG, Borer JS, Yoganathon A, Grunicemeier GL. Clinical evaluation of new heart valve prosthesis: update of objective performance criteria. Ann Thorac Surg. 2014;98:1865–74.
18. Butchart EG, Ionescu A, Payne N, et al. A new scoring system to determine thromboembolic risk after heart valve replacement. Circulation. 2003;108(Suppl II):II-68.
19. Akins CW, Buckley MJ, Daggett WM, et al. Risk of reoperative valve replacement for failed mitral and aortic bioprostheses. Ann Thorac Surg. 1998;65:1545.
20. Stassano P, Di Tommaso L, Monaco M, et al. Aortic valve replacement: a prospective randomized evaluation of mechanical versus biological valves in patients ages 55 to 70 years. J Am Coll Cardiol. 2009;54:1862.
21. Bloomfield P, Weathley J, Prescott RJ, Miller HC. Twelve-year comparison of a Bjork-Shiley mechanical valve with porcine bioprostheses. N Engl J Med. 1991;324:573.
22. Hammermeister K, Sethi GK, Henderson WG, et al. Outcomes 15 years after valve replacement with a mechanical versus a bioprosthetic valve: final report of the Veterans Affairs randomized trial. J Am Coll Cardiol. 2000;36:1152.

23. Forcillo J, El Hamamsy I, Stevens LM, et al. The perimount valve in the aortic position: twenty-year experience with patients under 60 years old. Ann Thorac Surg. 2014;97:1526–32.
24. Vongpatanasin W, Hillis LD, Lange RA. Prosthetic heart valves. N Engl J Med. 1996;335:407.
25. Borger MA, Carson SM, Ivanov J, et al. Stentless aortic valves are hemodynamically superior to stented valves during mid-term follow-up: a large retrospective study. Ann Thorac Surg. 2005;80:2180.
26. Maselli D, Pizio R, Bruno LP, Di Bella I, De Gasperis C. Left ventricular mass reduction after aortic valve replacement: homografts, stentless and stented valves. Ann Thorac Surg. 1999;67(4):966–71.
27. Svensson LG, Adams DH, Bonow RO, et al. Aortic valve and ascending aorta guidelines for management and quality measures. Ann Thorac Surg. 2013;95(6 Suppl):S1–66.
28. Foghsgaard S, Bruun N, Kjaergard H. Outcome of aortic homograft implantation in 24 cases of severe infective endocarditis. Scand J Infect Dis. 2008;40(3):216–20.
29. McGiffin DC, Kirklin JK. The impact of aortic valve homografts on the treatment of aortic prosthetic valve endocarditis. Semin Thorac Cardiovasc Surg. 1995;7(1):25–31.
30. El-Hamamsy I, Clark L, Stevens LM, Sarang Z, Melina G, Takkenberg JJ, Yacoub MH. Late outcomes following freestyle versus homograft aortic root replacement: results from a prospective randomized trial. J Am Coll Cardiol. 2010;55(4):368–76.
31. Oury JH. Clinical aspects of the Ross procedure: indications and contraindications. Semin Thorac Cardiovasc Surg. 1996;8(4):328–35.
32. Elkins RC, Thompson DM, Lane MM, et al. Ross operation: 16-year experience. J Thorac Cardiovasc Surg. 2008;136:623–30.
33. Mazine A, et al. Outcomes of the Ross Procedure versus mechanical aortic valve replacement: propensity-matched cohort study. Circulation. 2016;134:576–85.
34. Schmidtke C, et al. Up to seven years of experience with the Ross procedure in patients >60 years of age. J Am Coll Cardiol. 2000;36:1173–7.
35. Williams IA, et al. Ross procedure in infants and toddlers followed into childhood. Circulation. 2005;112:390–5.
36. Bowdish ME, et al. The Ross procedure: an excellent option in the right hands. Ann Transl Med. 2016;4(23):471.
37. David T. Reoperations after the Ross procedure. Circulation. 2010;122:1139–40.
38. Carrel T. The Ross procedure is under-used although long-term results show superior results to those obtained following mechanical aortic valve replacement. Ann Transl Med. 2016;4(Suppl 1):S21.
39. Nicks R, Cartmill T, Bernstein L. Hypoplasia of the aortic root—the problem of aortic valve replacement. Thorax. 1970;25:339–46.
40. Manouguian S, Seybold-Epting W. Patch enlargement of the aortic valve ring by extending the aortic incision into the anterior mitral leaflet—new operative technique. J Thorac Cardiovasc Surg. 1979;78:402–12.
41. Konno S, Imai Y, Iida Y, et al. A new method for prosthetic valve replacement in congenital aortic stenosis associated with hypoplasia of the aortic valve ring. J Thorac Cardiovasc Surg. 1975;70:909–17.
42. Popma JJ, Adams DH, Reardon MJ, et al. Transcatheter aortic valve replacement using a self-expanding bioprosthesis in patients with severe aortic stenosis at extreme risk for surgery. J Am Coll Cardiol. 2014;63(19):1972–81.
43. Smith CR, Leon MB, Mack MJ, et al. Transcatheter versus surgical aortic-valve replacement in high-risk patients. N Engl J Med. 2011;364(23):2187–98.
44. Kodali SK, Williams MR, Smith CR, et al. Two-year outcomes after transcatheter or surgical aortic-valve replacement. N Engl J Med. 2012;366(18):1686–95.
45. Movahed MR, Hepner AD, Ahmadi-Kashani M. Echocardiographic prevalence of bicuspid aortic valve in the population. Heart Lung Circ. 2006;15:297.
46. De Kerchove L, Boodhwani M, Glineur D, et al. Valve sparing-root replacement with the reimplantation technique to increase the durability of bicuspid aortic valve repair. J Thorac Cardiovasc Surg. 2011;142:143.
47. David TE. Aortic valve repair and aortic valve-sparing operations. In: Cohn LH, Adams DH, editors. Cardiac surgery in the adult, 5th ed. New York, NY: McGraw-Hill. http://accesssurgery.mhmedical.com.ezproxyhost.library.tmc.edu/content.aspx?bookid=2157&sectionid=164292095.
48. Enriquez-Sarano M, Schaff HV, Orszulak TA, Tajik AJ, Bailey KR, Frye RL. Valve repair improves the outcome of surgery for mitral regurgitation. A multivariate analysis. Circulation. 1995;91(4):1022–8.
49. DiBardino DJ, ElBardissi AW, RS MC, et al. Four decades of experience with mitral valve repair: analysis of differential indications, technical evolution, and long-term outcome. J Thorac Cardiovasc Surg. 2010;139(1):76–84.
50. Glower DD, Landolfo KP, Davis RD, et al. Comparison of open mitral commissurotomy with mitral valve replacement with or without chordal preservation in patients with mitral stenosis. Circulation. 1998;98(19 Suppl):II120–3.
51. Gillinov AM, Cosgrove DM, Blackstone EH, et al. Durability of mitral valve repair for degenerative disease. J Thorac Cardiovasc Surg. 1998;116:734–43.
52. Gillinov AM, Cosgrove DM, Shiota T, et al. Cosgrove-Edwards annulo-plasty system: midterm results. Ann Thorac Surg. 2000;69:717.
53. Shekar PS, Couper GS, Cohn LH. Mitral valve re-repair. J Heart Valve Dis. 2005;14:583.
54. Brinster DR, Unic D, D'Ambra MN, et al. Mid-term results of the edge to edge technique for complex mitral repair. Ann Thorac Surg. 2006;81:1612.
55. Braunberger E, Deloche A, Berrebi A, et al. Very long-term results (more than 20 years) of valve repair with Carpentier's techniques in nonrheumatic mitral valve insufficiency. Circulation. 2001;104(Suppl I):I-8–I-11.
56. Tabata M, Ghanta RK, Shekar PS, Cohn LH. Early and midterm outcomes of folding valvuloplasty without leaflet resection for myxomatous mitral valve disease. Ann Thorac Surg. 2008;86:1288.
57. Suri RM, Orszulak TA. Triangular resection for repair of mitral regurgitation due to degenerative disease. Op Tech Thorac Cardiovasc Surg. 2005;10:194–9.
58. Gazoni LM, Fedoruk LM, Kern JA, et al. A simplified approach to degenerative disease: triangular resections of the mitral valve. Ann Thorac Surg. 2007;83:1658–65.
59. Von Oppel UO, Mohr FW. Chordal replacement for both minimally invasive and conventional mitral valve surgery using premeasured Gore-Tex loops. Ann Thorac Surg. 2000;70:2166–8.
60. Gillinov AM, Banbury MK. Pre-measured artificial chordae for mitral valve repair. Ann Thorac Surg. 2007;84:2127–9.
61. Smedira NG, Selman R, Cosgrove DM, et al. Repair of anterior leaflet prolapse: chordal transfer is superior to chordal shortening. J Thorac Cardiovasc Surg. 1996;112:287.
62. Maisano F, Torracca L, Oppizzi M, et al. The edge-to-edge technique: a simplified method to correct mitral insufficiency. Eur J Cardiothorac Surg. 1998;13:240.
63. Alfieri O, Maisano F, De Bonis M, et al. The double-orifice technique in mitral valve repair: a simple solution for complex problems. J Thorac Cardiovasc Surg. 2001;122:674.
64. Bhudia SK, McCarthy PM, Smedira NG. Edge-to-edge (Alfieri) mitral repair: results in diverse clinical settings. Ann Thorac Surg. 2004;77:1598.
65. Maisano F, La Canna G, Colombo A, Alfieri O. The evolution from surgery to percutaneous mitral valve interventions: the role of the edge-to-edge technique. J Am Coll Cardiol. 2011;58:2174.

66. Glower D, et al. EVEREST II randomized clinical trial: predictors of mitral valve replacement in de novo surgery or after the Mitraclip procedure. J Thorac Cardiovasc Surg. 2012;143:S60–3.
67. Feldman T, et al. Percutaneous repair or surgery for mitral regurgitation. N Engl J Med. 2011;364:1395–406.
68. Shuhaiber J, Anderson RJ. Meta-analysis of clinical outcomes following surgical mitral valve repair or replacement. Eur J Cardiothorac Surg. 2007;31(2):267–75.
69. Acker MA, Parides MK, Perrault LP, et al. Mitral-valve repair versus replacement for severe ischemic mitral regurgitation. N Engl J Med. 2014;370(1):23–32.
70. Kaneko T, Aranki S, Javed Q, et al. Mechanical versus bioprosthetic mitral valve replacement in patients <65 years old. J Thorac Cardiovasc Surg. 2014;147(1):117–26.
71. Cohn LH, Collins JJ Jr, Rizzo RJ, Adams DH, Couper GS, Aranki SF. Twenty-year follow-up of the Hancock modified orifice porcine aortic valve. Ann Thorac Surg. 1998;66(6 Suppl):S30–4.
72. Corbineau H, Du Haut Cilly FB, Langanay T, Verhoye JP, Leguerrier A. Structural durability in Carpentier Edwards Standard bioprosthesis in the mitral position: a 20-year experience. J Heart Valve Dis. 2001;10(4):443–8.
73. Jamieson WR, Burr LH, Munro AI, Miyagishima RT. Carpentier-Edwards standard porcine bioprosthesis: a 21-year experience. Ann Thorac Surg. 1998;66(6 Suppl):S40–3.
74. Khan SS, Chaux A, Blanche C, et al. A 20-year experience with the Hancock porcine xenograft in the elderly. Ann Thorac Surg. 1998;66(6 Suppl):S35–9.
75. van Doorn CA, Stoodley KD, Saunders NR, Nair RU, Davies GA, Watson DA. Mitral valve replacement with the Carpentier-Edwards standard bioprosthesis: performance into the second decade. Eur J Cardiothorac Surg. 1995;9(5):253–8.
76. Pupello DF, Bessone LN, Hiro SP, et al. Bioprosthetic valve longevity in the elderly: an 18-year longitudinal study. Ann Thorac Surg. 1995;60(2 Suppl):S270–4; discussion S275
77. Jamieson WR, Tyers GF, Janusz MT, et al. Age as a determinant for selection of porcine bioprostheses for cardiac valve replacement: experience with Carpentier-Edwards standard bioprosthesis. Can J Cardiol. 1991;7(4):181–8.
78. David TE, Armstrong S, Sun Z. Left ventricular function after mitral valve surgery. J Heart Valve Dis. 1995;4(Suppl 2):S175–80.
79. Yun KL, Sintek CF, Miller DC, et al. Randomized trial comparing partial versus complete chordal-sparing mitral valve replacement: effects on left ventricular volume and function. J Thorac Cardiovasc Surg. 2002;123(4):707–14.
80. David TE. Mitral valve replacement with preservation of chordae tendinae: rationale and technical considerations. Ann Thorac Surg. 1986;41(6):680–2.
81. Cannegieter SC, Rosendaal FR, Wintzen AR, van der Meer FJ, Vandenbroucke JP, Briet E. Optimal oral anticoagulant therapy in patients with mechanical heart valves. N Engl J Med. 1995;333(1):11–7.
82. Heras M, Chesebro JH, Fuster V, et al. High risk of thromboemboli early after bioprosthetic cardiac valve replacement. J Am Coll Cardiol. 1995;25(5):1111–9.
83. Jegaden O, Eker A, Delahaye F, et al. Thromboembolic risk and late survival after mitral valve replacement with the St. Jude Medical valve. Ann Thorac Surg. 1994;58(6):1721–8. discussion 1727-1728
84. Meurin P, Tabet JY, Weber H, Renaud N, Ben Driss A. Low-molecular-weight heparin as a bridging anticoagulant early after mechanical heart valve replacement. Circulation. 2006;113(4):564–9.
85. Laffort P, Roudaut R, Roques X, et al. Early and long-term (one-year) effects of the association of aspirin and oral anticoagulant on thrombi and morbidity after replacement of the mitral valve with the St. Jude medical prosthesis: a clinical and transesophageal echocardiographic study. J Am Coll Cardiol. 2000;35(3):739–46.
86. Yamak B, Iscan Z, Mavitas B, et al. Low-dose oral anticoagulation and antiplatelet therapy with St. Jude Medical heart valve prosthesis. J Heart Valve Dis. 1999;8(6):665–73.
87. Braunwald E. Valvular heart diseases. Philadelphia: Saunders; 2001.
88. Cheung A, Webb JG, Barbanti M, et al. 5-Year experience with transcatheter transapical mitral valve-in-valve implantation for bioprosthetic valve dysfunction. J Am Coll Cardiol. 2013;61(17):1759–66.
89. Seiffert M, Conradi L, Baldus S, et al. Transcatheter mitral valve-in-valve implantation in patients with degenerated bioprostheses. JACC Cardiovasc Interv. 2012;5:341–9.
90. Webb JG, Wood DA, Ye J, et al. Transcatheter valve-in-valve implantation for failed bioprosthetic heart valves. Circulation. 2010;121:1848–57.
91. Wilbring M, Alexiou K, Tugtekin SM, et al. Transapical transcatheter valve-in-valve implantation for deteriorated mitral valve bioprostheses. Ann Thorac Surg. 2013;95:111–7.
92. Descoutures F, Himbert D, Maisano F, et al. Transcatheter valve-in-ring implantation after failure of surgical mitral repair. Eur J Cardiothorac Surg. 2013;44:e8–15.
93. Kilic A, et al. Trends and outcomes of tricuspid valve surgery in North America: an analysis of more than 50,000 patients from the Society of Thoracic Surgeons Database. Ann Thorac Surg. 2013;96:1546–52.
94. Ejiofor J, et al. Surgical outcomes of isolated tricuspid valve procedures: repair versus replacement. Ann Cardiothorac Surg. 2017;6(3):214–22.
95. Clinicaltrials.gov. Percutaneous Treatment of Tricuspid Valve Regurgitation With the TriCinch System™—Full Text View—ClinicalTrials.gov [online]. 2017. https://www.clinicaltrials.gov/ct2/show/NCT02098200.
96. Campelo-Parada F, et al. First-in-man experience of a novel transcatheter repair system for treating severe tricuspid regurgiatation. J Am Coll Cardiol. 2015;66:2475–83.
97. Rogers J, et al. The tricuspid valve: current perspective and evolving management of tricuspid regurgitation. Circulation. 2009;119:2718–25.
98. Clinicaltrials.gov. Evaluating the benefit of concurrent tricuspid valve repair during mitral surgery—Full Text View—ClinicalTrials.gov [online]. 2017. https://www.clinicaltrials.gov/ct2/show/NCT02675244.

Heart Disease in Pregnancy

12

Stephanie A. Coulter, Jeanney Lew, and Benjamin Jenny

Epidemiology of Cardiovascular Disease in Pregnancy

Cardiovascular disease (CVD) in pregnancy is relatively rare, affecting only 1–4% of pregnancies in the United States [1]. CVD includes congenital heart disease, acquired heart disease, and myocardial diseases. Worldwide, the most common causes of maternal death are hemorrhage and hypertensive disorders of pregnancy. Hypertensive disorders occur in 6–8% of all pregnancies [2] and contribute to CVD in pregnancy. Since 2006 in the United States, maternal deaths due to hemorrhage, hypertensive disorders of pregnancy, and anesthesia complications have decreased, and deaths attributed to cardiovascular conditions have increased [3]. CVD, specifically cardiomyopathy, is now the leading cause of maternal death in the United States and the United Kingdom [4]. In 2014, the overall US maternal mortality ratio was 17.2 per 100,000 births; this ratio is heavily influenced by race and advanced maternal age [3]. Maternal mortality ratios were 12.0 for non-Hispanic white women, 38.9 for non-Hispanic black women, and 11.7 for Hispanic women. Advanced maternal age due to voluntary postponement of pregnancy and improvements in fertility treatment have led to a greater prevalence of hypertension, valvular heart disease (VHD), diabetes, obesity, and preeclampsia in pregnancy [3]. Pregnancy-related mortality ratios increase with maternal age for all US women and within all age groups; in fact, 25% of all maternal deaths occur in women older than 35 years [3]. In a separate US nationwide inpatient study, women older than 45 years were significantly more likely to experience severe maternal morbidity and mortality than were women younger than 35 [5].

More importantly, surgical and medical improvements in the treatment of congenital heart disease (CHD) have allowed the highest-risk women to survive into the childbearing years [6]. CHD is now the most common form of CVD seen in pregnancy in the United States and western Europe, accounting for about 80% of CVD cases and 20% of maternal deaths [7]. Outside of Europe and North America, CHD represents only 9–19% of CVD. In developing countries, rheumatic heart disease (RHD) is the most common cause of CVD in pregnancy, causing 60–90% of CVD in pregnancy [8, 9].

Hemodynamic Adaptations of the Cardiovascular System in Pregnancy

The maternal cardiovascular system in pregnancy undergoes a rapid, robust, and reversible expansion to meet the growing metabolic and hemodynamic needs of the fetus. Systemic vascular resistance (SVR), a significant contributor to maternal cardiac afterload, declines 35–40% during pregnancy [10]. The decrease in SVR is detectable by the fifth week of gestation and before placentation, which begins between weeks 6 and 8 [11]. The SVR levels reach a plateau by week 16 and persist at that level until delivery. The decline in SVR is initially related to hormonal activation of renal vasodilation [12, 13] and maintained by uteroplacental shunting, which peaks at the end of the second trimester [10]. Mediators of vasodilation in pregnancy include enhanced production of endothelial nitric oxide [14] and placental prostacyclin [15]. Activation of the renin-angiotensin-aldosterone system early in pregnancy leads to increased sodium and water retention and causes an increase in preload as the stroke volume increases to a maximum of 40% above baseline by 34 weeks of gestation [16]. Starting around 20 weeks through 32 weeks, the heart rate increases to a maximum of 10–20 (16 average) beats per minute. The early increase in stroke volume augmented by the later rise

S. A. Coulter (✉)
Cardiovascular Education, Texas Heart Institute, Houston, TX, USA

Department of Cardiology, Baylor St. Lukes Medical Center, Houston, TX, USA
e-mail: scoulter@texasheart.org; SCoulter@thi.or

J. Lew · B. Jenny
Department of Cardiovascular Surgery, Texas Heart Institute, Houston, TX, USA

B. A. Carabello (ed.), *Valvular Heart Disease*, Cardiovascular Medicine, https://doi.org/10.1007/978-1-4471-2840-3_12

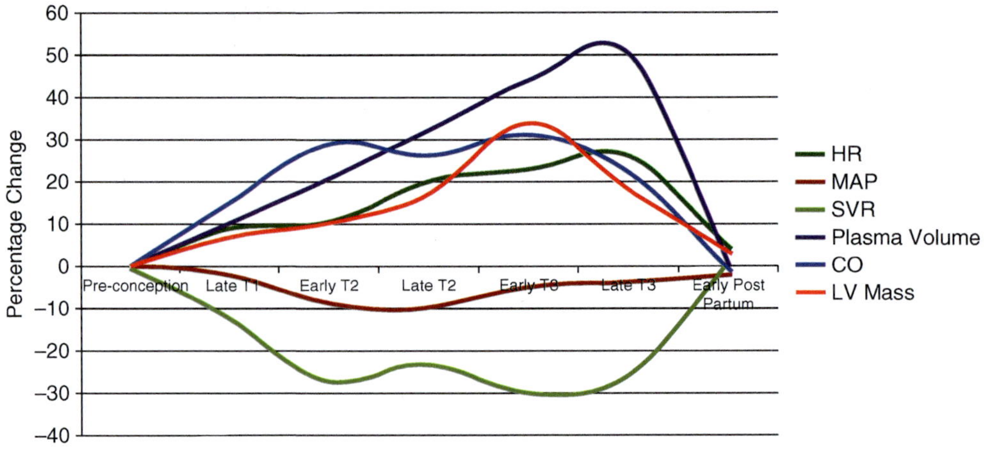

Fig. 12.1 Physiological changes in the cardiovascular system during pregnancy. From: Ashrafi R, Curtis SL. Heart Disease and Pregnancy. Cardiol Ther. 2017 Dec;6(2):157–173. Open Access, Springer Healthcare

in heart rate is responsible for a 30–45% increase in the cardiac output by the early third trimester (Fig. 12.1). A meta-analysis of 39 studies showed an average increase in cardiac output of 1.5 L/min (31%), a decline in SVR (30%), and a decrease in mean arterial pressure in pregnant women compared to values in nonpregnant women. In the early postpartum period, cardiac output returns to prepregnancy values [17]. Systolic and diastolic blood pressure (BP) decreases by up to 10mmHg early in gestation and remain below baseline levels through the second trimester. However, BP returns to baseline levels as the blood volume increases in the third trimester [18–20]. The decrease in BP parallels the decline in SVR [21]. Left ventricular mass is slightly increased during pregnancy to accommodate the rise in stroke volume. Left ventricular contractility and systolic function are relatively unchanged in pregnancy [17]. Maternal hemodynamic adaptation to twin pregnancy includes a further 15% volume expansion and a 5% increase in heart rate compared with singleton pregnancies [22].

Hemodynamic fluctuations are a part of normal labor and delivery. Pain, elevated heart rate, and catecholamine surge augment the cardiac output by 25–30% during the first stage of labor and up to 80% immediately postpartum [23, 24]. Maternal position, supine versus left lateral, also affects the venous return and thus the cardiac output. Volume shifts occur as uterine contractions autotransfuse 300–500 cm^3 of blood from the uterine sinusoids into the systemic circulation [25]. Postpartum hemodynamics are affected by analgesic drugs, bleeding, and infection and peak within 24–72 h after delivery. Marked hemodynamic changes during pregnancy, labor, and the postpartum period increase the burden to the maternal circulation, particularly in women with preexisting cardiomyopathy, VHD, or CHD. The time course of clinical deterioration in susceptible women parallels the rise in hemodynamic burden by the late second trimester, during, or just after delivery.

Maternal Risk Assessment

The risk of pregnancy in women with CVD depends on the clinical status of the patient and the specific cardiac defect. Lesion-specific risk assessment, discussed below, may be limited by validation based on small or retrospective studies. Three prospective maternal risk scores have been developed in larger populations with diverse CVD and include general and lesion-specific risk when available. Risk assessment will guide pregnancy and labor management plans.

The modified World Health Organization (WHO) risk classification [26], Cardiac Disease in Pregnancy (CARPREG) [27], and the ZAHARA (Zwangerschap bij vrouwen met een Aangeboren HARtAfwijking-II, translated as pregnancy in women with congenital heart disease II) [28] are maternal risk scoring systems. The modified WHO risk classification is based on expert consensus and incorporates known maternal risk factors and gives contraindications to pregnancy; it was endorsed by the ESC 2011 guidelines [29] on the management of CVD during pregnancy.

The CARPREG risk score is the most widely used and validated maternal risk score. In an observational cohort of 252 pregnant women with acquired and congenital heart disease (CHD), 4 predictors of an adverse maternal cardiac event were identified:

- Left heart obstruction (mitral valve area <2 cm^2, aortic valve area [AVA] <1.5 cm^2, or left ventricular outflow tract [LVOT] obstruction >30 mmHg)
- History of a cardiac event (congestive heart failure, transient ischemic attack or stroke, arrhythmia)
- Cyanosis or NYHA functional class III or IV
- Systolic ventricular function <40%

A prospective validation study of 562 women and 617 pregnancies assessed the accuracy of the prediction model

[8]. Maternal cardiac events, pulmonary edema, arrhythmia, stroke, or cardiac death occurred in 13% of pregnancies. Pregnancies with 0, 1, and >1 points had adverse cardiac event rates of 3, 39, and 66%. The agreement between the predicted and the observed event rates was excellent. Neonatal complications (death, intrauterine growth retardation [IUGR], preterm delivery, respiratory distress, or intraventricular hemorrhage) occurred in 17% of pregnancies and were associated with poor maternal functional class or cyanosis, left heart obstruction, anticoagulation, smoking, and multiple gestations. Adverse neonatal events occurred in a third of mothers (age <20 or >35 years) who smoked or received anticoagulants with a risk score ≥1 compared to the 11% rate in age-matched controls [27]. The CARPREG score may be associated with a higher rate of late cardiovascular events after pregnancy [30]. Late cardiac events (>6 months postpartum)—death, pulmonary edema, arrhythmia, and stroke—were evaluated in the CARPREG cohort of 318 women with 405 pregnancies (median follow-up, 2.6 years). Late cardiac events occurred in 12% of pregnancies and increased to 27% in women with cardiac complications during pregnancy. In women with 0, 1, >1 risk predictors, the 5-year late cardiac event rates were 7, 23, and 44%.

The ZAHARA score is a weighted score prediction model based on a retrospective observational cohort of 1302 pregnancies in 714 women with CHD exclusively (many complex). The ZAHARA score has not been validated. Cardiac complications, obstetric complications, and neonatal outcomes were assessed independently. Additive risk was assigned to women with the following factors:

- Mechanical heart valve (4.25 points)
- Severe left heart obstruction (mean pressure gradient >50 mmHg or AVA <1.0 cm^2) (2.50 points)
- History of arrhythmias (1.50 points)
- History of cardiac medication use before pregnancy (1.50 points)
- History of cyanotic heart disease (uncorrected or corrected) (1.00 points)
- Moderate-to-severe pulmonary or systemic atrioventricular valve regurgitation (0.75)
- Symptomatic heart failure before pregnancy (NYHA class ≥II) (0.75 points)

Scoring is based on five categories of cardiovascular risk (Table 12.1).

Table 12.1 ZAHARA scoring systems for estimating the risk of a cardiac complication during pregnancy

Points	Number of pregnancies	CV risk (%)
0–0.5	828	2.9
0.51–1.50	280	7.5
1.51–2.50	126	17.5
2.51–3.50	58	43.1
>3.51	10	70.0

CV cardiovascular

Data from: Ashrafi R, Curtis SL. Heart Disease and Pregnancy. Cardiol Ther. 2017 Dec;6(2):157–173

The most prevalent obstetric complications in the ZAHARA cohort were hypertensive complications (12.2%). Arrhythmias (4.7%) and heart failure (1.6%) were the most common cardiac complications. The most frequently encountered neonatal outcomes, which complicated 25% of completed pregnancies, were premature birth (12%), small for gestational age (14%), and mortality (4%). Maternal cardiac complications and neonatal outcomes were highly correlated ($r = 0.85$, $P = 0.002$). Adverse neonatal outcome correlated with cyanotic heart disease (corrected/uncorrected) ($P = 0.0003$), mechanical valve replacement ($P = 0.03$), maternal smoking ($P = 0.007$), multiple gestation ($P = 0.0014$), and the use of cardiac medication ($P = 0.0009$). The ZAHARA study identified the following additional independent predictors of adverse cardiac complications during pregnancy in women with CVD: moderate or severe systemic or pulmonary AV valve regurgitation, mechanical valve prosthesis, and "at birth" cyanotic CHD.

The predictors and risk scores derived from CARPREG (which included women with acquired heart disease and CHD) and ZAHARA (which included only women with CHD) are population dependent. The CARPREG score reportedly overestimated risk in other CHD cohorts [31–33], suggesting that women with acquired heart disease and arrhythmia may be at greater risk of cardiac events. Important maternal risk characteristics, including pulmonary hypertension and dilated aorta, were not included in CARPREG or ZAHARA because they were underrepresented in these studies. Right ventricular systolic dysfunction and/or severe pulmonary regurgitation have been reported as additional independent risk factors for adverse maternal and fetal events in women with CVD [34].

The modified WHO risk classification is the maternal risk assessment recommended by the European Society of Cardiology (ESC) guidelines on the management of CVD during pregnancy [29]. The modified WHO risk classification performed superiorly to both CARPREG and ZAHARA risk scores in a prospective evaluation of cardiovascular risk in 213 pregnancies in 203 women with CHD [26]. The WHO risk classification is based on expert consensus and incorporates all known specific maternal cardiac risk factors, congenital and acquired, and integrates them with other comorbidities [35, 36]. Risk is additive; therefore, for each individual, the risk of a pregnancy may move up a class if there are additional risk factors. The modified WHO classification divides women into four classes, ranging from low to high risk.

- Modified WHO risk class I conditions are associated with no detectable increased risk of maternal mortality and no/mild increase in morbidity. This category includes uncomplicated, small or mild pulmonic stenosis, patent ductus arteriosus, mitral valve prolapse, and successfully repaired simple lesions. Cardiology follow-up during pregnancy may be limited to 1–2 visits.
- Modified WHO risk class II conditions are of low to moderate risk and are associated with a small increased risk of maternal mortality or a moderate increase in morbidity. Conditions include arrhythmias, unrepaired atrial septal defect (ASD) or ventricular septal defect (VSD) and repaired tetralogy of Fallot (TOF). Cardiology follow-up is recommended every trimester.
- Modified WHO risk class II to III conditions can fall either into class II or III depending on individual circumstances and, thus, require individualized assessment. These conditions include native or tissue valvular heart disease (VHD), repaired coarctation, an ascending aorta diameter <45 mm associated with bicuspid aortic valve (BAV), mild left ventricular dysfunction, and HCM. Cardiology and obstetric follow-up recommendations range from every trimester to monthly.
- Modified WHO risk class III conditions are associated with significantly increased risk of maternal mortality or severe morbidity. Expert counseling is recommended to individualize maternal and fetal risk in pregnancy. Cyanosis with prepregnancy resting arterial oxygen saturation <85% is associated with only a 12% chance of a live birth. This class includes mechanical valve, systemic right ventricle, Fontan circulation, unrepaired cyanotic heart disease, complex CHD, BAV with ascending aortic diameter of 45–50 mm, and MFS with aortic dilatation 40–45 mm. The complication risk is high, and frequent (monthly or bimonthly) cardiac and obstetric monitoring is needed throughout pregnancy, childbirth, and the postpartum period.
- Modified WHO risk class IV includes cardiac conditions in which pregnancy is contraindicated due to the extremely high risk of maternal mortality or severe morbidity. If pregnancy occurs, termination is advised and should be discussed. If the pregnancy is terminated, appropriate intervention to correct severe left heart obstruction (mitral or aortic stenosis or coarctation) or severe dilatation of the aorta should be performed before pregnancy is attempted again. If the pregnancy continues, monthly or bimonthly cardiology and obstetric follow-up is recommended, as for class III patients.

Fetal Risk Assessment

Limited data for fetal risk have been derived from small cohorts or registry studies of pregnancies in women with CHD, VHD, or both [27, 37]. Neonatal or fetal complications occur in 20–25% of pregnancies in women with CVD. Fetal death occurs in 1–4% of pregnancies in women with CVD [26, 28]. Miscarriage rates are higher in women with complex CHD [29]. Fetal and neonatal complications include death, preterm delivery, decreased birth weight or IUGR, and intraventricular hemorrhage. Maternal predictors of fetal complications include maternal NYHA functional class III or IV, left heart obstruction, mechanical heart valves, anticoagulation use, smoking, cyanosis, multiple gestations, and maternal age <20 years or >35 years [8, 29, 32, 34]. No fetal risk score has been established. Although maternal and fetal risks correlate, maternal risk scores do not adequately predict fetal risk [26].

Congenital Heart Disease and Pulmonary Hypertension in Pregnancy

Maternal High-Risk (III–IV) Conditions

General Recommendations

Women with CHD will usually have a diagnosis before pregnancy. Assessment of prepregnancy risk is imperative. Medical and surgical history, functional status, echocardiography, and oxygen saturation should be evaluated by an interdisciplinary expert team before pregnancy. Women with pulmonary hypertension, severe obstructive valvular heart disease or coarctation, depressed left ventricular or right ventricular function, aortic dilatation in MFS or bicuspid aortopathy, poor functional class, or cyanosis are at the greatest maternal and fetal risk during pregnancy. Risk in pregnancy depends on the specific cardiac defect but increases as the disease becomes more complex. Overall, 80% of pregnancies occurring in women with CHD will complete, whereas 15% will miscarry. Of the completed pregnancies, 12% of women will have cardiac complications, including congestive heart failure, arrhythmia, stroke, and death [30]. Neonatal mortality approaches 13% in mothers with pulmonary hypertension (mean pulmonary artery pressure >25 mmHg) [38] and 88% when maternal cyanosis (oxygen saturation <85%) [39] is present. Women in the highest risk group, WHO IV, should be informed of the extreme maternal risk in pregnancy and offered effective permanent birth control. In cases of severe pulmonary hypertension, pregnancy termination is recommended and should be offered. If the pregnancy is continued, supplemental oxygen, anticoagulation, and specific therapies targeting the etiology of pulmonary hypertension may be required.

Pulmonary Hypertension

Pulmonary hypertension encompasses a group of diverse diseases defined by a mean pulmonary artery pressure at rest >25 mmHg or 30 mmHg on exercise in the absence of a left-to-right shunt. Mild pulmonary arterial hypertension can also be defined as a pulmonary artery systolic pressure of ~36–50 mmHg. The WHO classifies patients into the following five groups based on etiology [40]: Group 1, idiopathic or inheritable pulmonary artery hypertension; Group 2, pulmonary hypertension secondary to congenital and left heart disease (elevated pulmonary capillary wedge pressure); Group 3, pulmonary hypertension due to chronic lung disease or hypoxemia; Group 4, chronic thromboembolic pulmonary hypertension; and Group 5, pulmonary hypertension of unclear or multiple etiologies. Pulmonary hypertension of any etiology, when severe, is poorly tolerated in pregnancy. Pulmonary hypertension in pregnant women is most commonly related to CHD, as advances in treatment of CHD have increased the number of women surviving into the childbearing age [6]. The risk of maternal death is increased, even in the presence of mild pulmonary hypertension. In the United Kingdom, maternal mortality data suggest that pregnancy can be associated with progression of pulmonary hypertension [7]. Maternal deaths are a result of pulmonary thrombosis, pulmonary hypertensive crisis and right heart failure usually in the last trimester or after delivery as pulmonary blood flow increases and the hormonal milieu of pregnancy activates the clotting cascade. General anesthesia, late hospitalization, and increasing severity of pulmonary hypertension are risk factors for maternal death in pulmonary hypertension [38].

Eisenmenger Syndrome

Eisenmenger syndrome—the triad of systemic-to-pulmonary shunt, pulmonary arterial hypertension, and cyanosis—is the most severe form of shunt-related pulmonary hypertension. Eisenmenger syndrome is caused by unrestrictive left-to-right heart shunting of volume and pressure increases the pulmonary blood volume and pulmonary pressure. Altered pulmonary volume/pressure, in turn, disrupts the pulmonary vascular endothelium and results in long-term fixed pulmonary arteriolar hypertension [41]. The increased pulmonary vascular resistance eventually reduces the left-to-right flow across the intracardiac shunt, with eventual right-to-left shunting and resultant cyanosis. In pregnancy, the natural reduction in maternal SVR increases the right-to-left shunt flow, decreases pulmonary blood flow, and increases cyanosis. Asymptomatic women with compensated cardiac defects and mild-to-moderate pulmonary hypertension may clinically deteriorate during the later stages of pregnancy or immediately postpartum. Maternal mortality is due to sudden arrhythmia-related death, progressive heart failure, or pulmonary hemorrhage, and ranges from 17 to 50% in patients with severe pulmonary hypertension and Eisenmenger syndrome [1, 38, 39, 42]. The size of the shunt and the ratio of the SVR to pulmonary vascular resistance determine the volume of the left-to-right shunt flow in VSD. The development of pulmonary hypertension is related to the volume and duration of pulmonary shunt flow in ASD, VSD, and patent ductus arteriosis (PDA), but transmitted systemic pressures contribute and augment the pulmonary arteriolar endothelial damage in VSD and PDA. Even with a large ASD, the pulmonary pressures do not increase until adulthood, whereas pulmonary hypertension develops early in large nonrestrictive VSD and PDA [43, 44]. Eisenmenger syndrome occurs in only 10% of unrepaired ASDs and in 50% of unrepaired VSDs, but it's seen in nearly all patients with unrepaired truncus arteriosus [45]. In nonpregnant adults with Eisenmenger syndrome, life expectancy is reduced by 20 years in those with simple cardiac shunts but by 40 years in those with more complicated defects when compared to healthy adults [46]. Pregnancy is contraindicated in patients with Eisenmenger syndrome, and termination is recommended.

Cyanotic Heart Disease Without Pulmonary Hypertension

Most cases of cyanotic heart disease will be repaired or palliated in childhood, before childbearing age is reached. Possible cyanotic congenital lesions without pulmonary hypertension include unrepaired TOF, pulmonary atresia with aortopulmonary collaterals, some single ventricular lesions, tricuspid atresia, Ebstein's anomaly with right-to-left shunts via an ASD, and congenitally corrected transposition of the great arteries (TGA) with VSD or ASD [39]. Right-to-left intracardiac or extracardiac shunts result in hypoxemia, erythrocytosis, and cyanosis. Cyanosis causes fetal loss, prematurity and fetal growth restriction [47, 48]. The degree of maternal hypoxemia is the most important predictor of fetal outcome. Only 12% of fetuses survive to live birth when maternal cyanosis or resting oxygen saturation is <85%. Fetal survival is >90% when maternal oxygen saturation is >90% [39]. Maternal complications occur in up to 30% of cyanotic pregnancies and include arrhythmias, heart failure, pulmonary or arterial thrombosis, and IE. Pregnancy is contraindicated if cyanosis (oxygen saturation <85% at rest) is present as fetal loss is likely and maternal risk is high. Termination is recommended if pregnancy occurs. For resting oxygen saturation >90%, the risk of fetal loss remains increased, and women should be counseled. The decrease in maternal SVR in pregnancy may increase the right-to-left shunt flow and increase maternal cyanosis. For women with mild cyanosis without pulmonary hypertension, completed pregnancy may be possible. The ESC guidelines on the management of CVD in pregnancy recommend exercise oxygen saturation testing for patients with resting saturation >85% but <90%. If saturation declines with exercise, pregnancy should be avoided as fetal prognosis is poor [29].

Severe Left Ventricular Outflow Tract Obstruction

Severe LVOT obstruction from any etiology in pregnancy poses high maternal and fetal risk. Pregnancy is contraindicated, and termination is recommended. Women with severe LVOT obstruction should undergo repair before pregnancy.

Maternal Low- and Moderate-Risk (I, II, III) Conditions

Women with repaired and unrepaired defects in the absence of cyanosis, pulmonary hypertension, or mechanical valve replacement may tolerate pregnancy well as long as ventricular function is preserved and the functional class is good. Prepregnancy assessment with echocardiography and careful follow-up during each trimester is advised.

Atrial Septal Defect

An ASD, a persistent interatrial communication, is the most common repaired or unrepaired lesion in pregnant women with CHD [47, 49]. The reported birth prevalence is approximately 2 per 1000 live births [47, 50–52].

The most common ASD involves the secundum septum (fossa ovalis) and accounts for 70% of ASDs. The secundum ASD is twice as common in females as in males. A secundum ASD <8 mm in diameter usually closes spontaneously during childhood. The primum ASD (15–20% of ASDs) occurs because the septum primum fails to merge with the endocardial cushion during fetal development. Primum defects tend to be larger than secundum ASDs and are commonly associated with cleft mitral valve and VSD. The sinus venosus ASD, accounting for 5–10% of ASDs, usually involves the superior venosus septum and is almost always associated with anomalous drainage of the right superior pulmonary vein into the right atrium, which increases the volume of the left-to-right shunt [53]. The last type of ASD, the unroofed or coronary sinus ASD, is rare, accounting for <1% of ASDs. Primum, sinus venosus, and coronary sinus ASDs do not close spontaneously and cannot be closed percutaneously.

The clinical manifestations of an unrepaired ASD are related to defect location, ASD size, and the presence of other congenital defects. Atrial arrhythmias, exercise intolerance, fatigue, and late right heart failure may result from larger atrial shunts. Paradoxic embolization can occur, even in small ASDs, with a reported rate up to 5%. The presence of an ASD during the reproductive years is rarely associated with severe pulmonary hypertension and is generally well tolerated in pregnancy. Many pregnant women remain asymptomatic; those with significant shunts may develop a detectable systolic pulmonary flow murmur with pregnancy because of the pregnancy-related increase in intravascular volume. Closure of a symptomatic or large asymptomatic ASD is recommended before pregnancy to prevent right heart failure, atrial arrhythmia, and paradoxic embolization. Closure of asymptomatic small ASDs is not indicated pregnancy to prevent paradoxic embolization [29]. Risk of thromboembolism in pregnant women with ASD is decreased by preventing venous stasis (via ambulation or compression stockings), restricting the use of long-term intravenous catheters, and using prophylactic anticoagulation in the immobilized. Percutaneous closure of secundum ASD during pregnancy is very rarely indicated. Pregnant women with repaired ASD are not at increased maternal or fetal risk [29]

Ventricular Septal Defects

VSD is the second most common form of CHD with a prevalence of 3–3.5 per 1000 live births, which represents 10% of CHD in adults [54]. VSDs are most commonly perimembranous (80%), muscular (5–20%), inlet (8%), or infundibular (6%). Muscular VSDs often close during childhood. The functional size of the defect, the presence of associated congenital conditions, and the ratio of systemic-to-pulmonary vascular resistance determines the severity of the left-to-right shunt, the resultant increase in right ventricular volume, and the degree of pulmonary overcirculation. In adults, most VSDs occur as an isolated defect but also occur with ASD (35%), PDA (22%), right aortic arch (13%), TGA, or TOF. Small VSDs, usually with an orifice dimension ≤25% of the aortic annulus diameter, are restrictive to both pressure and volume and are well tolerated in pregnancy. Moderate-size defects, measuring 25–75% of the aortic annulus diameter, allow a moderately sized left-to-right volume shunt but no or minimal evidence of pulmonary hypertension. These defects are also relatively well tolerated in pregnancy. Large defects, ≥75% of the aortic annulus diameter, lead to a large unrestricted shunt volume, left ventricular volume overload, and pulmonary hypertension. The maternal risk of heart failure and arrhythmias is high in women with a large VSD with pulmonary hypertension, a history of ventricular dysfunction, moderate or greater pulmonic stenosis, or arrhythmias.

Women with successfully repaired VSDs with normal ventricular function are not at increased maternal or fetal risk with pregnancy. Prepregnancy evaluation by echocardiography to assess residual VSD, ventricular function, and pulmonary pressures is recommended. Children of women with VSD have a greater risk of CHD (3–7%). The risk of endocarditis is 11% for unrepaired VSD, but the rates are halved after successful repair. Subacute bacterial endocarditis in unrepaired VSD is not related to defect size [55].

Atrioventricular Septal Defects

Atrioventricular (AV) septal or AV canal defects are a complex congenital heart defect involving the development of the endocardial cushion and are associated with defects involving the AV valves and the AV septum. Representing around 5% of CHD, AVSDs have a prevalence of 0.3–0.4 per 1000 live births [50, 54]. Down syndrome (trisomy 21) is strongly associated with AVSD and is seen in 40–50% of AVSD cases

[56]. Maternal diabetes and obesity may be associated with nonsyndromic AVSDs [57]. AVSD involves both the atrial primum septum and the ventricular inlet septum in half the cases and is referred to as a complete AV canal defect. Otherwise, AVSD may be isolated to the atrial primum septum and is called an incomplete AV canal. Abnormalities of the AV valve are variable and include a common or cleft AV valve. AV valve regurgitation is common and contributes to symptoms. When the AV canal is complete, there is left-to-right shunting at both the atrial and ventricular levels, which produces a marked intracardiac shunt, leading to early heart failure and pulmonary hypertension in all cases. Surgical correction has enabled survival into the reproductive years. Residual shunt, AV valve regurgitation, and pulmonary pressures must be evaluated before pregnancy to assess maternal and fetal risk with pregnancy. Women with moderate or less residual AV valve regurgitation and normal left ventricular function after repair tolerate pregnancy well and are considered WHO category risk II. If ventricular function is abnormal (ejection fraction [EF] < 60% but >30%) and AV valve regurgitation is severe, surgical correction with mitral valve repair is recommended before pregnancy [58]. Worsening heart failure, arrhythmia, and perinatal mortality are consequences of pregnancy in AVSD with severe AV regurgitation and ventricular dysfunction [59]. For women with AVSD and pulmonary hypertension, pregnancy is contraindicated.

Coarctation of the Aorta

Coarctation of the aorta is defined as a significant narrowing of the proximal thoracic aorta at the insertion of the ductus arteriosum distal to the left subclavian artery. Aortic obstruction leads to systemic hypertension, early coronary artery disease, stroke, heart failure, aneurysm formation, and aortic dissection and rupture in unrepaired coarctation of the aorta [60, 61]. Genetic factors contribute to the pathogenesis of coarctation. Half of all cases of coarctation are associated with BAV and, almost one-fifth of patients with Turner syndrome have coarctation of the aorta [62]. Significant coarctation or recurrent coarctation after surgical or catheter repair with outflow obstruction (peak-to-peak gradient >20 mmHg or <20 mmHg with evidence of collateral flow) should be corrected before pregnancy. After successful repair of coarctation, pregnancy is well tolerated and is categorized as a WHO class II risk. Women with residual coarctation gradient, aortic aneurysm or residual hypertension are at increased risk of aortic rupture and rupture of cerebral aneurysm during pregnancy or delivery. During pregnancy, close BP monitoring and treatment of hypertension are recommended.

Pulmonary Valve Stenosis and Regurgitation

Pulmonary valve disease is a common congenital heart defect with a slight female prevalence and occurs in 7% of CHD cases [63–65]. Pulmonary stenosis also occurs in association with other congenital defects including TOF, congenital rubella syndrome, and Noonan, Williams, Alagille, and LEOPARD syndromes. Pulmonary stenosis may occur at the valve, subvalvular, or supravalvular position. Valvular pulmonary stenosis is usually an isolated lesion with a benign clinical course, and patients are expected to survive to adulthood. Bicuspid pulmonary valves occur in less than 20% of cases [66]. Dysplastic pulmonary valves are common in Noonan syndrome [67]. If stenosis is severe, pulmonary blood flow may be limited with exertion resulting in exercise-induced fatigue, dyspnea, syncope, or chest pain, and eventual symptomatic right heart failure. Women with severe pulmonary stenosis (peak pulmonary valve gradient >64 mmHg) are at increased risk of right heart failure and possible fetal compromise and should undergo valvuloplasty or valve replacement before pregnancy [68–70]. A normal pregnancy is expected following surgical or balloon repair of a congenital pulmonary valve stenosis with little residual obstruction or regurgitation. Pulmonary stenosis in the absence of right heart failure is well tolerated in pregnancy [71]. Percutaneous pulmonary valvotomy during pregnancy can reduce risk in symptomatic women with severe pulmonary stenosis [72]. Although no maternal complications were reported among 100 pregnant women with repaired and unrepaired pulmonary stenosis, fetal complications include fetal demise (0.8%), perinatal death (4.1%), premature delivery (14.5%), and recurrent CHD (2.8%) stenosis. Moderate or severe pulmonary regurgitation is usually a complication of repaired TOF or occurs after pulmonary valvotomy for childhood pulmonary stenosis. Severe pulmonary regurgitation may be associated with right ventricular dilatation or systolic dysfunction. Overall, pulmonary regurgitation, even when severe, is well tolerated in pregnancy. The risk of right heart failure during pregnancy is increased in women with severe pulmonary regurgitation and any one of the following: multiple gestations, right ventricular systolic dysfunction, right ventricular hypertrophy, or branch pulmonary stenosis [73]. In these circumstances, pulmonary valve replacement with a biologic prosthesis is recommended before pregnancy.

Ebstein's Anomaly of the Tricuspid Valve

Ebstein's anomaly is a congenital developmental defect involving the tricuspid valve and the right ventricle. It occurs in 1 in 20,000 births with equal frequency in males and females [74–76]. The risk of Ebstein's anomaly is increased in fetuses exposed to lithium early in gestation. Ebstein's anomaly occurs in conjunction with a patent foramen ovale (PFO) or secundum ASD in about 80% of cases [77] and is also associated less frequently with VSD, PDA, BAV, and L-TGA. An accessory conduction pathway (e.g., Wolff-Parkinson-White) in 6–36% of patients with Ebstein's anomaly predisposes to symptomatic tachycardia [78]. Apical displacement of the septal and posterior tricuspid valve leaflets into the right ventricle in Ebstein's anomaly (septal leaflet displacement ≥2 cm or 0.8 cm/m^2 >anterior mitral leaflet attachment) divides the right ventricle into two chambers: a superior "atrialized" thin, non-contracting right ventricle chamber above the tricuspid valve and a smaller distal right ventricular pumping chamber below the valve. Variable amounts of tricuspid regurgitation and right ventricle dysfunction are consequences of Ebstein's anomaly. Bidirectional shunting across the PFO or ASD can cause cyanosis without pulmonary hypertension. In women with Ebstein's anomaly without cyanosis or heart failure, pregnancy is well tolerated (WHO risk class II). Women with right ventricle failure and severe tricuspid regurgitation should undergo tricuspid valve repair before pregnancy. During pregnancy, the severity of the tricuspid regurgitation and the functional capacity of the right ventricle determine the hemodynamic burden and the outcome [79, 80]. Arrhythmias and right heart failure are associated with a worse prognosis [80] as premature delivery and fetal mortality are increased [79]. Women with Ebstein's anomaly and interatrial shunting may develop right-to-left shunt and cyanosis during pregnancy. Paradoxic embolic risk is also increased in pregnancy [29]. Isolated severe tricuspid regurgitation can be managed with diuretics if needed during pregnancy.

Tetralogy of Fallot

TOF is a cyanotic congenital heart defect with 4 components: a malpositioned (rightward) aorta that overrides the ventricular septum, a large malaligned VSD, infundibular subpulmonary pulmonary stenosis, and right ventricular hypertrophy. Because of the malaligned aorta and VSD, the pulmonary artery may be underdeveloped, and the aortic root may be dilated, which may cause aortic insufficiency (AI). The prevalence of TOF is about 4–5 per 10,000 live births and accounts for 7–10 % of CHD [50, 81]. Children with TOF usually present with symptoms of agitation and cyanosis within the first year of life [82]. Cyanosis is dependent on the degree of right ventricular outflow tract (RVOT) obstruction (infundibular right ventricular hypertrophy and pulmonary stenosis). Patients with mild RVOT stenosis may remain "pink" and go undiagnosed until late adolescence or early adulthood when they present with evidence of pulmonary overcirculation secondary to the large unrestricted VSD. Prenatal diagnosis is common as widespread screening ultrasonography has improved [83]. Intracardiac surgical repair of TOF is typically performed before 6 months of age [84]. Residual defects, right ventricular systolic function, and pulmonary insufficiency affect late prognosis. Severe pulmonary insufficiency with moderate right ventricle dilatation or right ventricle systolic dysfunction should be repaired before pregnancy. Women with repaired TOF tolerate pregnancy well (WHO risk class II). Cardiac arrhythmias, heart failure, VTE, and endocarditis may occur in up to 12% of pregnancies in women with repaired TOF [85].

Transposition of the Great Arteries

Transposition of the great arteries (TGA) is a congenital heart defect in which the aorta arises from the right ventricle and the pulmonary artery arises from the left ventricle. The great vessels are transposed with the pulmonary artery positioned posterior to the aorta. Orientation of the ventricles determines the physiology and prognosis. In the most common form, dextro-TGA (D-TGA), the left ventricle is aligned leftward producing two parallel circulations. Systemic venous blood recirculates via the right ventricle and the aorta to the peripheral tissues, whereas the oxygenated blood recirculates through the left ventricle and the pulmonary artery to the lungs. Cyanosis is present at birth with oxygenation dependent on intracardiac shunting (via an ASD, PFO, or VSD) or flow through a PDA. In levo-TGA (L-TGA), the left and right ventricles are "inverted" with the left ventricle rightward and the venous and arterial circuits "physiologically corrected" and arranged in series, which avoids cyanosis unless other cardiac defects are present. However, the systemic ventricle in L-TGA is the less resilient morphologic right ventricle, and patients are at risk of progressive right ventricle dysfunction and right heart failure as adults.

D Transposition of the Great Arteries

D-TGA occurs in 2.3–4.7 per 10,000 live births; it accounts for less than 3% of all CHD but is seen in up to 20% of cyanotic CHD [50, 81]. VSD is present in 50% of patients with D-TGA. LVOT obstruction due to pulmonary stenosis or pulmonary atresia occurs in 25% of D-TGA cases. Antenatal diagnosis is difficult even with fetal echocardiography, and diagnosis is usually made by echocardiogram in a cyanotic newborn with respiratory distress. Without surgical correction, mortality is 90% in the first year of life [86]. Atrial switch procedures, either Senning or Mustard, were widely used from the mid-1960s to the 1980s to surgically repair D-TGA and allowed children to survive into adulthood. Redirecting the venous atrial inflow corrected the cyanosis and provided for circulation in series at the expense of allowing the morphologic right ventricle to remain the systemic ventricle. Long-term complications include eventual right ventricular dysfunction, atrial arrhythmias, and atrial baffle obstruction [87–89]. The arterial switch operation (ASO), in widespread use since 1990, is a surgical procedure for correcting the anatomy and involves reorienting the left ventricle as the systemic ventricle and restoring the cardiac circulation in series. Improved ASO techniques, in which the coronaries are reimplanted onto the root of the native pulmonary artery, have decreased the perioperative mortality in uncomplicated D-TGA to near 0% [90]. Long-term complications of the ASO involve coronary arterial insufficiency in as many as 12% at 15 years after correction [91], neo-aortic root dilatation (Z score –3) in up to 50% at 10 years, and moderate to severe neo-aortic insufficiency in 8–15% at 20 years [92].

The data on pregnancy after ASO are limited, but successful pregnancies have been reported [93, 94]. In a retrospective review of women who underwent ASO for D-TGA, aortic valve regurgitation worsened in 11 of 21 (52%) pregnant women and in 0 of 15 nonpregnant controls followed for 100 months [95]. Cardiac events in patients with D-TGA were common in both pregnant and nonpregnant women (62% vs. 53%, nonsignificant) with worsening ventricular function in both groups (29% and 27%). Premature birth (38%) and small for gestational age (38%) were adverse fetal outcomes reported in the offspring of women with D-TGA who underwent arterial switch procedures.

Women with D-TGA treated with ASO may be at greater long-term risk of systemic right ventricular deterioration during and after pregnancy than those who were surgically corrected with ASO in whom the systemic ventricle is the left ventricle [96]. An irreversible decline in right ventricular function has been described in 10% of pregnancies after atrial switch procedures. Women with moderate or greater right ventricle dysfunction or severe systemic AV valve regurgitation (TR) are at greatest risk of worsening right ventricle function and should be advised against pregnancy.

L-Transposition of the Great Arteries

L-TGA is also known as congenitally corrected transposition of the great vessels. L-TGA is rare and occurs in <1% of CHD with a prevalence of 0.02–0.07 per 1000 live births [97, 98]. Associated cardiac defects occur in 80–90% of patients with L-TGA: VSD, 70–80%; pulmonary stenosis, 30–60%; and Ebstein-like tricuspid valve anomaly, 20–53% [99, 100]. In patients without associated cardiac defects (20% of L-TGA patients), survival into adulthood without correction and often without symptoms is the rule. These women tolerate pregnancy well. The risk of AV block is increased in L-TGA patients, and careful use of AV nodal agents is advised. The risk in pregnancy depends on the severity of the associated defects, the systemic ventricular function, systemic tricuspid valve regurgitation, and the severity of the RVOT obstruction as it relates to the VSD size. In 2 studies of pregnant women with L-TGA, live births were seen in 27 of 45 (60%) [101] and 50 of 60 (83%) pregnancies [102]. Four women developed heart failure and one woman had a stroke. Prepregnancy evaluation and counseling are required. Patients with L-TGA and right ventricle systolic function <40%, severe tricuspid regurgitation, or NYHA functional class III or IV should be advised against pregnancy [29, 99, 100].

Fontan Circulation

The Fontan procedure is a palliative surgical procedure performed in patients with functional or anatomic single-ventricle: hypoplastic left heart syndrome, tricuspid atresia, pulmonary atresia with intact ventricular septum, and double-inlet left ventricle [69, 103]. An extracardiac conduit is created surgically to bypass circulation from the vena cava (cavopulmonary) or the right atrial appendage (atriopulmonary) directly to the pulmonary artery. The Fontan procedure separates venous from arterial cardiac circulation into series while eliminating a sub-pulmonic ventricle. Fontan physiology is characterized by reduced cardiac output and chronically increased systemic venous pressures [104]. Complication rates after the Fontan procedure are frequent, and 15-to 20-year survival rates range from 60 to 85% [105, 106]. Survival into reproductive age is possible with good functional capacity. Women with successful Fontan circulation and a well-performing systemic ventricle, preserved contractile reserve, and high functional class may have the cardiac reserve required to accommodate the hemodynamic burden of pregnancy. Any pregnancy in a patient with a Fontan circulation is high risk (WHO risk class III or IV). Data are limited on pregnancy after a Fontan procedure. Outcomes from 33 pregnancies in patients with Fontan from two US centers and 25 pregnancies from a literature review have been reported. Spontaneous abortion, preterm labor, IUGR, and fetal demise [29] suggest that the uteroplacental blood flow may be compromised in mothers with Fontan physiology. Maternal complications include postpartum hemorrhage (in up to 50%), atrial arrhythmias, and ventricular dysfunction. Pregnancy in patients with Fontan circulation must be carefully considered, as successful pregnancies are possible only in selected patients. A comprehensive cardiovascular evaluation with an adult CHD specialist is recommended to identify suboptimal Fontan physiology and risk. Patients with poor functional class (NYHA III or IV), systemic ventricular function <40%, moderate to severe AV valve regurgitation, cyanosis with room air saturation <90%, or a history of arrhythmia, venous thromboembolism, heart failure, or protein-losing enteropathy should be advised against pregnancy [32], and termination is recommended.

Aortopathy

Aortic disorders primarily affecting the thoracic ascending aorta predispose patients to aortic aneurysm formation, aortic dissection, and aortic rupture. The most common inheritable aortopathies are associated with BAV, MFS, and Loeys-Dietz, Turner, and Ehlers Danlos syndromes. The congenital defects, coarctation of the aorta and TOF, are also associated with aortic aneurysm formation. Pregnancy increases the risk of aortic dissection and rupture in patients with preexisting aortic pathology. Dissection, although rare in pregnancy, is an important cause of maternal mortality [4]. Dissection occurs most frequently in the last trimester of pregnancy (50% of cases) or early postpartum (33%) due to the hemodynamic and hormonal changes associated with the end of pregnancy [107–109].

Because aortic pathology is silent until it becomes catastrophic, screening high-risk individuals—those with prior dissection, with Marfan, Loeys-Dietz, Ehlers Danlos, or Turner syndromes, and those with a family history of familial aortopathy—is the key to successfully preventing aortic dissection or rupture during or after pregnancy.

Marfan Syndrome

MFS is an autosomal dominant disorder affecting connective tissue with a reported incidence of 1 in 3000–5000 individuals [110, 111]. Of patients with MFS, 90% carry a fibrillin (FBN1) genetic mutation that is responsible for the clinical characteristics of MFS: aortic root dilatation/dissection, ectopia lentis, skeletal findings (kyphoscoliosis, pectus, arachnodactyly), mitral valve prolapse, dural ectasia, pneumothorax, and skin striae [112, 113]. Aortic root dilatation and lens ectopia are the cardinal features of MFS. Aortic aneurysmal dilatation, AI, aortic dissection, and aortic rupture are the primary causes of major morbidity and mortality in MFS. According to the revised Ghent criteria, patients with MFS must have aortic root dilatation, a family history of aortic root dilatation, or a FBN1 mutation [113, 114]. Aortic measurements in women of short stature should be indexed to body surface area. In MFS patients with a normal aortic root size (<20% of MFS patients), the risk of aortic dissection or other cardiac complications during pregnancy is 1% [115]. The risk of aortic dissection increases with increasing aortic diameter in MFS. The risk of major aortic complications during pregnancy appears to be low when the aortic root diameter is <4.0 cm [116]. Pregnant patients with MFS are at increased risk for aortic dissection if the aortic diameter exceeds 4 cm and if the diameter changes (>5 mm) during pregnancy [117–119]. In pregnant women with MFS and an aortic diameter >4.0 cm, half will have an aortic rupture or life-threatening aneurysm growth or will require prophylactic aortic surgery during pregnancy. Women with MFS and a history of aortic dissection are at greater risk of recurrent dissection with pregnancy and should be discouraged from getting pregnant [120].

Elective repair of aortic root enlargement >4.0 cm in MFS patients before conception is recommended by the American College of Cardiology/AHA/American Association of Thoracic Surgeons guidelines [121]. After successful surgical correction of the ascending aorta, there is a residual risk of aortic dissection in the remaining aorta during subsequent pregnancies [117, 120, 122]. All women with MFS should undergo monthly or bimonthly cardiovascular and echocardiographic monitoring throughout pregnancy and for at least 4 weeks postpartum [29, 117, 121, 123].

Treatment with beta-blockers, labetolol, or metoprolol tartrate is recommended throughout pregnancy to reduce arterial shear stresses, control heart rate, and decrease the risk of aneurysmal dilatation and dissection [29, 82, 117, 121, 123]. Strict BP control in all pregnant women with MFS is advised. Angiotensin-converting enzyme (ACE) inhibitors and angiotensin receptor blockers (ARBs) are contraindicated in pregnancy. Calcium channel antagonists should be avoided as limited evidence suggests an increase in aortic complications with their use [124]. Delivery should occur in a center with emergency cardiovascular surgery services.

Pregnant women with MFS who develop chest pain should undergo a thorough evaluation that includes aortic imaging for suspected aortic complications. Magnetic resonance imaging without gadolinium is recommended over computed tomographic imaging to avoid exposing the fetus to ionizing radiation. Aortic dissection in pregnancy poses a grave risk to both mother and fetus. Surgical treatment recommendations are the same as in nonpregnant MFS patients. For ascending aortic dissections during the first or second trimester, urgent surgical repair with aggressive fetal monitoring is recommended. Fetal loss is a common complication of hypothermia and cardiopulmonary bypass [125]. In the third trimester, when ascending aortic dissection occurs, urgent cesarean section with concomitant aortic repair appears to offer the best chance for survival for the unborn child and the mother. Medical therapy or stent grafting if anatomy is amendable is preferred in MFS patients who develop descending aortic dissection during pregnancy [121].The long-term rate of aortic dilatation may be increased in MFS patients after pregnancy compared to MFS women who have never been pregnant (0.36 vs. 0.14 mm per year), among those with baseline aortic diameter ≥40 mm [120].

Bicuspid Aortic Valve

Aortopathy, dilatation of any or all segments of the proximal aorta from the aortic root to the aortic arch, is present in approximately half of patients with BAV [126]. The two major complications of bicuspid aortopathy are aortic aneurysm formation and aortic dissection. The risk of aortic dissection risk is relatively low compared to the risk in MFS, with an incidence of 0.1% per patient-year of follow-up in a Toronto study involving 642 BAV patients [119, 127]. In another study, no dissections occurred in patients with an aortic diameter <4.5 cm and only two dissections occurred overall among 416 patients with BAV who were followed for 16 ± 7 years, yielding an incidence of 3.1 cases per 10,000 person-years [128].

Maximal aortic dilatation usually involves the distal ascending aorta, which is not well visualized with standard transthoracic echocardiography. Assessment of ascending aortic size by computed tomography or magnetic resonance imaging is recommended before pregnancy in patients with BAV. Baseline aortic diameter predicts aneurysm expansion in BAV patients [128, 129].

The risks of pregnancy in BAV with aortopathy have not been evaluated. In women with BAV, the hemodynamic and hormonal changes in pregnancy pose a risk of aortic dilatation and dissection. Women with BAV and aortic dilatation are at risk of spontaneous aortic dissection, usually in the third trimester or after delivery, especially if there is an associated aortic coarctation [130]. Guidelines for preconception prophylactic aortic repair for women with BAV have not been established. In nonpregnant patients with ascending aortic aneurysm, aortic repair is indicated when the aortic root or ascending aorta diameter is >5 cm or if the rate of increase is ≥5 mm per year [121]. The threshold for recommending ascending aortic repair in patients with BAV aortopathy before pregnancy varies. The 2010 ESC guidelines for managing adult CHD [68] and the ESC guidelines for managing CVD in pregnancy [29] recommend prepregnancy prophylactic ascending aorta repair in patients with BAV and aortic size >5 cm. However, the 2010 ACC/AHA thoracic aortic guidelines recommend an aortic diameter threshold >4.5 cm for aortic repair if aortic dilatation is progressive and/or there is progression of aortic regurgitation [121]. The consensus is that pregnancy should be avoided in women with BAV and aortic dilatation >5 cm. During pregnancy in patients with BAV and aortopathy, strict BP control with a beta-blocker is warranted.

Ehlers Danlos Syndrome

Type IV Ehlers Danlos syndrome is an autosomal dominant defect in type III collagen (COL3A1 gene) characterized by tissue fragility, which predisposes women to arterial, gastrointestinal, and uterine rupture [121]. According to the 2011 ESC guidelines on managing CVD in pregnancy [29], pregnancy is an absolute contraindication in women with type IV Ehlers Danlos syndrome. Celiprolol is recommended in pregnant and nonpregnant patients with type IV Ehlers Danlos syndrome to reduce the risk of high-risk dissections [121].

Turner Syndrome

Turner syndrome is characterized by short stature, skeletal abnormalities, primary ovarian failure, and BAV with and without coarctation in females caused by a loss of at least part of the X chromosome. The true prevalence is not known as mild cases may go undetected [131]. The reported incidence is approximately 1 in 2000 to 1 in 2500 live female births [132, 133] Abnormalities of the aortic valve and/or the aorta associated with Turner syndrome are responsible for the morbidity and mortality; BAV is present in up to 30% and coarctation in 18% [134–136]. The risk of aortic dissection is 100x greater in women with Turner syndrome than in normal females [137]. Aortic root dilatation, defined as an aortic size index (ASI) >2.0 cm/m^2 (which is >95th percentile), is a predictor of aortic dissection in patients with Turner syndrome. Aortic dissection or rupture leads to increased cardiovascular mortality usually during the third and fourth decade of life [138, 139]. The ESC guidelines for treating CVD in pregnancy recommend prophylactic aortic repair for those at the greatest risk of rupture/dissection: ASI >2.7 cm/m^2 [29]. Risk of aortic dissection or rupture is increased with coarctation, BAV, and maternal hypertension [137]. The prevalence of hypertension is 30–50% in patients with Turner syndrome, which also increases the risk of stroke. Infertility is the rule in Turner syndrome, but spontaneous pregnancies occur occasionally. In vitro fertilization with oocyte donation has increased the rate of pregnancy in Turner syndrome. Pregnancy increases the risk of aortic complications, and the maternal death risk is reported to be as high as 2–11% [29, 140]. Preeclampsia risk is also increased during pregnancy, and treatment of hypertension with beta receptor antagonists is recommended.

Valvular Heart Disease in Pregnancy

Worldwide, the most common cause of VHD in pregnancy is RHD [141, 142]. In the United States and Canada, RHD now causes less than a quarter of heart disease in pregnant women [8, 143]. Declining rates of RHD in developed countries have made congenital causes of VHD more common. Overall, stenotic VHD carries a greater risk in pregnancy than regurgitant VHD according to the WHO [35, 144] scoring systems of maternal risk in pregnancy. Left-sided valve lesions have a greater rate of adverse events than do right-sided ones. Severe LVOT obstruction almost exclusively due to mitral or aortic stenosis is one of four predictors of a maternal adverse event in pregnancy [29]: VHD with left heart obstruction, mechanical heart valves, anticoagulation in pregnancy, and poor NYHA functional class contribute significantly to neonatal complications including fetal death, preterm delivery, IUGR, reduced birth weight, and respiratory distress syndrome [29]. During pregnancy, increases in stroke volume, heart rate, and cardiac output by the second trimester can cause symptomatic decompensation in women with known and unknown VHD. The maternal hemodynamic adaptations to pregnancy may unmask a previously unrecognized valvular heart condition. Complication rates vary by the type and severity of VHD.

Women with known VHD benefit from preconception cardiac evaluation. Women with moderate or high-risk VHD should be followed at a center with a multidisciplinary team of cardiologists, maternal-fetal medicine specialists, obstetric anesthesiologists, and cardiac surgeons. Preconception medical and surgical history, assessment of functional status, an electrocardiogram, and a detailed transthoracic echocardiogram are recommended [145]. Echocardiography should determine the specific valve abnormality (stenotic, regurgitant, or mixed), the number and location of affected valves, and the severity of the valvular abnormalities. Evaluation of left and right ventricular systolic and diastolic function, estimation of the pulmonary artery pressure, and identification of other associated cardiac defects make the preconception echocardiogram vital in planning a future pregnancy [145]. Cardiac magnetic resonance imaging may also be useful in the prepregnancy evaluation of women with VHD and suspected aortopathy or right ventricle dysfunction for assessing aortic pathology as well as right ventricle volumes and function.

For women with advanced VHD who require valve replacement, a detailed discussion of the risks and benefits of surgical options with a specialized cardiovascular team before conception is recommended. All prosthetic valve types are associated with increased maternal and fetal risks during pregnancy. Mechanical valves require lifelong anticoagulation to prevent valve thrombosis and thromboembolic events and significantly increase maternal and fetal complications in pregnancy. Biologic valves generally do not require anticoagulation but have limited durability. Prosthetic valves placed in women of childbearing age will require a repeat valve intervention, which has a mortality of 0–5% depending on the valve position and degree of emergency [29]. The trade-off between the potential for reintervention for bioprosthetic deterioration and the risk associated with pregnancy and long-term anticoagulation should guide the discussion with the patient before pregnancy [146, 147]. The choice of specific prosthesis in a woman who desires pregnancy should be made only after extensive discussion and evaluation of specific patient risk. The desire for pregnancy is a class IIb indication for a biologic valve in the 2007 ESC guidelines on the management of VHD and a class Ic indication in the 2014 ACC/AHA Guidelines [58, 145].

Cardiac Surgery During Pregnancy

Cardiac surgery during pregnancy is high risk and should be reserved for women with severe intractable heart failure symptoms unresponsive to medical therapy [145]. The maternal mortality rate (3–6%) with cardiac surgery is similar to that in nonpregnant women, but the extreme emergency of cardiovascular surgery during pregnancy combined with the added risk of emergency delivery in many cases increases poor maternal outcomes [1, 125]. Maternal mortality occurs in 9% of surgical valve procedures but in 22% of aortic or arterial dissections and pulmonary embolectomies [1]. Fetal-neonatal risks of maternal surgery during pregnancy are high and unpredictable. The risk of fetal death during cardiac surgery is 20–30% [1]. The duration of pregnancy at the time of surgery does not appear to influence the fetal-neonatal outcomes [125].

Fetal outcome in cardiac surgery during pregnancy is related to reduced uteroplacental flow, which is compounded by uterine contractions, fetal bradycardia, and fetal lactic acidosis related to the fetal stress response [1, 148]. Techniques to improve fetal outcomes include increasing cardiopulmonary bypass flow rates above 2.5 L/min per m^2 and maintaining mean arterial pressures >70 mmHg. Continuous fetal monitoring is imperative as prolonged fetal bradycardia (<80 beats per minute) that is unresponsive to increasing flow rates during cardiac surgery is an indication for cesarean delivery if the fetus is viable. Hypothermia during cardiac surgery does not appear to increase fetal risk [1], but rewarming may induce preterm labor [125, 149].Timing of cardiac surgery during pregnancy is difficult to predict. Optimizing fetal and maternal clinical outcomes is the goal. The safest period for cardiac surgery is likely during weeks 20–28 of pregnancy, which limits the risk of fetopathy during early pregnancy and premature delivery and the increased maternal risk during the later stages of pregnancy [150]. Delaying cardiac surgery to 26–28 weeks gestation allows for fetal maturation, increased fetal viability, and better fetal neurologic outcomes. Performing a cesarean delivery before cardiac surgery after 26 weeks gestation has been recommended [29, 125], and successful cesarean delivery at the time of cardiac surgery has been reported [151].

Mitral Stenosis

Mitral stenosis is the most common cause of VHD in pregnancy worldwide and is almost always a distant consequence of acute rheumatic fever, although most patients do not recall the acute rheumatic reaction [152, 153]. A streptococcal infection [154] in childhood can trigger an exaggerated immune reaction that can lead acutely to a clinical syndrome of arthritis (in 35–66% of cases) and pancarditis (in 30–80% of cases) with pericarditis, myocarditis, and valvulitis [155]. The spectrum of valve inflammation without active infection varies geographically and temporally. Pure mitral regurgitation is the valvular abnormality commonly seen in the 2 decades after acute rheumatic fever. These patients have pliable non-scarred leaflets, elongated chordae, and mitral leaflet prolapse. Many (47%) of these valves have pathologic evidence of active valvular inflammation [156]. Over time, pure mitral stenosis or mixed mitral stenosis and mitral regurgitation develop as the commissures fuse, the subvalvular structures fibrose and retract, and the leaflets become calcified and immobilized predominantly at the tips with relative preservation of the motion at the base of the leaflet. Inflammatory reactions and leaflet prolapse are no longer seen. As this progresses, diastolic mitral leaflet motion becomes restricted causing mitral stenosis with and without mitral regurgitation. Rapid progression from mitral regurgitation to stenosis in endemic areas may be related to the lack of antibiotic use, recurrent streptococcal infection, or a more virulent strain of streptococci [156]. Long-term permanent valve damage associated with acute rheumatic fever is called RHD. The mitral valve is involved in almost all cases of RHD, and the aortic valve is affected in 20–30% of cases [157]. Females account for two-thirds of all RHD cases [158]. RHD is endemic in the poor and underdeveloped nations of Oceania, South Asia, and central sub-Saharan Africa. Globally, 33.4 million estimated cases of RHD were diagnosed in 2015, with more than 319,000 deaths [159]. Since 1990, mortality secondary to RHD has declined worldwide by an estimated 48%. [158]. RHD accounts for 55–88% of the cardiac disease in pregnant women in developing nations [141, 142] but less than 25% of the cardiac disease in US and Canadian pregnancies [8, 28, 143]. Mitral stenosis with and without mitral regurgitation accounted for 42% of VHD and only 11% of all heart disease cases in the European Registry on Pregnancy and Heart Disease from 2007 to 2011 [28]. Mixed mitral valve disease occurs at a similar frequency in pregnant women as does mitral stenosis and shares a similar maternal and fetal complication pattern [28, 160]. Maternal and fetal complications correlate with the severity of mitral stenosis in pregnancy [37, 160] (Table 12.2). Mild mitral stenosis (mitral valve area >1.5 cm^2) is well tolerated in pregnancy, whereas moderate or severe mitral stenosis (mitral valve area <1.5 cm^2) is poorly tolerated. Mitral stenosis obstructs left ventricular filling and creates a gradient across the mitral valve. As the diastolic gradient across the valve increases, left atrial and pulmonary venous pressures increase. In mid-to-late pregnancy and especially during labor, the rise in stroke volume and heart rate augment the elevation of the left atrial pressure and increase the risk of congestive heart failure and atrial fibrillation in women with known or unknown mitral stenosis. The hypercoagulability associated with pregnancy further increases the risk of stroke in patients with mitral stenosis and atrial fibrillation.

In developed countries, maternal mortality in mitral stenosis is low, ranging from 0 to 3% [37, 160]. In a report from sub-Saharan Africa, the maternal mortality among 46 pregnant women with rheumatic mixed mitral valve disease was high at 32%; this finding may reflect the lack of antenatal diagnosis and reduced surgical resources [142]. Congestive heart failure and arrhythmia are the most common maternal complications of mitral stenosis. Overall, congestive heart failure occurs in 31–36% of pregnancies among women with variable degrees of mitral stenosis [37, 160, 161]. Atrial fibrillation provokes acute deterioration with congestive heart failure in up to 20% of mitral stenosis cases in pregnancy as the elevated heart rate associated with atrial fibrillation reduces the diastolic filling time and increases the transmitral gradients [160]. Women with mild mitral stenosis in pregnancy have significant rates of congestive heart failure (20%) and arrhythmia (8%) as the stroke volume and heart rate increases in pregnancy may unmask previously asymptomatic mitral stenosis. Symptoms in women with mild mitral stenosis are usually not severe and can be easily managed. Women with moderate and severe mitral stenosis have the greatest risk of congestive heart failure and arrhythmia in pregnancy (Table 12.2). Heart failure in women with moderate to severe mitral stenosis is progressive and increases maternal mortality [29]. All women with moderate or severe mitral stenosis regardless of symptoms should avoid pregnancy, and valve intervention should be performed before conception. Percutaneous mitral commissurotomy is preferred for those with favorable valve morphology [29, 145].

Fetal complications in women with moderate or severe mitral stenosis include fetal demise (1–3%), preterm labor (20–30%), and fetal growth restriction (5–20%) [29].

The management of mitral stenosis in pregnancy depends on its severity. Clinical and echocardiographic follow-up is recommended every trimester and before delivery in women with mild mitral stenosis. For women with moderate-severe

Table 12.2 Pregnancy outcomes in women with mitral stenosis

Severity of MS	Number of pregnancies	Congestive heart failure	Arrhythmia	Preterm delivery	Small for gestational age or IUGR	Fetal demise
Mild MS MVA >1.5 cm^2	61	20%	8%	11%	8%	2%
Moderate or severe MS MVA <1.5 cm^2	65	51%	20%	31%	18%	5%

IUGR intrauterine growth restriction, *MS* mitral stenosis, *MVA* mitral valve area
Data from [37, 160]

mitral stenosis, monthly or bimonthly clinical and echocardiographic follow-up is recommended. Transmitral gradients and the pulmonary artery systolic pressures will increase during pregnancy because of the elevated stroke volume and heart rate. Mitral valve areas estimated by planimetry or by the pressure half time are less load-dependent and can be followed throughout pregnancy. The 2011 ESC guidelines for the management of CVD in pregnancy recommend activity restriction and β1 selective antagonists in symptomatic women and in those with pulmonary pressures greater than 50 mmHg [29]. In pregnant women with moderate or severe mitral stenosis, the normal augmentation of cardiac output may be blunted due to the obstruction to left ventricle filling. Reduction in heart rate with activity restriction and beta-antagonists may improve the diastolic filling time, reduce the left atrial pressure, and increase the cardiac output. Careful titration of the beta-blocker to symptoms and heart rate is important in patients with severe mitral stenosis who effectively have a fixed obstruction to inflow and in whom the heart rate augments the necessary increase in cardiac output. Diuretics can be used in women with persistent symptoms. Anticoagulant use is indicated in women with mitral stenosis with atrial fibrillation, left atrial thrombus, or previous thromboembolic event [145, 162]. Using low-molecular-weight heparin (LMWH) or intravenous unfractionated heparin (UFH) avoids the teratogenic risk and fetopathy associated with warfarin.

Aortic Stenosis

Aortic stenosis in women of childbearing age is predominantly caused by a congenital defect in valve development, usually a BAV. Women with unicuspid aortic valves usually progress to severe valvular stenosis and require valvular repair before puberty. BAV is the most common congenital abnormality and occurs in 1–2% of the general population. Although BAV is more common in men by an estimated 2–4:1 margin, it is seen in approximately 5 in 1000 females [163]. A normal aortic valve has three semilunar valve cusps, whereas a BAV typically comprises two leaflet cusps of unequal size [164]. A genetic cause for BAV is supported by the high rate (9%) of BAV in first-degree relatives [165], familial clustering (36% of patients with BAV have multiple first-degree relatives with BAV), and the association of BAV with known genetic abnormalities such as Turner (XO), Shone, and DiGeorge syndromes. First-degree relatives of patients with a BAV should be screened for the presence of this abnormality [121, 166]. Although it may go undetected for decades, BAV can cause serious complications in more than one-third of patients [127, 128].

Aortic stenosis is the most common complication of BAV. Stenosis is caused by premature fibrosis and leaflet calcification, which is increased in cusps with asymmetry or in those in an anteroposterior position [167]. Tobacco use and abnormal lipid profiles have been associated with progression of aortic stenosis in BAV patients [168].

Before pregnancy, aortic stenosis may be asymptomatic, and the diagnosis may be unknown. The augmented cardiac output associated with pregnancy will increase both the transaortic gradient [169] and the audible systolic ejection murmur. Echocardiography is important to discriminate aortic stenosis from the flow murmur associated with pregnancy. Echocardiography will indicate the valvular pathology and associated lesions (coarctation or PDA) and provide the resting transaortic stroke volume, the peak and mean aortic gradients, and an estimated AVA by the continuity equation. The AVA and the stroke volume should be indexed to body surface area to correct for different body sizes.

Severe aortic stenosis in pregnancy is rare [170]. Patients may be asymptomatic despite having severe aortic stenosis [58]. The 2011ESC guidelines on the management of CVD in pregnancy [29] recommend exercise testing before conception to confirm exercise tolerance, provoke symptoms or arrhythmia, and assess the BP response. All patients with severe symptomatic aortic stenosis should avoid pregnancy and undergo valve replacement or valvuloplasty before conception according to both the 2011 ESC guidelines and the 2014 AHA/ACC valve disease guidelines. In asymptomatic women with severe aortic stenosis who have normal ventricular function and good exercise tolerance, the 2011 ESC guidelines do not advise against pregnancy, whereas the 2014 AHA/ACC valve disease guidelines do advise against pregnancy. Aortic surgery is recommended if the aortic root is >5 cm. Mild and moderate aortic stenosis is generally well tolerated in pregnancy [29, 171]. Severe aortic stenosis (AVA <1.0 cm^2, mean aortic gradient ≥40 mmHg, and a peak gradient ≥4 m/s or 64 mmHg) increases the maternal risk of arrhythmia (3–25%) and heart failure (10%) [172]. Mortality is rare [37, 58, 171, 172].

Fetal complications of maternal moderate or severe aortic stenosis include preterm birth (28–44%), IUGR (27–33%), and low birth weight (25%) [37, 171].

Aortic Insufficiency

AI during the childbearing years is usually a consequence of BAV, endocarditis, or rheumatic valve disease. AI secondary to BAV may be associated with cusp prolapse, fibrotic retraction of the leaflets, or dilatation of the aortic root. Isolated severe AI complicating BAV [127, 173] leads to aortic valve replacement in approximately 2–6% of BAV patients during long-term follow-up. AI may be more common than aortic stenosis in younger patients with BAV who also have a greater risk of endocarditis and aortopathy [163, 174]. AI associated with rheumatic valve disease is characterized by significant mitral valve disease, and the mitral pathology dominates the clinical sequelae and risk [175].

Acute AI resulting from IE, aortic dissection, or trauma causes heart failure and low forward cardiac output. Acute AI is very poorly tolerated during and before pregnancy and requires urgent diagnosis and emergent aortic valve surgery.

Patients with chronic AI often have a long, asymptomatic phase as left ventricle compensation to the diastolic pressure and volume load leads to progressive increases in left ventricular end-diastolic volume with eccentric and concentric hypertrophy. The reduced SVR and the increased heart rate during pregnancy decrease the regurgitant volume of AI. Thus, AI from any cause, without associated enlargement of the ascending aorta (>4.5 cm), is generally well tolerated in pregnancy if left ventricular function and contractile reserve are normal [8, 32, 162]. Symptoms (even mild or transient), left ventricle size (at end systole indexed to BSA), and left ventricular systolic function are the most important predictors of complications in patients with severe AI [145, 176]. Asymptomatic women with moderate or severe AI and normal left ventricular systolic function who otherwise do not meet the criteria for valve surgery should not be referred for prophylactic aortic valve surgery before pregnancy [145, 162]. Left ventricular dysfunction increases the risk of heart failure (25%) and mortality in nonpregnant women with severe AI [176]. Mortality for symptomatic nonpregnant patients with severe AI exceeds 10% overall and is approximately 25% for patients with NYHA class III or IV symptoms [152]. Therefore, women with severe AI with symptoms or left ventricular dysfunction should be referred preferably for aortic valve repair over valve replacement before pregnancy [29]. Pregnancy in women with severe AI and LVEF <30% is not advised due to the very high risk of maternal complications [29]. Women with moderate or severe AI who become pregnant may be treated medically with diuretics and calcium channel blocking vasodilators [145]. ACE inhibitors and ARB vasodilators are contraindicated during pregnancy. Treatment of hypertension is effective in reducing the regurgitant AI volume. Cardiac surgery during pregnancy should be reserved only for women with refractory (NYHA III or IV) heart failure because of the significant fetal risk associated with surgery [145]. If the fetus is viable, cesarean delivery before aortic valve surgery is recommended [29, 177].

Mitral Regurgitation

Mitral regurgitation in women of childbearing age is usually related to myxomatous mitral valve prolapse, rheumatic valve disease, or rarely CHD. The reduction in SVR associated with pregnancy decreases the volume of mitral regurgitation during pregnancy. Asymptomatic women with variable degrees of mitral regurgitation tolerate pregnancy well if the left ventricular systolic function and pulmonary systolic pressures are normal [8, 32]. There is no evidence that severe mitral regurgitation accelerates left ventricle dysfunction in women during pregnancy [145]. Women with symptoms and severe mitral regurgitation should undergo corrective mitral surgery before pregnancy [178, 179]. Mitral repair is preferred over mitral valve replacement if the mitral anatomy is suitable to a durable repair. Pregnancy is contraindicated in women with severe mitral regurgitation and LVEF <30% or significant pulmonary hypertension [29]. During pregnancy, treatment with diuretics and calcium channel blocking vasodilators may control symptoms. Cardiac surgery is rarely required during pregnancy to treat cardiogenic shock and low cardiac forward output associated with severe mitral regurgitation.

Prosthetic Valve Replacement

Pregnancy can be successful in women with VHD after prosthetic valve replacement. Pregnancy risk is related to the type (mechanical or biologic) and position (mitral, aortic, tricuspid, or pulmonic) of the prosthetic valve, left ventricular systolic function, pulmonary arterial pressures, maternal functional class, and the presence of other associated cardiac defects. The hemodynamic and coagulation adaptations to pregnancy can lead to heart failure and valve thrombosis in susceptible patients with prosthetic valves during pregnancy. A preconception clinical evaluation with echocardiogram and electrocardiogram is strongly recommended. An assessment of baseline valve function, let ventricular systolic function, and pulmonary artery pressure allows for comparison during pregnancy [145]. Gradients are expected to increase with the increase in stroke volume and heart rate during pregnancy. Women with a prosthetic valve and LVEF <30%, significant pulmonary hypertension, or symptoms of NYHA class III or IV are classified as modified WHO risk class IV. Pregnancy is contraindicated in these patients, and pregnancy termination may be warranted.

Bioprosthetic Valves

Bioprosthetic valves offer excellent hemodynamic performance and do not require anticoagulants (AC) other than low-dose aspirin unless other thromboembolic risks (e.g., atrial fibrillation, deep vein thrombosis, valve thrombosis) are present. However, a bioprosthetic valve is less durable than a mechanical valve [145]. Bioprosthetic structural deterioration occurs more frequently in the mitral than the aortic or tricuspid position [145]. Structural deterioration also occurs earlier and more frequently in younger patients [180]. The 15-year rate of reoperation due to structural deterioration is 22% for patients 50 years old, 30% for patients 40 years old, and 50% for patients 20 years old at the time of bioprosthetic implantation [180]. Women who undergo prosthetic valve replacement in the childbearing years are expected to require a valvular reintervention (repeat valve replacement or valvotomy) during their lifetime, with an expected mortality of 0–5% depending on the valve position and timing of the procedure (emergent vs. nonemergent) [29]. Pregnancy has been reported to accelerate bioprosthetic structural deterioration [162, 181, 182], but more contemporary, larger studies have not confirmed this finding [183, 184]. Having bioprosthetic valves is considered to be a modified maternal risk class II, suggesting a small increased risk of maternal mortality or a moderate increase in morbidity [35]. Pregnancy in women with bioprosthetic valves is generally well tolerated. The data addressing the maternal and fetal risks in patients with bioprosthetic valves are limited. In a contemporary meta-analysis of 11 trials including 59 pregnancies in women with a bioprosthetic valve implanted from 1997 to 2012, no maternal deaths or thromboembolic events were reported; there were two perinatal deaths in 47 births and 14 pregnancy losses among 59 pregnancies [185]. Among 134 pregnancies in women with bioprosthetic valves who were prospectively followed in the ROPAC study, maternal mortality was 1.5%, and freedom from a serious adverse event during pregnancy did not differ from the group without a valve replacement (79% vs. 78%) [186]. Maternal risk is related to prosthetic valve function and left ventricular systolic function [187], and left ventricular dysfunction increases the risk of heart failure and arrhythmia during pregnancy.

The AHA/ACC guidelines for patients with valvular heart disease recommend low-dose aspirin (75–100 mg daily) during the second and third trimesters for pregnant patients with any type of prosthetic valve to reduce the rate of thromboembolic events [145].

Mechanical Valves

Mechanical valves offer excellent hemodynamic performance and long-term durability but require strict anticoagulation plus low-dose aspirin to prevent valve thrombosis and thromboembolic events [145]. The relative hypercoagulable state of pregnancy is associated with an increased thromboembolic risk in patients with mechanical valves [188], and the ideal anticoagulation regimen has not been determined in pregnancy [162, 170]. The risk of mechanical valve thrombosis and systemic embolization is related to valve type (ball and cage has a greater risk than tilting disc), valve size (<21 mm), valve position (mitral has a greater risk than aortic), the number of prosthetic valves (multiple has a greater risk than single), the anticoagulation regimen, atrial fibrillation, heart failure symptoms, and a history of thromboembolic events. Mechanical valve replacement is considered a modified WHO risk class III, indicating significantly increased risk of maternal mortality or severe morbidity [36]. Monthly or bimonthly cardiology and obstetric clinical follow-up with individualized and frequent anticoagulant monitoring is recommended during pregnancy [29] in patients with mechanical heart valves. Maternal complications associated with mechanical valve replacement include maternal death, valve thrombosis with valvular obstruction and systemic thromboembolism, heart failure, arrhythmia (including atrial fibrillation), hemolysis, endocarditis, and bleeding secondary to anticoagulation. Fetal risks dominate the sequelae with anticoagulation and include perinatal fetal loss and miscarriage, warfarin embryopathy, fetal hemorrhage, and small gestational weight. All anticoagulants are associated with increased fetal loss and miscarriage.

Anticoagulation During Pregnancy

Anticoagulation with continuous vitamin K antagonist (VKA) (warfarin) is the most reliable and effective approach for preventing maternal thromboembolic complications in pregnancy, with a 2–4% rate of pregnancy-related valve thromboembolic complications [189, 190].

The risk of valve thrombosis was 3.6% with oral VKA used throughout pregnancy, 9.2% with a sequential strategy of UFH during the first trimester followed by VKA in the second and third trimester, and 33% with UFH used throughout pregnancy. Maternal mortality due mostly to valve thrombosis was 2%, 4%, and 15% in these three groups, respectively [191]. UFH and LMWH are associated with greater risk of prosthetic valve thrombosis and systemic embolization than warfarin in pregnancy, but they do not cross the placenta and thus are not associated with embryopathy, significant fetal loss, or fetal hemorrhage. LMWH is preferred over UFH because of better bioavailability, more predictable anticoagulation levels, lower rates of valve thrombosis, and less bone loss, bleeding, and thrombocytopenia [192–194]. The dosage of LMWH required to keep the anti-Xa levels in the therapeutic range in pregnancy is markedly elevated because of increased renal clearance and a larger volume of distribution [195]. New oral direct thrombin inhibitors or anti-Xa anticoagulants are not approved in patients with VHD and are contraindicated in patients with mechanical prosthetic valves because of the increased risk of valve thrombosis compared to warfarin in nonpregnant patients [196–198].

Warfarin is associated with severe fetal complications especially when administered after 5 weeks gestation [162] and through the first trimester. Fetal embryopathy with characteristic fetal bone and cartilage anomalies (chondromalacia punctata with stippled epiphyses and nasal and limb hypoplasia) occur in 5–10% of fetuses exposed primarily during the first trimester [29, 162, 166, 189–191, 193, 199].

Miscarriage due to fetal loss before 20 weeks gestation occurs in approximately 30% of cases [162, 186], whereas late fetal loss after 20 weeks gestation may occur in another 10%. Fetal hemorrhage is another devastating complication of warfarin exposure during pregnancy [186, 191, 193]. Fetal embryopathy and fetal loss secondary to warfarin appear to be dose dependent; the incidence at low doses (≤5 mg daily) is 2.6 and 8% at higher doses (>5 mg daily) [200]. International normalized ratio (INR) ranges are recommended to target effective anticoagulation levels to specific patient risk. The INR target varies according to the valve site, valve type, and other risk factors for thromboembolic events (e.g., atrial fibrillation, multiple prosthetic valves, prior thromboembolism, or valve thrombosis).

In patients with mechanical bileaflet or current-generation single-tilting disc mechanical valves in the aortic position who have no additional risk factors for thromboembolism, the INR target is >2.5. However the On-X mechanical valve is approved for a target INR of 1.5 in non-pregnant patients. Whether that target pertains safely in pregnancy is unknown but it may allow for lower warfarin dosing and thus less risk of embryopathy. If a patient has additional risk factors for thromboembolism or an older generation ball and cage type AVR is present, the target INR is >3.0. The target INR for any mechanical valve in the mitral position is >3.0. Careful and frequent monitoring is important as fluctuations in the INR are associated with an increased risk of thromboembolic complications (low INR) and bleeding in patients (high INR) with mechanical heart valves. Pregnancy increases the variability in the INR because of changes in VKA drug availability, the volume of drug distribution, liver function, and food intake.

Low-dose daily aspirin is recommended in addition to VKA during the second and third trimesters to prevent valve thrombosis and thromboembolism in patients with mechanical valve replacement [145].

Treatment strategies in pregnancy are designed to minimize fetal and maternal complications of anticoagulation, although adequate randomized studies comparing different regimens are not available. In the available studies, live birth rates were the highest (92%) in an anticoagulation strategy using only LMWH throughout pregnancy, intermediate (80%) with a sequential strategy of LMWH during the first trimester followed by VKA in trimesters two and three, and lowest (65%) when VKA was used throughout pregnancy [189]. Unfortunately, maternal risk of thromboembolic complications with LMWH in pregnancy has been estimated as high as 12%, and many of these events are associated with poor dosing compliance or inadequate monitoring of anti-Xa activity [189, 192, 201].

In pregnant patients with no additional risk for thromboembolic events, a strategy that minimizes exposure to warfarin in the first trimester is recommended [145]. In women with a stable therapeutic INR on a dose of warfarin ≤5 mg daily, warfarin may be continued until 36 weeks gestation. If the stable warfarin dose is >5 mg daily or if the patient wants to limit fetal exposure to warfarin during the first trimester, dose-adjusted subcutaneous LMWH administered twice daily from 5 to 12 weeks is a more expensive but acceptable alternative. Monitoring of anti-Xa activity with LMWH is recommended to a target level of 1.0–1.2 units/mL for mitral valve prosthesis and 0.8–1.0 units/mL for aortic valve prosthesis at 4–6 h postdose. When LMWH is not available, another anticoagulant option is dose-adjusted, continuously administered, intravenous UFH from 5 to 12 weeks gestation. Subcutaneous administration of UFH may be offered if LMWH or inhospital continuous intravenous UFH is not available, but not all experts recommend this strategy. Monitoring of the activated partial thromboplastin time (aPTT) to a target of 2× control levels is recommended 6 h after subcutaneous UFH administration or randomly drawn if UFH is given continuously [145]. Conversion to VKA during the second trimester and up to 36 weeks gestation with careful INR monitoring is recommended. For patients at increased maternal risk of thrombosis or systemic embolization, a strategy of continuous warfarin until 36 weeks of gestation is recommended.

Peripartum Management of Anticoagulation for Mechanical Valves

For women receiving VKA up to 36 weeks of gestation, it is recommended to transition to a pre-planned delivery strategy of a shorter-acting and potentially reversible anticoagulant regimen to minimize the risks of maternal and fetal hemorrhage. The risk of valve thrombosis and systemic embolization must be balanced by the risk of obstetric hemorrhage and regional anesthesia in consultation with the care team of obstetricians, anesthesiologist, and cardiologist after discussion with the patient. VKA can be switched to subcutaneous LMWH twice daily until 12–24 h before planned delivery. Intravenous UFH can then be administered until hours before delivery. Reversal of anticoagulation from VKA with fresh-frozen plasma or intravenous prothrombin complex is an option in an obstetrical emergency. Administration of low-dose (1–2 mg) oral vitamin K may be beneficial as the effect of fresh-frozen plasma or prothrombin complex has a shorter half-life than the effects of VKA therapy [145]. Anticoagulation can be resumed postpartum after the bleeding risk has diminished.

Management of Valve Thrombosis During Pregnancy

Mechanical left-sided valve obstruction may present as a life-threatening emergency with high mortality and requires urgent treatment with either fibrinolytic therapy or surgical intervention [202–207]. In patients with symptoms of new or worsening dyspnea or a systemic embolic event, transthoracic echocardiography or flouoroscopy should be followed by transesophageal echocardiogram to better visualize the mechanical valve and assess for possible IE or acute thrombosis. Fibrinolysis is the therapy of choice for right-sided prosthetic valve thrombosis [58]. High-risk features of left-sided mechanical valve thrombosis are severe symptoms (NYHA functional class III or IV) and a mobile thrombus >0.3 cm in diameter or any thrombus with an area ≥1.0 cm^2. Unstable patients require fibrinolytic therapy or surgery. Surgery is usually indicated in nonpregnant patients with left-sided mechanical valve thrombosis because compared with thrombolysis, surgery has increased efficacy, less bleeding, and a reduction in embolic complications associated with a large thrombus burden. The overall 30-day mortality rate with surgery is 10–15% but <5% in patients with less severe NYHA class (I/II) symptoms [204, 207, 208]. Before 2013, the results of traditional fibrinolytic therapy showed an overall 30-day mortality rate of 7% and a hemodynamic success rate of 75%, but the thromboembolism rate was 13% and the major bleeding rate was 6% (intracerebral hemorrhage, 3%) [202–207].

Fetal loss with cardiovascular surgery is high, and surgery should be reserved for patients in whom fibrinolysis failed or is contraindicated. Most fibrinolytic agents do not cross the placenta; therefore, fetal hemorrhage risk is not increased, but there is a risk of placental hemorrhage. A new strategy is echocardiogram-guided, low-dose, slow-infusion fibrinolytic treatment with 25 mg tissue-type plasminogen activator (t-PA) infused over 6 hours without a bolus; the data are promising but limited (success rates >90%, embolic event rates <2%, and major bleeding rates <2%). After the t-PA infusion is completed, UFH is administered via a 70 IU/kg bolus followed by an infusion of 16 IU/h (up to 1000 IU/h) with a target aPTT of 1.5–2.0 times the mean reference range [209]. Repeat fibrinolytic protocol (once every 24 h up to six times to a maximum total dose of 150 mg) is guided by the following indicators of fibrinolytic success: resolution of clinical symptoms and echocardiographic resolution of the increased transvalvular gradient or a reduction by >50% in the thrombus area or length [209]. The 2017 AHA/ACC focused update of the 2014 AHA/ACC guideline for the management of patients with VHD [145] suggested a role for low-dose, slow-infusion fibrinolysis for patients with mechanical valve thrombosis. Intravenous UFH is recommended in stable patients with mechanical valve thrombosis associated with subtherapeutic anticoagulation.

Cardiomyopathy in Pregnancy

Preexisting Cardiomyopathy

Heart failure during pregnancy is rare and most frequently occurs in women with preexisting cardiomyopathy (idiopathic, infectious, valvular, and cardiotoxic drug-associated [adriamycin, herceptin, and cocaine]) with decompensation due to the physiologic hemodynamic burden of increased cardiac output during the later stages of pregnancy. If cardiomyopathy was not diagnosed before pregnancy, the timing of presentation during pregnancy helps to predict the cause of the cardiomyopathy. Dilated cardiomyopathy and secondary cardiomyopathy usually present within the second trimester. Later presentation is more characteristic of peripartum cardiomyopathy (PPCM). Women with primary or dilated cardiomyopathy present with symptoms of congestive heart failure and evidence of left ventricular systolic dysfunction without evidence of abnormal hypertrophy or VHD. Women with NYHA class II–IV symptoms and left ventricular systolic function <45% are at the greatest risk for decompensation and are thus advised to avoid pregnancy. Women with LVEF <20% are at the highest risk of maternal mortality, and pregnancy termination should be recommended.

Hypertrophic Cardiomyopathy

HCM is an autosomal dominant genetic cardiomyopathy caused by mutations in one of several sarcomere genes. HCM is characterized by left ventricular hypertrophy occurring in the absence of left ventricular hypertension (e.g., systemic hypertension, aortic stenosis pressure, aortic insufficiency, or VSD). In most patients with HCM, left ventricular hypertrophy develops during the adolescent period [210], and hypertrophy measurements do not change once early adulthood is reached. Abnormalities of diastolic function precede the development of hypertrophy and serve as phenotypic markers of HCM in at-risk family members. Symptoms of HCM are related to the pattern of hypertrophy, the presence and severity of LVOT obstruction, the severity of diastolic dysfunction, the presence and ventricular rate of arrhythmia-atrial fibrillation, and late systolic dysfunction.

Symptoms and Risk Stratification

Women with HCM may present with new-onset symptoms of congestive heart failure, arrhythmia, or an asymptomatic murmur of LVOT obstruction (augmented by Valsalva maneuver) in pregnancy. Echocardiographic evidence of otherwise unexplained hypertrophy of any pattern (diffuse, asymmetric, or apical) is diagnostic of HCM. A family history of HCM may be present but is not mandatory as genetic mutations may be sporadic. Although rare, patients with HCM have an increased risk of death from sudden cardiac death (SCD), heart failure, and stroke. SCD risk stratification is recommended in all patients with HCM. High-risk features of SCD in HCM include a history of sudden cardiac arrest or ventricular arrhythmia, severe hypertrophy (>3 cm), a family history of SCD, unexplained syncope [211], and non-sustained ventricular tachycardia (most commonly defined as ≥3 beats at 120 beats per minute), especially in patients younger than 30 years old [210, 212–214]. The degree of resting LVOT obstruction as well as the age at presentation (<30 years) are also relative markers of SCD risk [215].

Women with HCM usually tolerate pregnancy well. The increased stroke volume associated with pregnancy acts to decrease the risk of LVOT obstruction by increasing left ventricular volumes. Women with symptoms before pregnancy and those with high resting LVOT gradients are at greater risk of symptomatic deterioration in pregnancy and need specialized cardiac care.

Management

Beta-blockers are useful in women with HCM to slow the maternal heart rate, blunt the inotropic response to catecholamines, increase left ventricular volumes, and decrease the risk for atrial fibrillation. Beta-blockers reduce the risk of resting and exercise-related LVOT obstruction and mitral regurgitation related to systolic anterior motion of the mitral valve. Verapamil can be substituted when beta-blockers are not well tolerated. If atrial fibrillation occurs in pregnancy and is poorly tolerated, electrical cardioversion is the preferred treatment. There is little risk to the fetus during electrical cardioversion as the amniotic fluid acts as an insulator. Maternal hemodynamic instability poses the greatest risk to the fetus. Women with high-risk ventricular arrhythmia require specialized electrophysiologic management and possible automatic implantable cardiac defibrillation placement.

Mode of Delivery

Low-risk women with HCM should be allowed to have a spontaneous labor and a normal vaginal delivery. Symptomatic or high-risk women with HCM should have a planned, controlled delivery. Pain, volume losses, and epidural anesthesia may increase the risk of LVOT obstruction.

Acquired-Peripartum Cardiomyopathy

Definition and Diagnosis

In 1971, Demakis proposed the original diagnostic criteria for PPCM, which included symptoms of heart failure within the last month or within 5 months of delivery in the absence of demonstrable heart disease or other cause for heart failure [216]. Since then, the definition of PPCM has evolved. Advances in cardiac imaging techniques have helped to demonstrate the primary cardiomyopathic etiology in PPCM, and newer definitions of PPCM require a depression of left ventricular systolic function to below 45% [217].

The timing of symptom presentation has been debated as a diagnostic criterion in PPCM. Symptoms of heart failure arise from the severity of left ventricular dysfunction and the rapidity of its decline. Because young, healthy pregnant women can accommodate a decline in cardiac function without significant symptoms, early less severe forms of PPCM may have been overlooked and thus undertreated by applying traditional criteria. More importantly, women with onset of symptoms earlier than the last month of pregnancy would be excluded from the traditional PPCM diagnosis. A comparison of risk and outcomes between women who present with pregnancy-induced cardiomyopathy early ($n = 23$; mean, 32 weeks gestation) versus late or the traditional definition ($n = 100$; mean, 38 weeks gestation) suggests that women with early cardiomyopathy may share a common etiology, risk, and prognosis when compared with women who meet the traditional definition of PPCM [218].

A broad definition of PPCM is recommended although no distinct definition is used globally. In the 2011 guidelines for management of CVD in pregnancy, the ESC recommended a definition for PPCM: symptomatic heart failure with depression of left ventricular systolic function that develops within the last months of, and up to 6 months after, pregnancy in women without known CVD [29, 219].

The diagnosis of PPCM is one of exclusion. Initial definitions of PPCM relied exclusively on clinical findings of congestive heart failure in pregnant or postpartum women who presented within the window of assumed risk. In the past, congenital cardiac defects, pericardial disease, occult valvular abnormalities, hypertensive diastolic dysfunction, and the subjectivity of symptoms led to false classifications of PPCM. In 1997, a National Heart, Lung, and Blood Institute working group added strict criteria to the diagnosis of PPCM including left ventricular dysfunction and now a LVEF <45% [220]. Noninvasive imaging with echocardiography, cardiac computed tomography, or cardiac magnetic resonance is necessary to exclude occult causes of heart failure in women in whom the hemodynamic demands of pregnancy have been superimposed on chronic cardiac disorders. These techniques can also be used to define the hemodynamics during pregnancy, including cardiac output, preload (right or left atrial pressures), and right ventricular afterload (right ventricular or pulmonary arterial systolic pressure).

Biomarkers in Peripartum Cardiomyopathy

Currently, no specific biomarkers for PPCM are available. The diagnosis of PPCM is often delayed and complicated by the overlap of symptoms of heart failure—fatigue, edema, and shortness of breath—with normal pregnancy-associated symptoms. Specific biomarkers could help distinguish PPCM patients early and expedite a quick diagnosis and initiation of treatment. N-terminal (NT)-proBNP and troponin T are nonspecific markers of structural heart disease and elevated filling pressures, and their levels are increased in hypertension/left ventricular hypertrophy and in heart failure/cardiomyopathy. NT-proBNP levels were significantly higher in 38 PPCM patients than in healthy postpartum controls [221]. However, it has not been established whether

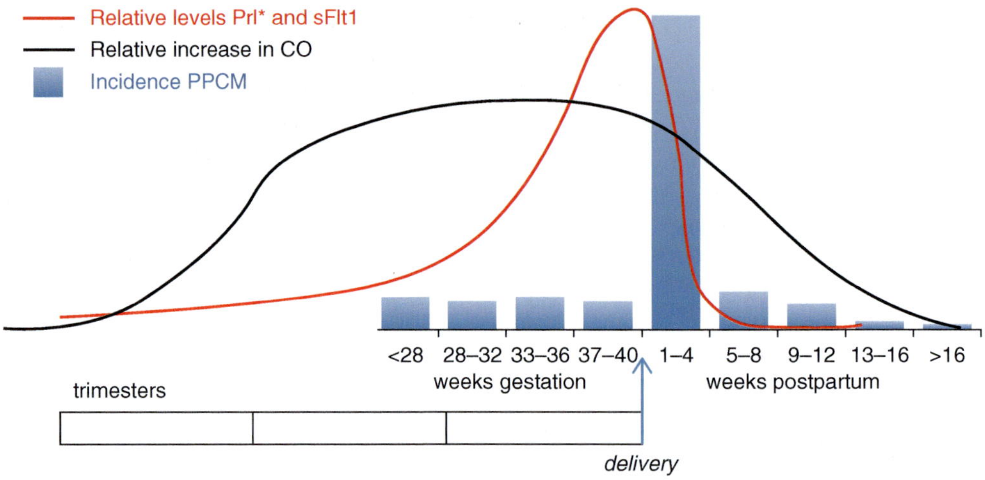

Fig. 12.2 Comparison of timing during and after pregnancy of hemodynamic changes, exemplified as cardiac output (CO; in black), elevations in prolactin and soluble Fms-like tyrosine kinase 1 (sFlt1) hormones (red), and incidence of peripartum cardiomyopathy (PPCM; blue bars). *Prl levels stay elevated in women who nurse. From: Arany Z, Elkayam. Peripartum cardiomyopathy. Circulation 2016;133:1397-1409. Free Access ©2016 American Heart Association, Inc.

NT-proBNP levels distinguish congestive heart failure secondary to PPCM from symptoms secondary to volume overload or structural heart disease. Increased cardiac troponin T levels (>0.4 ng/mL) within 2 weeks of PPCM onset have also been shown to predict persistent left ventricular dysfunction and lower LVEF at 6-month follow-up ($P < 0.001$) [222]. Because increased troponin T levels are not specific for PPCM, the clinical diagnostic utility of troponin T in PPCM is not expected. Two biomarkers are potentially specific for PPCM: micro-RNA-146a and sFlt (see etiology below). Their levels may reflect mechanistic alterations in prolactin processing that have been demonstrated in women with PPCM [223] (Fig. 12.2).

Incidence and Associated Conditions

The incidence of PPCM in populations around the world varies greatly according to geography and socioeconomic class. Overall, the incidence of PPCM is about 1 in 3000 pregnancies [224, 225]. Ascertainment bias with reporting based on clinical symptoms alone overestimates the risk. Shortness of breath, peripheral edema, and palpitations are common nonspecific symptoms in pregnancy; therefore, milder expressions of PPCM are likely underdiagnosed. Baseline characteristics of women with PPCM, however, are remarkably similar. Women who develop PPCM are frequently older, of African ancestry, and have preeclampsia, hypertension, and multiple gestations. [218, 226–228].

Age

Increasing age is strongly associated with PPCM; half of all PPCM cases occur in women over 30 years old [224, 229, 230]. Moreover, age >40 years is associated with a 10-fold increased risk of PPCM compared to age under 20 years [229, 230].

Geography and Race

The reported incidence of PPCM varies geographically [219, 231]. The incidence of PPCM in the United States varies from 1 in 968 to 1 in 4000 live births [229]. The incidence has increased from 8.5 cases per 10,000 live births in 2004 to 11.8 cases per 10,000 live births in 2011. This increase is attributed to increased awareness, access to diagnostic imaging, advanced maternal age, and multiple gestation pregnancies [229]. Japan has the lowest reported rate of PPCM at 1 in 20,000 live births, whereas Nigeria and Haiti have the highest rate at 1 in 100 live births [228, 232, 233]. Cultural rituals may contribute to the high risk of PPCM in Nigeria, where it is customary in the postpartum period to consume large amounts of salt, which promotes fluid overload and hypertension [234]. Genetic predisposition has not been well studied, but race appears to affect the risk of PPCM. The prevalence of PPCM is higher in women in Africa and women with African ancestry in Haiti and in the United States. In the United States, African American (AA) women have a higher prevalence of PPCM, a greater burden of gestational hypertension, more severe disease, and greater morbidity than white women [235, 236].

Preeclampsia and Hypertension

Hypertension, pregnancy-induced hypertension, and preeclampsia are increased in many cohorts of PPCM patients [218, 226, 237]. Historically, women with preeclampsia or eclampsia were purposefully excluded in many PPCM studies to avoid misclassification of preeclampsia-associated pulmonary edema as PPCM. Preeclampsia, but not gestational hypertension, induces subclinical abnormalities of diastolic function as measured by echocardiographic indices of myocardial strain and myocardial performance index, and these abnormalities persist after normalization of BP [238,

239]. Volume overload during pregnancy or at delivery may trigger overt congestive heart failure without systolic dysfunction. PPCM rarely occurs in women with preeclampsia or hypertension disorders of pregnancy (<10%). However, preeclampsia and hypertension in pregnancy frequently coexist in women who develop PPCM. Demakis and Rahimtoola [240], in their classic 1971 description of PPCM, reported that "toxemia," an older term for preeclampsia, was detected in 22% of affected women. Preeclampsia has often been cited as an independent risk factor for the development of PPCM [241, 242], but not all clinical studies support this conclusion [243]. In a global meta-analysis of 22 studies involving 979 women with PPCM, the prevalence of preeclampsia was 22%, which is 4–5 times the average expected rate in the general population. The rate of hypertension during pregnancy in this large blended cohort of PPCM was 37% [226]. No geographic or racial differences were detected [244]. The findings in a US review of 535 women with PPCM in 6 states supported the association between PPCM and preeclampsia, with a 29% prevalence of preeclampsia and a 47% prevalence of hypertension [245]. In a single-center study of 75 PPCM cases, one-third were associated with preeclampsia, which is markedly more than the population rate of 3–5% [246]. These studies suggest that preeclampsia is associated with a predisposition to PPCM through a shared pathophysiologic mechanism that is independent of race and geography.

Parity

Multiparity has traditionally been considered a risk factor for PPCM [247]. However, in most US studies, PPCM developed in conjunction with the first or second pregnancy in 50% of patients [218, 248]. Therefore, these data do not support a strong association between multiparity and PPCM in the United States.

Multiple Gestations

Pregnancies associated with multiple gestations, twins or less commonly triplets, are sharply associated with a greater risk of PPCM. In the global meta-analysis of PPCM described above, the rate of twin gestation was 9%, which is three times the expected rate (3%) in women without PPCM [226]. Twin pregnancy has also been associated with a greater risk of preeclampsia, and this association may hint at an underlying placental etiology (see below) [249]. Overall, in cohort studies of women with PPCM, the frequency of multiple gestations ranges between 4% and 13% [218, 226].

Etiology

Hemodynamics

PPCM has a unique time course of symptom onset, with the peak incidence occurring within 1 month of delivery in more than 80% of cases. Normal pregnancy is associated with up to a 50% increase in cardiac output as a result of a 15% increase in heart rate, a 30% reduction in SVR, and a 15–25% increase in stroke volume. These hemodynamic accommodations to pregnancy plateau by the end of the second trimester. Patients with preexisting cardiac disease develop signs and symptoms of heart failure as the hemodynamic demands increase, usually within the second trimester [161]. Pregnancies in mothers with a preexisting cardiac structure abnormality are at even greater risk of clinical deterioration when multiple fetuses are present, given the even larger hemodynamic burden to the maternal heart. The symptoms of PPCM do not develop along this timeline, and thus the increase in hemodynamic cardiac output is unlikely to be the primary precipitant of PPCM.

Genetics

Genetics is unlikely to be the primary mechanistic cause of PPCM because most women with PPCM have no family history of PPCM or dilated cardiomyopathy. Furthermore, women with PPCM in whom left ventricular function recovers after delivery rarely develop a recurrence of clinical heart failure or PPCM with subsequent pregnancies. The increased prevalence of PPCM in women in Africa and in black women of African descent in the United States and Haiti provide clues that a genetic susceptibility may predispose a subset of women to develop PPCM. In the United States, 40% of PPCM cases occur in black women, and, in some series, the prevalence in black women is 3- to 14-fold greater than in white women [250]. Black women also have a worse prognosis, lower recovery rates, and delays in left ventricular recovery [235, 251]. A single genetic polymorphism involving the guanine nucleotide-binding proteinsβ-3 subunit (*GNB3/TT*) has a prevalence of 50% in black women and 10% in white women and is associated with increased rates of hypertension, decreased plasma renin activity, and abnormalities of cardiac remodeling [252–255]. The Investigations of Pregnancy-Associated Cardiomyopathy (IPAC) investigators compared left ventricular recovery at 6 and 12 months in black and white women with and without the *GNB3 TT* polymorphism. Black women with the *GNB3* variant had less left ventricular recovery than did white women with and without the variant [256].

Evidence that genetics are involved in PPCM also comes from familial clusters of PPCM and dilated cardiomyopathy and [250, 257–260] female genetic carriers of the X-linked cardiomyopathies, Becker, Duchenne, and Danon, who demonstrate an increased risk of PPCM [261–263]. Additionally, whole genome sequencing of 41 patients with PPCM identified a single-gene polymorphism near the *PTHLH* gene that may link the genomics with abnormalities of vascular homeostasis [264, 265].

Abnormalities of the genes coding for myofibril proteins, specifically the sarcomere protein, titin (*TTN*), have been described in two rare pedigree cohorts of patients with

PPCM and familial dilated cardiomyopathy [250, 257]. Truncating variants involving the *TTN* gene were also found in 10% of 172 women with PPCM who were screened for high-impact nonsense, frameshift, and splicing variants of 43 genes associated with familial dilated cardiomyopathy. PPCM participants from the IPAC study [266] with the *TTN* variant had a lower EF at 6 and 12 months than those without the *TTN* variant. *TTN* variants were noted in both black and white women. Of note, the *TTN* variant was tenfold greater in nonhypertensive patients than in those with hypertension. These findings suggest that PPCM in the absence of hypertension may derive from a separate, more genetic pathophysiologic mechanism than that observed in the presence of hypertension [263]. Overall, 15% of women with PPCM and 17% of sporadic dilated cardiomyopathy patients from another cohort exhibited important similar genetic variants, further contributing to the role of genetic susceptibility in PPCM [263].

Hormonal Vascular Theory

In two seminal papers, investigators have expanded the proposed mechanism of PPCM to include a link between late gestational placental and maternal hormone secretion and vascular injury in susceptible hosts [267, 268].

Hormones secreted at the end of pregnancy—prolactin by the pituitary and a soluble variant of the vascular endothelial growth factor (VEGF) receptor 1(soluble fms-like tyrosine kinase—*sflt1*) by the placenta—have potent antiangiogenic properties that can lead to endothelial cell apoptosis and a decline in myocardial vascularity in susceptible hosts. Evidence in humans that angiogenesis inhibition may induce cardiomyopathy is suggested by the cardiac dysfunction reported with the use of VEGF neutralizing antibodies in treating human cancers [269]. Two murine models of PPCM have been induced by knockout of specific myocyte transcriptional factors, *STAT3* [267] and cardiac-specific deletion of proliferator-activated receptor-gamma coactivator-1α (*PGC-1α*) [268]. Additionally, *STAT3* has been shown to be reduced in patients with end-stage dilated cardiomyopathy [270]. Through similar pathways, deletion of these nuclear transcription factors allows the overexpression of reactive oxygen species and a subsequent increase in cathepsin D [267, 268, 271].

Cathepsin D cleaves the hormone prolactin to an antiangiogenic 17 kDa prolactin fragment that has been shown to enhance the secretion of a miR146a, which, in turn, leads to endothelial apoptosis, altered energy metabolism, reduced myocardial vascularity, myocardial dysfunction, and eventual cardiomyopathy [223, 272]. Cardiomyopathy could not be provoked in nonpregnant female or male mice, suggesting a mechanistic pathway specific to the development of PPCM. However, cardiomyopathy could be provoked in the nulliparous PGC1α-deficient mice administered sFlt; this evidence suggests that late gestational antiangiogenic placental hormones can directly trigger cardiomyopathy. In the second model, depletion of PGC-1α also leads to vascular injury through the loss of a proangiogenic VEGF-mediated pathway. Evidence that a toxic late gestational hormonal milieu causes maternal cardiomyopathy is supported by the observation that hormonal blockade reverses the cardiomyopathy. Reversal of PPCM in murine models has been achieved by inhibiting prolactin secretion via bromocriptine alone in the STAT3 model [267] and with bromocriptine combined with VEGF in the PGC-1α model [268]. Partial reversal of murine PPCM (improved contractile function and partial rescue of capillary density) has been demonstrated with administration of antisense oligonucleotides to silence miRNA 146a without the suppression of lactation, which occurs as a consequence of bromocriptine treatment. Of note, circulating levels of mi R146a have been shown to be increased in women with PPCM, and levels decline in women treated with bromocriptine. SFlt1 levels, which are usually increased in women with PPCM, correlated with congestive heart failure symptoms and outcome in women with PPCM who were enrolled in the IPAC study [249, 268].

Excess placental sFlt1 secretion in women with preeclampsia [273] and multiple gestations [249] highlights the epidemiologic association between preeclampsia, twin or multiple gestations, and PPCM [274]. Removal of vasculotoxic placental hormones after delivery may also explain the rapid reversal of cardiomyopathy seen in the majority of patients with PPCM compared to other forms of cardiomyopathy. In late pregnancy, an angiogenic balance is necessary to allow the safe separation of the uteroplacental circulation while protecting maternal myocytes from vascular injury. Abnormalities in this balance in susceptible women can lead to the development of PPCM and influence its severity through the proposed hormonal vascular injury hypothesis described above.

Prognosis and Complications

PPCM confers risk to the mother and the neonate. Maternal risks include death, cardiovascular arrest, the need for heart transplantation or mechanical circulatory support, fulminant heart failure, and thromboembolic events [275–277]. In a retrospective review of 535 women diagnosed with PPCM from 2003 to 2007 in the United States, 36% experienced a major maternal adverse event [229]. In the recent prospective IPAC study, which enrolled 100 US women from multiple centers and followed their clinical and echocardiographic course for 12 months, the prognosis of women with PPCM was better. Only 13% of IPAC subjects had a major event or persistent cardiomyopathy with EF <35% [251]. Overall, more than 50% of women recover completely, with relief of symptoms and recovery of LV systolic function within six months [218, 248].

Mortality

PPCM is now the leading cause of maternal death in California (causing 23% of maternal deaths) [278]. Maternal mortality estimates in PPCM vary according to race and length of follow-up; the estimates range from 3 to 28% [218, 248, 279–281]. US maternal inhospital mortality rates secondary to PPCM are low at 1.3% [229], 4% at 1 year in the IPAC study [251], and 11–16% over 7–8 years of follow-up [282]. Adverse prognostic factors for maternal death include higher NYHA class [283], EF <25–30% [251], black race [281, 284], and age >30–35 years [245, 282].

Obstetric and Neonatal Outcomes

Cesarean delivery was performed for obstetrical indications in 40% of 123 PPCM patients [218]. Stillbirths are more common in mothers with PPCM, occurring in 3.8% of 535 pregnancies [229]. Of the 100 women with PPCM prospectively followed in the IPAC study, there were two stillbirths, one neonatal death, and four newborns with congenital anomalies. Mean birth weight, intrauterine growth, and Apgar scores [241] are lower in neonates born to women with PPCM and may be a consequence of the 25% rate of preterm birth (<37 weeks) seen in PPCM. Delivery decisions should involve a team of maternal fetal specialists, pediatricians, and cardiologists. Early delivery should be restricted to cases of impending maternal or fetal loss since it has not been shown to improve maternal or fetal outcomes.

Thromboembolic Events

Thromboembolic events are more common in women with PPCM than in those with idiopathic or virally mediated cardiomyopathy [228, 257, 285]. The hypercoagulable state of pregnancy may potentiate the risk of left ventricular thrombus formation in women with severe cardiomyopathy and reduced cardiac output. In one study, thromboembolic complications were the most common adverse event associated with PPCM, occurring in 6.6% of patients [229].

Left Ventricular Recovery

Myocardial recovery is greater in women with PPCM than in nonperipartum women with cardiomyopathy [228, 285]. Nevertheless, recovery of left ventricular function (EF >50%) is heterogeneous in women with PPCM [275]. Partial or complete recovery in PPCM occurs in 40–72% of affected women [223, 228, 285, 286]. In the IPAC study, only 13% of women with PPCM had severe persistent cardiomyopathy or major adverse events (death, transplant, left ventricular assist device [LVAD]) at 1 year; 15% experienced a partial recovery; and 72% recovered completely [286]. Although most who recover left ventricular function do so within 6 months, up to one-third of women may have delayed recovery [228]. Of the women who recover left ventricular function, three-quarters have an EF >45% by 2 months from presentation, suggesting that recovery occurs early in most women [223]. In a US retrospective single-center study of data from January 1986-December 2016, African American women with PPCM were younger than non-African American women with PPCM, had more advanced left ventricular dysfunction with a lower EF at presentation (39.5% vs. 56.5%, respectively), and were twice as likely to fail to recover (43.0% vs. 24.2%) [211, 236].

In two retrospective studies of predominantly African-American women [280], recovery of left ventricular function was low with only 23–30% of women achieving an EF >50% at 6 months. In a larger more contemporary study, full recovery of EF was noted in 59% of black women and 77% of white women by 1 year [286]. Recovery may be poorer in black women because of later disease presentation (>6 weeks postpartum in 50% of black women vs. 22% in white women) and a higher prevalence of hypertension (70% in black women vs. 34% in white women) [286].

Predictors of Recovery

Overall EF at presentation is the best predictor of left ventricular recovery. Determinants of poor recovery include LVEF <30% at diagnosis [286], left ventricular internal diameter end diastole (LVIDD) >5.6–6.0 cm [223, 286], late diagnosis [257, 286], presence of left ventricular thrombus [223], and black race [223, 257, 286]. In the IPAC study, no woman achieved a full recovery at 1 year when the LVIDD was >6 cm and the EF was <0.3 at presentation, whereas full recovery occurred in 91% of women in whom the LVIDD was <6 cm and the EF was >0.3 at presentation [286]. In this cohort, echocardiography was performed at baseline, 2, 6, and 12 months after presentation, and recovery was predicted in 86% of women with a baseline LVEF $\geq$0.30 compared with only 37% of those with an LVEF <0.30 ($p < 0.001$) [286]. In 187 women with PPCM, the EF at presentation predicted failure to recover EF by echocardiogram at 6 months. For those with an EF of 10–19%, 63% failed to recover (EF >50%) compared to 32% of women with an EF of 20–29% and 21% of those with an EF at presentation of >30% [227]. Failure to achieve a LVEF $\geq$30% was seen in 30% of patients with an EF of 10–19% and 13% of patients with an EF of 20–29% at presentation [227].

Recurrence in Subsequent Pregnancies

Since PPCM usually occurs in a first or second pregnancy, the risk of PPCM in a subsequent pregnancy is important. Relapse is greatest in women who do not recover left ventricular systolic function. In a review of 191 recurrent pregnancies in women with PPCM, the risk of relapse (decline in left ventricular function) was almost twice as great for women who failed to recover left ventricular function than in those who had full recovery (48% vs. 27%). The mortality rate in the group who failed to recover was 16%, whereas no deaths were reported in women with full left ventricular recovery [287]. In a smaller study of 28 women with subsequent pregnancy after complete recovery of left ventricular systolic function, no maternal deaths occurred. In 16 women without complete recovery who had a subsequent pregnancy, the mortality rate was 19%. Congestive heart failure developed in 44% and a decline in EF >20% was measured in 25 [288]. Reduction in contractile reserve measured by dobutamine stress echocardiography in recovered patients suggests persistent subclinical myocardial abnormalities [263]. The best predictor of left ventricular deterioration and death with recurrent pregnancy is prepregnancy LVEF. Normalization of EF, however, does not predict a risk-free subsequent pregnancy. Women with persistent left ventricular dysfunction who want a subsequent pregnancy should be advised of the grave risk and counseled to avoid pregnancy, continue standard heart failure medications, and wait for normalization of left ventricular function before becoming pregnant [287]. Women with complete recovery after PPCM in whom normal left ventricular function persists after medication weaning can be counseled that risk of maternal death is likely zero but that deterioration of LVEF may occur. Long-term outcomes in women with relapse are not known. Careful monitoring of symptoms and left ventricular function by echocardiography are strongly recommended during and after pregnancy.

Treatment

Pharmacologic Therapies

The treatment recommendation for PPCM follows the guidelines for the treatment of other causes of cardiomyopathy because evidence-based clinical data are lacking for treating heart failure during or after pregnancy. Treatment escalation is tailored individually to the severity of symptoms at presentation. The recommended treatment for symptomatic heart failure in PPCM is to optimize oxygenation via supplemental oxygen, mechanical ventilation, and very rarely venoarterial extracorporeal membrane oxygenation or even extracorporeal mechanical oxygenation. Interventions to reduce preload and optimize cardiac contractility are emphasized as afterload reduction is a natural consequence of the low resistance placental circuit in pregnancy. Standard cardiomyopathy drug treatment includes the potential use of diuretics, intravenous or oral vasodilators, intravenous inotropes, ACE inhibitors, ARBs, beta-blockers, inhibitors of mineralocorticoid activity, and digoxin. Drug treatment in patients with PPCM requires knowledge of the drug's unique risks during pregnancy and lactation, when detrimental effects are known.

Diuretics are recommended to reduce preload-pulmonary capillary wedge pressures to relieve symptoms and to maximize oxygenation. The use of diuretics before delivery may impair placental perfusion and potentially harm the fetus; therefore, the lowest dosage possible is recommended. Improvement in stroke volume and cardiac output may require inotropic drugs, vasopressors, and rarely mechanical circulatory support. Digoxin use is safe in pregnancy, but its usefulness in the treatment of systolic heart failure is uncertain. Its use is acceptable in persistently symptomatic women during pregnancy and lactation, but levels should be checked as pregnancy increases digoxin clearance [289].

Pharmacologic antagonism of the neurohormonal axis is recommended for longer-term improvement in left ventricular contractility in PPCM patients, according to the guidelines for use in cardiomyopathy for other causes. Inhibiting the adrenergic, angiotensin, and mineralocorticoid pathways in nonpregnant women with symptomatic heart failure has been shown to reduce symptoms, improve hemodynamics and left ventricular contractility, stimulate left ventricular remodeling, and, most importantly, prolong survival.

1. *Beta-blockers*

   Controlled studies on the use of beta-blockers in PPCM have not been performed. However, beta-blockade is recommended in all women with symptomatic PPCM, but dosages should be carefully titrated to avoid short-term worsening of cardiac output. In the United States, 3 beta-blockers have been approved for treating congestive heart failure: carvedilol, bisoprolol, and metoprolol tartrate. Data on their efficacy in pregnancy and their risk to the fetus are limited.

   Antepartum use of the cardioselective β1-antagonists (metoprolol tartrate or bisoprolol) are preferred over the nonselective beta-blockers (propralolol) as they interfere less with the β2-mediated effects on uterine tone [290] which can potentially lead to uterine contractions and preterm labor. The mixed alpha and nonselective beta-antagonist, labetolol, has been used extensively antepartum in the treatment of hypertension, and carvedilol shares a similar receptor affinity. The antepartum use of atenolol has been associated with IUGR [291] and should be avoided.

2. *Inhibitors of angiotensin and mineralocorticoid activity*

   Treatment with ACE inhibitors or ARBs is restricted to use in women who are no longer pregnant because of the risk of teratogenicity in all trimesters to the fetus [292]. During pregnancy, substitution with nitrates and hydralazine is recommended especially for black or African American women in whom this combination has been shown to be beneficial in nonpregnant patients with congestive heart failure and in pregnant women with severe hypertension [29, 219, 293, 294]. Doses should be introduced gradually as postpartum women tend to have low SVR, which can lead to hypotension especially with concomitant diuretic use. ACE inhibitors are excreted in low levels into breast milk; treatment with enalapril, captopril, quinapril, or benazepril is preferred as safety in infants has been established [295]. Because there are no data on ARBs or angiotensin receptor-Neprilysin inhibitor safety during breastfeeding, their use is not recommended.

Mineralocorticoid (aldosterone) receptor antagonists (spironolactone, eplerenone) are also recommended for use in postpartum mothers to improve symptoms and increase life-expectancy. The antiandrogenic effects of spironolactone may theoretically lead to feminization of the fetus [292]. Eplerenone has no antiandrogenic effects, but its safety in pregnancy is unknown. The excretion of aldactone into breast mild is negligible, and the American Academy of Pediatrics rates it as compatible with breast feeding [289].

3. *Anticoagulation*

PPCM increases the risk of venothromboembolism and intracardiac thrombus secondary to the hypercoagulable state of pregnancy coupled with stasis from the reduction in stroke volume associated with left ventricular dysfunction. The risk of thromboembolic events is highest in the first 4 weeks of the postpartum period due to the release of tissue thromboplastin after placental separation. Bedrest compounds the exaggerated hypercoagulable state and is not recommended. The reported rate for stroke in PPCM ranges from 1.5 to 12%, and the rate for acute lower extremity arterial occlusion is 1.5% [276, 277]. In symptomatic women with severe left ventricular dysfunction and PPCM, intracardiac thrombus was visualized by echocardiography in 12–30% of cases [276, 277]. In the absence of atrial fibrillation, no data are available to guide the recommendation of antithrombotic therapy as primary prevention to reduce thromboembolic events in symptomatic women with severe left ventricular dysfunction secondary to PPCM. Careful evaluation of the left ventricle apex for thrombus with contrast echocardiography is recommended at initial and follow-up screening if the LVEF is severely depressed and if the apex is incompletely visualized by standard echocardiographic views. Primary prevention of thromboembolic events with anticoagulants is recommended if atrial fibrillation or left ventricular thrombus is detected. The choice of anticoagulant in pregnancy is discussed elsewhere, but since PPCM occurs late in pregnancy, heparin (antepartum) and warfarin (postpartum) are the preferred treatments. Patients treated with bromocriptine may be at greater risk of stroke [296] and myocardial infarction [297], and anticoagulation should be considered prophylactically in bromocriptine-treated patients [298]. For all other PPCM patients with severe left ventricular systolic function without atrial fibrillation or left ventricle thrombus, antiplatelet and anticoagulant treatments are not currently warranted.

4. *Novel treatments*

Evidence that a cleaved 16-kDa angiostatic and pro-apoptotic form of prolactin may mediate PPCM pathophysiology has led to interest in treating PPCM patients with bromocriptine, which inhibits prolactin secretion. Bromocriptine, approved for the treatment of galactorrhea and certain pituitary tumors, was deemed to be safe to the fetus in 1982 [299], but the US Food and Drug Administration withdrew its approval for the suppression of lactation in 1995 because of safety concerns after reports of adverse maternal vascular events such as stroke and myocardial infarction [300].

Bromocriptine has been shown to prevent the onset of PPCM in mice [267]. Individual patients with acute PPCM have been successfully treated with bromocriptine added to standard heart failure therapy. In a single-center study in South Africa, 20 women with severe PPCM were randomized within 24 h of presentation to standard cardiomyopathy therapy or standard therapy plus bromocriptine (2.5 mg twice daily for 2 weeks followed by once daily for 6 weeks). Bromocriptine-treated patients showed improvement in NYHA class and recovery of LVEF at 6 months. No thrombotic complications were observed. Mortality in this cohort was high (25%); however, only one bromocriptine-treated patient died, whereas 4 women in the standard therapy group died [301]. In a German multicenter study, 63 patients with PPCM and EF <35% were randomized to short-term (7 days) bromocriptine (2.5 mg daily) or long-term (8 weeks) bromocriptine (5 mg daily for 2 weeks followed by 2.5 mg daily) added to standard cardiomyopathy treatment. No placebo group was included. Full recovery (LVEF ≥50%) was nonsignificantly higher in the long-term treatment group (52% vs. 68%). No patient in the study died or needed heart transplantation or LVAD placement [302]. Without a placebo group, it is unclear if the observed improvement in outcomes is related to treatment (in both groups) with bromocriptine or to this group being a lower-risk cohort of PPCM patients. Bromocriptine use in refractory cases may be considered as the potential benefit to myocardial recovery may outweigh a small thromboembolic risk. Larger placebo-controlled trials are needed to establish the safety and efficacy of bromocriptine treatment before its use can be recommended [267, 303, 304].

Immunosuppression and immunoglobulin infusion therapies are not recommended for treating PPCM [219]. In the absence of biopsy-proven giant cell myocarditis, immunosuppression is not warranted as the efficacy is unproven and the side effects may be significant [305, 306]. In a retrospective study of 6 women with PPCM, the rate of left ventricular recovery at 6 months was greater in women treated with intravenous immunoglobulin than in 11 historical controls (26% vs. 13%) [307]. However, the small sample size and the high probability of recovery with standard treatments limit the generalizability of this therapy to common practice [219, 305].

5. *Treatment after recovery of left ventricular function*

   There are no data on the long-term treatment of women with PPCM. Experts generally agree that continued therapy with standard heart failure medications, including β-blockade, ACE inhibition, and mineralocorticoid antagonism, is warranted for a minimum of 12 months as some PPCM patients showed ongoing improvement in cardiac function up to 5 years after diagnosis [308]. In a small study of 15 women with recovery of left ventricular function, no deterioration in function occurred over 2 years after withdrawal of long-term medications [248]. Limited MRI studies do not show persistent subclinical myocardial damage in recovered PPCM women [309]. For those with persistently reduced left ventricular function, standard heart failure therapy should be continued indefinitely. Subclinical cellular abnormalities may persist as suggested by abnormalities in contractile reserve demonstrated by dobutamine echocardiography in women with recovered PPCM [279], reports of left ventricle deterioration after recovery [275], and the increased risk of recurrence in subsequent pregnancies. Full medical therapy is recommended for 6 months after full recovery. Medications should be weaned one at a time, and close clinical and echocardiographic monitoring should be maintained during weaning and continued annually.

Devices

Because left ventricular systolic function normalizes or improves within 6 to 12 months in most PPCM patients, an implantable cardioverter defibrillator (ICD) and cardiac resynchronization therapy may not be necessary long term for preventing SCD and treating left ventricular dyssynchrony [219]. For women with SCD or sustained ventricular arrhythmias, secondary prevention with an automated ICD is recommended per the guidelines [310]. The risk of lethal tachyarrhythmia in women with PPCM and severely depressed left ventricular systolic function is unknown. Death in patients with PPCM usually accompanies symptomatic deterioration of left ventricular function. A wearable cardioverter defibrillator (WCD) may be an alternative to implantable devices as a primary prevention strategy in PPCM. The use of a WCD is recommended as a bridge-to-decision for 3–6 months with serial echocardiographic assessments of left ventricular function. Discontinuation of WCD is recommended when the LVEF improves to >35%, which follows the guidelines for nonpregnancy cardiomyopathy [310]. ICD placement should be deferred for primary prevention for at least 3 months and possibly 6 months after presentation to allow ventricular recovery while optimizing medical therapy.

Mechanical Circulatory Support

Newer percutaneous mechanical support options, as well as the more widely available intra-aortic balloon counterpulsation pump are short-term percutaneous interventional options available to improve cardiac output and maternal hemodynamics when profound and refractory cardiovascular shock is present. These devices can be used as a bridge to recovery with weaning as left ventricular function improves [311, 312]. Rarely, these devices can be used to bridge to a more durable LVAD if continued circulatory support is required. Transplantation was ultimately required in 48% of women with PPCM who required a mechanical assist device in a registry study [313]. Recovery of left ventricular function after LVAD was rare (6%) [313] in women with PPCM. Transplantation was required in up to 25% of women with PPCM in a series from 1987 to 2010 [266] but in only 1% of more recent IPAC participants [251]. Transplant outcomes are lower for women with PPCM than for all other female transplant recipients with lower graft and age-adjusted survival, which may be related to younger age and higher rates of inhospital and 1-year posttransplant rejection [266].

Delivery

Limited data are available to guide the timing and mode of delivery in PPCM [219]. Scheduled delivery in an institution with a multidisciplinary team comprising cardiology, obstetric, anesthesiology, and neonatology services [219] is advised. Maternal hemodynamic instability requires urgent cesarean delivery. Scheduled cesarean delivery is preferred for women with advanced heart failure requiring inotropic therapy or mechanical circulatory support [219]. For stable women with PPCM, the balance between the individual maternal and fetal risks and the benefits of early delivery should be carefully considered by the multidisciplinary team and the patient. Early delivery is not required if the maternal (cervical status, placental position, cardiovascular status) and fetal (viability, lung maturity, growth) conditions are stable [219]. The mode of delivery in stable patients is dictated by the obstetrical conditions (failure of labor to progress, placenta previa, fetal intolerance of labor) [219, 284].

Breastfeeding

Breastfeeding in PPCM has become a controversial topic with the implication that prolactin may influence the pathophysiology of PPCM. Breastfeeding prolongs the exposure of the postpartum mother to increased prolactin. In developing nations, breastfeeding is important to infant survival [314]. Furthermore, the immunological, nutritional, and developmental neonatal benefits of breastfeeding have been well established, and limiting the beneficial effects of breastfeeding requires solid evidence of efficacy. Despite this and with no evidence of benefit, the 2010 ESC group suggested that breastfeeding be avoided because of the potential effects of prolactin [315]. However, breastfeeding was not associated with a reduction in left ventricular recovery in the IPAC study [251], and breastfeeding women had improved outcomes over those who did not breastfeed in a retrospective internet-based study.

Overall, given the benefits of breastfeeding some experts have recommended that women who are clinically stable should not be discouraged from breastfeeding as long as it is compatible with their heart failure medications [316]. If a mother decides to breastfeed, we suggest avoiding ARBs due to the lack of safety data [316].

Contraception

Women with PPCM or a history of PPCM should receive counseling regarding the risk of recurrence and family planning and contraception options. Women with persistent left ventricular dysfunction (EF <50%) or LVEF <25% at diagnosis should avoid future pregnancy due to the increased risk of recurrence. Sterilization of the patient or her partner is recommended. Alternatively, nonestrogen contraceptive implants or intrauterine devices are effective contraception and do not increase the thromboembolic risk [317, 318].

Hypertension in Pregnancy

Hypertensive disorders complicate up to 15% of pregnancies in the United States and are responsible for 10–15% of all US maternal deaths [319]. National guidelines can aid in recognizing and managing hypertension in pregnancy to reduce morbidity and mortality. The increased morbidity related to hypertensive disorders of pregnancy is presumed to be associated with the development of severe hypertension [320]. Hypertension in pregnancy increases the maternal risk of abruptio placenta, stroke, intracerebral hemorrhage, preeclampsia, organ failure, and death. Maternal hypertension also increases the fetal risk of CHD, IUGR, preterm labor, and intrauterine death [290, 321, 322].

Circulatory changes begin early in pregnancy. SVR declines, resulting in increased stroke volume and cardiac output. However, systolic BP remains relatively unchanged. In contrast, diastolic BP has a bimodal trend. Diastolic BP decreases an average of 10 mmHg in the second trimester due to decreased SVR and then returns to prepregnancy levels during the third trimester because of the increased blood volume and stroke volume [323].

Hypertension Categories

Hypertensive disorders of pregnancy can be classified into four categories: chronic hypertension, gestational hypertension, preeclampsia-eclampsia, and preeclampsia superimposed upon underlying chronic hypertension [324]. Diagnosis generally depends on gestational age at the time of presentation and the presence of proteinuria or on end-organ damage. Distinguishing preeclampsia from other causes of hypertension can be difficult but is essential to maternal and fetal outcomes [325].

The Sprint Study [326] showed a significant reduction in stroke, myocardial infarction, and heart failure with antihypertension treatment in adults with BP above 130/90 when the BP was targeted to <120/80 mmHg. On the basis of these compelling results, the definition of hypertension in nonpregnant adults was revised to stricter standards in 2017; normal BP in nonpregnant adults is now defined as systolic BP <120 mmHg and diastolic <80 mmHg [327]. The category of prehypertension has been eliminated, and the group with mildly elevated systolic BP (120–129 mmHg) but normal diastolic BP (<80 mmHg) was reclassified as having elevated BP. Hypertension in nonpregnant adults is now defined as follows:

- Stage 1—Systolic 130–139 mmHg or diastolic 80–89 mmHg
- Stage 2—Systolic at least 140 mmHg or diastolic at least 90 mmHg

Chronic Hypertension

Chronic hypertension in pregnancy remains defined as BP ≥140/90 mmHg, recorded before pregnancy and before 20 weeks of gestation, or persisting longer than 12 weeks postpartum [328]. Chronic hypertension is uncommon in pregnancy and occurs in only 0.5–3% of hypertensive pregnant women [328]. The incidence of this disorder is higher in women who are older, obese, or black [329]. Chronic hypertension increases morbidity and is associated with superimposed preeclampsia, placenta abruption, prematurity, fetal growth restriction, and CHD [290, 321, 322]. Severe chronic hypertension can result in stroke, heart failure, acute renal failure, hypertensive encephalopathy, and cerebral hemorrhage. Patients at risk should be evaluated before pregnancy [328], and all teratogenic medications, such as ACE inhibitors, ARBs, and direct renin inhibitors, should be replaced before conception [330].

Gestational Hypertension

Gestational hypertension is a temporary increase in BP during pregnancy; it is defined as elevated BP (systolic BP >140 mmHg or a diastolic BP >90 mmHg) that develops after 20 weeks of gestation in the absence of proteinuria or other diagnostic features of preeclampsia. It is the most common cause of hypertension in pregnancy and occurs in 6–17% of nulliparous women and in 2–4% of multiparous women [331–333]. Adverse perinatal outcomes are significantly higher in severe gestational hypertension than in mild preeclampsia [331]. Women with gestational hypertension who develop end-organ dysfunction or proteinuria will be reclassified as having preeclampsia. Women with persistent hypertension 12 weeks postpartum will subsequently be diagnosed as having chronic hypertension. The highest prevalence of gestational hypertension occurs in women with a history of preeclampsia in a previous pregnancy, women with multifetal pregnancy, and women who are obese or overweight [328, 334]. The rate of recurrence of gestational hypertension in subsequent pregnancies is at least 20%.

Preeclampsia

Preeclampsia is a pregnancy-specific clinical syndrome of new onset hypertension in a previously normotensive pregnant woman with proteinuria or end-organ dysfunction with or without proteinuria that usually occurs after 20 weeks gestation. Overall, preeclampsia complicates 5–7% of all pregnancies but may occur in up to 25% of pregnancies with preexisting hypertension. Preeclampsia is defined as BP >140/90 mmHg, with proteinuria >0.3 g in a 24-h urine collection or as organ dysfunction defined by a platelet count <100,000/mm^3, a creatinine level >1.1 mg/dL, transaminitis, congestive heart failure, or neurologic symptoms [335]. Eclampsia is diagnosed when seizures occur.

The cause of preeclampsia is poorly understood. Placental, immunologic, and genetic factors lead to systemic endothelial dysfunction, and circulation abnormalities might result in hypoperfusion, hypoxemia, and ischemia of the placenta. Risk factors include first pregnancy, multiple pregnancies, obesity, diabetes mellitus, a history of chronic hypertension, and a family history of mothers with preeclampsia. Preeclampsia can have an early or late onset. Late-onset preeclampsia (prevalence, 5% of cases) occurs within 48 h after delivery. The early-onset condition (<34 weeks of gestation) tends to be more severe. Management of preeclampsia relies on proper recognition of the condition. Definitive therapy is delivery of the placenta; however, conservative management may be pursued in selected cases, particularly if the condition occurs early in gestation (allowing maximal time for the fetus to mature). Rates of recurrent preeclampsia with subsequent pregnancies are much lower than for gestational hypertension at 5% versus 20% [336, 337].

Preeclampsia Superimposed on Chronic or Gestational Hypertension

Establishing the diagnosis of preeclampsia superimposed on chronic hypertension or gestational hypertension can be difficult [328]. Preeclampsia should be suspected in women who have a sudden increase in BP and proteinuria, or who develop transaminitis, thrombocytopenia, or symptoms of end-organ damage such as visual changes, right upper quadrant pain, and heart failure. Up to 25% of women with preexisting hypertension (either chronic or gestational) develop preeclampsia. The risk that gestational hypertension will progress to preeclampsia is increased if hypertension develops before 34 weeks of gestation, with uric acid levels >5.2 mg/dL, and when mean systolic BP is >135 mmHg on ambulatory 24-h BP monitoring [338, 339]. Doppler velocimetry measurements of fetoplacental flow are abnormal in preeclampsia and normal in gestational or chronic hypertension [340].

General Principles of Hypertension

Measurement of Blood Pressure

The accurate measurement of BP in pregnancy is essential in guiding medical decisions that affect both mother and fetus. The timing and method of BP measurement affect the accuracy of the results, which depend on proper patient position, BP device used, and cuff size and placement [327, 341].

BP may be measured by a mercury-based sphygmomanometer or by approved, validated, and calibrated automated oscillometric brachial (upper arm) BP devices (AOBP). Mercury-based auscultatory devices are used less frequently due to concerns for mercury toxicity, but improvements in AOBP device accuracy have increased their use in medical offices and home monitoring [342, 343]. BP screening in pregnancy is performed in the office and may be confirmed or monitored by home or ambulatory measurements. BP measurements in the office may be 5–10 mmHg higher than measurements made by ambulatory or home BP monitoring. Multiple in-office measurements by either device or by AOBP while the patient is unattended and alone approach the accuracy of ambulatory or home-obtained readings [344, 345]. The BP should be measured for screening of hypertension in the office with the quiet patient *seated* with feet uncrossed on the floor and with the arm supported at the level of the heart (midpoint of the sternum) while at rest for 5 min. Measurement of BP in left lateral recumbency may be used if a seated BP is not feasible [343]. The BP readings should be documented on at least two occasions at least 4 hours apart. An average of at least two BP measurements with 1–2 min rest between measurements is recommended in the diagnosis of adults with hypertension [327] and is useful to discriminate patients with reactive “white-coat” hypertension or high in-office readings that do not meet the diagnostic criteria for hypertension based on out-of-office readings. Home BP monitoring is useful to establish and confirm the presence of hypertension in patients with elevated in-office BP. Avoidance of caffeine and exercise for 30 min is recommended before BP measurement as they may increase BP.

BP cuff size affects the accuracy of BP measurement. BP cuffs that are too small may falsely increase the systolic BP by 10–50 mmHg in obese subjects. The cuff should encircle 80% of the forearm with the width of the bladder 40% of the arm circumference. A large adult cuff, for arm circumferences 35–44 cm, or a thigh cuff, for those 45–52 cm, may be required in obese women [343].

An accurate auscultatory assessment of BP depends on the skill and technique of the operator. The cuff should be inflated 20–30 mmHg above the systolic pressure where the radial or brachial pulse disappears from palpation [346]. The cuff should be deflated slowly at a rate of 2–3 mmHg per second [347] until the first audible sound is heard by either the bell or the diaphragm of the stethoscope placed lightly over the brachial artery (Korotkoff phase 1). This pressure is the systolic BP. As the cuff is deflated below the systolic pressure, the pulse continues to be heard until there is abrupt muffling (phase IV) followed by complete disappearance of sound (phase V) [348]. The pressure at which the auscultatory sounds first disappear is the diastolic BP [343]. However, if sounds remain audible with the cuff deflated, which can happen in pregnant women due to elevated stroke volume and low SVR, then Korotkoff phase IV should be used [343, 346].

Maternal Evaluation with Hypertension

Once hypertension in pregnancy has been diagnosed, an investigation for evidence of preeclampsia (proteinuria or end-organ damage) and secondary causes of hypertension is recommended.

Routine baseline tests for pregnant women with hypertension include [349] the following:

- Quantitative analysis of proteinuria by using a urine protein-to-creatinine ratio ≥0.26 mg protein/mg creatinine (30 mg/mmol) on a random urine sample
- Urine culture
- Glomerular filtration rate or serum creatinine
- Electrolyte testing
- Fasting glucose levels
- Thyroid function test
- Possible electrocardiogram

Causes of secondary hypertension such as chronic kidney disease, hyperthyroidism, primary hyperaldosteronism (low serum potassium, low plasma renin activity), and renovascular hypertension (high renin activity) may be evident on these baseline screening tests. If coarctation of the aorta is suspected, a cardiology referral and an echocardiogram should be requested.

Quantification of urinary protein excretion is recommended to differentiate preeclampsia from other causes of hypertension in pregnancy because the diagnosis of preeclampsia has both prognostic and therapeutic consequences. Results from a urine dipstick test are not sensitive or specific enough for diagnostic purposes. False negative results occur with low urine specific gravity (<1.010), hypertonic or acidic urine, or nonalbumin proteinuria. A positive urine dipstick result requires confirmation as false positives can also occur.

If proteinuria is present, preeclampsia should be suspected, and a quantitative 24-hour examination of urine protein excretion, as well as serum uric acid levels, platelet count, and liver function tests are recommended. Diagnosing preeclampsia may be difficult, and any signs or symptoms of end-organ dysfunction (new onset of cerebral or visual disturbances or epigastric or right upper-quadrant pain) in a woman with hypertension without proteinuria should be treated as preeclampsia [350] as up to 10% of women with clinical or histological signs of preeclampsia do not have proteinuria [351].

Given the risks of these hypertensive conditions, frequent prenatal visits with careful monitoring of BP and proteinuria are essential. Home monitoring of maternal BP is also advisable [242].

Fetal Evaluation in Mothers With Hypertension

Fetal well-being should be assessed with a biophysical profile or nonstress test with amniotic fluid estimation. A sonographic estimation of fetal weight is recommended. Umbilical artery Doppler velocimetry is reserved for fetuses with growth restriction [328].

Congenital Heart Disease

Pregnant women with chronic hypertension appear to have an 80% greater risk of having offspring with CHD than do normotensive pregnant women (relative risk [RR], 1.8; 95% confidence interval [CI], 1.5–2.2) [322]. Pharmacologic treatment of hypertension appears to increase this risk (RR, 2.0; 95% CI, 1.5–2.7). The risk remained 40% higher in untreated women with chronic hypertension than in normotensive pregnant women, suggesting that the elevated risk may be related to the hypertension itself and possibly worsened with pharmacologic treatment (RR, 1.4; 95% CI, 1.2–1.7) [322]. It is not clear if the pharmacologic treatment increases the CHD risk or whether it is related to the severity of hypertension (which triggered pharmacologic treatment). It is also possible that hypertension in pregnancy and CHD share similar risk factors.

Blood Pressure Severity and Treatment Targets

BP elevation in pregnancy is divided into categories based on BP severity and evidence of preeclampsia. Compared with nonpregnant individuals, BP in pregnant women is considered normal at a higher level (<140/90 mmHg);

mild-to-moderate hypertension is classified as BP ranging from 140 to 159 mmHg systolic and 90 to 109 mmHg diastolic, and severe hypertension is reported as BP greater than 160/110 mmHg. Treatment strategies are based on these categories and the presence of preeclampsia.

Treatment of severe hypertension has well-established maternal benefits including a reduction in stroke risk and maternal complications in patients with and without evidence of maternal end-organ damage or proteinuria [352]. The 2011 ESC task force for the management of CVD in pregnancy recommends emergent inhospital management of systolic BP >170 mmHg or diastolic BP >110 mmHg [29]. Pharmacologic treatments with intravenous labetolol or intravenous nicardipine are recommended before initiating intravenous hydralazine. If BP is not responsive to parenteral labetolol or nicardipine, the temporary use of sodium nitroprusside in hypertensive crisis may be required to control BP quickly. Prolonged use of sodium nitroprusside is associated with fetal cyanide poisoning as accumulation of its metabolite, thiocyanate, is excreted into the fetal urine [353]. In women with preeclampsia and congestive heart failure, nitroglycerin infusion is recommended [29].

The data for treating mild-to-moderate and moderate hypertension (140–159/90–109 mmHg) in pregnancy are controversial [354, 355]. Most women with hypertension in pregnancy have mild-to-moderate disease and are at low risk of cardiovascular or neonatal complications. The short-term benefit of temporary treatment of hypertension during a relatively short duration in pregnancy must be balanced against the potential direct risk to the fetus from the medications as well as the risk of BP overtreatment with a resultant decrease in placental perfusion and low birth weight or fetal maldevelopment. Women with treated chronic essential hypertension who become pregnant may have a decrease in BP during the first half of pregnancy due to the natural decrease in SVR with pregnancy and may not require any medications. In a 2002 meta-regression analysis of antihypertension treatment related to any diagnostic category of pregnancy hypertension, a reduction in maternal mean arterial BP by 10 mmHg was associated with a slight (176-g) decrease in birth weight [351].

A 2014 meta-analysis of 49 trials of antihypertensive therapy revealed a 50% lower incidence of severe maternal hypertension, with no differences in the rates of abruption, IUGR, preeclampsia, or prematurity, in treated patients with mild-to-moderate hypertension in pregnancy than in those who were not treated [57, 356].

The 2015 CHIPS (Control of Hypertension in Pregnancy Study) trial examined the strategy of tight (diastolic target <85 mmHg) vs. less-tight (diastolic target <100 mmHg) BP control in 981 pregnant women with nonsevere chronic or gestational hypertension [354]. The mean difference in BP between groups was 4.6 mmHg for diastolic BP and 5.8 mmHg for systolic BP. Overall, maternal hypertension treatment reduced the occurrence of severe maternal hypertension during pregnancy but did not increase the risk of delivery of a small-for- gestational-age infant or cause excess fetal risk. Women randomized to less-tight control who developed severe hypertension had a higher rate of preterm delivery and lower infant birth weight and a higher rate of serious maternal morbidity due to preeclampsia and HELLP syndrome [355].

A recent post hoc analysis of women treated before 24 weeks gestation in the CHIPS trial demonstrated that early tight BP control (diastolic BP <85 mmHg) was associated with a decrease in iatrogenic preterm birth and a decrease in the development of severe maternal hypertension at all gestational ages but particularly before 28 weeks [357]. The benefit of tight control of diastolic BP before 24 weeks was offset by an increased rate of newborn weights below the 10th percentile [357] with no overall effect on perinatal death or morbidity. The authors concluded that in women with nonsevere chronic or gestational hypertension, tighter control of diastolic BP (<85 mmHg) at all gestational ages is preferred to optimize maternal and perinatal outcomes.

Despite these studies detailing maternal benefit in treatment of uncomplicated mild-to-moderate hypertension in pregnancy, medical societies remain conservative in their treatment recommendations [358]. The treatment threshold of systolic BP >140 mmHg and diastolic BP >90 mmHg are recommended in the select group of pregnant women at highest risk of complications: gestational hypertension with or without proteinuria, chronic hypertension with proteinuria, and in all women with preeclampsia or those with subclinical signs or symptoms of end-organ damage at any time during pregnancy.

Treatment of Hypertension in Preeclampsia

Delivery is the definitive maternal treatment of preeclampsia. Before delivery in preeclampsia, the mother is at risk of seizures, placental abruption, thrombocytopenia, cerebral and liver hemorrhage, pulmonary edema, acute renal injury, and death. After delivery of the fetus and the placenta, the maternal risk declines rapidly within hours. The fetal risk in preeclampsia is determined by the gestational age at the onset of preeclampsia and the fetal maturity at the time of delivery. Fetal loss and IUGR are increased in preeclampsia. Treatment of hypertension in preeclampsia may be indicated to allow fetal maturation in the absence of significant maternal end-organ damage. Hypertension treatment does not alter the pathophysiology or the time course in preeclampsia as abnormalities in the placental vasculature lead to reduced uteroplacental perfusion, which directly leads to the release of factors that cause diffuse endothelial dysfunction and eventual multiorgan failure.

Treatment of severe hypertension (>160 mmHg/110 mmHg) in preeclampsia with intravenous medications is recommended to prevent maternal stroke, intracranial hemorrhage, seizures, and heart failure. Severe systolic hypertension appears to be more predictive of adverse maternal cerebral stroke events than diastolic hypertension in preeclampsia or eclampsia [359]. Stroke was hemorrhagic in 25 of 27 cases (93%) with a maternal mortality of 54%. Systolic BP was >155 mmHg in all stroke patients before the stroke symptoms developed, whereas diastolic BP was >110 mmHg in only 12%. In this study, almost half of strokes occurred during magnesium infusion. Thus, it may be prudent to shift the focus toward managing systolic rather than diastolic BP thresholds (>150 mmHg) in women with severe preeclampsia or eclampsia in whom a magnesium drip is not protective. Optimal treatment goals have not been studied. Consensus thresholds for treatment are also not well delineated, but several sources and most physicians recommend treatment in women with preeclampsia when BP is greater than 150/100 mmHg, especially if delivery is delayed for fetal reasons. The 2011 ESC Task Force for the management of CVD in pregnancy recommends treatment of hypertension when systolic BP is >140 mmHg and diastolic BP is >90 mmHg or when signs or symptoms of end-organ damage are evident at any time during pregnancy [29]. Some clinicians advocate for withholding hypertension treatment until systolic BP is >160 mmHg or diastolic BP is ≥105–110 mmHg [335, 359]. However, most women with preeclampsia will develop neurologic symptoms when mean arterial pressure exceeds 110 mmHg at which point antihypertensive treatment should be initiated. If symptoms of neurologic (confusion, headache, visual changes) or cardiac (shortness of breath, chest discomfort) decompensation occur with moderately elevated BP, the hypertension should be treated acutely. Asymptomatic women with preeclampsia and mild hypertension (BP <140/90) can be cared for without medications according to ACOG.

High-quality clinical trials are needed to clarify the parameters for antihypertensive use in women with preeclampsia. At present, reliable evidence to support practice recommendations is lacking because the available trials are limited by several factors, including differences in BP measurement techniques, diagnostic criteria, etiology of hypertension, and target BP.

Treatment of Hypertension

All antihypertensive agents cross the placenta. The clinical efficacy and fetal risk of hypertension medications in pregnancy have not been assessed in a randomized clinical trial; only retrospective and anecdotal data are available for guiding treatment decisions in hypertension in pregnancy. Furthermore, because antihypertensive treatment of chronic hypertension during pregnancy is associated with a twofold increase in the risk of CHD in offspring, the use of antihypertensive medications should be limited to prevent maternal cardiovascular morbidity and mortality during pregnancy. The medications should be chosen on the basis of their safety profiles. The antihypertensive drugs considered to be safe in pregnancy include alpha methyldopa, beta-blockers (especially labetalol), calcium channel blockers, and hydralazine [360].

Nonpharmacologic Management and Prevention of Hypertension in Pregnancy

Nonpharmacologic treatment is advised in women with uncomplicated hypertension in pregnancy when the systolic BP is <150 mmHg or the diastolic BP is <100 mmHg. Women with chronic hypertension who become pregnant should discontinue use of diuretics, ACE inhibitors, ARBs, and direct renin inhibitors before pregnancy or as soon as pregnancy is detected. BP during the first half of pregnancy may decline as SVR decreases naturally with pregnancy. BP should be monitored, but pharmacologic treatment may not be required until the later stages of pregnancy. Dietary salt restriction is not advised as intravascular volume depletion may result [29]. Weight loss during pregnancy is not advised, even in obese women, as it can lead to reduced neonatal weights. Weight gain in pregnancy should follow established guidelines [361]. Physical activity should not be restricted in most pregnant women with stable chronic hypertension [362, 363]. In fact, ACOG recommends continued moderate exercise during pregnancy in women with well-controlled chronic hypertension and no complications who exercised before pregnancy [335, 350]. Activity restriction may be advised in women with hypertension and preeclampsia to improve uteroplacental blood flow and to prevent severe fluctuations in BP, although this approach has not been shown to improve maternal or fetal outcomes. Daily calcium supplementation of at least 1 g has reduced the risk of preeclampsia by 50%, but the benefit in preventing other hypertensive disorders in pregnancy has not been established [364]. Low-dose aspirin is advised by the AHA and the American Stroke Association for use in pregnant women with hypertension or a previous pregnancy associated with hypertension to reduce the risk of preeclampsia [365].

Pharmacologic Antihypertension Treatment Options

The following antihypertensive medication classes are effective in pregnancy and have acceptable safety profiles based on long clinical use and retrospective analysis. Drug selection for treatment is based on individual patient characteristics including the severity and acuity of the hypertension.

Alpha Methyl Dopa

Alpha methyl dopa is a weak centrally acting oral antihypertensive used almost only during pregnancy; it has a favorable safety profile in the fetus based on decades of use in pregnancy [366, 367]. It has a latency of 3–6 h to onset. Higher doses may be required to control BP, but the sedative effects at high doses may limit its use. Alpha methyl dopa is also safe for use in lactation.

Calcium Channel Blockers

The use of long-acting oral nifedipine is recommended over short-acting nifedipine, amlodipine (the newer calcium channel blocker) [368], and the nonhydropyridines, diltiazem and verapamil. Long-acting nifedipine (30–120 mg/day) has a good safety record in pregnancy [369], but the data on the use of other calcium channel blockers in pregnancy are limited. Nicardipine, a parenterally available dihydropyridine calcium channel blocker, is used for short-term treatment of severe hypertension. The initial dose of 5 mg/h can be increased to a maximum of 15 mg/h. The two major limitations of long-acting nifedipine are a longer onset of action, which precludes rapid titration, and a longer serum elimination half-life (3–6 h).

Beta-Blockers

As a class, beta-blockers are generally considered safe in pregnancy and have been extensively reviewed above in the section on treatment of cardiomyopathy. Labetolol has a unique mix of alpha and beta antagonism and is thought to preserve uteroplacental blood flow better than traditional beta-blockers [370–372]. Labetolol has a long history of safety in pregnancy and a rapid onset of action (<5 min), which makes it the preferred beta-blocker for treatment of acute (intravenous) hypertensive emergencies [373]. Carvedilol shares a similar mechanism of action with labetolol, but its use in pregnancy has not been well studied.

Hydralazine

Hydralazine is a direct arteriolar vasodilator that can be administrated orally or parenterally. It is widely used parenterally to treat acute severe hypertension in pregnant women with preeclampsia [374]. Additionally, hydralazine can be used as an intravenous bolus (10–20 mg) with an onset of action within 10–30 min. Sudden drops in BP may occur, and careful BP monitoring in an intensive care unit is recommended. Reflex tachycardia is common, and coadministration with labetolol may be beneficial. Oral hydralazine has a relatively short half-life (<8 h) and leads to rebound hypertension and poorly controlled BP.

Thiazide Diuretics

Thiazide diuretics are useful in controlling mildly elevated BP in nonpregnant adults. The use of thiazide diuretics in pregnancy is associated with a reduced blood volume and the potential for decreased placental perfusion when initiated during pregnancy. Thiazides are not recommended for use in pregnancy unless the patient has symptoms of or is at risk of heart failure.

Arrhythmias in Pregnancy

Arrhythmias are one of the most common cardiovascular complications during pregnancy and may affect women with or without preexisting cardiac disorders [375]. Any type of arrhythmia may manifest; however, most are benign, do not require therapy, and resolve after delivery [376, 377].

Although the exact mechanism is unclear, multiple physiologic adaptations occur during pregnancy that may predispose women to develop arrhythmias [29]. The pregnancy-associated expansion in total body plasma volume leads to cardiac dilatation and subsequent activation of stretch-activated ion channels and cardiomyocyte depolarization [378]. Higher levels of circulating estrogen may also contribute to increased automaticity from upregulation of myocardial alpha-adrenergic receptors [379]. Autonomic changes such as increases in resting heart rate and cardiac output in pregnant women have also been associated with a higher risk of tachyarrhythmias [380].

The following general principles apply to managing arrhythmias during pregnancy: (1) most do not require pharmacologic therapy unless intolerable symptoms develop; (2) hemodynamically unstable tachyarrhythmias should be treated with emergent electrical cardioversion; and (3) if pharmacologic therapy is needed, avoid using it during the first trimester if possible, and choose drugs that are safe in pregnant women, using the lowest doses possible [381].

Supraventricular Arrhythmias

Atrial Premature Beats

Atrial premature beats, which result from benign ectopic activity, are common and occur in more than 50% of pregnant women [377]. Patients with atrial premature beats may be asymptomatic or present with palpitations, which do not require treatment unless intolerable to the patient. Those requiring therapy may respond well to cardioselective beta-blockers such as metoprolol.

Paroxysmal Supraventricular Reentrant Tachycardia

Paroxysmal supraventricular tachycardia (PSVT) is a form of reentrant tachycardia common in pregnant women and most frequently occurs during the third trimester or the postpartum period [382]. It is relatively uncommon for new-onset PSVT to develop during pregnancy (~3.9% risk), but women with a previous diagnosis of PSVT are more prone to exacerbation of symptoms during pregnancy (22%) [383]. The most common mechanism is reentry within the atrioventricular node (AVNRT), followed by atrioventricular reentry via an accessory pathway (AVRT) [383]. Supraventricular tachycardia (SVT) may be associated with adverse maternal and fetal outcomes [384]. Vagal maneuvers are the first-line intervention for acute termination of SVT in pregnant women [375, 385]. If the vagal maneuvers fail, adenosine is the drug of choice for highly symptomatic patients [375, 381]. Non-first-line agents that may be used for acute termination of SVT include intravenous metoprolol, verapamil, and procainamide [385, 386]. Intravenous amiodarone is reserved for life-threatening SVT when alternative agents have failed [385]. For ongoing management, digoxin, flecainide, metoprolol, propafenone, propranolol, sotalol, and verapamil are used [375, 387]. First-line agents for long-term prophylaxis include metoprolol, propranolol, and digoxin.

Atrial Tachycardia

Focal atrial tachycardia is rare during pregnancy but may be seen in the absence of structural heart disease [388]. This arrhythmia is notoriously difficult to manage due to resistance to drugs and recurrence after electrical cardioversion. Treatment recommendations include rate control with beta-blockers, digoxin, or non-dihydropyridine calcium channel blocker and possible catheter ablation in patients with intolerable symptoms and drug resistance [29].

Atrial Fibrillation and Flutter

Atrial fibrillation and atrial flutter are rare in the absence of structural heart disease, hyperthyroidism, or other risk factors [376], but may occur as lone atrial fibrillation in women with structurally normal hearts [389]. Principles of management mirror those for nonpregnant patients except for certain nuances such as choice and use of pharmacologic agents.

Rate Control

Metoprolol, verapamil, and digoxin are appropriate agents for ventricular rate control. However, in practice, metoprolol tends to be the agent of choice due to its history of safe use in pregnant women [29]. Digoxin appears less effective on its own than beta-blockers, especially during exertion [29, 390].

Rhythm Control

Quinidine and procainamide are reasonable options for pharmacologic rhythm control. However, quinidine has a longer history of safe use in pregnant women.

Anticoagulation

Anticoagulation is an important consideration in pregnant women with atrial fibrillation who are at increased risk of thromboembolic complications. In addition to the baseline hypercoagulable state of pregnancy, atrial fibrillation tends to occur in women with other risk factors such as mitral stenosis and mechanical heart valves. Decisions and specific regimens for anticoagulation are individualized according to the thromboembolism risk. Thromboembolism prophylaxis is recommended throughout pregnancy in women with a CHADS2 score ≥2 [29]. Women with low thrombotic risk and lone atrial fibrillation that spontaneously resolves or is cardioverted within 48 h do not require long-term anticoagulation [391].

Ventricular Arrhythmias

Ventricular Premature Beats

Ventricular premature beats are common during pregnancy, occurring in approximately 50–60% of pregnant women with and without structural heart disease [377]. Most patients do not require treatment, but if symptoms are intolerable, cardioselective beta-blockers may be used.

Ventricular Tachycardia

Ventricular tachycardia (VT) and ventricular fibrillation are rare during pregnancy [29]. Most cases of VT occur in women with preexisting structural heart disease; however, idiopathic VT may occur in those with normal hearts [392, 393].

Idiopathic VT tends to have a benign prognosis with low risk of degeneration into an unstable rhythm [392, 393]. The most common pattern is right ventricular outflow tract tachycardia, which tends to be catecholamine-triggered [393] and may be treated with beta-blockers or sotalol. The less common idiopathic left VT may respond to calcium channel blockade with verapamil [394].

Bradyarrhythmias and Conduction Defects

Bradycardia

Normal pregnancy is associated with increases in maternal resting heart rate and cardiac output. Sinus bradycardia is very uncommon, but transient episodes may occur in the setting of vagal maneuvers. Rarely, inferior vena cava compression by the gravid uterus can result in paradoxical bradycardia known as supine hypotensive syndrome of pregnancy [29, 395]. Although sinus bradycardia rarely requires intervention, women with persistent symptoms may need temporary pacing [29].

Atrioventricular Block

First-degree atrioventricular block can be seen in structurally normal hearts. Prognosis is benign and progression to complete heart block is unlikely [29]. Second- and third-degree heart blocks are much less common and are usually associated with underlying heart disease. Of note, pregnancy may unmask previously undiagnosed congenital atrioventricular block in up to 30% of patients [29]. Symptomatic complete heart block should be managed with temporary pacing [395].

Fetal Arrhythmias

Fetal arrhythmias are identified in approximately 1–2% of pregnancies [396, 397]. Most are self-limited ectopic beats. However, even uncomplicated fetal arrhythmias carry the potential to evolve into more dangerous tachyarrhythmias [398].

Fetal Ectopy

Ectopic beats are the most common cause of irregular fetal rhythm; premature atrial contractions are more common than ventricular contractions [397]. Once considered benign, fetal ectopic beats are now seen as potential markers of more severe conditions such as atrioventricular block [399] or CHD [398, 400]. Therefore, the presence of complicated features or risk factors for cardiac disease should prompt investigation. Complicated fetal ectopy is defined as (A) frequent ectopy (bigeminy, trigeminy, or >3–5 beats per minute); (B) ectopy persisting for more than 1–2 weeks; or (C) ectopy of uncertain etiology (e.g., atrial vs. ventricular origin) [401]. Fetal echocardiogram should be obtained to evaluate cardiac structure and function in these situations [401].

Fetal Tachyarrhythmias (Heart Rate >180)

Transient sinus tachycardia occurring with fetal movements is normal during later gestational ages. However, prolonged sinus tachycardia should raise concern for fetal distress secondary to hypoxia, infection, or various metabolic issues such as thyrotoxicosis [396].

AVRT is the most common fetal tachyarrhythmia, accounting for up to 90% of cases [397, 402]. The most common mechanism involves initiation by a premature atrial contraction with reentry through persistent atrioventricular connections, which are normally lost during fetal development [403, 404]. Transplacental digoxin (oral or intravenous given to the mother) has historically been the pharmacologic treatment of choice for fetal SVT. However, recent studies and meta-analyses have shown that flecainide may be a more effective first-line agent with higher rates of SVT termination [405, 406].

Atrial flutter, which is also associated with persistent atrioventricular connections, is the second most common fetal tachyarrhythmia (~30%) [397, 407]. Sotalol is the most effective treatment for fetal atrial flutter termination [397, 408]. In contrast, fetal atrial fibrillation is extremely rare and, if present, should raise concern for CHD or VHD. Management of atrial fibrillation may include rate control with digoxin or propranolol or cardioversion with sotalol [409] or flecainide [410].

Ventricular tachyarrhythmias (and ventricular fibrillation) are rare in the fetus; thus, no definitive management guidelines exist. However, treatment with intravenous magnesium sulfate, propranolol, or amiodarone are options [397].

The presence of fetal tachyarrhythmia warrants immediate cardiology evaluation to identify CHD and prevent fatal complications of sustained tachycardia including fetal distress, systolic dysfunction, and cardiovascular collapse resulting in nonimmune hydrops fetalis [398, 400].

Hydrops Fetalis

Nonimmune hydrops fetalis is a dreaded complication of sustained fetal tachycardia; mortality ranges from 50% to nearly 100% [411, 412]. Hydrops fetalis is a state of decompensated heart failure that manifests with subcutaneous edema, ascites, and pleural and pericardial effusions. Importantly, signs of evolving hydrops may occur within 24 h of onset of sustained tachycardia [397]. Therefore, identifying these signs and terminating tachycardia are of utmost importance. Unfortunately, once hydrops has developed, achieving therapeutic fetal digoxin levels becomes more difficult because of impaired transplacental transfer [410]. Sotalol and flecainide, which both have excellent transplacental transfer, concentrate in amniotic fluid without accumulating in the fetus and have been more effective than digoxin in terminating SVT in hydropic fetuses [405, 408, 410]. Alternatively, direct fetal intramuscular digoxin has also been used to raise drug levels [413].

Fetal Bradycardia (Heart Rate <110)

Fetal bradycardia is defined as heart rate below 110 beats per minute [414]. The most common cause is complete heart block (CHB), which is associated with CHD in approximately 50% of cases [415]. Another important cause of fetal CHB is maternal autoantibody-mediated (SSA/Ro and SSB/La) damage to the fetal conduction system [397, 399, 416]. Approximately 2% of pregnancies in SSA or SSB antibody-positive women will be complicated by fetal AV block, and women with previous pregnancies complicated by CHB are at 10–15 times higher risk of recurrence [417, 418]. SSA/SSB autoantibodies have also been associated with transient sinus bradycardia and structural heart disorders [419]. The prognosis of fetal CHB depends on the etiology; AV block secondary to CHD has the worst prognosis with mortality exceeding 80% [420]. Management of CHB requires pacemaker placement after delivery, but timing of placement may vary [421, 422].

Brief periods of sinus bradycardia are commonly seen during normal pregnancy, especially during the second trimester, but may be indicative of more concerning issues such as fetal hypotension or hypoxia. Sinus bradycardia and second-degree AV block have also been associated with congenital long-QT syndrome [423, 424].

Pharmacologic Antiarrhythmic Therapy

All antiarrhythmic drugs have the potential to cross the placenta and cause fetal adverse effects [375, 425]. Large randomized controlled trials on the safety of these drugs during pregnancy and lactation are lacking, and safety recommendations are based primarily on historical experience, case reports, observational studies, and animal studies [395]. Therefore, while several antiarrhythmic drugs have historically been well tolerated in pregnant women with relatively low fetal risk, most fall into the FDA pregnancy category C. Their use is generally reserved for those with significant symptoms and should be avoided during the first trimester if possible, when teratogenic risk is highest [375, 395, 396]. Most antiarrhythmic medications are excreted in breast milk to varying degrees, but most are still compatible with breastfeeding.

Class I: Sodium Channel Blockers

The class IA antiarrhythmic medications including quinidine, procainamide, and disopyramide have historically been used to treat various atrial and ventricular arrhythmias but are seldom used today. All carry proarrhythmic potential from QT_C prolongation and require hospitalization for continuous cardiac monitoring and serial drug level measurements [381]. Among these drugs, quinidine has the longest history of use in pregnant women [381]. Quinidine and procainamide are both present in fetal serum and excreted in breast milk at low levels thought to be safe in breastfeeding [425, 426]. Disopyramide and its anticholinergic metabolites are transmitted to breastfed infants [427]. Although case reports have not identified adverse effects in nursing infants, other drugs are preferred [427, 428]. If disopyramide therapy is required, breastfed infants should be monitored for anticholinergic symptoms.

Class IB antiarrhythmics, lidocaine and mexiletine, have been used to treat ventricular arrhythmias and appear to be well tolerated during pregnancy. Lidocaine in particular has a long history of safe use in pregnant women, has a low degree of excretion into breast milk, and is poorly absorbed by breastfed infants [429, 430]. Although data on mexiletine are more limited, risks of harm seem unlikely due to its low concentration in breast milk and large volume of distribution [431].

Class IC drugs, flecainide and propafenone, have been used to treat maternal and fetal supraventricular and ventricular arrhythmias. However, this class of drugs has been associated with increased mortality in patients with prior myocardial infarction and should not be used in this population [432]. Flecainide and propafenone are present in low levels in breast milk and are considered compatible with breastfeeding with careful monitoring [433, 434].

Class II: Beta-Blockers

Beta-blockers have been used to treat SVT and are first-line agents for ventricular rate control in atrial fibrillation. Their use is discussed above in the pharmacologic treatment of PPCM.

Class III: Potassium Channel Blockers

The class III antiarrhythmics have been used to treat a wide spectrum of arrhythmias. All carry proarrhythmic potential through QT_C prolongation and require close monitoring. Sotalol is a pregnancy category B agent and has been used safely in pregnant women. It possesses additional beta-antagonist properties and therefore has the same theoretical risk profile associated with other beta-blocking agents.

Amiodarone has been used to treat ventricular and supraventricular arrhythmias and has been safely used in pregnant women. However, adverse effects include fetal hypothyroidism, neurotoxicity, and neurodevelopmental abnormalities [435, 436]. Therefore, amiodarone falls into pregnancy category D and is contraindicated except for life-threatening arrhythmias resistant to alternative agents. Amiodarone and its active metabolites are excreted in breast milk and may be associated with high concentrations and significant ingestion by nursing infants [435]. Therefore, although not preferred, amiodarone may be considered with close cardiac and thyroid monitoring [435].

Data on dofetilide and ibutilide are limited. Both are category C drugs, but it is unknown whether these agents are excreted in breast milk. Dronedarone is structurally similar to amiodarone in structure and has been used to treat atrial fibrillation [437]. In addition, dronedarone has been associated with fetal abnormalities in animal studies; it is considered a category X drug and is contraindicated during pregnancy and breastfeeding.

Class IV: Calcium Channel Blockers

The non-dihydropyridine calcium channel blockers verapamil and diltiazem are considered category C drugs and have been used to treat maternal and fetal SVT. Although they have been used safely in pregnant women, fetal hypotension, bradycardia, and heart block have been reported [438]. Verapamil and diltiazem are both present in low concentrations in breast milk and are considered compatible with breastfeeding [439].

Miscellaneous Antiarrhythmic Drugs

Adenosine has been safely used during pregnancy and breastfeeding and is considered the drug of choice for acute termination of SVT in pregnancy [381, 440].

Digoxin, a category C drug, has a long history of safe use during pregnancy. It has traditionally been considered the first-line agent for treating a variety of maternal and fetal arrhythmias. However, newer data suggest that other agents may be more effective for certain maternal and fetal arrhythmias, especially with hydrops fetalis.

Nonpharmacologic Interventions

Electrical Cardioversion

Hemodynamically unstable tachyarrhythmias should be managed with emergent electrical cardioversion, which can be safely performed during all stages of pregnancy as minimal electrical energy reaches the fetus [375, 441, 442]. Elective electrical cardioversion may be considered in women with persistent drug-refractory tachyarrhythmias.

Radiofrequency Catheter Ablation

Ideally, catheter ablation procedures should be delayed until after delivery to avoid potential risks of fetal radiation exposure such as malignancy and developmental abnormalities [443]. However, if needed, catheter ablation with radiation-minimizing precautions may be a reasonable option for drug-refractory arrhythmias causing intolerable symptoms [375]. Studies have determined that radiation doses <50 mGy confer negligible risk [29]. Typical ablation procedures result in very low fetal radiation doses (<1 mGy) [444] and, in some cases, can be performed with minimal or no radiation [445]. However, the risk of adverse effects is not zero, and fluoroscopy procedures should be considered a last resort.

Device Implantation

The presence of a preexisting ICD does not appear to increase the risk of ICD discharge or fetal harm [446]. New ICD implantation is preferably performed after delivery. However, pacemaker placement during pregnancy has been safely performed using echocardiographic guidance and radiation-minimizing techniques [447].

References

1. Weiss BM, von Segesser LK, Alon E, Seifert B, Turina MI. Outcome of cardiovascular surgery and pregnancy: a systematic review of the period 1984–1996. Am J Obstet Gynecol. 1998;179:1643–53.
2. Peters RM, Flack JM. Hypertensive disorders of pregnancy. J Obstet Gynecol Neonatal Nurs. 2004;33:209–20.
3. Creanga AA, Berg CJ, Syverson C, Seed K, Bruce FC, Callaghan WM. Pregnancy-related mortality in the United States, 2006–2010. Obstet Gynecol. 2015;125:5–12.
4. Al-Foudri H, Kevelighan E, Catling S. CEMACH 2003–5 saving mothers' lives: lessons for anaesthetists. Contin Educ Anaesth Crit Care Pain. 2010;10:81–7.
5. Nevo O, Soustiel JF, Thaler I. Maternal cerebral blood flow during normal pregnancy: a cross-sectional study. Am J Obstet Gynecol. 2010;203:475.e1–6.
6. Khairy P, Ionescu-Ittu R, Mackie AS, Abrahamowicz M, Pilote L, Marelli AJ. Changing mortality in congenital heart disease. J Am Coll Cardiol. 2010;56:1149–57.
7. Confidential Enquiry into Maternal and Child Health. Why mothers die 2000–2002—executive summary and key findings—the sixth report of confidential enquiries into maternal deaths in the United Kingdom. London, UK: RCOG Press; 2004.
8. Siu SC, Sermer M, Colman JM, et al. Prospective multicenter study of pregnancy outcomes in women with heart disease. Circulation. 2001;104:515–21.
9. Stangl V, Schad J, Gossing G, Borges A, Baumann G, Stangl K. Maternal heart disease and pregnancy outcome: a single-centre experience. Eur J Heart Fail. 2008;10:855–60.
10. Chapman AB, Abraham WT, Zamudio S, et al. Temporal relationships between hormonal and hemodynamic changes in early human pregnancy. Kidney Int. 1998;54:2056–63.
11. Trudinger B. Fetal-placental circulation and placentation in normal and hypertensive pregnancies. In: Jacobsen H, Striker G, Klahr S, editors. The principles and practice of nephrology, 2nd ed. 1995. p. 431–5.
12. August P, Lenz T, Ales KL, et al. Longitudinal study of the renin-angiotensin-aldosterone system in hypertensive pregnant women: deviations related to the development of superimposed preeclampsia. Am J Obstet Gynecol. 1990;163:1612–21.
13. Sealey JE, Itskovitz-Eldor J, Rubattu S, et al. Estradiol- and progesterone-related increases in the renin-aldosterone system: studies during ovarian stimulation and early pregnancy. J Clin Endocrinol Metab. 1994;79:258–64.
14. Weiner CP, Thompson LP. Nitric oxide and pregnancy. Semin Perinatol. 1997;21:367–80.
15. Knock GA, Poston L. Bradykinin-mediated relaxation of isolated maternal resistance arteries in normal pregnancy and preeclampsia. Am J Obstet Gynecol. 1996;175:1668–74.
16. Pritchard JA. Changes in the blood volume during pregnancy and delivery. Anesthesiology. 1965;26:393–9.
17. Meah VL, Cockcroft JR, Backx K, Shave R, Stohr EJ. Cardiac output and related haemodynamics during pregnancy: a series of meta-analyses. Heart. 2016;102:518–26.
18. Grindheim G, Estensen ME, Langesaeter E, Rosseland LA, Toska K. Changes in blood pressure during healthy pregnancy: a longitudinal cohort study. J Hypertens. 2012;30:342–50.
19. Hermida RC, Ayala DE, Mojon A, Iglesias M. High sensitivity test for the early diagnosis of gestational hypertension and preeclampsia. II. Circadian blood pressure variability in health and hypertensive pregnant women. J Perinat Med. 1997;25:153–67.
20. MacGillivray I, Rose GA, Rowe B. Blood pressure survey in pregnancy. Clin Sci. 1969;37:395–407.
21. Lang RM, Pridjian G, Feldman T, Neumann A, Lindheimer M, Borow KM. Left ventricular mechanics in preeclampsia. Am Heart J. 1991;121:1768–75.
22. Kametas NA, McAuliffe F, Krampl E, Chambers J, Nicolaides KH. Maternal cardiac function in twin pregnancy. Obstet Gynecol. 2003;102:806–15.
23. Froen JF, Moyland RA, Saugstad OD, Stray-Pedersen B. Maternal health in sudden intrauterine unexplained death: do urinary tract infections protect the fetus? Obstet Gynecol. 2002;100:909–15.
24. Robson SC, Dunlop W, Moore M, Hunter S. Combined Doppler and echocardiographic measurement of cardiac output: theory and application in pregnancy. Br J Obstet Gynaecol. 1987;94:1014–27.
25. Campbell DM, MacGillivray I. Comparison of maternal response in first and second pregnancies in relation to baby weight. J Obstet Gynaecol Br Commonw. 1972;79:684–93.

26. Balci A, Sollie-Szarynska KM, van der Bijl AG, et al. Prospective validation and assessment of cardiovascular and offspring risk models for pregnant women with congenital heart disease. Heart. 2014;100:1373–81.
27. Siu SC, Colman JM, Sorensen S, et al. Adverse neonatal and cardiac outcomes are more common in pregnant women with cardiac disease. Circulation. 2002;105:2179–84.
28. Roos-Hesselink JW, Ruys TP, Stein JI, et al. Outcome of pregnancy in patients with structural or ischaemic heart disease: results of a registry of the European Society of Cardiology. Eur Heart J. 2013;34:657–65.
29. European Society of Gynecology, Association for European Paediatric Cardiology, German Society for Gender Medicine, et al. ESC Guidelines on the management of cardiovascular diseases during pregnancy: the Task Force on the Management of Cardiovascular Diseases during Pregnancy of the European Society of Cardiology (ESC). Eur Heart J. 2011;32:3147–97.
30. Balint OH, Siu SC, Mason J, et al. Cardiac outcomes after pregnancy in women with congenital heart disease. Heart. 2010;96:1656–61.
31. Curtis SL, Marsden-Williams J, Sullivan C, et al. Current trends in the management of heart disease in pregnancy. Int J Cardiol. 2009;133:62–9.
32. Drenthen W, Boersma E, Balci A, et al. Predictors of pregnancy complications in women with congenital heart disease. Eur Heart J. 2010;31:2124–32.
33. Ford AA, Wylie BJ, Waksmonski CA, Simpson LL. Maternal congenital cardiac disease: outcomes of pregnancy in a single tertiary care center. Obstet Gynecol. 2008;112:828–33.
34. Khairy P, Ouyang DW, Fernandes SM, Lee-Parritz A, Economy KE, Landzberg MJ. Pregnancy outcomes in women with congenital heart disease. Circulation. 2006;113:517–24.
35. Thorne S, MacGregor A, Nelson-Piercy C. Risks of contraception and pregnancy in heart disease. Heart. 2006;92:1520–5.
36. Thorne S, Nelson-Piercy C, MacGregor A, et al. Pregnancy and contraception in heart disease and pulmonary arterial hypertension. J Fam Plann Reprod Health Care. 2006;32:75–81.
37. Hameed A, Karaalp IS, Tummala PP, et al. The effect of valvular heart disease on maternal and fetal outcome of pregnancy. J Am Coll Cardiol. 2001;37:893–9.
38. Bedard E, Dimopoulos K, Gatzoulis MA. Has there been any progress made on pregnancy outcomes among women with pulmonary arterial hypertension? Eur Heart J. 2009;30:256–65.
39. Presbitero P, Somerville J, Stone S, Aruta E, Spiegelhalter D, Rabajoli F. Pregnancy in cyanotic congenital heart disease. Outcome of mother and fetus. Circulation. 1994;89:2673–6.
40. Simonneau G, Gatzoulis MA, Adatia I, et al. Updated clinical classification of pulmonary hypertension. J Am Coll Cardiol. 2013;62:D34–41.
41. Miller VM, Aarhus LL, Vanhoutte PM. Modulation of endothelium-dependent responses by chronic alterations of blood flow. Am J Physiol. 1986;251:H520–7.
42. Saha A, Balakrishnan KG, Jaiswal PK, et al. Prognosis for patients with Eisenmenger syndrome of various aetiology. Int J Cardiol. 1994;45:199–207.
43. Hopkins WE. The remarkable right ventricle of patients with Eisenmenger syndrome. Coron Artery Dis. 2005;16:19–25.
44. Hopkins WE, Waggoner AD. Severe pulmonary hypertension without right ventricular failure: the unique hearts of patients with Eisenmenger syndrome. Am J Cardiol. 2002;89:34–8.
45. Granton JT, Rabinovitch M. Pulmonary arterial hypertension in congenital heart disease. Cardiol Clin. 2002;20:441–57. vii
46. Diller GP, Dimopoulos K, Broberg CS, et al. Presentation, survival prospects, and predictors of death in Eisenmenger syndrome: a combined retrospective and case-control study. Eur Heart J. 2006;27:1737–42.
47. Perloff JK, Marelli A. Perloff's clinical recognition of congenital heart disease. 6th ed. Philadelphia: Saunders; 2012.
48. Schmaltz AA, Neudorf U, Winkler UH. Outcome of pregnancy in women with congenital heart disease. Cardiol Young. 1999;9:88–96.
49. Zuber M, Gautschi N, Oechslin E, Widmer V, Kiowski W, Jenni R. Outcome of pregnancy in women with congenital shunt lesions. Heart. 1999;81:271–5.
50. Reller MD, Strickland MJ, Riehle-Colarusso T, Mahle WT, Correa A. Prevalence of congenital heart defects in metropolitan Atlanta, 1998–2005. J Pediatr. 2008;153:807–13.
51. Schwedler G, Lindinger A, Lange PE, et al. Frequency and spectrum of congenital heart defects among live births in Germany : a study of the Competence Network for Congenital Heart Defects. Clin Res Cardiol. 2011;100:1111–7.
52. van der Linde D, Konings EE, Slager MA, et al. Birth prevalence of congenital heart disease worldwide: a systematic review and meta-analysis. J Am Coll Cardiol. 2011;58:2241–7.
53. Attenhofer Jost CH, Connolly HM, Danielson GK, et al. Sinus venosus atrial septal defect: long-term postoperative outcome for 115 patients. Circulation. 2005;112:1953–8.
54. Hoffman JI, Kaplan S. The incidence of congenital heart disease. J Am Coll Cardiol. 2002;39:1890–900.
55. Gersony WM, Hayes CJ, Driscoll DJ, et al. Bacterial endocarditis in patients with aortic stenosis, pulmonary stenosis, or ventricular septal defect. Circulation. 1993;87:I121–6.
56. Korenberg JR, Bradley C, Disteche CM. Down syndrome: molecular mapping of the congenital heart disease and duodenal stenosis. Am J Hum Genet. 1992;50:294–302.
57. Agopian AJ, Moulik M, Gupta-Malhotra M, Marengo LK, Mitchell LE. Descriptive epidemiology of non-syndromic complete atrioventricular canal defects. Paediatr Perinat Epidemiol. 2012;26:515–24.
58. Vahanian A, Baumgartner H, Bax J, et al. Guidelines on the management of valvular heart disease: The Task Force on the Management of Valvular Heart Disease of the European Society of Cardiology. Eur Heart J. 2007;28:230–68.
59. Drenthen W, Pieper PG, van der Tuuk K, et al. Cardiac complications relating to pregnancy and recurrence of disease in the offspring of women with atrioventricular septal defects. Eur Heart J. 2005;26:2581–7.
60. Brown ML, Burkhart HM, Connolly HM, et al. Coarctation of the aorta: lifelong surveillance is mandatory following surgical repair. J Am Coll Cardiol. 2013;62:1020–5.
61. Stewart AB, Ahmed R, Travill CM, Newman CG. Coarctation of the aorta life and health 20-44 years after surgical repair. Br Heart J. 1993;69:65–70.
62. Wong SC, Burgess T, Cheung M, Zacharin M. The prevalence of turner syndrome in girls presenting with coarctation of the aorta. J Pediatr. 2014;164:259–63.
63. Rocchini AP, Emmanouilides GC. Moss and Adams heart disease in infants, children, and adolescents. 5th ed. Baltimore: Williams & Wilkins; 1995.
64. Samanek M, Slavik Z, Zborilova B, Hrobonova V, Voriskova M, Skovranek J. Prevalence, treatment, and outcome of heart disease in live-born children: a prospective analysis of 91,823 live-born children. Pediatr Cardiol. 1989;10:205–11.
65. Stephensen SS, Sigfusson G, Eiriksson H, et al. Congenital cardiac malformations in Iceland from 1990 through 1999. Cardiol Young. 2004;14:396–401.
66. Keith JD, Rowe RD, Vlad P. Heart disease in infancy and childhood. 3rd ed. New York: MacMillan; 1978.
67. Koretzky ED, Moller JH, Korns ME, Schwartz CJ, Edwards JE. Congenital pulmonary stenosis resulting from dysplasia of valve. Circulation. 1969;40:43–53.

68. Baumgartner H, Bonhoeffer P, De Groot NM, et al. ESC Guidelines for the management of grown-up congenital heart disease (new version 2010). Eur Heart J. 2010;31:2915–57.
69. Warnes CA, Williams RG, Bashore TM, et al. ACC/AHA 2008 Guidelines for the Management of Adults with Congenital Heart Disease: a report of the American College of Cardiology/American Heart Association Task Force on Practice Guidelines (writing committee to develop guidelines on the management of adults with congenital heart disease). Circulation. 2008;118:e714–833.
70. Hayes CJ, Gersony WM, Driscoll DJ, et al. Second natural history study of congenital heart defects. Results of treatment of patients with pulmonary valvar stenosis. Circulation. 1993;87:I28–37.
71. Drenthen W, Pieper PG, Roos-Hesselink JW, et al. Non-cardiac complications during pregnancy in women with isolated congenital pulmonary valvar stenosis. Heart. 2006;92:1838–43.
72. Presbitero P, Prever SB, Brusca A. Interventional cardiology in pregnancy. Eur Heart J. 1996;17:182–8.
73. Greutmann M, Von Klemperer K, Brooks R, Peebles D, O'Brien P, Walker F. Pregnancy outcome in women with congenital heart disease and residual haemodynamic lesions of the right ventricular outflow tract. Eur Heart J. 2010;31:1764–70.
74. Correa-Villasenor A, Ferencz C, Neill CA, Wilson PD, Boughman JA. Ebstein's malformation of the tricuspid valve: genetic and environmental factors. The Baltimore-Washington Infant Study Group Teratology. 1994;50:137–47.
75. Lupo PJ, Langlois PH, Mitchell LE. Epidemiology of Ebstein anomaly: prevalence and patterns in Texas, 1999–2005. Am J Med Genet A. 2011;155A:1007–14.
76. Pradat P, Francannet C, Harris JA, Robert E. The epidemiology of cardiovascular defects, Part I: a study based on data from three large registries of congenital malformations. Pediatr Cardiol. 2003;24:195–221.
77. Attenhofer Jost CH, Connolly HM, O'Leary PW, Warnes CA, Tajik AJ, Seward JB. Left heart lesions in patients with Ebstein anomaly. Mayo Clin Proc. 2005;80:361–8.
78. Attenhofer Jost CH, Connolly HM, Dearani JA, Edwards WD, Danielson GK. Ebstein's anomaly. Circulation. 2007;115:277–85.
79. Connolly HM, Warnes CA. Ebstein's anomaly: outcome of pregnancy. J Am Coll Cardiol. 1994;23:1194–8.
80. Donnelly JE, Brown JM, Radford DJ. Pregnancy outcome and Ebstein's anomaly. Br Heart J. 1991;66:368–71.
81. Centers for Disease Control and Prevention. Improved national prevalence estimates for 18 selected major birth defects—United States, 1999–2001. MMWR Morb Mortal Wkly Rep. 2006;54:1301–5.
82. Report of the New England Regional Infant Cardiac Program. Pediatrics. 1980;65:375–461.
83. Bhat AH, Kehl DW, Tacy TA, Moon-Grady AJ, Hornberger LK. Diagnosis of tetralogy of Fallot and its variants in the late first and early second trimester: details of initial assessment and comparison with later fetal diagnosis. Echocardiography. 2013;30:81–7.
84. Al Habib HF, Jacobs JP, Mavroudis C, et al. Contemporary patterns of management of tetralogy of Fallot: data from the Society of Thoracic Surgeons Database. Ann Thorac Surg. 2010;90:813–9; discussion 819–20
85. Veldtman GR, Connolly HM, Grogan M, Ammash NM, Warnes CA. Outcomes of pregnancy in women with tetralogy of Fallot. J Am Coll Cardiol. 2004;44:174–80.
86. Wernovsky G. Transposition of the great arteries. In: Allen HD, Shaddy RE, Driscoll DJ, Feltes TF, editors. Moss and Adams' heart disease in infants, children, and adolescents: including the fetus and young adult. 7th ed. Philadelphia: Wolters Kluwer Health/Lipincott Williams & Wilkins; 2008.
87. Buch J, Wennevold A, Jacobsen JR, Hvid-Jacobsen K, Lauridsen P. Long-term follow-up of right ventricular function after Mustard operation for transposition of the great arteries. Scand J Thorac Cardiovasc Surg. 1988;22:197–202.
88. Derrick GP, Josen M, Vogel M, Henein MY, Shinebourne EA, Redington AN. Abnormalities of right ventricular long axis function after atrial repair of transposition of the great arteries. Heart. 2001;86:203–6.
89. Fulton DR, Fyler DC. D-Transposition of the great arteries. In: Keane JF, Lock JE, Fyler DC, editors. Nadas' pediatric cardiology. 2nd ed. Philadelphia: Saunders Elsevier; 2001.
90. Hutter PA, Kreb DL, Mantel SF, Hitchcock JF, Meijboom EJ, Bennink GB. Twenty-five years' experience with the arterial switch operation. J Thorac Cardiovasc Surg. 2002;124:790–7.
91. Legendre A, Losay J, Touchot-Kone A, et al. Coronary events after arterial switch operation for transposition of the great arteries. Circulation. 2003;108(Suppl 1):II186–90.
92. Schwartz ML, Gauvreau K, del Nido P, Mayer JE, Colan SD. Long-term predictors of aortic root dilation and aortic regurgitation after arterial switch operation. Circulation. 2004;110:II128–32.
93. Ploeg M, Drenthen W, van Dijk A, Pieper PG. Successful pregnancy after an arterial switch procedure for complete transposition of the great arteries. BJOG. 2006;113:243–4.
94. Tobler D, Fernandes SM, Wald RM, et al. Pregnancy outcomes in women with transposition of the great arteries and arterial switch operation. Am J Cardiol. 2010;106:417–20.
95. Cataldo S, Doohan M, Rice K, Trinder J, Stuart AG, Curtis SL. Pregnancy following Mustard or Senning correction of transposition of the great arteries: a retrospective study. BJOG. 2016;123:807–13.
96. Horer J, Schreiber C, Cleuziou J, et al. Improvement in long-term survival after hospital discharge but not in freedom from reoperation after the change from atrial to arterial switch for transposition of the great arteries. J Thorac Cardiovasc Surg. 2009;137:347–54.
97. Ferencz C, Rubin JD, McCarter RJ, et al. Congenital heart disease: prevalence at livebirth. The Baltimore-Washington Infant Study. Am J Epidemiol. 1985;121:31–6.
98. Samanek M, Voriskova M. Congenital heart disease among 815,569 children born between 1980 and 1990 and their 15-year survival: a prospective Bohemia survival study. Pediatr Cardiol. 1999;20:411–7.
99. Hornung TS, Calder L. Congenitally corrected transposition of the great arteries. Heart. 2010;96:1154–61.
100. Warnes CA. Transposition of the great arteries. Circulation. 2006;114:2699–709.
101. Therrien J, Barnes I, Somerville J. Outcome of pregnancy in patients with congenitally corrected transposition of the great arteries. Am J Cardiol. 1999;84:820–4.
102. Connolly HM, Grogan M, Warnes CA. Pregnancy among women with congenitally corrected transposition of great arteries. J Am Coll Cardiol. 1999;33:1692–5.
103. Fontan F, Baudet E. Surgical repair of tricuspid atresia. Thorax. 1971;26:240–8.
104. Gewillig M. The Fontan circulation. Heart. 2005;91:839–46.
105. Driscoll DJ, Offord KP, Feldt RH, Schaff HV, Puga FJ, Danielson GK. Five- to fifteen-year follow-up after Fontan operation. Circulation. 1992;85:469–96.
106. Khairy P, Fernandes SM, Mayer JE Jr, et al. Long-term survival, modes of death, and predictors of mortality in patients with Fontan surgery. Circulation. 2008;117:85–92.
107. Elkayam U, Ostrzega E, Shotan A, Mehra A. Cardiovascular problems in pregnant women with the Marfan syndrome. Ann Intern Med. 1995;123:117–22.
108. Manalo-Estrella P, Barker AE. Histopathologic findings in human aortic media associated with pregnancy. Arch Pathol. 1967;83:336–41.
109. Meijboom LJ, Nollen GJ, Merchant N, et al. Frequency of coronary ostial aneurysms after aortic root surgery in patients with the Marfan syndrome. Am J Cardiol. 2002;89:1135–8.

110. Judge DP, Dietz HC. Marfan's syndrome. Lancet. 2005;366:1965–76.
111. Ramirez F, Godfrey M, Lee B. Marfan syndrome and related disorders. In: Scriver CR, Beaudet AL, Sly WS, Childs B, Valle D, Kinzler KW, editors. The metabolic and molecular basis of inherited disease. New York: McGraw Hill; 1995.
112. Collod-Beroud G, Le Bourdelles S, Ades L, et al. Update of the UMD-FBN1 mutation database and creation of an FBN1 polymorphism database. Hum Mutat. 2003;22:199–208.
113. Loeys BL, Dietz HC, Braverman AC, et al. The revised Ghent nosology for the Marfan syndrome. J Med Genet. 2010;47:476–85.
114. Radonic T, de Witte P, Groenink M, et al. Critical appraisal of the revised Ghent criteria for diagnosis of Marfan syndrome. Clin Genet. 2011;80:346–53.
115. Pyeritz RE. Maternal and fetal complications of pregnancy in the Marfan syndrome. Am J Med. 1981;71:784–90.
116. Therrien J, Gatzoulis M, Graham T, et al. Canadian Cardiovascular Society consensus conference 2001 update: recommendations for the management of adults with congenital heart disease—Part II. Can J Cardiol. 2001;17:1029–50.
117. Rossiter JP, Repke JT, Morales AJ, Murphy EA, Pyeritz RE. A prospective longitudinal evaluation of pregnancy in the Marfan syndrome. Am J Obstet Gynecol. 1995;173:1599–606.
118. Deanfield J, Thaulow E, Warnes C, et al. Management of grown up congenital heart disease. Eur Heart J. 2003;24:1035–84.
119. Immer FF, Bansi AG, Immer-Bansi AS, et al. Aortic dissection in pregnancy: analysis of risk factors and outcome. Ann Thorac Surg. 2003;76:309–14.
120. Meijboom LJ, Vos FE, Timmermans J, Boers GH, Zwinderman AH, Mulder BJ. Pregnancy and aortic root growth in the Marfan syndrome: a prospective study. Eur Heart J. 2005;26:914–20.
121. Hiratzka LF, Bakris GL, Beckman JA, et al. ACCF/AHA/AATS/ACR/ASA/SCA/SCAI/SIR/STS/SVM guidelines for the diagnosis and management of patients with Thoracic Aortic Disease: a report of the American College of Cardiology Foundation/American Heart Association Task Force on Practice Guidelines, American Association for Thoracic Surgery, American College of Radiology, American Stroke Association, Society of Cardiovascular Anesthesiologists, Society for Cardiovascular Angiography and Interventions, Society of Interventional Radiology, Society of Thoracic Surgeons, and Society for Vascular Medicine. Circulation. 2010;121:e266–369.
122. Bonow RO, Carabello BA, Chatterjee K, et al. Focused update incorporated into the ACC/AHA 2006 guidelines for the management of patients with valvular heart disease: a report of the American College of Cardiology/American Heart Association Task Force on Practice Guidelines (Writing Committee to Revise the 1998 Guidelines for the Management of Patients With Valvular Heart Disease): endorsed by the Society of Cardiovascular Anesthesiologists, Society for Cardiovascular Angiography and Interventions, and Society of Thoracic Surgeons. Circulation. 2008;118:e523–661.
123. Lipscomb KJ, Smith JC, Clarke B, Donnai P, Harris R. Outcome of pregnancy in women with Marfan's syndrome. Br J Obstet Gynaecol. 1997;104:201–6.
124. Doyle JJ, Doyle AJ, Wilson NK, et al. A deleterious gene-by-environment interaction imposed by calcium channel blockers in Marfan syndrome. Elife. 2015;4.
125. Parry AJ, Westaby S. Cardiopulmonary bypass during pregnancy. Ann Thorac Surg. 1996;61:1865–9.
126. Siu SC, Silversides CK. Bicuspid aortic valve disease. J Am Coll Cardiol. 2010;55:2789–800.
127. Tzemos N, Therrien J, Yip J, et al. Outcomes in adults with bicuspid aortic valves. JAMA. 2008;300:1317–25.
128. Michelena HI, Khanna AD, Mahoney D, et al. Incidence of aortic complications in patients with bicuspid aortic valves. JAMA. 2011;306:1104–12.
129. Shimada I, Rooney SJ, Pagano D, et al. Prediction of thoracic aortic aneurysm expansion: validation of formulae describing growth. Ann Thorac Surg. 1999;67:1968–70; discussion 1979–80
130. Anderson RA, Fineron PW. Aortic dissection in pregnancy: importance of pregnancy-induced changes in the vessel wall and bicuspid aortic valve in pathogenesis. Br J Obstet Gynaecol. 1994;101:1085–8.
131. Gunther DF, Eugster E, Zagar AJ, Bryant CG, Davenport ML, Quigley CA. Ascertainment bias in Turner syndrome: new insights from girls who were diagnosed incidentally in prenatal life. Pediatrics. 2004;114:640–4.
132. Bondy CA, Turner Syndrome Study G. Care of girls and women with Turner syndrome: a guideline of the Turner Syndrome Study Group. J Clin Endocrinol Metab. 2007;92:10–25.
133. Nielsen J, Wohlert M. Chromosome abnormalities found among 34,910 newborn children: results from a 13-year incidence study in Arhus, Denmark. Hum Genet. 1991;87:81–3.
134. Cramer JW, Bartz PJ, Simpson PM, Zangwill SD. The spectrum of congenital heart disease and outcomes after surgical repair among children with Turner syndrome: a single-center review. Pediatr Cardiol. 2014;35:253–60.
135. Gotzsche CO, Krag-Olsen B, Nielsen J, Sorensen KE, Kristensen BO. Prevalence of cardiovascular malformations and association with karyotypes in Turner's syndrome. Arch Dis Child. 1994;71:433–6.
136. Sachdev V, Matura LA, Sidenko S, et al. Aortic valve disease in Turner syndrome. J Am Coll Cardiol. 2008;51:1904–9.
137. Carlson M, Airhart N, Lopez L, Silberbach M. Moderate aortic enlargement and bicuspid aortic valve are associated with aortic dissection in Turner syndrome: report of the international turner syndrome aortic dissection registry. Circulation. 2012;126:2220–6.
138. Lin AE, Lippe B, Rosenfeld RG. Further delineation of aortic dilation, dissection, and rupture in patients with Turner syndrome. Pediatrics. 1998;102:e12.
139. Matura LA, Ho VB, Rosing DR, Bondy CA. Aortic dilatation and dissection in Turner syndrome. Circulation. 2007;116:1663–70.
140. Karnis MF, Zimon AE, Lalwani SI, Timmreck LS, Klipstein S, Reindollar RH. Risk of death in pregnancy achieved through oocyte donation in patients with Turner syndrome: a national survey. Fertil Steril. 2003;80:498–501.
141. Avila WS, Rossi EG, Ramires JA, et al. Pregnancy in patients with heart disease: experience with 1,000 cases. Clin Cardiol. 2003;26:135–42.
142. Diao M, Kane A, Ndiaye MB, et al. Pregnancy in women with heart disease in sub-Saharan Africa. Arch Cardiovasc Dis. 2011;104:370–4.
143. Kuklina E, Callaghan W. Chronic heart disease and severe obstetric morbidity among hospitalisations for pregnancy in the USA: 1995–2006. BJOG. 2011;118:345–52.
144. Siu SC, Sermer M, Harrison DA, et al. Risk and predictors for pregnancy-related complications in women with heart disease. Circulation. 1997;96:2789–94.
145. Nishimura RA, Otto CM, Bonow RO, et al. 2014 AHA/ACC guideline for the management of patients with valvular heart disease: a report of the American College of Cardiology/American Heart Association Task Force on Practice Guidelines. J Am Coll Cardiol. 2014;63:e57–185.
146. Chikwe J, Chiang YP, Egorova NN, Itagaki S, Adams DH. Survival and outcomes following bioprosthetic vs mechanical mitral valve replacement in patients aged 50 to 69 years. JAMA. 2015;313:1435–42.
147. McClure RS, McGurk S, Cevasco M, et al. Late outcomes comparison of nonelderly patients with stented bioprosthetic and mechanical valves in the aortic position: a propensity-matched analysis. J Thorac Cardiovasc Surg. 2014;148:1931–9.

148. Chambers CE, Clark SL. Cardiac surgery during pregnancy. Clin Obstet Gynecol. 1994;37:316–23.
149. Pomini F, Mercogliano D, Cavalletti C, Caruso A, Pomini P. Cardiopulmonary bypass in pregnancy. Ann Thorac Surg. 1996;61:259–68.
150. Becker RM. Intracardiac surgery in pregnant women. Ann Thorac Surg. 1983;36:453–8.
151. Martin MC, Pernoll ML, Boruszak AN, Jones JW, LoCicero J 3rd. Cesarean section while on cardiac bypass: report of a case. Obstet Gynecol. 1981;57:41S–5S.
152. Rheumatic fever and rheumatic heart disease. World Health Organ Tech Rep Ser. 2004;923:1–122, back cover.
153. Selzer A, Cohn KE. Natural history of mitral stenosis: a review. Circulation. 1972;45:878–90.
154. Zuhlke LJ, Beaton A, Engel ME, et al. Group A Streptococcus, acute rheumatic fever and rheumatic heart disease: epidemiology and clinical considerations. Curr Treat Options Cardiovasc Med. 2017;19:15.
155. Gewitz MH, Baltimore RS, Tani LY, et al. Revision of the Jones Criteria for the diagnosis of acute rheumatic fever in the era of Doppler echocardiography: a scientific statement from the American Heart Association. Circulation. 2015;131:1806–18.
156. Marcus RH, Sareli P, Pocock WA, Barlow JB. The spectrum of severe rheumatic mitral valve disease in a developing country. Correlations among clinical presentation, surgical pathologic findings, and hemodynamic sequelae. Ann Intern Med. 1994;120:177–83.
157. Bland EF, Duckett JT. Rheumatic fever and rheumatic heart disease; a twenty year report on 1000 patients followed since childhood. Circulation. 1951;4:836–43.
158. Zuhlke L, Engel ME, Karthikeyan G, et al. Characteristics, complications, and gaps in evidence-based interventions in rheumatic heart disease: the Global Rheumatic Heart Disease Registry (the REMEDY study). Eur Heart J. 2015;36:1115–22.
159. Watkins DA, Johnson CO, Colquhoun SM, et al. Global, regional, and national burden of rheumatic heart disease, 1990–2015. N Engl J Med. 2017;377:713–22.
160. Silversides CK, Colman JM, Sermer M, Siu SC. Cardiac risk in pregnant women with rheumatic mitral stenosis. Am J Cardiol. 2003;91:1382–5.
161. Ruys TP, Roos-Hesselink JW, Hall R, et al. Heart failure in pregnant women with cardiac disease: data from the ROPAC. Heart. 2014;100:231–8.
162. Elkayam U, Bitar F. Valvular heart disease and pregnancy Part I: Native valves. J Am Coll Cardiol. 2005;46:223–30.
163. Roberts WC. The congenitally bicuspid aortic valve. A study of 85 autopsy cases. Am J Cardiol. 1970;26:72–83.
164. Eisenberg LM, Markwald RR. Molecular regulation of atrioventricular valvuloseptal morphogenesis. Circ Res. 1995;77:1–6.
165. Huntington K, Hunter AG, Chan KL. A prospective study to assess the frequency of familial clustering of congenital bicuspid aortic valve. J Am Coll Cardiol. 1997;30:1809–12.
166. Joint Task Force on the Management of Valvular Heart Disease of the European Society of Cardiology European Association for Cardio-Thoracic Surgery, Vahanian A, et al. Guidelines on the management of valvular heart disease (version 2012). Eur Heart J. 2012;33:2451–96.
167. Ward C. Clinical significance of the bicuspid aortic valve. Heart. 2000;83:81–5.
168. Chan KL, Ghani M, Woodend K, Burwash IG. Case-controlled study to assess risk factors for aortic stenosis in congenitally bicuspid aortic valve. Am J Cardiol. 2001;88:690–3.
169. Silversides CK, Colman JM, Sermer M, Farine D, Siu SC. Early and intermediate-term outcomes of pregnancy with congenital aortic stenosis. Am J Cardiol. 2003;91:1386–9.
170. Easterling TR, Chadwick HS, Otto CM, Benedetti TJ. Aortic stenosis in pregnancy. Obstet Gynecol. 1988;72:113–8.
171. Lao TT, Sermer M, MaGee L, Farine D, Colman JM. Congenital aortic stenosis and pregnancy—a reappraisal. Am J Obstet Gynecol. 1993;169:540–5.
172. Yap SC, Drenthen W, Pieper PG, et al. Risk of complications during pregnancy in women with congenital aortic stenosis. Int J Cardiol. 2008;126:240–6.
173. Roberts WC, Morrow AG, McIntosh CL, Jones M, Epstein SE. Congenitally bicuspid aortic valve causing severe, pure aortic regurgitation without superimposed infective endocarditis. Analysis of 13 patients requiring aortic valve replacement. Am J Cardiol. 1981;47:206–9.
174. Pachulski RT, Chan KL. Progression of aortic valve dysfunction in 51 adult patients with congenital bicuspid aortic valve: assessment and follow up by Doppler echocardiography. Br Heart J. 1993;69:237–40.
175. Remenyi B, Wilson N, Steer A, et al. World Heart Federation criteria for echocardiographic diagnosis of rheumatic heart disease—an evidence-based guideline. Nat Rev Cardiol. 2012;9:297–309.
176. Dujardin KS, Enriquez-Sarano M, Schaff HV, Bailey KR, Seward JB, Tajik AJ. Mortality and morbidity of aortic regurgitation in clinical practice. A long-term follow-up study. Circulation. 1999;99:1851–7.
177. John AS, Gurley F, Schaff HV, et al. Cardiopulmonary bypass during pregnancy. Ann Thorac Surg. 2011;91:1191–6.
178. De Santo LS, Romano G, Della Corte A, et al. Mitral mechanical replacement in young rheumatic women: analysis of long-term survival, valve-related complications, and pregnancy outcomes over a 3707-patient-year follow-up. J Thorac Cardiovasc Surg. 2005;130:13–9.
179. Vural KM, Ozatik MA, Uncu H, et al. Pregnancy after mechanical mitral valve replacement. J Heart Valve Dis. 2003;12:370–6.
180. Bourguignon T, Bouquiaux-Stablo AL, Candolfi P, et al. Very long-term outcomes of the Carpentier-Edwards Perimount valve in aortic position. Ann Thorac Surg. 2015;99:831–7.
181. Badduke BR, Jamieson WR, Miyagishima RT, et al. Pregnancy and childbearing in a population with biologic valvular prostheses. J Thorac Cardiovasc Surg. 1991;102:179–86.
182. Sbarouni E, Oakley CM. Outcome of pregnancy in women with valve prostheses. Br Heart J. 1994;71:196–201.
183. El SF, Hassan W, Latroche B, et al. Pregnancy has no effect on the rate of structural deterioration of bioprosthetic valves: long-term 18-year follow up results. J Heart Valve Dis. 2005;14:481–5.
184. North RA, Sadler L, Stewart AW, McCowan LM, Kerr AR, White HD. Long-term survival and valve-related complications in young women with cardiac valve replacements. Circulation. 1999;99:2669–76.
185. Lawley CM, Lain SJ, Algert CS, Ford JB, Figtree GA, Roberts CL. Prosthetic heart valves in pregnancy, outcomes for women and their babies: a systematic review and meta-analysis. BJOG. 2015;122:1446–55.
186. van Hagen IM, Roos-Hesselink JW, Ruys TP, et al. Pregnancy in women with a mechanical heart valve: data of the European Society of Cardiology Registry of Pregnancy and Cardiac Disease (ROPAC). Circulation. 2015;132:132–42.
187. Vongpatanasin W, Hillis LD, Lange RA. Prosthetic heart valves. N Engl J Med. 1996;335:407–16.
188. Elkayam U, Singh H, Irani A, Akhter MW. Anticoagulation in pregnant women with prosthetic heart valves. J Cardiovasc Pharmacol Ther. 2004;9:107–15.
189. D'Souza R, Ostro J, Shah PS, et al. Anticoagulation for pregnant women with mechanical heart valves: a systematic review and meta-analysis. Eur Heart J. 2017;38:1509–16.

190. Huttel E, Padberg S, Meister R, Beck E, Schaefer C. Pregnancy outcome of first trimester exposure to the vitamin K antagonist phenprocoumon depends on duration of treatment. Thromb Haemost. 2017;117:870–9.
191. Chan WS, Anand S, Ginsberg JS. Anticoagulation of pregnant women with mechanical heart valves: a systematic review of the literature. Arch Intern Med. 2000;160:191–6.
192. Abildgaard U, Sandset PM, Hammerstrom J, Gjestvang FT, Tveit A. Management of pregnant women with mechanical heart valve prosthesis: thromboprophylaxis with low molecular weight heparin. Thromb Res. 2009;124:262–7.
193. McLintock C, McCowan LM, North RA. Maternal complications and pregnancy outcome in women with mechanical prosthetic heart valves treated with enoxaparin. BJOG. 2009;116:1585–92.
194. Saeed CR, Frank JB, Pravin M, Aziz RH, Serasheini M, Dominique TG. A prospective trial showing the safety of adjusted-dose enoxaparin for thromboprophylaxis of pregnant women with mechanical prosthetic heart valves. Clin Appl Thromb Hemost. 2011;17:313–9.
195. Barbour LA, Oja JL, Schultz LK. A prospective trial that demonstrates that dalteparin requirements increase in pregnancy to maintain therapeutic levels of anticoagulation. Am J Obstet Gynecol. 2004;191:1024–9.
196. Eikelboom JW, Connolly SJ, Brueckmann M, et al. Dabigatran versus warfarin in patients with mechanical heart valves. N Engl J Med. 2013;369:1206–14.
197. U.S. Food and Drug Administration. FDA Drug Safety Communication: Pradaxa (dabigatran etexilate mesylate) should not be used in patients with mechanical prosthetic heart valves. https://www.fda.gov/Drugs/DrugSafety/ucm332912.htm. Accessed 3 Aug 2018.
198. Van de Werf F, Brueckmann M, Connolly SJ, et al. A comparison of dabigatran etexilate with warfarin in patients with mechanical heart valves: THE Randomized, phase II study to evaluate the safety and pharmacokinetics of oral dabigatran etexilate in patients after heart valve replacement (RE-ALIGN). Am Heart J. 2012;163:931–937.e1.
199. Quinn J, Von Klemperer K, Brooks R, Peebles D, Walker F, Cohen H. Use of high intensity adjusted dose low molecular weight heparin in women with mechanical heart valves during pregnancy: a single-center experience. Haematologica. 2009;94:1608–12.
200. Steinberg ZL, Dominguez-Islas CP, Otto CM, Stout KK, Krieger EV. Maternal and fetal outcomes of anticoagulation in pregnant women with mechanical heart valves. J Am Coll Cardiol. 2017;69:2681–91.
201. Yinon Y, Siu SC, Warshafsky C, et al. Use of low molecular weight heparin in pregnant women with mechanical heart valves. Am J Cardiol. 2009;104:1259–63.
202. Caceres-Loriga FM, Perez-Lopez H, Morlans-Hernandez K, et al. Thrombolysis as first choice therapy in prosthetic heart valve thrombosis. A study of 68 patients. J Thromb Thrombolysis. 2006;21:185–90.
203. Karthikeyan G, Math RS, Mathew N, et al. Accelerated infusion of streptokinase for the treatment of left-sided prosthetic valve thrombosis: a randomized controlled trial. Circulation. 2009;120:1108–14.
204. Keuleers S, Herijgers P, Herregods MC, et al. Comparison of thrombolysis versus surgery as a first line therapy for prosthetic heart valve thrombosis. Am J Cardiol. 2011;107:275–9.
205. Nagy A, Denes M, Lengyel M. Predictors of the outcome of thrombolytic therapy in prosthetic mitral valve thrombosis: a study of 62 events. J Heart Valve Dis. 2009;18:268–75.
206. Ozkan M, Gunduz S, Biteker M, et al. Comparison of different TEE-guided thrombolytic regimens for prosthetic valve thrombosis: the TROIA trial. JACC Cardiovasc Imaging. 2013;6:206–16.
207. Roudaut R, Lafitte S, Roudaut MF, et al. Management of prosthetic heart valve obstruction: fibrinolysis versus surgery. Early results and long-term follow-up in a single-centre study of 263 cases. Arch Cardiovasc Dis. 2009;102:269–77.
208. Karthikeyan G, Senguttuvan NB, Joseph J, Devasenapathy N, Bahl VK, Airan B. Urgent surgery compared with fibrinolytic therapy for the treatment of left-sided prosthetic heart valve thrombosis: a systematic review and meta-analysis of observational studies. Eur Heart J. 2013;34:1557–66.
209. Ozkan M, Cakal B, Karakoyun S, et al. Thrombolytic therapy for the treatment of prosthetic heart valve thrombosis in pregnancy with low-dose, slow infusion of tissue-type plasminogen activator. Circulation. 2013;128:532–40.
210. Maron BJ. Hypertrophic cardiomyopathy: a systematic review. JAMA. 2002;287:1308–20.
211. Sliwa K, Mebazaa A, Hilfiker-Kleiner D, et al. Clinical characteristics of patients from the worldwide registry on peripartum cardiomyopathy (PPCM): EURObservational Research Programme in conjunction with the Heart Failure Association of the European Society of Cardiology Study Group on PPCM. Eur J Heart Fail. 2017;19:1131–41.
212. Monserrat L, Elliott PM, Gimeno JR, Sharma S, Penas-Lado M, McKenna WJ. Non-sustained ventricular tachycardia in hypertrophic cardiomyopathy: an independent marker of sudden death risk in young patients. J Am Coll Cardiol. 2003;42:873–9.
213. Spirito P, Rapezzi C, Autore C, et al. Prognosis of asymptomatic patients with hypertrophic cardiomyopathy and nonsustained ventricular tachycardia. Circulation. 1994;90:2743–7.
214. Yetman AT, Hamilton RM, Benson LN, McCrindle BW. Long-term outcome and prognostic determinants in children with hypertrophic cardiomyopathy. J Am Coll Cardiol. 1998;32:1943–50.
215. Nienaber CA, Hiller S, Spielmann RP, Geiger M, Kuck KH. Syncope in hypertrophic cardiomyopathy: multivariate analysis of prognostic determinants. J Am Coll Cardiol. 1990;15:948–55.
216. Demakis JG, Rahimtoola SH, Sutton GC, et al. Natural course of peripartum cardiomyopathy. Circulation. 1971;44:1053–61.
217. Pearson VL, Rothwell NJ, Toulmond S. Excitotoxic brain damage in the rat induces interleukin-1beta protein in microglia and astrocytes: correlation with the progression of cell death. Glia. 1999;25:311–23.
218. Elkayam U, Akhter MW, Singh H, et al. Pregnancy-associated cardiomyopathy: clinical characteristics and a comparison between early and late presentation. Circulation. 2005;111:2050–5.
219. Sliwa K, Hilfiker-Kleiner D, Petrie MC, et al. Current state of knowledge on aetiology, diagnosis, management, and therapy of peripartum cardiomyopathy: a position statement from the Heart Failure Association of the European Society of Cardiology Working Group on peripartum cardiomyopathy. Eur J Heart Fail. 2010;12:767–78.
220. Hibbard JU, Lindheimer M, Lang RM. A modified definition for peripartum cardiomyopathy and prognosis based on echocardiography. Obstet Gynecol. 1999;94:311–6.
221. Forster O, Hilfiker-Kleiner D, Ansari AA, et al. Reversal of IFN-gamma, oxLDL and prolactin serum levels correlate with clinical improvement in patients with peripartum cardiomyopathy. Eur J Heart Fail. 2008;10:861–8.
222. Hu CL, Li YB, Zou YG, et al. Troponin T measurement can predict persistent left ventricular dysfunction in peripartum cardiomyopathy. Heart. 2007;93:488–90.
223. Halkein J, Tabruyn SP, Ricke-Hoch M, et al. MicroRNA-146a is a therapeutic target and biomarker for peripartum cardiomyopathy. J Clin Invest. 2013;123:2143–54.
224. Brar SS, Khan SS, Sandhu GK, et al. Incidence, mortality, and racial differences in peripartum cardiomyopathy. Am J Cardiol. 2007;100:302–4.

225. Deneux-Tharaux C, Berg C, Bouvier-Colle MH, et al. Underreporting of pregnancy-related mortality in the United States and Europe. Obstet Gynecol. 2005;106:684–92.
226. Bello N, Rendon ISH, Arany Z. The relationship between preeclampsia and peripartum cardiomyopathy: a systematic review and meta-analysis. J Am Coll Cardiol. 2013;62:1715–23.
227. Homans DC. Peripartum cardiomyopathy. N Engl J Med. 1985;312:1432–7.
228. Seftel H, Susser M. Maternity and myocardial failure in African women. Br Heart J. 1961;23:43–52.
229. Kolte D, Khera S, Aronow WS, et al. Temporal trends in incidence and outcomes of peripartum cardiomyopathy in the United States: a nationwide population-based study. J Am Heart Assoc. 2014;3:e001056.
230. Mielniczuk LM, Williams K, Davis DR, et al. Frequency of peripartum cardiomyopathy. Am J Cardiol. 2006;97:1765–8.
231. Pearson GD, Veille JC, Rahimtoola S, et al. Peripartum cardiomyopathy: National Heart, Lung, and Blood Institute and Office of Rare Diseases (National Institutes of Health) workshop recommendations and review. JAMA. 2000;283:1183–8.
232. Isezuo SA, Abubakar SA. Epidemiologic profile of peripartum cardiomyopathy in a tertiary care hospital. Ethn Dis. 2007;17:228–33.
233. Sliwa K, Damasceno A, Mayosi BM. Epidemiology and etiology of cardiomyopathy in Africa. Circulation. 2005;112:3577–83.
234. Sanderson JE, Adesanya CO, Anjorin FI, Parry EH. Postpartum cardiac failure—heart failure due to volume overload? Am Heart J. 1979;97:613–21.
235. Goland S, Modi K, Hatamizadeh P, Elkayam U. Differences in clinical profile of African-American women with peripartum cardiomyopathy in the United States. J Card Fail. 2013;19:214–8.
236. Irizarry OC, Levine LD, Lewey J, et al. Comparison of clinical characteristics and outcomes of peripartum cardiomyopathy between African American and non-African American women. JAMA Cardiol. 2017;2:1256–60.
237. Barasa A, Rosengren A, Sandstrom TZ, Ladfors L, Schaufelberger M. Heart failure in late pregnancy and postpartum: Incidence and long-term mortality in Sweden from 1997 to 2010. J Card Fail. 2017;23:370–8.
238. Melchiorre K, Sutherland GR, Baltabaeva A, Liberati M, Thilaganathan B. Maternal cardiac dysfunction and remodeling in women with preeclampsia at term. Hypertension. 2011;57:85–93.
239. Melchiorre K, Sutherland GR, Liberati M, Thilaganathan B. Preeclampsia is associated with persistent postpartum cardiovascular impairment. Hypertension. 2011;58:709–15.
240. Demakis JG, Rahimtoola SH. Peripartum cardiomyopathy. Circulation. 1971;44:964–8.
241. Gunderson EP, Croen LA, Chiang V, Yoshida CK, Walton D, Go AS. Epidemiology of peripartum cardiomyopathy: incidence, predictors, and outcomes. Obstet Gynecol. 2011;118:583–91.
242. Zuspan FP, Rayburn WF. Blood pressure self-monitoring during pregnancy: practical considerations. Am J Obstet Gynecol. 1991;164:2–6.
243. Felker GM, Jaeger CJ, Klodas E, et al. Myocarditis and long-term survival in peripartum cardiomyopathy. Am Heart J. 2000;140:785–91.
244. Ntusi NB, Mayosi BM. Aetiology and risk factors of peripartum cardiomyopathy: a systematic review. Int J Cardiol. 2009;131:168–79.
245. Kao DP, Hsich E, Lindenfeld J. Characteristics, adverse events, and racial differences among delivering mothers with peripartum cardiomyopathy. JACC Heart Fail. 2013;1:409–16.
246. Redman CW, Sargent IL. Latest advances in understanding preeclampsia. Science. 2005;308:1592–4.
247. Sliwa K, Fett J, Elkayam U. Peripartum cardiomyopathy. Lancet. 2006;368:687–93.
248. Amos AM, Jaber WA, Russell SD. Improved outcomes in peripartum cardiomyopathy with contemporary. Am Heart J. 2006;152:509–13.
249. Bdolah Y, Lam C, Rajakumar A, et al. Twin pregnancy and the risk of preeclampsia: bigger placenta or relative ischemia? Am J Obstet Gynecol. 2008;198:428e1–6.
250. van Spaendonck-Zwarts KY, Posafalvi A, van den Berg MP, et al. Titin gene mutations are common in families with both peripartum cardiomyopathy and dilated cardiomyopathy. Eur Heart J. 2014;35:2165–73.
251. McNamara DM, Elkayam U, Alharethi R, et al. Clinical outcomes for peripartum cardiomyopathy in North America: results of the IPAC study (Investigations of Pregnancy-Associated Cardiomyopathy). J Am Coll Cardiol. 2015;66:905–14.
252. Meirhaeghe A, Bauters C, Helbecque N, et al. The human G-protein beta3 subunit C825T polymorphism is associated with coronary artery vasoconstriction. Eur Heart J. 2001;22:845–8.
253. Schunkert H, Hense HW, Doring A, Riegger GA, Siffert W. Association between a polymorphism in the G protein beta3 subunit gene and lower renin and elevated diastolic blood pressure levels. Hypertension. 1998;32:510–3.
254. Siffert W. G-protein beta3 subunit 825T allele and hypertension. Curr Hypertens Rep. 2003;5:47–53.
255. Siffert W, Rosskopf D, Siffert G, et al. Association of a human G-protein beta3 subunit variant with hypertension. Nat Genet. 1998;18:45–8.
256. Sheppard R, Hsich E, Damp J, et al. GNB3 C825T polymorphism and myocardial recovery in peripartum cardiomyopathy: results of the multicenter investigations of pregnancy-associated cardiomyopathy study. Circ Heart Fail. 2016;9:e002683.
257. Morales A, Painter T, Li R, et al. Rare variant mutations in pregnancy-associated or peripartum cardiomyopathy. Circulation. 2010;121:2176–82.
258. Ntusi NB, Wonkam A, Shaboodien G, Badri M, Mayosi BM. Frequency and clinical genetics of familial dilated cardiomyopathy in Cape Town: implications for the evaluation of patients with unexplained cardiomyopathy. S Afr Med J. 2011;101:394–8.
259. Pearl W. Familial occurrence of peripartum cardiomyopathy. Am Heart J. 1995;129:421–2.
260. van Spaendonck-Zwarts KY, van Tintelen JP, van Veldhuisen DJ, et al. Peripartum cardiomyopathy as a part of familial dilated cardiomyopathy. Circulation. 2010;121:2169–75.
261. Cheng VE, Prior DL. Peripartum cardiomyopathy in a previously asymptomatic carrier of Duchenne muscular dystrophy. Heart Lung Circ. 2013;22:677–81.
262. Politano L, Nigro V, Nigro G, et al. Development of cardiomyopathy in female carriers of Duchenne and Becker muscular dystrophies. JAMA. 1996;275:1335–8.
263. Ware JS, Li J, Mazaika E, et al. Shared genetic predisposition in peripartum and dilated cardiomyopathies. N Engl J Med. 2016;374:233–41.
264. Bakre MM, Zhu Y, Yin H, et al. Parathyroid hormone-related peptide is a naturally occurring, protein kinase A-dependent angiogenesis inhibitor. Nat Med. 2002;8:995–1003.
265. Horne BD, Rasmusson KD, Alharethi R, et al. Genome-wide significance and replication of the chromosome 12p11.22 locus near the PTHLH gene for peripartum cardiomyopathy. Circ Cardiovasc Genet. 2011;4:359–66.
266. Rasmusson K, Brunisholz K, Budge D, et al. Peripartum cardiomyopathy: post-transplant outcomes from the United Network for Organ Sharing Database. J Heart Lung Transplant. 2012;31:180–6.
267. Hilfiker-Kleiner D, Kaminski K, Podewski E, et al. A cathepsin D-cleaved 16 kDa form of prolactin mediates postpartum cardiomyopathy. Cell. 2007;128:589–600.
268. Patten IS, Rana S, Shahul S, et al. Cardiac angiogenic imbalance leads to peripartum cardiomyopathy. Nature. 2012;485:333–8.

269. Uraizee I, Cheng S, Moslehi J. Reversible cardiomyopathy associated with sunitinib and sorafenib. N Engl J Med. 2011;365:1649–50.
270. Ng DC, Court NW, dos Remedios CG, Bogoyevitch MA. Activation of signal transducer and activator of transcription (STAT) pathways in failing human hearts. Cardiovasc Res. 2003;57:333–46.
271. Arany Z, Foo SY, Ma Y, et al. HIF-independent regulation of VEGF and angiogenesis by the transcriptional coactivator PGC-1alpha. Nature. 2008;451:1008–12.
272. Bajou K, Herkenne S, Thijssen VL, et al. PAI-1 mediates the antiangiogenic and profibrinolytic effects of 16K prolactin. Nat Med. 2014;20:741–7.
273. Powe CE, Levine RJ, Karumanchi SA. Preeclampsia, a disease of the maternal endothelium: the role of antiangiogenic factors and implications for later cardiovascular disease. Circulation. 2011;123:2856–69.
274. Levine RJ, Maynard SE, Qian C, et al. Circulating angiogenic factors and the risk of preeclampsia. N Engl J Med. 2004;350:672–83.
275. Goland S, Modi K, Bitar F, et al. Clinical profile and predictors of complications in peripartum cardiomyopathy. J Card Fail. 2009;15:645–50.
276. Kane A, Mbaye M, Ndiaye MB, et al. [Evolution and thromboembolic complications of the idiopathic peripartal cardiomyopathy at Dakar University Hospital: forward-looking study about 33 cases]. J Gynecol Obstet Biol Reprod (Paris). 2010;39:484–9.
277. Simeon IA. Echocardiographic profile of peripartum cardiomyopathy in a tertiary care hospital in sokoto, Nigeria. Indian Heart J. 2006;58:234–8.
278. Main EK, McCain CL, Morton CH, Holtby S, Lawton ES. Pregnancy-related mortality in California: causes, characteristics, and improvement opportunities. Obstet Gynecol. 2015;125:938–47.
279. Lampert MB, Weinert L, Hibbard J, Korcarz C, Lindheimer M, Lang RM. Contractile reserve in patients with peripartum cardiomyopathy and recovered left ventricular function. Am J Obstet Gynecol. 1997;176:189–95.
280. Pillarisetti J, Kondur A, Alani A, et al. Peripartum cardiomyopathy: predictors of recovery and current state of implantable cardioverter-defibrillator use. J Am Coll Cardiol. 2014;63:2831–9.
281. Sliwa K, Skudicky D, Bergemann A, Candy G, Puren A, Sareli P. Peripartum cardiomyopathy: analysis of clinical outcome, left ventricular function, plasma levels of cytokines and Fas/APO-1. J Am Coll Cardiol. 2000;35:701–5.
282. Harper MA, Meyer RE, Berg CJ. Peripartum cardiomyopathy: population-based birth prevalence and 7-year mortality. Obstet Gynecol. 2012;120:1013–9.
283. Sliwa K, Forster O, Libhaber E, et al. Peripartum cardiomyopathy: inflammatory markers as predictors of outcome in 100 prospectively studied patients. Eur Heart J. 2006;27:441–6.
284. Murali S, Baldisseri MR. Peripartum cardiomyopathy. Crit Care Med. 2005;33:S340–6.
285. Veille JC. Peripartum cardiomyopathies: a review. Am J Obstet Gynecol. 1984;148:805–18.
286. Grewal J, Siu SC, Ross HJ, et al. Pregnancy outcomes in women with dilated cardiomyopathy. J Am Coll Cardiol. 2009;55:45–52.
287. Elkayam U. Risk of subsequent pregnancy in women with a history of peripartum cardiomyopathy. J Am Coll Cardiol. 2014;64:1629–36.
288. Desai D, Moodley J, Naidoo D. Peripartum cardiomyopathy: experiences at King Edward VIII Hospital, Durban, South Africa and a review of the literature. Trop Doct. 1995;25:118–23.
289. American Academy of Pediatrics Committee on Drugs. Transfer of drugs and other chemicals into human milk. Pediatrics. 2001;108:776–89.
290. Sibai BM. Chronic hypertension in pregnancy. Obstet Gynecol. 2002;100:369–77.
291. Butters L, Kennedy S, Rubin PC. Atenolol in essential hypertension during pregnancy. BMJ. 1990;301:587–9.
292. Briggs GG, Freeman RK, Yatte SJ. Drugs in pregnancy and lactation. 8th ed. Philadelphia: Wolters Kluwer; 2008.
293. Kuzniar J, Skret A, Piela A, Szmigiel Z, Zaczek T. Hemodynamic effects of intravenous hydralazine in pregnant women with severe hypertension. Obstet Gynecol. 1985;66:453–8.
294. Vink GJ, Moodley J, Philpott RH. Effect of dihydralazine on the fetus in the treatment of maternal hypertension. Obstet Gynecol. 1980;55:519–22.
295. U.S. National Library of Medicine. Drugs and lactation database (LactMed). https://toxnet.nlm.nih.gov/cgi-bin/sis/htmlgen?LACTMED. Accessed 1 July 2014.
296. Iffy L, Lindenthal J, McArdle JJ, Ganesh V. Severe cerebral accidents postpartum in patients taking bromocriptine for milk suppression. Isr J Med Sci. 1996;32:309–12.
297. Loewe C, Dragovic LJ. Acute coronary artery thrombosis in a postpartum woman receiving bromocriptine. Am J Forensic Med Pathol. 1998;19:258–60.
298. Bouabdallaoui N, Mouquet F, Lebreton G, Demondion P, Le Jemtel TH, Ennezat PV. Current knowledge and recent development on management of peripartum cardiomyopathy. Eur Heart J Acute Cardiovasc Care. 2017;6:359–66.
299. Turkalj I, Braun P, Krupp P. Surveillance of bromocriptine in pregnancy. JAMA. 1982;247:1589–91.
300. U.S. Government Publishing Office. Sandoz Pharmaceuticals Corp.; Bromocriptine mesylate (Parlodel); Withdrawal of approval of the indication for the prevention of physiological lactation. Fed Regist. 1995;60:3404–5.
301. Sliwa K, Blauwet L, Tibazarwa K, et al. Evaluation of bromocriptine in the treatment of acute severe peripartum cardiomyopathy: a proof-of-concept pilot study. Circulation. 2010;121:1465–73.
302. Hilfiker-Kleiner D, Haghikia A, Berliner D, et al. Bromocriptine for the treatment of peripartum cardiomyopathy: a multicentre randomized study. Eur Heart J. 2017;38:2671–9.
303. Hilfiker-Kleiner D, Meyer GP, Schieffer E, et al. Recovery from postpartum cardiomyopathy in 2 patients by blocking prolactin release with bromocriptine. J Am Coll Cardiol. 2007;50:2354–5.
304. Jahns BG, Stein W, Hilfiker-Kleiner D, Pieske B, Emons G. Peripartum cardiomyopathy--a new treatment option by inhibition of prolactin secretion. Am J Obstet Gynecol. 2008;199:e5–6.
305. Lampert MB, Lang RM. Peripartum cardiomyopathy. Am Heart J. 1995;130:860–70.
306. Mason JW, O'Connell JB, Herskowitz A, et al. A clinical trial of immunosuppressive therapy for myocarditis. The Myocarditis Treatment Trial Investigators. N Engl J Med. 1995;333:269–75.
307. Bozkurt B, Villaneuva FS, Holubkov R, et al. Intravenous immune globulin in the therapy of peripartum cardiomyopathy. J Am Coll Cardiol. 1999;34:177–80.
308. Fett JD, Christie LG, Carraway RD, Murphy JG. Five-year prospective study of the incidence and prognosis of peripartum cardiomyopathy at a single institution. Mayo Clin Proc. 2005;80:1602–6.
309. Mouquet F, Lions C, de Groote P, et al. Characterisation of peripartum cardiomyopathy by cardiac magnetic resonance imaging. Eur Radiol. 2008;18:2765–9.
310. Al-Khatib SM, Stevenson WG, Ackerman MJ, et al. AHA/ACC/HRS guideline for management of patients with ventricular arrhythmias and the prevention of sudden cardiac death: a report of the American College of Cardiology/American Heart Association Task Force on Clinical Practice Guidelines and the Heart Rhythm Society. J Am Coll Cardiol. 2018;138:e272–391.

311. Zimmerman H, Coelho-Anderson R, Smith R, Nolan P, Copeland J. Bridge to recovery with a thoratec biventricular assist device for postpartum cardiomyopathy. ASAIO J. 2010;56:479–80.
312. Emmert MY, Pretre R, Ruschitzka F, Krahenmann F, Falk V, Wilhelm MJ. Peripartum cardiomyopathy with cardiogenic shock: recovery after prolactin inhibition and mechanical support. Ann Thorac Surg. 2011;91:274–6.
313. Loyaga-Rendon RY, Pamboukian SV, Tallaj JA, et al. Outcomes of patients with peripartum cardiomyopathy who received mechanical circulatory support. Data from the Interagency Registry for Mechanically Assisted Circulatory Support. Circ Heart Fail. 2014;7:300–9.
314. Mathur NB, Dhingra D. Breastfeeding. Indian J Pediatr. 2014;81:143–9.
315. Safirstein JG, Ro AS, Grandhi S, Wang L, Fett JD, Staniloae C. Predictors of left ventricular recovery in a cohort of peripartum cardiomyopathy patients recruited via the internet. Int J Cardiol. 2012;154:27–31.
316. Elkayam U. Clinical characteristics of peripartum cardiomyopathy in the United States: diagnosis, prognosis, and management. J Am Coll Cardiol. 2011;58:659–70.
317. Curtis KM, Tepper NK, Jatlaoui TC, et al. U.S. medical eligibility criteria for contraceptive use, 2016. MMWR Recomm Rep. 2016;65:1–103.
318. Tepper NK, Paulen ME, Marchbanks PA, Curtis KM. Safety of contraceptive use among women with peripartum cardiomyopathy: a systematic review. Contraception. 2010;82:95–101.
319. Lo JO, Mission JF, Caughey AB. Hypertensive disease of pregnancy and maternal mortality. Curr Opin Obstet Gynecol. 2013;25:124–32.
320. James PR, Nelson-Piercy C. Management of hypertension before, during, and after pregnancy. Heart. 2004;90:1499–504.
321. Sibai BM, Caritis SN, Hauth JC, et al. Preterm delivery in women with pregestational diabetes mellitus or chronic hypertension relative to women with uncomplicated pregnancies. The National institute of Child health and Human Development Maternal-Fetal Medicine Units Network. Am J Obstet Gynecol. 2000;183:1520–4.
322. Ramakrishnan A, Lee LJ, Mitchell LE, Agopian AJ. Maternal hypertension during pregnancy and the risk of congenital heart defects in offspring: a systematic review and meta-analysis. Pediatr Cardiol. 2015;36:1442–51.
323. Hall ME, George EM, Granger JP. The heart during pregnancy. Rev Esp Cardiol. 2011;64:1045–50.
324. The American College of Obstetricians and Gynecologists. Preeclampsia and high blood pressure during pregnancy. https://www.acog.org/Patients/FAQs/Preeclampsia-and-High-Blood-Pressure-During-Pregnancy. Accessed 20 June 2018.
325. The American College of Obstetricians and Gynecologists. Hypertension in pregnancy. https://www.acog.org/~/media/Task%20Force%20and%20Work%20Group%20Reports/public/HypertensioninPregnancy.pdf. Accessed 20 June 2018.
326. The SPRINT Research Group, A randomized trial of intensive versus standard blood-pressure control. N Engl J Med. 2017;377:2506.
327. Whelton PK, Carey RM, Aronow WS, et al. 2017 ACC/AHA/AAPA/ABC/ACPM/AGS/APhA/ASH/ASPC/NMA/PCNA Guideline for the Prevention, Detection, Evaluation, and Management of High Blood Pressure in Adults: A Report of the American College of Cardiology/American Heart Association Task Force on Clinical Practice Guidelines. J Am Coll Cardiol. 2018;71:e127–248.
328. Sibai BM. Diagnosis and management of chronic hypertension in pregnancy. Obstet Gynecol. 1991;78:451–61.
329. Sibai BM. Treatment of hypertension in pregnant women. N Engl J Med. 1996;335:257–65.
330. Al-Maawali A, Walfisch A, Koren G. Taking angiotensin-converting enzyme inhibitors during pregnancy: is it safe? Can Fam Physician. 2012;58:49–51.
331. Buchbinder A, Sibai BM, Caritis S, et al. Adverse perinatal outcomes are significantly higher in severe gestational hypertension than in mild preeclampsia. Am J Obstet Gynecol. 2002;186:66–71.
332. Hauth JC, Ewell MG, Levine RJ, et al. Pregnancy outcomes in healthy nulliparas who developed hypertension. Calcium for Preeclampsia Prevention Study Group. Obstet Gynecol. 2000;95:24–8.
333. Yoder SR, Thornburg LL, Bisognano JD. Hypertension in pregnancy and women of childbearing age. Am J Med. 2009;122:890–5.
334. Gaillard R, Steegers EA, Hofman A, Jaddoe VW. Associations of maternal obesity with blood pressure and the risks of gestational hypertensive disorders. The Generation R Study J Hypertens. 2011;29:937–44.
335. American College of Obstetricians and Gynecologists, Task Force on Hypertension in Pregnancy. Hypertension in pregnancy. Report of the American College of Obstetricians and Gynecologists' Task Force on Hypertension in Pregnancy. Obstet Gynecol. 2013;122:1122–31.
336. Hjartardottir S, Leifsson BG, Geirsson RT, Steinthorsdottir V. Recurrence of hypertensive disorder in second pregnancy. Am J Obstet Gynecol. 2006;194:916–20.
337. Brown MA, Mackenzie C, Dunsmuir W, et al. Can we predict recurrence of pre-eclampsia or gestational hypertension? BJOG. 2007;114:984–93.
338. Bellomo G, Venanzi S, Saronio P, Verdura C, Narducci PL. Prognostic significance of serum uric acid in women with gestational hypertension. Hypertension. 2011;58:704–8.
339. Melamed N, Ray JG, Hladunewich M, Cox B, Kingdom JC. Gestational hypertension and preeclampsia: are they the same disease? J Obstet Gynaecol Can. 2014;36:642–7.
340. Gyselaers W, Staelens A, Mesens T, et al. Maternal venous Doppler characteristics are abnormal in pre-eclampsia but not in gestational hypertension. Ultrasound Obstet Gynecol. 2015;45:421–6.
341. Beevers G, Lip GY, O'Brien E. ABC of hypertension: Blood pressure measurement. Part II—Conventional sphygmomanometry: technique of auscultatory blood pressure measurement. BMJ. 2001;322:1043–7.
342. Myers MG. A proposed algorithm for diagnosing hypertension using automated office blood pressure measurement. J Hypertens. 2010;28:703–8.
343. Pickering TG, Hall JE, Appel LJ, et al. Recommendations for blood pressure measurement in humans and experimental animals: Part 1: Blood pressure measurement in humans: a statement for professionals from the Subcommittee of Professional and Public Education of the American Heart Association Council on High Blood Pressure Research. Circulation. 2005;111:697–716.
344. Bakris GL. The implications of blood pressure measurement methods on treatment targets for blood pressure. Circulation. 2016;134:904–5.
345. Myers MG, Kaczorowski J, Dawes M, Godwin M. Automated office blood pressure measurement in primary care. Can Fam Physician. 2014;60:127–32.
346. ESH/ESC Task Force for the Management of Arterial Hypertension. 2013 Practice guidelines for the management of arterial hypertension of the European Society of Hypertension (ESH) and the European Society of Cardiology (ESC): ESH/ESC Task Force for the Management of Arterial Hypertension. J Hypertens. 2013;31:1925–38.
347. Tholl U, Forstner K, Anlauf M. Measuring blood pressure: pitfalls and recommendations. Nephrol Dial Transplant. 2004;19:766–70.
348. Leung AA, Nerenberg K, Daskalopoulou SS, et al. Hypertension Canada's 2016 Canadian Hypertension Education Program Guidelines for blood pressure measurement, diagnosis, assess-

ment of risk, prevention, and treatment of hypertension. Can J Cardiol. 2016;32:569–88.

349. Crowther CA, Bouwmeester AM, Ashurst HM. Does admission to hospital for bed rest prevent disease progression or improve fetal outcome in pregnancy complicated by non-proteinuric hypertension? Br J Obstet Gynaecol. 1992;99:13–7.
350. American College of Obstetricians and Gynecologists Committee on Obstetric Practice. ACOG Committee Opinion No. 421, November 2008: antibiotic prophylaxis for infective endocarditis. Obstet Gynecol. 2008;112:1193–4.
351. Sibai BM. Eclampsia. VI. Maternal-perinatal outcome in 254 consecutive cases. Am J Obstet Gynecol. 1990;163:1049–54. discussion 1054–5
352. Kilpatrick SJ, Abreo A, Greene N, et al. Severe maternal morbidity in a large cohort of women with acute severe intrapartum hypertension. Am J Obstet Gynecol. 2016;215:91.e91–7.
353. Coppage KH, Sibai BM. Treatment of hypertensive complications in pregnancy. Curr Pharm Des. 2005;11:749–57.
354. Magee LA, von Dadelszen P, Rey E, et al. Less-tight versus tight control of hypertension in pregnancy. N Engl J Med. 2015;372:407–17.
355. Magee LA, von Dadelszen P, Singer J, et al. The CHIPS randomized controlled trial (control of hypertension in pregnancy study): is severe hypertension just an elevated blood pressure? Hypertension. 2016;68:1153–9.
356. Webster LM, Conti-Ramsden F, Seed PT, Webb AJ, Nelson-Piercy C, Chappell LC. Impact of antihypertensive treatment on maternal and perinatal outcomes in pregnancy complicated by chronic hypertension: a systematic review and meta-analysis. J Am Heart Assoc. 2017;6(5).
357. Pels A, Mol BWJ, Singer J, et al. Influence of gestational age at initiation of antihypertensive therapy: Secondary analysis of CHIPS trial data (Control of Hypertension in Pregnancy Study). Hypertension. 2018;71:1170–7.
358. Mancia G, De Backer G, Dominiczak A, et al. 2007 ESH-ESC practice guidelines for the management of arterial hypertension: ESH-ESC task force on the management of arterial hypertension. J Hypertens. 2007;25:1751–62.
359. Martin JN Jr, Thigpen BD, Moore RC, Rose CH, Cushman J, May W. Stroke and severe preeclampsia and eclampsia: a paradigm shift focusing on systolic blood pressure. Obstet Gynecol. 2005;105:246–54.
360. Brown CM, Garovic VD. Drug treatment of hypertension in pregnancy. Drugs. 2014;74:283–96.
361. Leddy MA, Power ML, Schulkin J. The impact of maternal obesity on maternal and fetal health. Rev Obstet Gynecol. 2008;1:170–8.
362. Abdul Sultan A, West J, Tata LJ, Fleming KM, Nelson-Piercy C, Grainge MJ. Risk of first venous thromboembolism in pregnant women in hospital: population based cohort study from England. BMJ. 2013;347:f6099.
363. Meher S, Abalos E, Carroli G. Bed rest with or without hospitalisation for hypertension during pregnancy. Cochrane Database Syst Rev. 2005:CD003514.
364. Hofmeyr GJ, Atallah AN, Duley L. Calcium supplementation during pregnancy for preventing hypertensive disorders and related problems. Cochrane Database Syst Rev. 2006:CD001059.
365. Bushnell C, McCullough LD, Awad IA, et al. Guidelines for the prevention of stroke in women: a statement for healthcare professionals from the American Heart Association/American Stroke Association. Stroke. 2014;45:1545–88.
366. Cockburn J, Moar VA, Ounsted M, Redman CW. Final report of study on hypertension during pregnancy: the effects of specific treatment on the growth and development of the children. Lancet. 1982;1:647–9.
367. Magee LA, Group CS, von Dadelszen P, et al. Do labetalol and methyldopa have different effects on pregnancy outcome? Analysis of data from the Control of Hypertension In Pregnancy Study (CHIPS) trial. BJOG. 2016;123:1143–51.
368. Ahn HK, Nava-Ocampo AA, Han JY, et al. Exposure to amlodipine in the first trimester of pregnancy and during breastfeeding. Hypertens Pregnancy. 2007;26:179–87.
369. Smith P, Anthony J, Johanson R. Nifedipine in pregnancy. BJOG. 2000;107:299–307.
370. Molvi SN, Mir S, Rana VS, Jabeen F, Malik AR. Role of antihypertensive therapy in mild to moderate pregnancy-induced hypertension: a prospective randomized study comparing labetalol with alpha methyldopa. Arch Gynecol Obstet. 2012;285:1553–62.
371. WFt P, Hilleman DE, Levy PD, Rhoney DH, Varon J. A systematic review of nicardipine vs labetalol for the management of hypertensive crises. Am J Emerg Med. 2012;30:981–93.
372. Webster LM, Myers JE, Nelson-Piercy C, et al. Labetalol versus nifedipine as antihypertensive treatment for chronic hypertension in pregnancy: a randomized controlled trial. Hypertension. 2017;70:915–22.
373. Peacock WF, Varon J, Baumann BM, et al. CLUE: a randomized comparative effectiveness trial of IV nicardipine versus labetalol use in the emergency department. Crit Care. 2011;15:R157.
374. Committee on Obstetric Practice. Committee opinion no. 692: Emergent therapy for acute-onset, severe hypertension during pregnancy and the postpartum period. Obstet Gynecol. 2017;129:e90–5.
375. Page RL, Joglar JA, Caldwell MA, et al. 2015 ACC/AHA/HRS guideline for the management of adult patients with supraventricular tachycardia: a report of the American College of Cardiology/American Heart Association task force on clinical practice guidelines and the Heart Rhythm Society. J Am Coll Cardiol. 2016;67:e27–e115.
376. Li JM, Nguyen C, Joglar JA, Hamdan MH, Page RL. Frequency and outcome of arrhythmias complicating admission during pregnancy: experience from a high-volume and ethnically-diverse obstetric service. Clin Cardiol. 2008;31:538–41.
377. Shotan A, Ostrzega E, Mehra A, Johnson JV, Elkayam U. Incidence of arrhythmias in normal pregnancy and relation to palpitations, dizziness, and syncope. Am J Cardiol. 1997;79:1061–4.
378. Franz MR, Cima R, Wang D, Profitt D, Kurz R. Electrophysiological effects of myocardial stretch and mechanical determinants of stretch-activated arrhythmias. Circulation. 1992;86:968–78.
379. Roberts JM, Insel PA, Goldfien A. Regulation of myometrial adrenoreceptors and adrenergic response by sex steroids. Mol Pharmacol. 1981;20:52–8.
380. Soliman EZ, Elsalam MA, Li Y. The relationship between high resting heart rate and ventricular arrhythmogenesis in patients referred to ambulatory 24 h electrocardiographic recording. Europace. 2010;12:261–5.
381. Joglar JA, Page RL. Management of arrhythmia syndromes during pregnancy. Curr Opin Cardiol. 2014;29:36–44.
382. Li Y, Rabey KN, Schmitt D, Norton JN, Reynolds RP. Characteristics of vibration that alter cardiovascular parameters in mice. J Am Assoc Lab Anim Sci. 2015;54:372–7.
383. Lee SH, Chen SA, Wu TJ, et al. Effects of pregnancy on first onset and symptoms of paroxysmal supraventricular tachycardia. Am J Cardiol. 1995;76:675–8.
384. Silversides CK, Harris L, Haberer K, Sermer M, Colman JM, Siu SC. Recurrence rates of arrhythmias during pregnancy in women with previous tachyarrhythmia and impact on fetal and neonatal outcomes. Am J Cardiol. 2006;97:1206–12.
385. Ghosh N, Luk A, Derzko C, Dorian P, Chow CM. The acute treatment of maternal supraventricular tachycardias during pregnancy: a review of the literature. J Obstet Gynaecol Can. 2011;33:17–23.
386. Allen NM, Page RL. Procainamide administration during pregnancy. Clin Pharm. 1993;12:58–60.

387. Qasqas SA, McPherson C, Frishman WH, Elkayam U. Cardiovascular pharmacotherapeutic considerations during pregnancy and lactation. Cardiol Rev. 2004;12:201–21.
388. Doig JC, McComb JM, Reid DS. Incessant atrial tachycardia accelerated by pregnancy. Br Heart J. 1992;67:266–8.
389. DiCarlo-Meacham A, Dahlke J. Atrial fibrillation in pregnancy. Obstet Gynecol. 2011;117:489–92.
390. Rathore SS, Wang Y, Krumholz HM. Sex-based differences in the effect of digoxin for the treatment of heart failure. N Engl J Med. 2002;347:1403–11.
391. Goland S, Elkayam U. Anticoagulation in pregnancy. Cardiol Clin. 2012;30:395–405.
392. Brodsky M, Doria R, Allen B, Sato D, Thomas G, Sada M. New-onset ventricular tachycardia during pregnancy. Am Heart J. 1992;123:933–41.
393. Lemery R, Brugada P, Bella PD, Dugernier T, van den Dool A, Wellens HJ. Nonischemic ventricular tachycardia. Clinical course and long-term follow-up in patients without clinically overt heart disease. Circulation. 1989;79:990–9.
394. Cleary-Goldman J, Salva CR, Infeld JI, Robinson JN. Verapamil-sensitive idiopathic left ventricular tachycardia in pregnancy. J Matern Fetal Neonatal Med. 2003;14:132–5.
395. Page RL, Hamdan MH, Joglar JA. Arrhythmias occurring during pregnancy. Card Electrophysiol Rev. 2002;6:136–9.
396. Shenker L. Fetal cardiac arrhythmias. Obstet Gynecol Surv. 1979;34:561–72.
397. Strasburger JF, Wakai RT. Fetal cardiac arrhythmia detection and in utero therapy. Nat Rev Cardiol. 2010;7:277–90.
398. Copel JA, Liang RI, Demasio K, Ozeren S, Kleinman CS. The clinical significance of the irregular fetal heart rhythm. Am J Obstet Gynecol. 2000;182:813–7; discussion 817–9
399. Cuneo BF, Strasburger JF, Wakai RT, Ovadia M. Conduction system disease in fetuses evaluated for irregular cardiac rhythm. Fetal Diagn Ther. 2006;21:307–13.
400. Boldt T, Eronen M, Andersson S. Long-term outcome in fetuses with cardiac arrhythmias. Obstet Gynecol. 2003;102:1372–9.
401. Donofrio MT, Moon-Grady AJ, Hornberger LK, et al. Diagnosis and treatment of fetal cardiac disease: a scientific statement from the American Heart Association. Circulation. 2014;129:2183–242.
402. van Engelen AD, Weijtens O, Brenner JI, et al. Management outcome and follow-up of fetal tachycardia. J Am Coll Cardiol. 1994;24:1371–5.
403. Hahurij ND, Gittenberger-De Groot AC, Kolditz DP, et al. Accessory atrioventricular myocardial connections in the developing human heart: relevance for perinatal supraventricular tachycardias. Circulation. 2008;117:2850–8.
404. Wakai RT, Strasburger JF, Li Z, Deal BJ, Gotteiner NL. Magnetocardiographic rhythm patterns at initiation and termination of fetal supraventricular tachycardia. Circulation. 2003;107:307–12.
405. Alsaied T, Baskar S, Fares M, et al. First-line antiarrhythmic transplacental treatment for fetal tachyarrhythmia: a systematic review and meta-analysis. J Am Heart Assoc 2017;6.
406. Hill GD, Kovach JR, Saudek DE, Singh AK, Wehrheim K, Frommelt MA. Transplacental treatment of fetal tachycardia: a systematic review and meta-analysis. Prenat Diagn. 2017;37:1076–83.
407. Naheed ZJ, Strasburger JF, Deal BJ, Benson DW Jr, Gidding SS. Fetal tachycardia: mechanisms and predictors of hydrops fetalis. J Am Coll Cardiol. 1996;27:1736–40.
408. Oudijk MA, Ruskamp JM, Ververs FF, et al. Treatment of fetal tachycardia with sotalol: transplacental pharmacokinetics and pharmacodynamics. J Am Coll Cardiol. 2003;42:765–70.
409. Shah A, Moon-Grady A, Bhogal N, et al. Effectiveness of sotalol as first-line therapy for fetal supraventricular tachyarrhythmias. Am J Cardiol. 2012;109:1614–8.
410. Ebenroth ES, Cordes TM, Darragh RK. Second-line treatment of fetal supraventricular tachycardia using flecainide acetate. Pediatr Cardiol. 2001;22:483–7.
411. Castillo RA, Devoe LD, Hadi HA, Martin S, Geist D. Nonimmune hydrops fetalis: clinical experience and factors related to a poor outcome. Am J Obstet Gynecol. 1986;155:812–6.
412. Wy CA, Sajous CH, Loberiza F, Weiss MG. Outcome of infants with a diagnosis of hydrops fetalis in the 1990s. Am J Perinatol. 1999;16:561–7.
413. Parilla BV, Strasburger JF, Socol ML. Fetal supraventricular tachycardia complicated by hydrops fetalis: a role for direct fetal intramuscular therapy. Am J Perinatol. 1996;13:483–6.
414. The American College of Obstetricians and Gynecologists. ACOG Practice Bulletin No. 106: Intrapartum fetal heart rate monitoring: nomenclature, interpretation, and general management principles. Obstet Gynecol. 2009;114:192–202.
415. Schmidt KG, Ulmer HE, Silverman NH, Kleinman CS, Copel JA. Perinatal outcome of fetal complete atrioventricular block: a multicenter experience. J Am Coll Cardiol. 1991;17:1360–6.
416. Buyon JP, Winchester R. Congenital complete heart block. A human model of passively acquired autoimmune injury. Arthritis Rheum. 1990;33:609–14.
417. Buyon JP, Clancy RM, Friedman DM. Autoimmune associated congenital heart block: integration of clinical and research clues in the management of the maternal/foetal dyad at risk. J Intern Med. 2009;265:653–62.
418. Buyon JP, Hiebert R, Copel J, et al. Autoimmune-associated congenital heart block: demographics, mortality, morbidity and recurrence rates obtained from a national neonatal lupus registry. J Am Coll Cardiol. 1998;31:1658–66.
419. Ozkutlu S, Onderoglu L, Karagoz T, Celiker A, Sahiner UM. Isolated noncompaction of left ventricular myocardium with fetal sustained bradycardia due to sick sinus syndrome. Turk J Pediatr. 2006;48:383–6.
420. Glatz AC, Gaynor JW, Rhodes LA, et al. Outcome of high-risk neonates with congenital complete heart block paced in the first 24 hours after birth. J Thorac Cardiovasc Surg. 2008;136:767–73.
421. Berg C, Geipel A, Kohl T, et al. Atrioventricular block detected in fetal life: associated anomalies and potential prognostic markers. Ultrasound Obstet Gynecol. 2005;26:4–15.
422. Zhao H, Cuneo BF, Strasburger JF, Huhta JC, Gotteiner NL, Wakai RT. Electrophysiological characteristics of fetal atrioventricular block. J Am Coll Cardiol. 2008;51:77–84.
423. Hofbeck M, Ulmer H, Beinder E, Sieber E, Singer H. Prenatal findings in patients with prolonged QT interval in the neonatal period. Heart. 1997;77:198–204.
424. Mitchell JL, Cuneo BF, Etheridge SP, Horigome H, Weng HY, Benson DW. Fetal heart rate predictors of long QT syndrome. Circulation. 2012;126:2688–95.
425. Joglar JA, Page RL. Treatment of cardiac arrhythmias during pregnancy: safety considerations. Drug Saf. 1999;20:85–94.
426. Pittard WB 3rd, Glazier H. Procainamide excretion in human milk. J Pediatr. 1983;102:631–3.
427. Barnett DB, Hudson SA, McBurney A. Disopyramide and its N-monodesalkyl metabolite in breast milk. Br J Clin Pharmacol. 1982;14:310–2.
428. MacKintosh D, Buchanan N. Excretion of disopyramide in human breast milk. Br J Clin Pharmacol. 1985;19:856–7.
429. Ortega D, Viviand X, Lorec AM, Gamerre M, Martin C, Bruguerolle B. Excretion of lidocaine and bupivacaine in breast milk following epidural anesthesia for cesarean delivery. Acta Anaesthesiol Scand. 1999;43:394–7.
430. Zeisler JA, Gaarder TD, De Mesquita SA. Lidocaine excretion in breast milk. Drug Intell Clin Pharm. 1986;20:691–3.
431. Lewis AM, Patel L, Johnston A, Turner P. Mexiletine in human blood and breast milk. Postgrad Med J. 1981;57:546–7.

432. Echt DS, Liebson PR, Mitchell LB, et al. Mortality and morbidity in patients receiving encainide, flecainide, or placebo. The Cardiac Arrhythmia Suppression Trial. N Engl J Med. 1991;324:781–8.
433. Kulas J, Lunell NO, Rosing U, Steen B, Rane A. Atenolol and metoprolol. A comparison of their excretion into human breast milk. Acta Obstet Gynecol Scand Suppl. 1984;118:65–9.
434. Libardoni M, Piovan D, Busato E, Padrini R. Transfer of propafenone and 5-OH-propafenone to foetal plasma and maternal milk. Br J Clin Pharmacol. 1991;32:527–8.
435. Bartalena L, Bogazzi F, Braverman LE, Martino E. Effects of amiodarone administration during pregnancy on neonatal thyroid function and subsequent neurodevelopment. J Endocrinol Invest. 2001;24:116–30.
436. Plomp TA, Vulsma T, de Vijlder JJ. Use of amiodarone during pregnancy. Eur J Obstet Gynecol Reprod Biol. 1992;43:201–7.
437. Kozlowski D, Budrejko S, Lip GY, et al. Dronedarone: an overview. Ann Med. 2012;44:60–72.
438. Byerly WG, Hartmann A, Foster DE, Tannenbaum AK. Verapamil in the treatment of maternal paroxysmal supraventricular tachycardia. Ann Emerg Med. 1991;20:552–4.
439. Anderson P, Bondesson U, Mattiasson I, Johansson BW. Verapamil and norverapamil in plasma and breast milk during breast feeding. Eur J Clin Pharmacol. 1987;31:625–7.
440. Elkayam U, Goodwin TM. Adenosine therapy for supraventricular tachycardia during pregnancy. Am J Cardiol. 1995;75:521–3.
441. Page RL. Treatment of arrhythmias during pregnancy. Am Heart J. 1995;130:871–6.
442. Schroeder JS, Harrison DC. Repeated cardioversion during pregnancy. Treatment of refractory paroxysmal atrial tachycardia during 3 successive pregnancies. Am J Cardiol. 1971;27:445–6.
443. McCollough CH, Schueler BA, Atwell TD, et al. Radiation exposure and pregnancy: when should we be concerned? Radiographics. 2007;27:909–17; discussion 917–8
444. Damilakis J, Theocharopoulos N, Perisinakis K, et al. Conceptus radiation dose and risk from cardiac catheter ablation procedures. Circulation. 2001;104:893–7.
445. Szumowski L, Szufladowicz E, Orczykowski M, et al. Ablation of severe drug-resistant tachyarrhythmia during pregnancy. J Cardiovasc Electrophysiol. 2010;21:877–82.
446. Natale A, Davidson T, Geiger MJ, Newby K. Implantable cardioverter-defibrillators and pregnancy: a safe combination? Circulation. 1997;96:2808–12.
447. Jordaens LJ, Vandenbogaerde JF, Van de Bruaene P, De Buyzere M. Transesophageal echocardiography for insertion of a physiological pacemaker in early pregnancy. Pacing Clin Electrophysiol. 1990;13:955–7.

13 Evidenced-Based and Practical Management of Real-World Valvular Heart Disease

Blase A. Carabello

Introduction

The following valve cases represent "real world" clinical problems to be solved. In some cases the correct answer is predicated of solid evidence; in others there may be only a "best" answer but where experienced clinicians might differ in their response.

Case 1

The patient is a 76 y/o white male who is referred for the evaluation of a heart murmur found on a routine physical exam. The patient has been well. He is retired from an office job. His major physical activity is gardening which does not elicit symptoms of angina, dyspnea, or syncope. He has a history of hypertension treated with amlodipine. He denies diabetes, smoking, or excessive alcohol consumption.

Physical Examination

Pulse 66. BP 130/76. BMI 25

Neck: est. CVP 5 cm H_2O Carotid upstrokes delayed.

Chest clear

Cor: PMI sustained in the fifth IS MCL; 2/6 late peaking SEM, RUSB; S2 physiologically split

Ext: no edema

Q1. Based on the physical exam the patient: (pick 1 best answer)
   (A) Has pulmonic stenosis
   (B) Has aortic sclerosis
   (C) Has mild aortic stenosis
   (D) Has severe aortic stenosis

B. A. Carabello (✉)
Cardiology Division, Brody School of Medicine, East Carolina University, Greenville, NC, USA

Department of Cardiovascular Sciences, Vidant Medical Center, Greenville, NC, USA
e-mail: carabellob16@ecu.edu

Lab Exam

EKG: NSR; LVH

Hb: 14.1 g/dL

Creatinine: 1.1 mg/dL

Echocardiogram: heavily calcified aortic valve; EF: 65%; septal wall thickness: 13 mm; peak aortic jet velocity: 4.2 m/s; mean gradient 38 mmHg; AVA: 1.0 cm^2

BNP: 67 pg/mL

Q2. According to current guideline the degree of this patient's AS is:
   (A) Moderate
   (B) Indeterminate
   (C) Severe

Q3. You now:
   (A) Elect for follow-up in 6–12 months
   (B) Perform a formal exercise test
   (C) Refer for AVR
   (D) Refer for TAVR
   (E) A or B

You elect to treat the patient "medically" and he returns in 6 months. He denies symptoms but his wife thinks he is "slowing down"

Repeat echo finds

EF 60%; peak jet velocity 4.8 m/s; mean gradient 55 mmHg; AVA 0, 8 cm^2; BNP 143 pg/mL

Q4. At this time you
   (A) Repeat the exercise test
   (B) Refer for AVR
   (C) Refer for TAVR
   (D) Continue "medical management
   (E) A or B

B. A. Carabello (ed.), *Valvular Heart Disease*, Cardiovascular Medicine, https://doi.org/10.1007/978-1-4471-2840-3_13

Case 2

An 85 y/o white female is evaluated for the cause of her heart failure. She lives alone with support from her family. About 2 years ago she began noticing dyspnea on exertion which has progressed so that she can only walk 20 ft without stopping to rest. She notes two pillow orthopnea but denies PND, syncope, angina, or edema. Her family notes that she has become progressively forgetful over the past year, occasionally unable to identify family members.

Physical Examination

BP 123/67; pulse 75 BMI: 18

Unable to move from wheelchair to exam table without assistance

Neck: carotid upstrokes delayed; CVP 10 cm H_2O

Chest: scatted rales

Cor: 2/6 late peaking SEM

Ext: +1 edema

Lab Exam

Hb: 10.9 g/dL

Creatinine: 2.1 mg/dL

Albumen: 3.0 g/dL

Echo: EF 55%. Jet velocity: 4.6 m/s. Mean gradient 50 mmHg. AVA 0.7 cm^2

STS mortality risk 11%

Q5. As a member of the Heart Team evaluating the case you would recommend
- (A) SAVR
- (B) TAVR
- (C) Hospice
- (D) Balloon valvotomy as a bridge to TAVR
- (E) B, C, or D

Case 3

A 76 y/o man is evaluated for heart failure and a murmur. The patient has noted progressively worsening dyspnea on exertion over the past 2 years. He can no longer reach the bedroom of his second story home without resting half way to the top. He has begun to sleep on three pillows. He denies syncope or angina. He has been an orally controlled diabetic for 5 years. He is unhappy with these limitations and is anxious for relief.

Physical Examination

BP 94/56; pulse 82; BMI 22

Neck: carotid pulse slightly delayed; CVP 12 cm H_2O

Chest bibasilar rales

Cor: 2/6 mid-late peaking murmur

Ext: +2 edema

Lab Exam

Hb: 11 g/dL

Creatinine: 2.2 mg/dL

Echo: EF 20–25%. Peak jet velocity: 2.7 m/s; mean gradient 22 mmHg; AVA 0.8 cm^2

Q6. The patient's diagnosis is:
- (A) Severe aortic stenosis
- (B) Mild aortic stenosis
- (C) Aortic pseudo-stenosis
- (D) Aortic valve disease, severity unknown

Q7. The patient should now:
- (A) Undergoing valve CT calcium scoring
- (B) Inotropic stress testing
- (C) TAVR
- (D) Consideration for hospice
- (E) Guideline-directed heart failure therapy

The patient underwent echocardiography during dobutamine infusion. Peak jet velocity increased to 4.1 m/s; mean gradient increased to 39 mmHg and AVA was calculated as 0.9 cm^2.

Q8. Best management now is:
- (A) TAVR
- (B) SAVR
- (C) Guideline-directed therapy for heart failure
- (D) Hospice

Case 4

This 75 y/o woman was evaluated for dyspnea that has worsened over the past year. Currently she is limited in doing her housework and cannot vacuum a room without resting. She also notes occasional chest pressure when walking up a hill. She denies orthopnea, PND, or syncope. She denies smoking or diabetes but has a long history of moderately controlled hypertension. She was a former 30 pck/year smoker.

Physical Examination

BP 170/86; pulse 66; BMI 30
Neck: carotid upstrokes delayed; CVP 5 cm H_2O
Chest: clear
Cor: 3/6 late peaking SEM; single S2
Ext: no edema; absent pulses R foot

Lab Exam

Hb: 12.9 g/dL
Creatinine 1.6 mg/dL
Echo: EF 65%, LVH. Septal thickness 15 mm. Peak gradient 3.0 m/s. Mean gradient 30 mmHg. AVA 0.8 cm^2

Q9. At this point she should undergo:
(A) TAVR
(B) SAVR
(C) Valve calcium scoring
(D) Cardiac catheterization
(E) C&D

The patient underwent multi-detector CT scanning which found a high calcium score consistent with severe AS. At heart catheterization her mean aortic valve gradient was 32 mmHg, cardiac output 4.4 L/min, and calculated AVA of 0.8 cm^2. There was a 90% obstruction of the right coronary artery.

Q10. As a member of the heart team you would recommend:
(A) SAVR
(B) TAVR
(C) Balloon valvotomy
(D) Medical management for heart failure

Case 5

An 80 y/o man is evaluated for dyspnea on exertion. He began noting fatigue and dyspnea 1 year ago and it has progressed so that he can walk only about 20 yards without stopping for rest. He denies orthopnea, PND, syncope, angina, or edema. He had been a 50 pck/year smoker but quit 3 years ago. He has been an insulin-controlled diabetic for 5 years. He lives alone and enjoys gardening and playing with his grandchildren.

Physical Examination

BP 115/76; pulse 86 RR 16
Neck: carotid upstrokes delayed; CVP 6 cm H_2O
Chest: scattered wheezes
Cor: 3/6 late-peaking SEM
Ext: no edema. Absent pulses L foot

Lab Exam

FEV_{1sec}: 70% predicted
HB: 13 g/dL
Creatinine: 2.1 mg/dL
HB a1c: 6.1%
Echocardiogram: EF 55%; moderate LVH; peak jet velocity: 4.5 m/s. Mean gradient 48 mmHg AVA 0.7 cm^2; est RV systolic pressure 30 mmHg.

Q11. As a member of the heart team you would recommend
(A) SAVR
(B) TAVR
(C) Guideline-directed heart failure therapy
(D) Hospice care

He was discharged to home after an uneventful 4 day hospital course, receiving aspirin, clopidogrel, and insulin. His dyspnea improved dramatically over the next 2 months and his exercise tolerance improved to the level it had been 3 years previously. However over the next 3 months his dyspnea again worsened such that his exercise tolerance was reduced to that just prior to TAVR.

Physical Exam

BP 110/70; pulse 90; RR 14
Neck: carotid upstrokes delayed; CVP: 7 cm H_2O
Chest: clear
Cor: 3/6 late peaking SEM
Ext: +1 edema

Q12. You now:
(A) Suspect worsening COPD and begin a course of prednisone and bronchodilators.
(B) Suspect a cardiomyopathy and begin heart failure therapy.
(C) Suspect TAVR leaflet thrombosis and order a cardiac CT and echocardiogram.
(D) Suspect depression, reassure the patient and begin an SSRI.

Q13. An echocardiogram finds a transvalvular gradient of 40 mmHg and the CT scan finds TAVR leaflet thickening. You now recommend:
(A) Watchful waiting
(B) Urgent surgery
(C) Valve-in-valve TAVR
(D) Warfarin anticoagulation

Case 6

A 71 y/o woman presents with progressive fatigue and dyspnea on exertion. Her symptoms began about 2 months ago and have progressed such that she is unable to perform household chores such as vacuuming. Her dyspnea is associated with chest tightness that abates with rest. She denies orthopnea, PND, or syncope. She notes occasional blood in her stools.

Physical Examination

BP 110/62. Pulse 94
HEENT: conjunctival pallor without petechiae
Neck: carotid upstrokes delayed
Chest: clear
Cor: 3/6 SEM; 2/6 diastolic blowing murmur LUSB
Ext no edema
Rectal: +for occult blood

Lab Exam

Hb: 5 g/dL; MCV 65 fL
Serum Fe: 12 mcg/dL; ferritin 24 ng/mL
Creatinine 1.3 mg/dL BUN 13 mg/dL
Echocardiogram: EF 60%. Mild LVH; peak jet velocity: 4.7 m/s. Mean gradient 50 mmHg moderate aortic insufficiency; AVA 0.9 cm^2
Colonoscopy reveals multiple A-V malformations

Q14. Which is probably **not** true?
(A) Anemia may be creating a high output state leading to overestimation of AVA by jet velocity
(B) The aortic insufficiency alters the management of aortic stenosis
(C) She has acquired von Willebrand disease
(D) She should have a repeat echo after transfusion to better assess the severity of her valve disease

The patient's von Willebrand factor is 40% of normal. After 3 units of packed RBCs her Hb is 8 g/dL. Repeat echo finds a slightly reduced jet velocity 4.5 m/s.

Left heart catheterization finds a severe proximal complex LAD lesion.

Q15. She should:
(A) Have resection of her A-V malformations
(B) Undergo TAVR and coronary intervention
(C) Undergo SAVR and internal mammary artery bypass to LAD
(D) Have a trial of medical therapy for angina and heart failure

Case 7

This 39 y/o woman seeks a second opinion regarding her valve disease. She is an active professional whose passion is running marathon races. She notes that in her last competition, 3 months ago, she ran her best time ever, breaking the 4 h mark at 3:56:23. She has known of a heart murmur since childhood. Serial echocardiograms performed elsewhere found:

	Velocity (m/s)	Mean gradient (mmHg)	AVA (cm^2)	LV thickness (mm)
2010	2.6	14	1.7	9
2012	2.8	18	1.6	9
2014	3.0	24	1.4	9
2015	3.2	28	1.3	10
2016	3.5	33	1.2	11
NOW	3.7	37	1.1	11.5

Physical Examination

BP 110/64; pulse 54
Neck: carotid upstrokes mildly delayed. CVP 5 cm H_2O
Chest: clear
Cor: 3/6 Mid-late peaking SEM
Ext: no edema

Q16. The following are reasonable except:
(A) Continue running until data indicate "severe" AS
(B) No therapy but stop running
(C) Standard SAVR
(D) The Ross procedure

She indicates that cessation of marathon running is unacceptable to her and she wishes to proceed with valve replacement therapy. She wishes advice on the risks and benefits of various valve replacement strategies.

Q17. For mechanical vs. heterograft bioprostheses valves you advise that:
(A) Survival is better for mechanical valves compared to bioprostheses.
(B) Bleeding risk is higher for mechanical valves
(C) Valve deterioration is more likely for bioprostheses
(D) TAVR valve in valve will prolong life if the bioprosthesis fails
(E) A, B, and C
(F) All the above

Q18. The patient requests more information regarding homograft valves and the Ross procedure as she does not want to pursue lifelong warfarin therapy. You advise that:
(A) Homografts are more durable than heterografts
(B) The Ross procedure is inferior to homograft implantation
(C) Neither A or B

Case 8

The patient is a 50 y/o man who works in an office and has little time for exercise. He denies dyspnea on exertion, orthopnea, PND, angina, syncope, or edema. He was told of a heart murmur by his primary care giver and is referred for further evaluation. He denies hypertension, smoking, or diabetes.

Physical Examination

BP 110/76; pulse 80

Neck: carotid upstrokes normal; CVP 5 cm H_2O

Chest: clear

Cor: PMI displaced downward and to the left; 3/6 holosystolic apical murmur. S3

Ext: no edema

Echocardiogram: Enlarged LV and LA. EF 60%; end systolic dimension 38 mm. est RV systolic pressure: 30 mmHg. There is a flail P2 mitral leaflet and severe mitral regurgitation (MR) with systolic pulmonary vein flow reversal.

Q19. Sound management strategies include all **except:**
- (A) Referral for mitral repair to a center of repair excellence
- (B) Obtaining and BNP level and exercise test
- (C) Conservative "watchful waiting" with follow-up in 2 years
- (D) Referral for mitral valve replacement
- (E) C&D

Case 9

A 76 y/o man is seen for evaluation of heart failure. He suffered an anterior myocardial infarction 4 years previously for which he delayed seeking medical attention for several hours. An echocardiogram obtained 2 years ago found akinesis of the LV apex and anterior wall with an EF of 30%. He noted that over the past several weeks that he has become progressively more dyspneic, now unable to walk 30 ft to get the newspaper each morning. He now sleeps on 3 pillows instead of his usual 2. He denies chest pain or syncope but developed ankle edema about 2 weeks ago.

Current Medications

Furosemide 80 mg daily

Lisinopril 10 mg daily

Physical Examination

BP 130/72; pulse 80

Est CVP 12 cm H_2O

Chest: bibasilar rales

Cor: S3; 1/6 holosystolic apical murmur

Ext: +2 ankle edema

BNP: 845 ng/mL

Creatinine: 1.1 mg/dL

Echocardiogram: Moderate LV and LA enlargement. Anterior and apical akinesis with wall thinning in those regions. EF 25%. Est RV systolic pressure: 55 mmHg. Severe MR with both leaflets tethered, a central jet and ERO 0.4 cm^2.

Q20. A true statement regarding this patient is
- (A) Mitral surgery will prolong his life.
- (B) Mitral repair is favored over mitral valve replacement
- (C) He should undergo exercise testing to further define his pulmonary hypertension
- (D) Surgery is preferred over medical therapy.
- (E) His medical therapy should be up-titrated.

Case 10

The patient is a 42 y/o man seen by his primary care provider for general malaise and back pain. He has known of a heart murmur for several years but was told it was an "innocent" murmur. His physical activity has never been limited by heart disease and he worked out at a local gym nearly daily without difficulty until recently. He underwent routine teeth cleaning about 2 months ago. Over the past month he has noted a gradual decline in his health. He has become fatigued and noted occasional night sweats, anorexia and a 10 lb. weight loss. He is unable to work out at the gym where his activity is limited both by fatigue and dyspnea. He denies orthopnea, PND, syncope, angina, or edema. He denies intravenous drug use.

Physical Examination

BP 130/80; pulse 100; T 100.8 °F. RR 16

Skin: petechiae anterior chest

HEENT: conjunctival petechiae

Chest: clear

Cor: S1, S2 normal; 2/6 SEM radiating to the neck

Abd: soft non-tender; no organomegaly

Back: no flank or spinal tenderness

Lab Exam

Hb: 10.9 g/dL
WBCs: 11,600/μL; 85% neutrophils
Creatinine: 1.0 mg/dL
Echocardiogram: LV volume normal. EF 65%. Bicuspid aortic valve with mild leaflet restriction. Mean gradient 10 mmHg; 5 × 7 mm vegetation, non-coronary cusp.
4 of 4 blood cultures are + for Viridans group Streptococcus.

Q21. Which of the following is/are true?
(A) He should have received antibiotic prophylaxis for his dental procedure.
(B) He requires urgent aortic valve replacement.
(C) Back pain is an uncommon presenting symptom in infective endocarditis IE).
(D) Cardiac surgery and infectious disease should be consulted.

Case 11

A 28 y/o man presents to the emergency department with fever and malaise. He uses IV heroin regularly. Two weeks ago, he began noting chills and fever which he thought represented the "flu." Persistence of the symptoms caused him to seek medical attention. He notes fatigue and poor appetite but denies dyspnea, orthopnea, PND, angina, or edema.

Physical Examination

Ill appearing man but in no acute distress
BP 100/60; pulse 110; T 102.0 °F
Skin: Hot to the touch; no petechiae
Neck: CVP: 8 cm H_2O; pronounced v waves
Chest: scattered rales
Cor: S1 normal; 2/6 holosystolic murmur R lower sternal border; 1/6 diastolic blowing murmur, L upper sternal border
Abd: non-pulsatile liver

Lab Exam

Hb: 10 g/dL
WBC: 15,600/μL
Creatinine: 1.5 mg/dL
Blood cultures are drawn and are + for methicillin-resistant Staph aureus.

Echocardiogram: LV normal in size, EF 65%. 10 × 12 mm vegetation, aortic valve, mild aortic insufficiency; 8 × 8 mm vegetation tricuspid valve; moderate tricuspid insufficiency.

Q22. Which of the following statements are true?
(A) He is at moderate risk for vegetation embolization
(B) The risk of embolization is mitigated by antibiotic therapy
(C) He currently has a class I indication for surgery
(D) Early surgical therapy will improve his chance of survival
(E) All of the above

Antibiotic therapy with vancomycin is begun and his fever improves. On the third hospital day he notes difficulty in sleeping the night before due to orthopnea. Physical exam finds:
BP 90/60; pulse 110. RR 22; T 99.6 °F
CVP 8 cm H_2O
Chest bibasilar rales
Cor: soft S1, 1/6 diastolic blowing murmur

Q23. Which statement(s) is/are true
(A) Stat TEE is indicated
(B) A stat surgical consult is indicated
(C) Valve replacement after just 2 days of antibiotics will lead to a high reinfection rate
(D) The best pressor agent to use is norepinephrine
(E) A and B

Case 12

A 60 y/o man is followed for management of aortic insufficiency. He suffered an episode of IE 8 years previously, resulting in an aortic leaflet perforation but was hemodynamically stable at the time and did not undergo surgery. He denies symptoms, leads an active lifestyle, and plays singles tennis two times per week.

Physical Examination

BP 140/60; pulse 71
Neck: bounding carotid pulse. CVP 5 cm H_2O
Chest clear
COR: PMI prominently visible 3 cm L mid-clavicular line
2/6 diastolic rumble LUSB; Apical diastolic rumble
Ext: Quinke's pulse present
Serial echocardiograms: (all show severe AR of tricuspid perforated aortic valve):

	EF (%)	End diastolic dimension (cm)	End systolic dimension (cm)
12/2010	60	6.0	4.0
11/2011	60	6.1	4.1
12/2013	58	6.4	4.3
12/2014	58	6.5	4.4
Now	55	7.0	4.9

Q24. Reasonable options for the patient are
- (A) Begin an ACE inhibitor
- (B) Recommend AVR
- (C) Discuss TAVR options
- (D) Continue to observe his progress
- (E) B, C, and D

Case 13

The patient is a 55 y/o woman of Middle Eastern extraction seen for evaluation of dyspnea on exertion. As a child she was told she had had acute rheumatic fever and suffered from arthritis that kept her out of school for several weeks. Her symptoms eventually resolved and she was well until about 2 years ago when she noted progressive dyspnea while performing household chores. About 2 years ago she began sleeping on two pillows. She denies PND, syncope, hemoptysis, or angina. She complains about frequent palpitation. She notes the recent onset of peripheral edema. She has an 8-year history of insulin-controlled diabetes. She notes controlled hypertension. She suffered a stroke 5 years ago from which she has recovered completely. She was noted to be in sinus rhythm at the time of the stroke.

Physical Examination

BP 123/78; pulse 80 and regular
Neck: CVP 10 cm H_2O
Chest: bilateral rales
Cor; Loud S1; Increased P2, S2 followed by and opening snap 80 ms later, followed by a diastolic rumble
Ext: +2 pitting edema

Lab Exam

Hb: 12.3 g/dL
Creatinine: 3.3 mg/dL
Hb: a1c 7.3%
Echocardiogram: LV EF 55%. Moderate LA enlargement. Mitral valve, thickened, calcified, poorly mobile with mild to moderate MR. Est RV systolic pressure 68 mmHg. Est Wilkins score 10.

Q25. You would recommend:
- (A) A formal exercise tolerance test with echo estimation of RV pressure
- (B) Begin beta blockade
- (C) MVR
- (D) TEE; If no LAA clot, proceed to balloon mitral valvotomy

Case 14

A 45 y/o woman is evaluated for the acute onset of dyspnea. She has had similar self-limited episodes in the past but her current episode has persisted. Between acute episodes she is asymptomatic but lives a sedentary lifestyle and works as a bank teller.

Physical Examination

BP 110/80; pulse 177, irregularly, irregular
Neck: CVP 8 cm H_2O
Chest: bibasilar rales
COR: loud S1; no murmur
Ext: no edema
EKG: AF with rapid ventricular response
Chest X-ray: Double density R heart border

Q26. Proper management calls for:
- (A) Rate control. Anticoagulation with heparin
- (B) Rate control. Anticoagulation with apixaban
- (C) D/C cardioversion. Anticoagulation with dabigatran
- (D) Rate control followed by a loading dose of warfarin.

Case 15

A 60 y/o man is evaluated for dyspnea. He began noting difficulty in keeping pace with his wife on their evening walks about 6 months ago and his exercise tolerance has grown progressively worse since then. He has begun sleeping on two pillows. He denies angina, syncope or edema. He denies diabetes, smoking, or hypertension. An echocardiogram performed 3 years ago to evaluate a heart murmur found severe AR and a preserved EF. He was then lost to follow-up.

Physical Examination

BP: 120/60; pulse 79
Neck: CVP 9 cm H_2O; bounding carotid pulse
Chest: clear
Cor: prominent PMI anterior axillary line; 2/6 long diastolic blowing murmur LUSB; 1/6 apical diastolic rumble
EXT: trace edema
Echocardiogram; Severe AR. End diastolic dimension, 8.0 cm; end systolic dimension 6.8 cm; EF 30%

Q27. You would:
(A) Begin workup for cardiac transplant
(B) Recommend urgent AVR
(C) Begin guideline-directed heart failure therapy
(D) Begin heart failure therapy followed by AVR

Case 16

A 35 y/o man is seen for the recent onset of progressive dyspnea. Three years ago, he received a bileaflet mechanical heart valve for symptomatic unicuspid aortic stenosis. Surgery resulted in resolution of angina, his complaint at the time. Since then he received warfarin 8 mg/day with INR in therapeutic range 60% of the time. However, 3 weeks ago he ran out of his medications and has not had them refilled. His dyspnea has progressed so that he has dyspnea with minimal activity such as going to the bathroom.

Physical Examination

BP 90/70; pulse 102; RR 22
Neck: CVP 11 cm H_2O. Carotid upstrokes weak
Chest: Bibasilar rales
Cor: S1 normal; prosthetic clicks muted. No murmur
EXT: bilateral ankle edema

Lab Exam

INR 1.0
Hb 14 g/dL
Creatinine 1.4 mg/dL

Q28. The patient should undergo:
(A) Transthoracic echocardiography
(B) Transesophageal echocardiography
(C) Fluoroscopy
(D) Cardiac MRI
(E) A and B

TEE finds a 6 × 8 mm thrombus limiting leaflet motion. LV EF 30%. Peak jet velocity: 5.2 m/s.

Q29. Best management is:
(A) Urgent surgery
(B) Thrombolytic therapy
(C) Administration of unfractionated heparin
(D) Administration of low molecular weight heparin

Case 17

The patient is a 71 y/o woman evaluated for progressive dyspnea on exertion. She was told of heart murmur by her primary provider several years ago but was asymptomatic until 6 months ago. Since then she has noted becoming progressively short of breath performing routine housework. She denies syncope, orthopnea, PND, angina, or edema. She has never smoked and denies diabetes and hypertension.

Physical Examination

BP 110/70; Pulse 76 with occasional extra systoles. BMI 21
Neck: carotid upstrokes delayed; CVP 6 cm H_2O
Chest: clear
COR: 2/6 SEM RUSB; Apical systolic murmur. Following the pause after her extra-systoles, both murmurs intensify and the carotid pulse is augmented.

Lab Exam

Hb 14 g/dL
Creatinine 1.8 mg/dL

Q30. Her physical exam is most consistent with:
(A) Obstructive hypertrophic cardiomyopathy
(B) Aortic stenosis with Gallavardin's Phenomenon
(C) Aortic and pulmonic stenosis
(D) Aortic stenosis and mitral regurgitation
(E) Both B and D

Echocardiography finds: a severely calcified aortic, peak jet velocity 3.9 m/s; mean gradient 40 mmHg; AVA 0.9 cm^2. There is mitral prolapse of P2 with moderate MR. LV and LA mildly enlarged.

Q31. Best therapy would be:
(A) TAVR
(B) SAVR
(C) SAVR + mitral repair
(D) SAVR + MVR

Case 18

A 73 y/o man is evaluated for severe mitral regurgitation. The patient has known of a heart murmur for several years but was asymptomatic until 6 months ago when he began experiencing dyspnea playing golf. He carries his golf clubs and began noting dyspnea climbing to an uphill green that, in the past, had not caused him symptoms. He denies orthopnea, PND, angina, syncope, or edema. He is a lifelong nonsmoker and denies diabetes or hypertension.

Physical Examination

BP 118/82; pulse 76

Neck: carotid upstrokes normal; CVP 6 cm H_2O without prominent v waves

Chest: clear

Cor; PMI displaced downward and to the left. 3/6 holosystolic apical murmur

Ext: no edema

Lab Exam

Hb 14.1 g/dL

Creatinine 0.9 mg/dL

Echocardiogram: LV and LA enlargement. EF 60%. LV end systolic dimension 4.0 cm. Severe MR with a flail P2 segment. ERO 0.4 cm^2. Moderate tricuspid regurgitation. Est RV systolic pressure 30 mmHg. RV and RA slightly enlarged. Normal RV systolic function.

Mitral repair is planned.

Q32. Regarding this patient's tricuspid regurgitation:
- (A) Tricuspid surgery is not warranted since his TR will improve with successful mitral repair
- (B) Tricuspid repair will both reduce TR and prolong life
- (C) Tricuspid repair will reduce the risk of worsening TR later in life
- (D) The incidence of tricuspid repair during left-sided surgery has increased over the past decade
- (E) C and D

Case 19

The patient is a 30-year-old man referred for evaluation of a heart murmur. The murmur has been present since birth but he has not seen a health care professional since childhood. He now wishes to begin training for a marathon race and has begun running 4 miles/day. He runs an average 8 min mile without dyspnea. He denies angina, syncope, orthopnea, PND, or edema. Otherwise he is in excellent health and denies diabetes, hypertension, and other systemic illness.

Physical Examination

BP 100/60. Pulse 58

Neck: carotid upstrokes normal. CVP 4 cm H_2O

Chest: clear

COR: LUSB ejection click followed by a 3/6 SEM; Click disappears with inspiration

Ext: no edema

Lab Exam

Echocardiogram: Normal LV, LA, aortic, mitral, and tricuspid valves. There is doming of the pulmonic valve and peak jet velocity of 4.2 m/s.

Q33. You advise:
- (A) Proceed with his marathon training but to alert you if he notices symptoms
- (B) Undergo pulmonic balloon valvotomy
- (C) Undergo surgical pulmonary valve replacement
- (D) Undergo transcatheter pulmonary valve replacement

Case 20

A 40 y/o man is seen for his yearly follow-up visit after pulmonary balloon valvotomy as a child. He denies dyspnea on exertion and works out at a gym three times per week. He denies edema, ascites, orthopnea, PND, or angina. Five years ago he was noted to have moderate to severe pulmonic regurgitation and undergoes yearly cardiac MRI for quantification of RV volume and function.

Physical Examination

BP 110/70; pulse 72

Neck: CVP 8 cm H_2O. Prominent v waves noted

Chest: clear

COR: RV sternal lift. 3/6 long diastolic murmur heard throughout the precordium

EXT: no edema

Lab Exam

Hb: 14.6 g/dL

Creatinine: 1.0 mg/dL

	Serial MRI results				
	RVEDVI	RVESDI	RVEF (%)	RVRF (%)	LVEF (%)
2010	110	50	55	35	60
2012	122	56	54	36	62
2014	145	70	52	36	60
2016	145	70	52	36	60
Now	160	81	49	41	58

Q34. Based on these data:
(A) His regurgitant fraction of only 40% indicates that his PI is less than severe
(B) He should undergo transcatheter pulmonic valve replacement
(C) He should undergo surgical pulmonic valve replacement
(D) Valve replacement will, on average, add 5 years to his lifespan

Answers and Explanations

Q1. The answer is D, severe AS. The sustained PMI indicates that the lesion involves the LV excluding pulmonic stenosis as the murmur source. Although S2 remains split, the delay in the carotid upstrokes and the late peaking quality indicate severe disease.

Q2. The answer is C, severe AS. The ACC/AHA Guidelines [1] classify severe AS as a peak jet velocity of ≥4.0 m/s **OR** a mean gradient of 40 mmHg **OR** AVA of ≤1.0 cm^2. While data support the use of each of these measures in grading severity [2–4], they are often internally inconsistent with each other [5] (Fig. 13.1). He has 2 of the criteria for "severe" AS consistent with his physical exam.

Q3. The answer is E, either continued observation or perform a stress test. A key turning point in the natural history of aortic stenosis is the onset of symptoms, a Class I indication for AVR [1]. Because he appears to be asymptomatic, it would be acceptable to continue to observe him. However, because of the subjective nature of symptoms and the failure of many patients to recognize them, formal exercise testing is commonly employed to help establish symptom presence more objectively [6] and is recommended at a level IIa in the Guidelines.

Q4. The answer is E, either conclude that there is a change in his condition and refer for AVR or repeat the exercise test for more objective data. The report from the patient's spouse, the slight decline in EF and the increase in BNP [7] (Fig. 13.2) could be taken together as an indication that the patient is becoming symptomatic or further proof could be sought from exercise testing. Data are provided to calculate an STS risk score (1.1% mortality risk). Thus the patient does not currently qualify for TAVR although TAVR is likely to be approved for use in low risk patients.

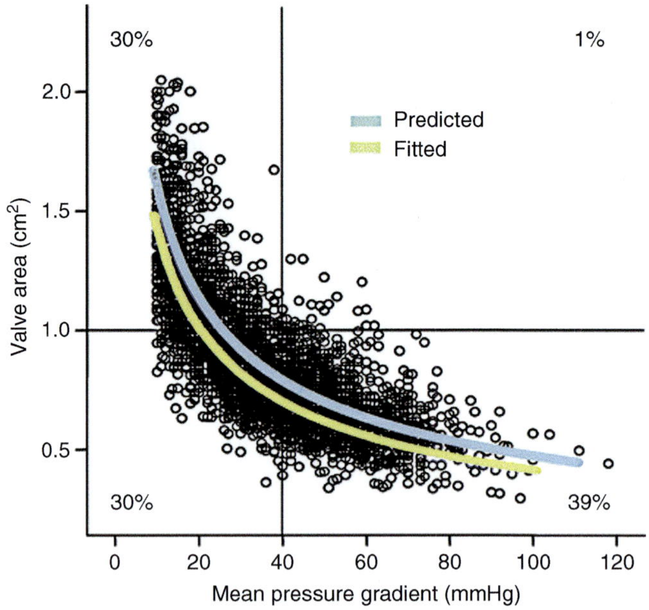

Fig. 13.1 Valve area is plotted against gradient from over 3000 patients as predicted by the Gorlin formula (blue line) and actual echocardiographic AVA (yellow line). Both are close to one another. Importantly, hundreds of patients fail to conform to both AVA and gradient benchmarks for "severe AS." From: Minners J, Allgeier M [5]. Reprinted with permission from Oxford University Press

Q5. The best answer is E, Consider TAVR, balloon valvotomy or hospice. Her STS score combined with obvious frailty [8] put her at prohibitive risk for SAVR. While TAVR would relieve her heart failure it is unclear if she could benefit enough or that her life expectancy would exceed a year so that TAVR could be futile therapy. Balloon valvotomy would be a reasonable choice, using it to gauge improvement in the non-cardiac aspects of her presentation that sometimes does improve with partial relief of AS [9]. This "real-world" case emphasizes the difficulties in decision-making in elderly patients.

Q6. The answer is D, severity unknown. Nearly all of the data presented are discordant. While the valve area suggests severe aortic stenosis, the murmur fails to peak late in systole, the carotid upstrokes are only mildly delayed and the peak jet velocity and gradient suggest only mild to moderate disease.

Q7. The answer is B, inotropic stress testing. Because aortic valve area is flow dependent [10] and because cardiac output is reduced in this patient, it is necessary to recalculate valve area at higher flow [11]. Infusion of an inotrope to increase flow can accomplish two goals. First it can separate true aortic stenosis from aortic pseudo-stenosis. In truly severe AS, increased flow increases gradient in parallel and valve area remains nearly constant [12]. Second, the presence of inotropic reserve helps risk stratify

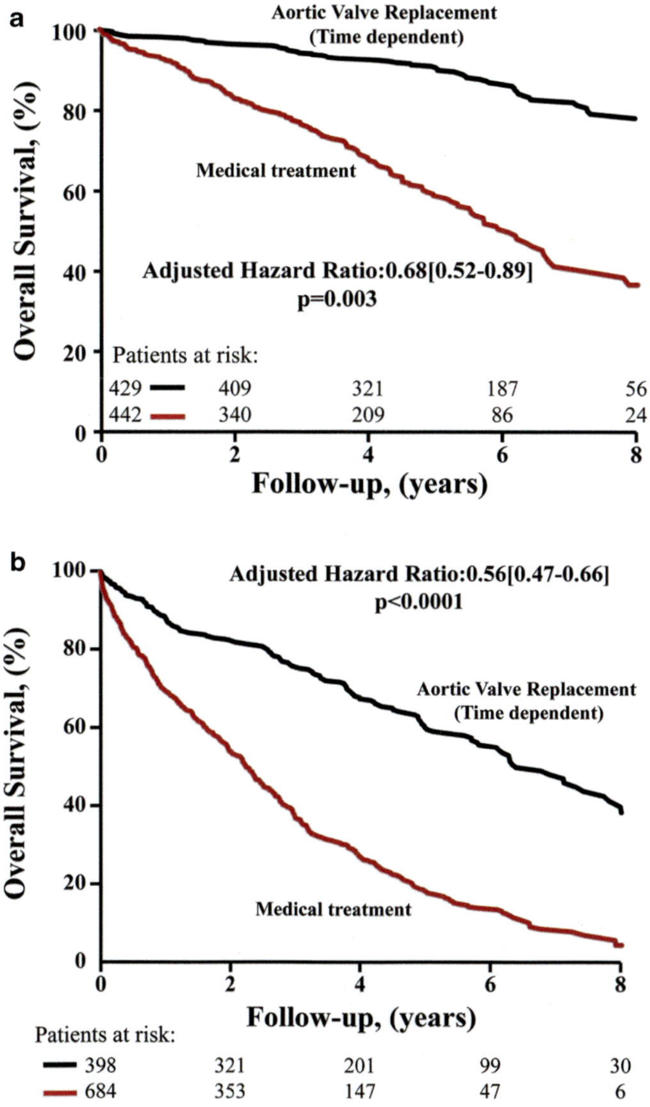

Fig. 13.2 Survival for aortic stenosis patients is plotted against the ratio of the patients' BNP and normal BNP, < than a ratio of 2;1 (black line) or greater than 2:1 (red line). Higher BNP/normal ratios were associated with worse outcomes for both surgically treated (upper panel) or medically treated (lower panel) patients. From: Clavel MA, et al. [7]. Reprinted with permission from Elsevier

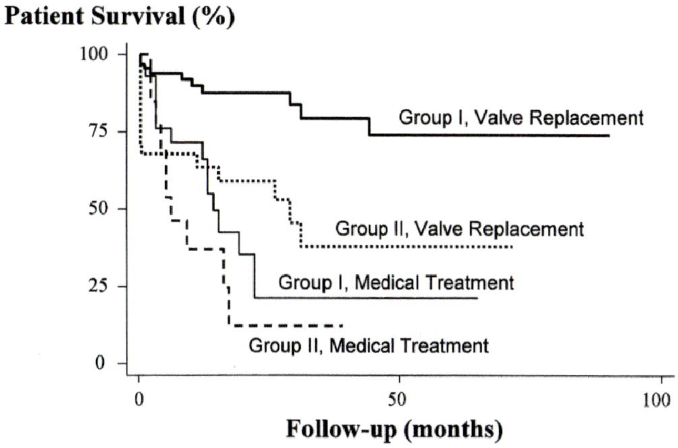

Fig. 13.3 Survival is plotted for AS patients with low ejection fraction for those that had inotropic reserve (group I) vs. those that did not (group II). Patients with inotropic reserve had 1/3 the operative risk and better long-term survival than those that did not. From: Monin JL, et al. [13]. Reprinted with permission from Wolters Kluwer Health, Inc.

patients for surgical aortic valve replacement. Patients that increase stroke volume by ≥20% with dobutamine infusion have 1/3 the operative risk of those who fail to augment [13] (Fig. 13.3). While valve calcium scoring can help distinguish true from aortic pseudo-stenosis [14] it remains preferable that patients generate a peak jet velocity of ≥4.0 m/s to qualify for TAVR and little is known about TAVR patients who fail to do this.

Q8. The answer is A, TAVR. His STS risk score is 5.5 but STS does not take into account this very high-risk group of low gradient, low, EF patients. However, his favorable response to dobutamine makes his risk acceptable and patients in this group have a better outcome with TAVR than with so-called medical therapy [15].

Q9. The answer is E, Calcium scoring and heart catheterization. The assessment of her AS severity is discordant with a physical exam and AVA consistent with severe AS but a jet velocity and gradient consistent with moderate AS. It is likely that she has low flow, low gradient, normal EF (paradoxical) AS [16]. In this condition, there is usually severe concentric LV hypertrophy reducing LV end diastolic volume. As such, a normal ejection fraction from a small volume yields a low stroke volume and thus a low gradient and low jet velocity. It is necessary to confirm the diagnosis of "severe" AS independently of standard echo parameters since they are discordant in this case. Valve calcium density correlates well with valve area and can be used to confirm AVA [17]. Because the EF is already normal, it is not clear what additional data will be garnered from inotropic challenge although dobutamine has been used in some cases. Because the patient has angina and peripheral vascular disease and because coronary disease is present in many patients with AS [18], she will require cardiac catheterization. Invasive hemodynamics during the procedure could help confirm that her AS is truly severe.

Q10. The answer is either A or B, SAVR or TAVR. Her STS risk calculated from the data available is 5.6, putting her at intermediate risk. Current guidelines indicate a IIa indication for TAVR [19–21] (although this will be upgraded to a class I in the future) which would leave her right coronary artery (RCA) unrevascularized. It could be approached percutaneously before or after TAVR or the RCA could be bypassed at the time of

SAVR. It is this kind of case where the heart team is crucial in weighing all the options.

Q11. The answer is B, TAVR. His data allow calculation of an STS risk score of 11.1 making him a high surgical risk. He therefore fulfills a class I indication for TAVR [19, 22, 23]. Heart failure therapy is not applicable to AS patients in general and his activities and life expectancy make hospice inappropriate.

Q12. The answer is C, suspect leaflet thrombosis and order CT and echo. Leaflet thrombosis occurs at varying intervals following both SAVR and TAVR but is more common with TAVR [24, 25] (Fig. 13.4). Both balloon expandable and self-expanding types of TAVR are affected. Up to 13% of TAVR patients show leaflet thickening and restricted motion on CT scan. In the majority of cases the finding is subclinical without a significant transvalvular gradient developing. However about 15% of patients with leaflet thickening have a gradient of ≥20 mmHg.

Q13. The answer is D, anticoagulation. Although no randomized trials are available, patients receiving anticoagulation had a much lower incidence of leaflet thrombosis

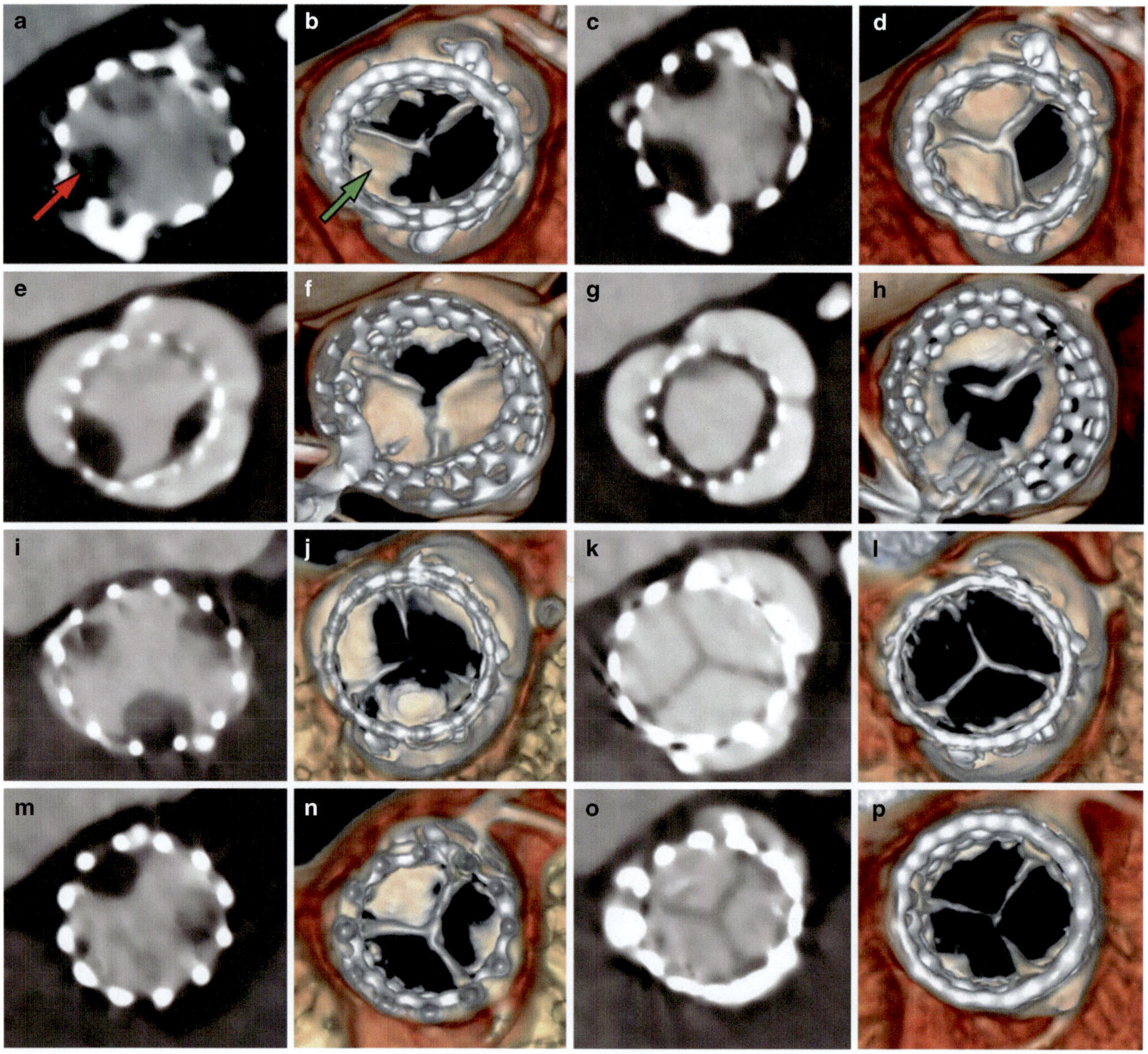

Fig. 13.4 Effect of dual antiplatelet therapy versus anticoagulation on hypoattenuating opacities and reduced leaflet motion. (**a–d**) Reduced leaflet motion at baseline, noted to have worsening hypoattenuating opacities and reduced leaflet motion with follow-up CT in a patient receiving dual antiplatelet therapy after transcatheter aortic valve replacement. Resolution of hypoattenuating opacities and restoration of normal leaflet motion with 3 months of anticoagulation with (**e–h**) warfarin, (**i–l**) rivaroxaban, and (**m–p**) apixaban. The red arrow indicates hypoattenuating opacities and the green arrow represents reduced leaflet mobility. From Chakravarty T, et al. [25]. Reprinted with permission from Elsevier

than did patients receiving aspirin and clopidogrel. Further, most patients resolved leaflet thickening once placed on anticoagulation with either warfarin or newer non-vitamin K antagonist anticoagulants [24, 25].

Q14. The answer is B. The natural history of mixed aortic valve disease is the same as it is for pure AS unless there is very severe aortic insufficiency (AI) and only mild AS [26] (Fig. 13.5). While the AI may increase the total stroke volume and thus increase the gradient, it is the total pressure load on the LV that directs the natural history of the disease not simply the valve area. Gastrointestinal bleeding in AS in often caused or worsened by shear stress at the stenotic valve that degrades von Willebrand factor (vwf) [27].

Q15. The answer is C, SAVR and bypass. Restoration of relatively normal valve architecture with either SAVR or TAVR substantially reduces GI bleeding while restoring vwf [27, 28]. Resection of AV malformations is rarely adequate or successful. Her STS risk is calculated as 1.5 by the data given and arterial bypass + SAVR is the most logical choice that would correct her symptoms. While there may be some concern for GI bleeding during anticoagulation for extracorporeal circulation, this concern is outweighed by the need to revascularize her LAD. She does in fact have severe symptomatic AS so that medical therapy is inappropriate.

Q16. The answer is A, continue running. Her AS nearly meets criteria for severe AS but even if it were considered moderate, recent guidelines counsel against long

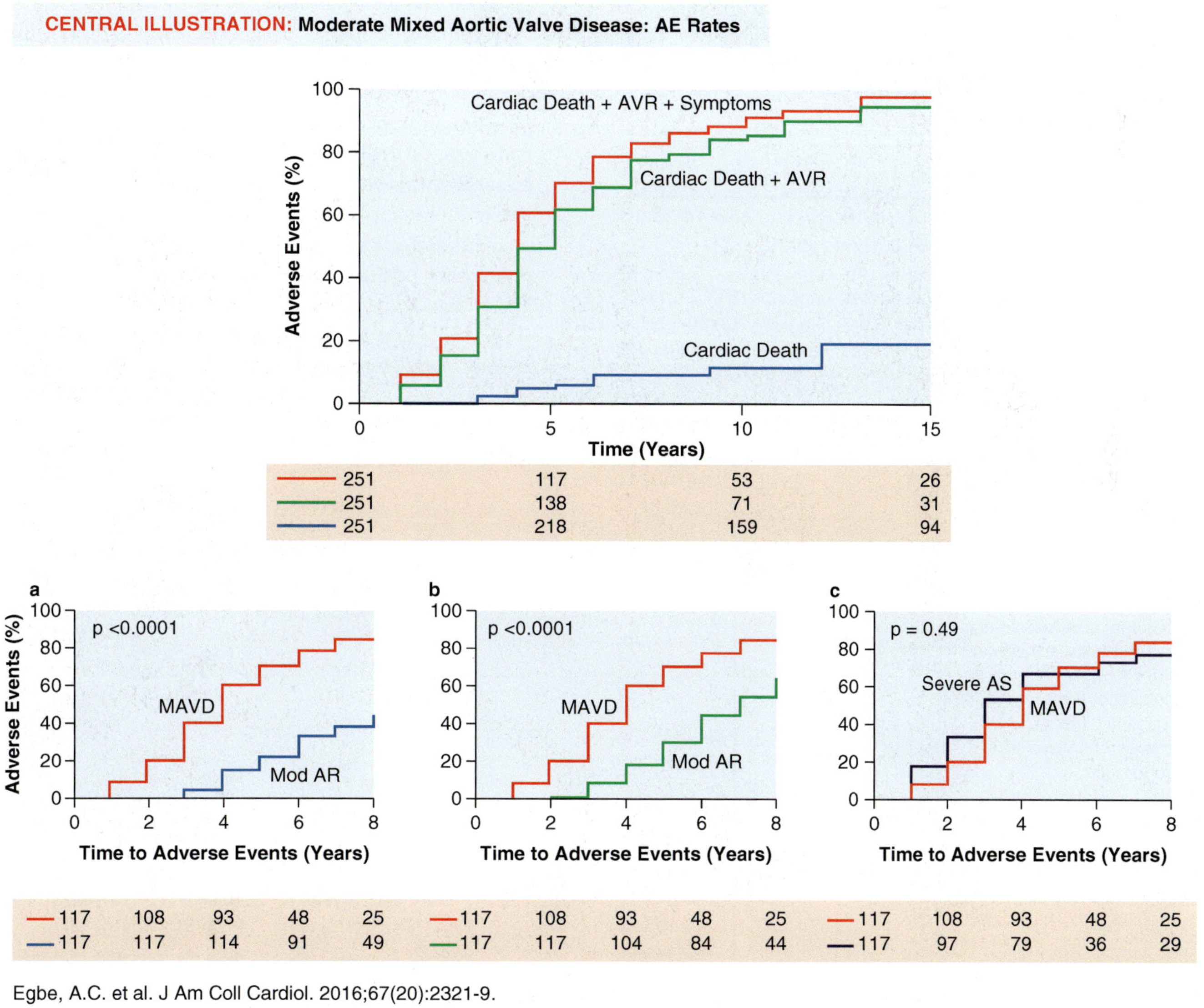

Fig. 13.5 Survival and adverse events are plotted for patients with mixed aortic valve disease (MAVD) (upper panel) and for moderate aortic regurgitation (AR), moderate aortic stenosis (AS) and severe AS. Mixed disease had the same natural history as severe aortic stenosis. From Egbe AC, et al. [26]. Reprinted with permission from Elsevier

distance running for competitive athletes [29]. While the definition of "competitive" is controversial it is clear that she has an aggressive approach to her sport and is unlikely to heed advice to stop in any case. Further her longitudinal data indicate steady, almost predictable progression of her AS making her a candidate for valve replacement class IIb [1].

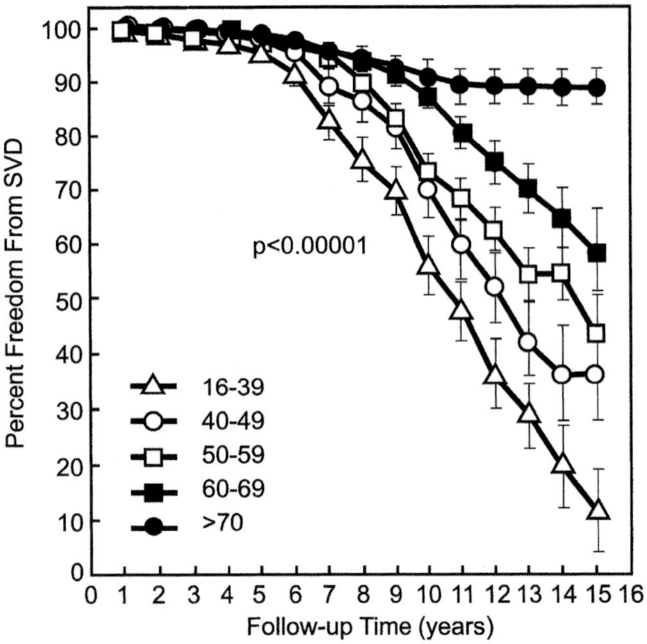

Fig. 13.6 Freedom from structural valve deterioration (SVD) for bioprostheses at patient age of implantation is shown. The earlier the age at implantation, the more rapid is SVD. From Hung L, Rahimtoola SH [32]. Reprinted with permission from Wolters Kluwer Health, Inc.

Q17. The answer is E: A, B, and C. Existing data indicated significantly longer survival with a mechanical valve than with a heterograft despite the higher risk of bleeding in a woman her age [30, 31]. The likelihood of structural valve deterioration with a bioprosthesis increases inversely with the age of the patient at implantation so the patient has a >50% chance of requiring valve re-replacement during her lifetime [32] (Fig. 13.6). Placing a TAVR valve inside a failed bioprosthesis is accepted practice for treating patients at high risk for reoperation. However, the durability of this procedure in young patients is unclear. Further if the initial prosthesis is small in size resulting in a valve-in-valve TAVR gradient >20 Hg, survival is reduced [33]. Thus it is impossible to know the effect of V-I-V TAVR on survival.

Q18. C, originally touted as a superior bioprosthesis, the homograft has fallen into relative disuse. Its durability does not appear superior to heterografts [34] and lack of availability of all sizes, more difficult implantation and more difficult reoperation if needed) have led to less use of this valve. The Ross operation in which the native pulmonary valve is transplanted into the aortic position and a homograft is placed in the low pressure pulmonary position remains controversial. In experienced hands it is superior to the homograft [34] (Fig. 13.7) and provides survival equal to that of a normal population in the first 2 decades after surgery

Fig. 13.7 Survival for a normal population, (black line), patients randomized to receive an aortic homograft (dotted line) vs. and autograft (Ross procedure, solid green line) is shown. Survival after the Ross procedure is similar to that of normal subjects and superior to that of homograft implantation. From El-Hamamsy I, et al. [34]. Reprinted with permission from Elsevier

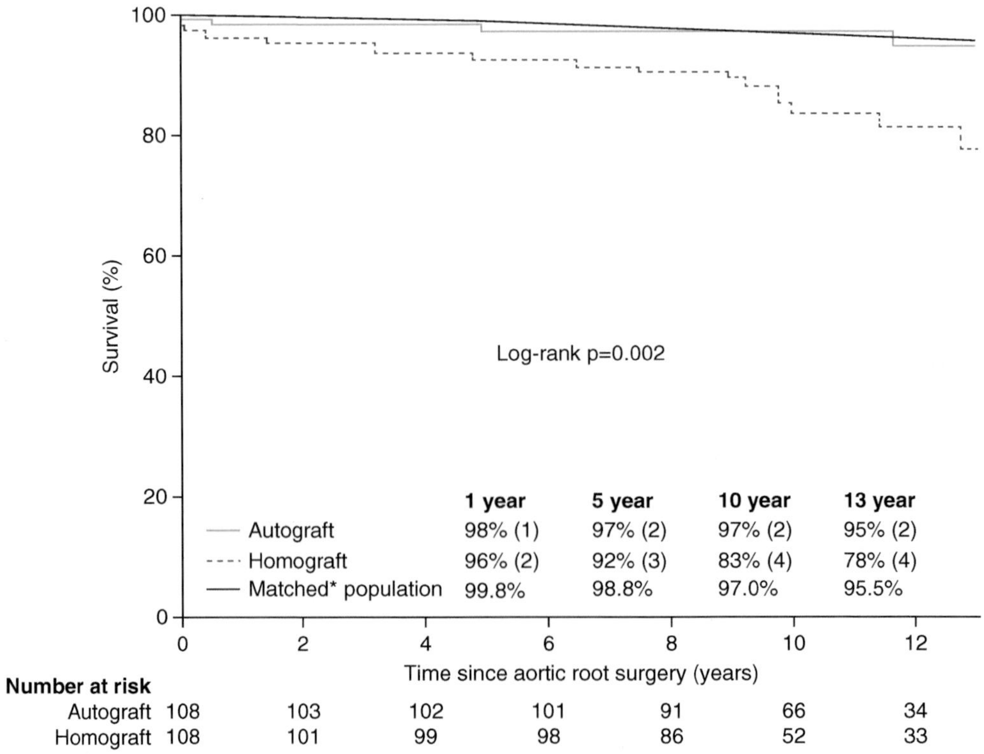

[34–36] but afterwards may show evidence of deterioration [35]. It may be an excellent operation for this young patient who wishes to avoid anticoagulation with warfarin.

Q19. The answer E, either continued observation for 2 years or referral for replacement. The patient has severe mitral regurgitation (MR) by all the data given. The natural history of MR is one of fairly rapid progression where patients with severe disease reach a trigger point for surgery at the rate of 8%/year [37] (Fig. 13.8) so that 2 years is too long for a follow-up visit. If this apparently asymptomatic patient is to have surgery mitral valve repair which should be accomplished by an experienced surgeon is safer and with better outcomes than replacement [38] (Fig. 13.9) such that replacement should not be contemplated at this point. The presence of symptoms forms an important turning point in the natural history of the disease [39] (Fig. 13.10). However the subjective nature of symptoms makes them an imperfect benchmark. Thus echocardiography, exercise testing, and biomarkers can be helpful in adding objective evidence of cardiac decompensation [40–43]. Triggers for mitral surgery based upon outcome data are the onset of symptoms [39] an ejection fraction falling toward 60% [40] ("normal" in MR is 65–70%) and an end systolic dimension increasing toward 40 mm [41]. Because our patient is already approaching those triggers, it is reasonable to refer the patient for mitral repair now instead of waiting for further deterioration [19].

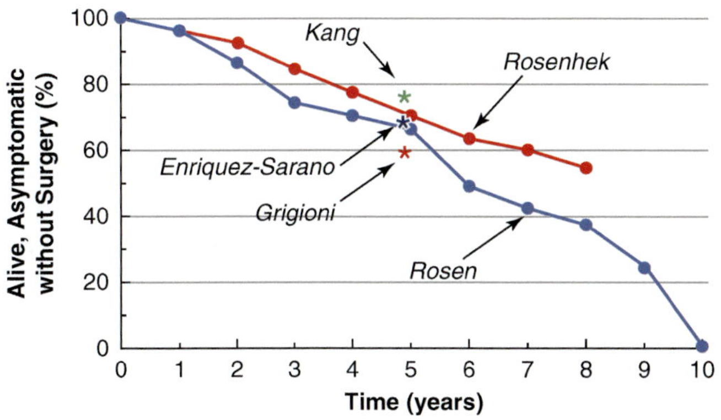

Fig. 13.8 The natural history of severe mitral regurgitation (complied by several authors, named on the graph) is shown. The pattern is remarkably concordant and shows that the per cent of patients alive, asymptomatic without surgery declines at a rate of about 8%/year. From Bonow RO [37]. Reprinted with permission from Elsevier

Q20. The answer is E, medical therapy should be up-titrated. The patient has secondary MR. It has been caused by tethering of the valve leaflets due to LV dilatation from his previous myocardial infarction (MI). His LV function is depressed from the MI and while MR is probably worsening his condition, the MR is a secondary problem and correcting it will not correct the underlying MI. As such there is no convincing evidence that surgical treatment of his MR will prolong his life [44–46]. While mitral repair is unquestionably the treatment of choice for primary MR, there is no proven benefit to surgical repair over replacement for secondary MR [46] (Fig. 13.11). This difference lies in the fact that in secondary MR the valve itself is normal. As such "repairs" include restrictive annuloplasty in an attempt to increase coaptation, an effort that often fails within a few months after surgery. Exercise testing would not add much to what we already know about his right-sided pressures. Medical therapy aggressively treating with ACE inhibitors (or ARBs) beta-blockers, mineralocorticoid antagonists and diuretics can lead to striking improvement and is first line therapy [47]. However in many cases (as this one) medical therapy is

Fig. 13.9 Survival of a normal population (gray line), MR patients undergoing mitral repair (black line) and those undergoing mitral replacement (dotted line) is shown. Survival after repair is similar to a normal population and superior to mitral valve replacement. From Vassileva CM, et al. [38]. Reprinted with permission from Wolters Kluwer Health, Inc.

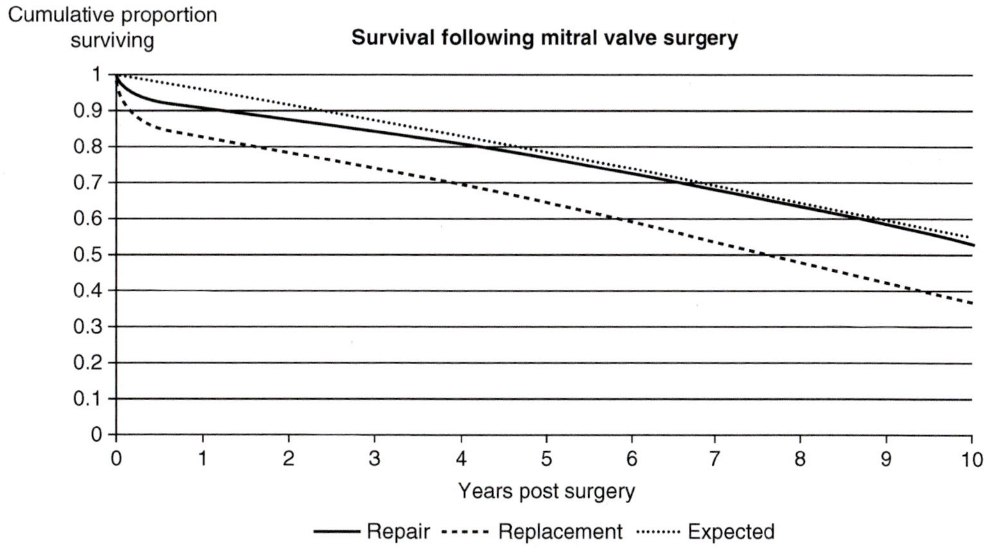

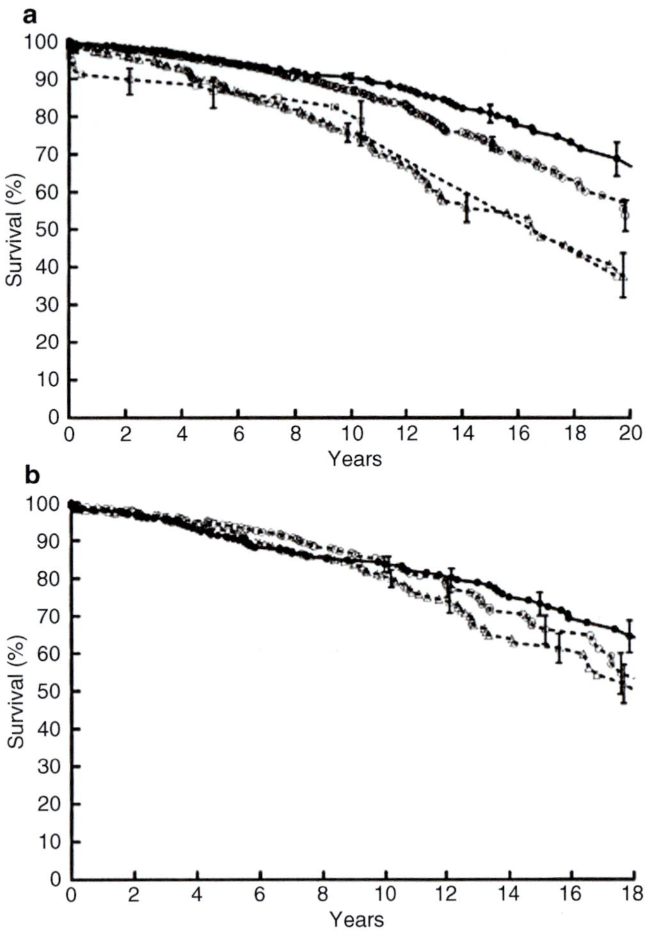

Fig. 13.10 Raw survival (**a**) and risk-adjusted survival (**b**) is shown for asymptomatic patients (closed circles), patients with Class II symptoms (open circles) and patients with Class III/IV symptoms (triangles). The presence of even mild symptoms had a negative effect on long term survival. From Gillinov AM, et al. [39]. Reprinted with permission from Elsevier

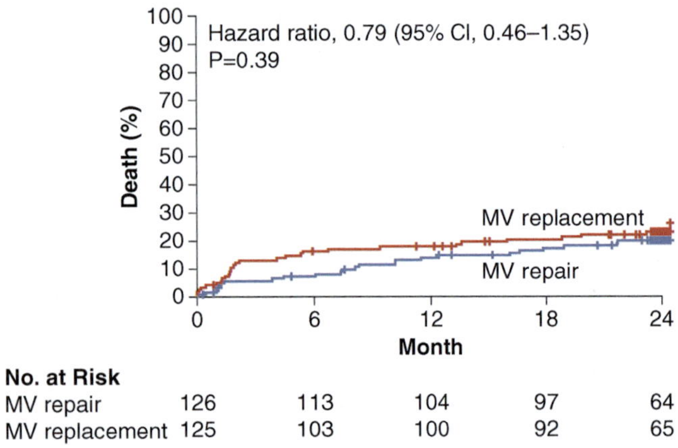

Fig. 13.11 Two year outcome is presented for patients with ischemic secondary MR undergoing mitral repair vs. replacement. There was no difference in survival which was poor with a 10%/year mortality. From Goldstein D, et al. [46]. Reprinted with permission from Massachusetts Medical Society

not aggressive enough. If medical therapy fails to achieve symptomatic improvement, surgery or percutaneous mitral repair may then be employed [19].

Q21. The answer is D, cardiac surgery and infectious disease should be consulted. Because of the wide variety of complex issues facing the patient with IE, such patients should be cared for by a heart team consisting of general cardiologists, imagers, cardiac surgeons and infectious disease specialists [1]. Arthritic complaints, especially back pain, are common in IE [48]. Because bacteremia occurs daily with eating and because of uncertainty that antibiotic prophylaxis is effective in preventing IE, prophylaxis is now only recommended for the highest risk patients undergoing dental procedures that involve gingival manipulation. These include patients with prosthetic heart valves, cardiac transplant patients, patients who have suffered a previous episode of IE, patients with uncorrected cyanotic congenital heart disease, and patients with corrected congenital heart disease where correction was afforded by use of prosthetic material or devices [1]. Our patient had none of these indications. While surgery for IE is occurring more liberally and earlier in the course of the disease, our patient has none of the current indications for surgery: (1) hemodynamic compromise; (2) multiple recurrent emboli; and (3) little likelihood of bacteriologic cure without surgery.

Q22. The answer is E. The aortic vegetation is of moderate size and has an approximately 15% risk of embolization [49]. However the risk of embolization diminishes once antibiotics are begun [49, 50]. The current class I indications for surgery in IE are hemodynamic instability, inability to affect a cure with antibiotics and infection with highly resistant organism including S aureus [1]. Although there are no large randomized trials, existing evidence indicates improved survival for early surgery especially in cases of S aureus infection [51, 52].

Q23. The answer is E. The patient has decompensated and manifests heart failure. The reduction in the intensity of S1 likely indicates either prolongation or the PR interval due to invasion of the conduction system and ring abscess formation, or pre-closure of the mitral valve due to severe aortic insufficiency. Because TEE is much more sensitive in diagnosing sub-aortic extension, it is indicated here [53]. The patient's rapid deterioration is an indication for surgery especially if there is now acute severe aortic insufficiency [54, 55]. While there is always concern about reinfection of newly implanted valves, the risk of reinfection is only 5–10%, low compared to the high risk of delay [54]. Pressor agents in general are poorly tolerated in acute AI. Vasoconstrictors increase AI severity without improving cardiac output.

Q24. The best answer is E. The patient has severe AI. While there was initial enthusiasm for the use of ACE inhibitors in the treatment of AI [56], a subsequent study found no benefit [57], leaving the issue unresolved. While the patient might be administered as ACE inhibitor there is little solid evidence benefit. Current guidelines [1] indicate symptoms [58] or an EF ≤50% or an end systolic dimension of 5.0–5.5 cm are triggers for AVR. However they also make provision for AVR if there is a progressive increase in cardiac size as our patient has. Additionally, a recent report suggests that these benchmarks cause us to operate too late on patients with chronic AI and that an end systolic dimension of 4.0–4.5 might be more appropriate [59]. Thus a recommendation of AVR now is reasonable. However while TAVR currently is reserved for AS patients wherein the calcified aortic annulus is used to secure the valve, newer valves [60] are apt for patients with AR and might become available before he reaches a trigger for AVR. Thus continued observation would also be reasonable.

Q25. The best answer is D, proceed to MBV. There would be little to be gained by exercise testing since she is already symptomatic and has pulmonary hypertension at rest. While beta blockade can occasionally be beneficial by reducing the transmitral gradient, it rarely improves exercise tolerance, and would be unlikely to help her class III symptoms [61]. Her STS risk score from the data presented is 8.5, a high surgical risk. Although her valve anatomy is sub-optimal for balloon valvotomy (BMV) [62] the Wilkins score is a relative one and does not preclude the procedure. It is reasonable to attempt BMV. If there is no clinical improvement, high-risk MVR could be addressed.

Q26. The answer is A, rate control; anticoagulation with heparin. By physical exam and chest x ray the patient has mitral stenosis (although her heart rate was too fast to be able to hear a murmur) and thus valvular atrial fibrillation (AF). This term has led to some confusion but is defined in current guidelines as having rheumatic mitral stenosis or a mechanical heart valve [1, 19]. Thus a patient with calcific AS and AF would not be considered to have valvular AF. Because of an extraordinary risk of systemic embolism in mitral stenosis patients with AF, aggressive anticoagulation is warranted [63]. A trial of dabigatran failed to offer protection equal to that of warfarin for mechanical heart valves; thus non-vitamin K antagonists are not used in valvular AF [64]. A loading dose of warfarin might make patients temporarily hypercoagulable by lowering levels of proteins S and C, although this may be more of hypothetical than actual concern [65]. Following rate control, warfarin is begun in tandem with heparin until an INR of 2.5–3.5 is reached.

Q27. The answer is D. Although the patient has far-advanced LV dysfunction from AR and prognosis is impaired there are several reasons for optimism. His LV dysfunction is probably relatively short lived because it was normal 3 years prior to the current presentation. The shorter the period of LV dysfunction, the better is the chance for recovery [66] (Fig. 13.12). Indeed patients with ejection fraction as low as 20% may have a better outcome with AVR than without it [67]. Further his STS risk from the data presented is only 1%. Finally he has heart failure and AR patients respond well to heart failure therapy. Even beta blockade which will prolong diastole, possibly worsening AR, may improve function in AR patients with heart failure [68]. Thus a short course of heart failure therapy followed by AVR seems reasonable.

Q28. The answer is E. TTE will allow for estimation of overall cardiac function and that valve thrombosis is present while TEE will better assess valve function and will also better assess clot burden [69, 70]. While fluoroscopy can assess leaflet motion and can be a

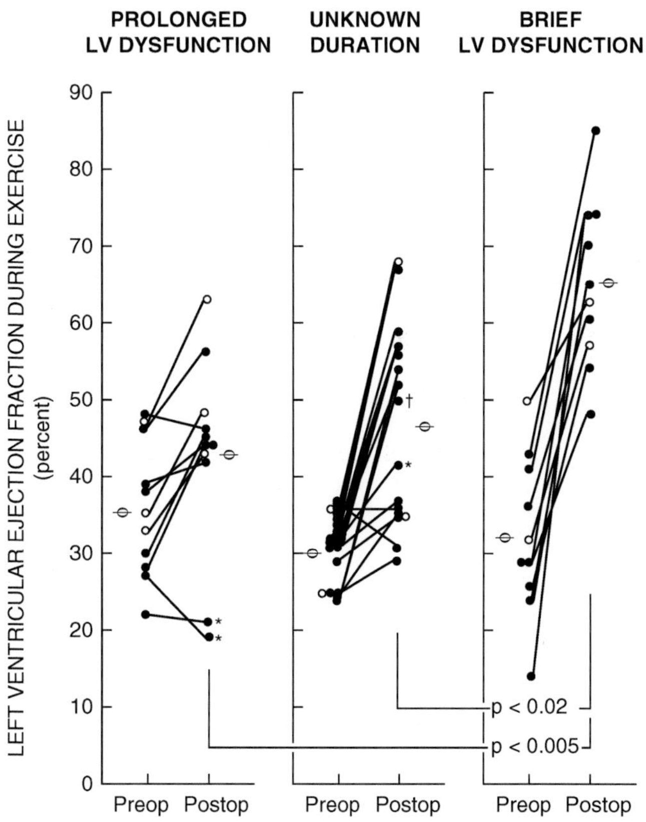

Fig. 13.12 Change in ejection fraction is shown for aortic insufficiency patients with LV dysfunction according to whether dysfunction was present for greater than or less than 18 months. Even severe LV dysfunction improved if it was present for a short period of time. From Bonow RO, et al. [66]. Reprinted with permission from Wolters Kluwer Health, Inc.

"quick" guide to the diagnosis, its diagnostic ability is limited compared to echocardiography.

Q29. The answer is A, surgery. While the clot burden is small, reducing the risk of thrombolytic-related embolization, the patient's advanced symptomatic status and obvious hemodynamic instability militate toward urgent surgery [1, 71, 72], where surgery has produced fewer embolic complications and better survival than thrombolytic therapy. Some have advocated for thrombolysis [73] in this circumstance. However if that therapy fails it obviously complicates bleeding potential for urgent surgery.

Q30. The answer is E, either Gallavardin's phenomenon or combined AS and MR. Following a long pause the murmur of AS is augmented by increased stroke volume due to increased LV filling and also increased contractility from altered calcium release. While these phenomena both also occur in MR, the longer filling time also allows for decrease in aortic pressure such the LV contracts against lower afterload and the murmur does not intensify. However in AS, the lower aortic pressure following the pause might not reduce afterload very much because much of the load is predicated on the AS. Thus augmentation of the murmur following a long pause in AS could be to apical radiation (Gallavardin's phenomenon) or the combination of AS + MR. That the carotid pulse augments following the pause occurs is AS but not hypertrophic cardiomyopathy where the pause would augment obstruction to outflow and weaken the pulse.

Q31. The answer is C. SAVR + mitral repair. While it may be hoped that MR severity will decrease after AVR reduces LV afterload, allowing preferential flow into the aorta and away from the mitral valve, this response is inconsistent [74] (Fig. 13.13). Mitral regurgitation most often fails to improve when there is anatomic mitral disease and a relatively low aortic gradient as is the case here. Her STS risk is 3.1, higher than average but not severe. Thus surgery, where both of her valve diseases can be treated, is preferable.

Q32. The answer is E. The fate of TR following successful left-sided surgery is remarkably uncertain. While it

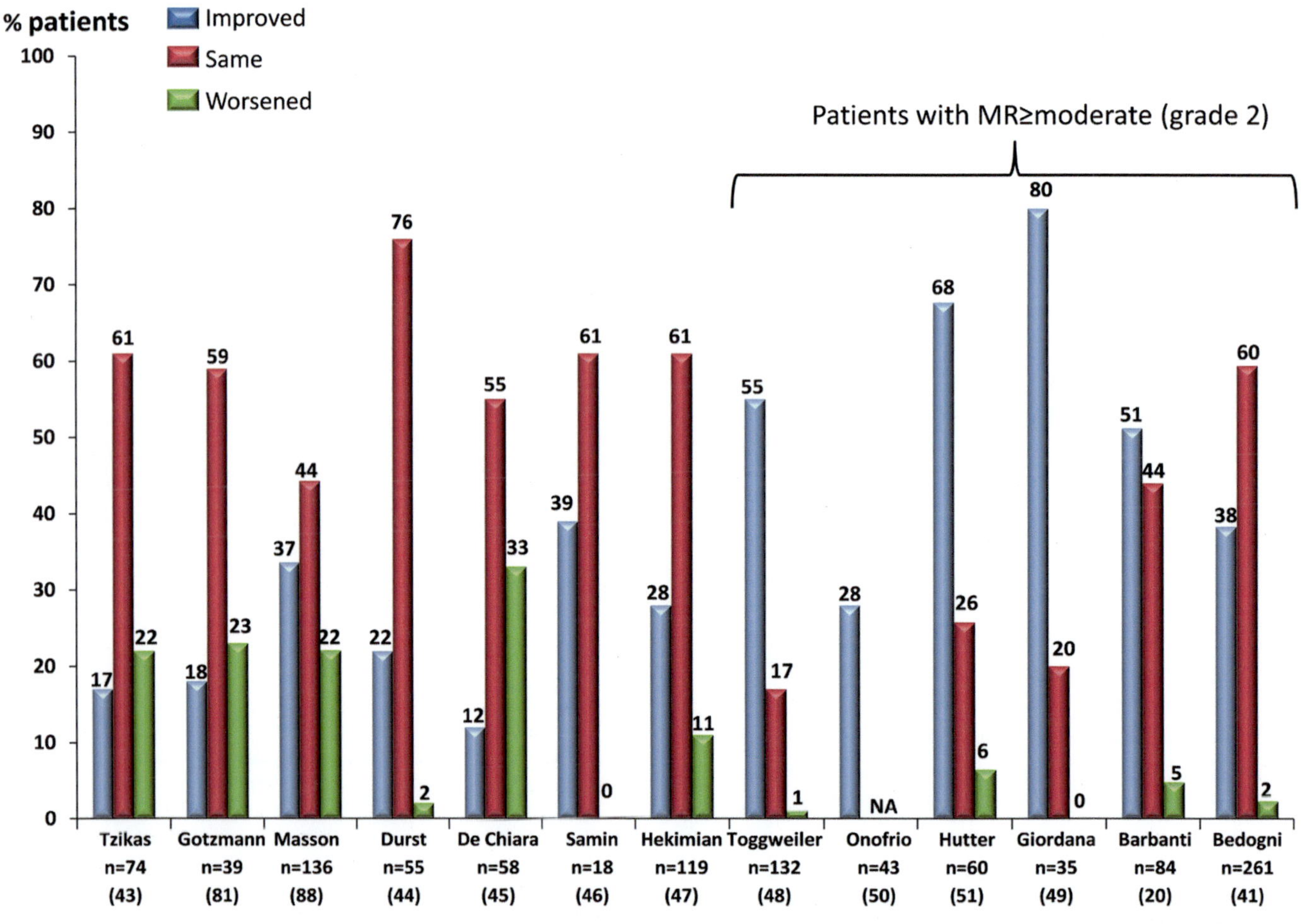

Fig. 13.13 The fate of MR following TAVR is shown as distilled from several studies (author noted at bottom of graph. While MR was unchanged for many patients is worsened in some and improved in others. From Nombela-Franco L, et al. [74]. Reprinted with permission from Elsevier

seems intuitive that correction of either LV pressure or volume overload would also unload the RV and improve TR, this response is quite variable [75, 76]. While studies show that tricuspid repair at time of left-side surgery reduces TR both early and late [75, 77, 78] (Fig. 13.14), there is no convincing mortality benefit to surgery for mild to moderate TR. Severe TR is routinely treated at the time of left-sided surgery, thus there is little data relating to untreated severe TR during left-sided surgery. In some cases tricuspid repair has reduced the risk of late onset heat failure [79]. Because of relatively high risk of repeat surgery to correct symptomatic TR following left-sided surgery [78], there is an increasing tendency to address even mild TR during the initial operation [80].

Q33. The answer is B, undergo balloon valvotomy. His peak transpulmonary gradient of 70 mmHg defines his PS as severe for which anything more than mild exercise is not recommended [81]. Correction of this degree of stenosis, irrespective of symptoms offers better survival than conservative management [82]. Because his valve leaflets are pliable (doming during systole), balloon valvotomy provides excellent results and is obviously less invasive than surgery.

Q34. The answer is C. Based upon his progressive RV dilatation, approaching a threshold where reverse remodeling is unlikely to occur [83], he should probably undergo surgical pulmonic valve replacement at this time to prevent irreversible RV damage. However there is no proof that surgery will prolong his life [84]. For left-sided lesions a regurgitant fraction (RF) of 50% is thought consistent with severe disease. However because lower resistance to forward flow reduces back flow in pulmonary regurgitation (PR), 40% RF is considered severe. In TAVR, the prosthesis gains purchase on the aortic annulus using the calcium present in AS, calcium lacking in PR. Thus percutaneous pulmonic valve replacement is a two-step process wherein a stent has to be placed into the pulmonary annulus or outflow tract and the valve deployed into the stent, a process for which there is little experience.

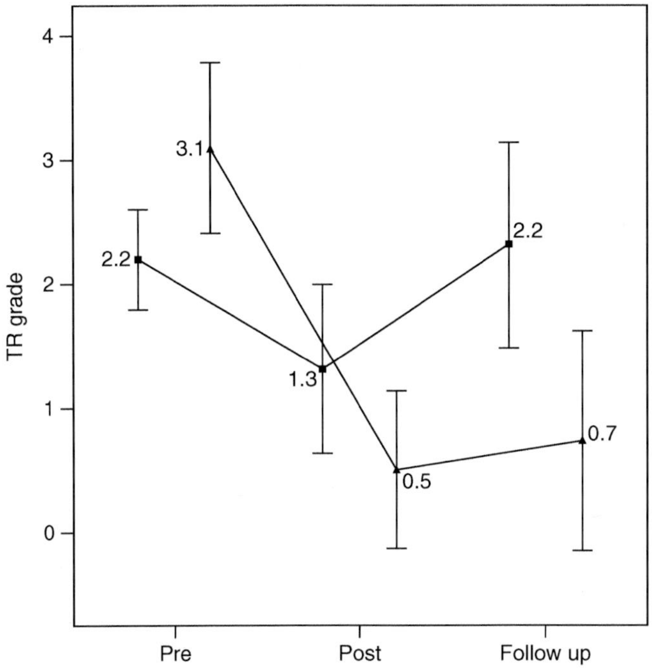

Fig. 13.14 The fate of tricuspid regurgitation (TR) following mitral valve surgery whether TR was addressed (closed triangles) or unattended (closed circles) at the time of the operation. Calafiore AM, et al. [75]. Reprinted with permission from Elsevier

References

1. Nishimura RA, Otto CM, Bonow RO, Carabello BA, et al. American College of Cardiology/American Heart Association Task Force on Practice Guidelines 2014 AHA/ACC guideline for the management of patients with valvular heart disease: a report of the American College of Cardiology/American Heart Association Task Force on Practice Guidelines. J Am Coll Cardiol. 2014;63(22):e57–185.
2. Otto CM, Burwash IG, Legget ME, et al. Prospective study of asymptomatic valvular aortic stenosis. Clinical, echocardiographic, and exercise predictors of outcome. Circulation. 1997;95(9):2262–70.
3. Berthelot-Richer M, Pibarot P, Capoulade R, et al. Discordant grading of aortic stenosis severity: echocardiographic predictors of survival benefit associated with aortic valve replacement. JACC Cardiovasc Imaging. 2016;9(7):797–805.
4. Baron SJ, Arnold SV, Herrmann HC, et al. Impact of ejection fraction and aortic valve gradient on outcomes of transcatheter aortic valve replacement. J Am Coll Cardiol. 2016;67(20):2349–58.
5. Minners J, Allgeier M, Gohlke-Baerwolf C, et al. Inconsistencies of echocardiographic criteria for the grading of aortic valve stenosis. Eur Heart J. 2008;29(8):1043–8.
6. Lancellotti P, Lebois F, Simon M, et al. Prognostic importance of quantitative exercise Doppler echocardiography in asymptomatic valvular aortic stenosis. Circulation. 2005;112:I377–82.
7. Clavel MA, Malouf J, Michelena HI, et al. B-type natriuretic peptide clinical activation in aortic stenosis: impact on long-term survival. J Am Coll Cardiol. 2014;63(19):2016–25.
8. Afilalo J, Lauck S, Kim DH, et al. Frailty in older adults undergoing aortic valve replacement: the FRAILTY-AVR Study. J Am Coll Cardiol. 2017;70(6):689–700.
9. Kefer J, Gapira JM, Pierard S, et al. Recovery after balloon aortic valvuloplasty in patients with aortic stenosis and impaired left ventricular function: predictors and prognostic implications. J Invasive Cardiol. 2013;25(5):235–41.
10. Carabello BA. Advances in the hemodynamic assessment of stenotic cardiac valves. J Am Coll Cardiol. 1987;10:912–9.
11. Blais C, Burwash IG, Mundigler G, et al. Projected valve area at normal flow rate improves the assessment of stenosis severity in patients with low-flow, low-gradient aortic stenosis: the multicenter TOPAS (Truly or Pseudo-Severe Aortic Stenosis) study. Circulation. 2006;113(5):711–21.

12. Nishimura RA, Grantham JA, Connolly HM, et al. Low-output, low-gradient aortic stenosis in patients with depressed left ventricular systolic function: the clinical utility of the dobutamine challenge in the catheterization laboratory. Circulation. 2002;106:809–13.
13. Monin JL, Quéré JP, Monchi M, et al. Low-gradient aortic stenosis: operative risk stratification and predictors for long-term outcome: a multicenter study using dobutamine stress hemodynamics. Circulation. 2003;108(3):319–2.
14. Tastet L, Enriquez-Sarano M, Capoulade R, et al. Impact of aortic valve calcification and sex on hemodynamic progression and clinical outcomes in AS. J Am Coll Cardiol. 2017;69:2096–8.
15. Herrmann HC, Pibarot P, Hueter I, et al. Predictors of mortality and outcomes of therapy in-low-flow severe aortic stenosis: a Placement of Aortic Transcatheter Valves (PARTNER) trial analysis. Circulation. 2013;127:2316–26.
16. Hachicha Z, Dumesnil JG, Bogaty P, Pibarot P. Paradoxical low-flow, low-gradient severe aortic stenosis despite preserved ejection fraction is associated with higher afterload and reduced survival. Circulation. 2007;115(22):2856–64.
17. Clavel MA, Messika-Zeitoun D, Pibarot P, et al. The complex nature of discordant severe calcified aortic valve disease grading: new insights from combined Doppler echocardiographic and computed tomographic study. J Am Coll Cardiol. 2013;62(24):2329–38.
18. Masson JB, Lee M, Boone RH, et al. Impact of coronary artery disease on outcomes after transcatheter aortic valve implantation. Catheteriz Cardiovasc Interv. 2010;76(2):165–73.
19. Nishimura RA, Otto CM, Bonow RO, Carabello BA, et al. 2017 AHA/ACC focused update of the 2014 AHA/ACC guideline for the management of patients with valvular heart disease: a report of the American College of Cardiology/American Heart Association Task Force on Clinical Practice Guidelines. J Am Coll Cardiol. 2017;70(2):252–89.
20. Leon MB, Smith CR, Mack MJ, et al. Transcatheter or surgical aortic-valve replacement in intermediate-risk patients. N Engl J Med. 2016 Apr 28;374(17):1609–20.
21. Reardon MJ, Van Mieghem NM, Popma JJ, et al. Surgical or transcatheter aortic-valve replacement in intermediate-risk patients. N Engl J Med. 2017;376(14):1321–13.
22. Smith CR, Leon MB, Mack MJ, et al. Transcatheter versus surgical aortic-valve replacement in high-risk patients. N Engl J Med. 2011;364(23):2187–98.
23. Adams DH, Popma JJ, Reardon MJ, et al. Transcatheter aortic-valve replacement with a self-expanding prosthesis. N Engl J Med. 2014;370(19):1790–8.
24. Makkar RR, Fontana G, Jilaihawi H, et al. Possible subclinical leaflet thrombosis in bioprosthetic aortic valves. N Engl J Med. 2015;373(21):2015–24.
25. Chakravarty T, Søndergaard L, Friedman J, et al. Subclinical leaflet thrombosis in surgical and transcatheter bioprosthetic aortic valves: an observational study. Lancet. 2017;389(10087):2383–92.
26. Egbe AC, Luis SA, Padang R, Warnes CA. Outcomes in moderate mixed aortic valve disease: is it time for a paradigm shift? J Am Coll Cardiol. 2016;67(20):2321–232.
27. Vincentelli A, Susen S, Le Tourneau T, et al. Acquired von Willebrand syndrome in aortic stenosis. N Engl J Med. 2003;349(4):343–9.
28. Abi-Akar R, El-Rassi I, Karam N, Jassar Y, Slim R, Jebara V. Treatment of Heyde's Syndrome by aortic valve replacement. Curr Cardiol Rev. 2011;7(1):47–9.
29. Mitten MJ, Zipes DP, Maron BJ, Bryant WJ. Eligibility and disqualification recommendations for competitive athletes with cardiovascular abnormalities: task force 15: legal aspects of medical eligibility and disqualification recommendations: a scientific statement from the American Heart Association and American College of Cardiology. J Am Coll Cardiol. 2015;66(21):2447–50.
30. Hammermeister K, Sethi GK, Henderson WG, et al. Outcomes 15 years after valve replacement with a mechanical versus a bioprosthetic valve: final report of the veterans affairs randomized trial. J Am Coll Cardiol. 2000;36(4):1152–8.
31. Weber A, Noureddine H, Englberger L, et al. Ten-year comparison of pericardial tissue valves versus mechanical prostheses for aortic valve replacement in patients younger than 60 years of age. J Thorac Cardiovasc Surg. 2012;144(5):1075–83.
32. Hung L, Rahimtoola SH. Prosthetic heart valves and pregnancy. Circulation. 2003;107(9):1240–6.
33. Webb JG, Mack MJ, White JM, et al. Transcatheter aortic valve implantation within degenerated aortic surgical bioprostheses: PARTNER 2 valve-in-valve registry. J Am Coll Cardiol. 2017;69(18):2253–26.
34. El-Hamamsy I, Eryigit ZG, Stevens LM, et al. Long-term outcomes after autograft versus homograft aortic root replacement in adults with aortic valve disease: a randomized controlled trial. Lancet. 2010;376:524–31.
35. Martin E, Mohammadi S, Jacques F, et al. Clinical outcomes following the Ross procedure in adults: a 25-year longitudinal study. J Am Coll Cardiol. 2017;70:1890–9.
36. David TE, David C, Woo A, et al. The Ross procedure: outcomes at 20 years. J Thorac Cardiovasc Surg. 2014;147:85–94.
37. Bonow RO. Chronic mitral regurgitation and aortic regurgitation: have indications for surgery changed? J Am Coll Cardiol. 2013;61(7):693–701.
38. Vassileva CM, Mishkel G, McNeely C, et al. Long-term survival of patients undergoing mitral valve repair and replacement: a longitudinal analysis of Medicare fee-for-service beneficiaries. Circulation. 2013;127(18):1870–6.
39. Gillinov AM, Mihaljevic T, Blackstone EH, et al. Should patients with severe degenerative mitral regurgitation delay surgery until symptoms develop? Ann Thorac Surg. 2010;90(2):481–8.
40. Enriquez-Sarano M, Tajik AJ, et al. Echocardiographic prediction of survival after surgical correction of organic mitral regurgitation. Circulation. 1994;90(2):830–7.
41. Tribouilloy C, Grigioni F, Avierinos JF, et al. Survival implication of left ventricular end-systolic diameter in mitral regurgitation due to flail leaflets a long-term follow-up multicenter study. J Am Coll Cardiol. 2009;54(21):1961–8.
42. Clavel MA, Tribouilloy C, Vanoverschelde JL, et al. Association of B-type natriuretic peptide with survival in patients with degenerative mitral regurgitation. J Am Coll Cardiol. 2016;68(12):1297–307.
43. Lancellotti P, Magne J. Stress testing for the evaluation of patients with mitral regurgitation. Curr Opin Cardiol. 2012;27:492–8.
44. Wu AH, Aaronson KD, Bolling SF, et al. Impact of mitral valve annuloplasty on mortality risk in patients with mitral regurgitation and left ventricular systolic dysfunction. J Am Coll Cardiol. 2005;45(3):381–7.
45. Fattouch K, Guccione F, Sampognaro R, et al. POINT: efficacy of adding mitral valve restrictive annuloplasty to coronary artery bypass grafting in patients with moderate ischemic mitral valve regurgitation: a randomized trial. J Thorac Cardiovasc Surg. 2009;138(2):278–85.
46. Goldstein D, Moskowitz AJ, Gelijns AC, et al. Two-year outcomes of surgical treatment of severe ischemic mitral regurgitation. N Engl J Med. 2016;374(4):344–53.
47. Stevenson LW, Bellil D, Grover-McKay M, et al. Effects of afterload reduction (diuretics and vasodilators) on left ventricular volume and mitral regurgitation in severe congestive heart failure secondary to ischemic or idiopathic dilated cardiomyopathy. Am J Cardiol. 1987;60(8):654–8.
48. González-Juanatey C, González-Gay MA, Llorca J, et al. Rheumatic manifestations of infective endocarditis in non-addicts. A 12-year study. Medicine (Baltimore). 2001;80(1):9–19.
49. Vilacosta I, Graupner C, San Román JA, et al. Risk of embolization after institution of antibiotic therapy for infective endocarditis. J Am Coll Cardiol. 2002;39(9):1489–95.

50. Heiro M, Nikoskelainen J, Engblom E, et al. Neurologic manifestations of infective endocarditis: a 17-year experience in a teaching hospital in Finland. Arch Intern Med. 2000;160(18):2781–7.
51. Remadi JP, Habib G, Nadji G, et al. Predictors of death and impact of surgery in Staphylococcus aureus infective endocarditis. Ann Thorac Surg. 2007;83(4):1295–302.
52. Kang DH, Kim YJ, Kim SH, Sun BJ, Kim DH, Yun SC, et al. Early surgery versus conventional treatment for infective endocarditis. N Engl J Med. 2012;366(26):2466–73.
53. Karalis DG, Bansal RC, Hauck AJ, et al. Transesophageal echocardiographic recognition of subaortic complications in aortic valve endocarditis. Clinical and surgical implications. Circulation. 1992;86(2):353–62.
54. Al Jubair K, Al Fagih MR, Ashmeg A, et al. Cardiac operations during active endocarditis. J Thorac Cardiovasc Surg. 1992;104(2):487–90.
55. Ao Habib G, Avierinos JF, Thuny F. Aortic valve endocarditis: is there an optimal surgical timing? Curr Opin Cardiol. 2007;22(2):77–83.
56. Scognamiglio R, Rahimtoola SH, Fasoli G, et al. Nifedipine in asymptomatic patients with severe aortic regurgitation and normal left ventricular function. N Engl J Med. 1994;331(11):689–94.
57. Evangelista A, Tornos P, Sambola A, et al. Long-term vasodilator therapy in patients with severe aortic regurgitation. N Engl J Med. 2005;353(13):1342–9.
58. Klodas E, Enriquez-Sarano M, Tajik AJ, et al. Optimizing timing of surgical correction in patients with severe aortic regurgitation: role of symptoms. J Am Coll Cardiol. 1997;30(3):746–52.
59. Mentias A, Feng K, Alashi A, et al. Long-term outcomes in patients with aortic regurgitation and preserved left ventricular ejection fraction. J Am Coll Cardiol. 2016;68(20):2144–53.
60. Figulla HR, Webb JG, Lauten A, Feldman T. The transcatheter valve technology pipeline for treatment of adult valvular heart disease. Eur Heart J. 2016;37(28):2226–39.
61. Ashcom TL, Johns JP, Bailey SR, Rubal BJ. Effects of chronic beta-blockade on rest and exercise hemodynamics in mitral stenosis. Catheter Cardiovasc Diagn. 1995;35(2):110–5.
62. Wilkins GT, Weyman AE, Abascal VM, Block PC, Palacios IF. Percutaneous balloon dilatation of the mitral valve: an analysis of echocardiographic variables related to outcome and the mechanism of dilatation. Br Heart J. 1988;60(4):299–308.
63. Pérez-Gómez F, Salvador A, Zumalde J, et al. Effect of antithrombotic therapy in patients with mitral stenosis and atrial fibrillation: a sub-analysis of NASPEAF randomized trial. Eur Heart J. 2006;27(8):960–7.
64. Eikelboom JW, Connolly SJ, Brueckmann M, et al. Dabigatran versus warfarin in patients with mechanical heart valves. N Engl J Med. 2013;369(13):1206–14.
65. Bungard TJ, Mutch J, Ritchie B. A randomized trial of restarting warfarin at maintenance versus loading doses following an elective procedure. J Thromb Thrombolysis. 2017;44(4):507–15.
66. Bonow RO, Rosing DR, Maron BJ, et al. Reversal of left ventricular dysfunction after aortic valve replacement for chronic aortic regurgitation: influence of duration of preoperative left ventricular dysfunction. Circulation. 1984;70(4):570–9.
67. Kamath AR, Varadarajan P, Turk R, et al. Survival in patients with severe aortic regurgitation and severe left ventricular dysfunction is improved by aortic valve replacement: results from a cohort of 166 patients with an ejection fraction < or =35%. Circulation. 2009;120(11 Suppl):S134–8.
68. Sampat U, Varadarajan P, Turk R, Kamath A, Khandhar S, Pai RG. Effect of beta-blocker therapy on survival in patients with severe aortic regurgitation results from a cohort of 756 patients. J Am Coll Cardiol. 2009;54:452–7.
69. Barbetseas J, Nagueh SF, Pitsavos C, et al. Differentiating thrombus from pannus formation in obstructed mechanical prosthetic valves: an evaluation of clinical, transthoracic and transesophageal echocardiographic parameters. J Am Coll Cardiol. 1998;32(5):1410–7.
70. Tong AT, Roudaut R, Ozkan M, et al. Prosthetic Valve Thrombolysis-Role of Transesophageal Echocardiography (PRO-TEE) Registry Investigators. Transesophageal echocardiography improves risk assessment of thrombolysis of prosthetic valve thrombosis: results of the international PRO-TEE registry. J Am Coll Cardiol. 2004;43(1):77–84.
71. Roudaut R, Lafitte S, Roudaut MF, et al. Management of prosthetic heart valve obstruction: fibrinolysis versus surgery. Early results and long-term follow-up in a single-centre study of 263 cases. Arch Cardiovasc Dis. 2009;102(4):269–77.
72. Karthikeyan G, Senguttuvan NB, Joseph J, et al. Urgent surgery compared with fibrinolytic therapy for the treatment of left-sided prosthetic heart valve thrombosis: a systematic review and meta-analysis of observational studies. Eur Heart J. 2013;34(21):1557–66.
73. Keuleers S, Herijgers P, Herregods MC, et al. Comparison of thrombolysis versus surgery as a first line therapy for prosthetic heart valve thrombosis. Am J Cardiol. 2011;107(2):275–9.
74. Nombela-Franco L, Ribeiro HB, Urena M, et al. Significant mitral regurgitation left untreated at the time of aortic valve replacement: a comprehensive review of a frequent entity in the transcatheter aortic valve replacement era. J Am Coll Cardiol. 2014;63(24):2643–58.
75. Calafiore AM, Gallina S, Iac AL, et al. Mitral valve surgery for functional mitral regurgitation: should moderate-or-more tricuspid regurgitation be treated? A propensity score analysis. Ann Thorac Surg. 2009;87(3):698–703.
76. Kusajima K, Fujita T, Hata H, Shimahara Y, Miura S, Kobayashi J. Long-term echocardiographic follow-up of untreated 2+ functional tricuspid regurgitation in patients undergoing mitral valve surgery. Interact Cardiovasc Thorac Surg. 2016;23(1):96–103.
77. Kim JB, Yoo DG, Kim GS, et al. Mild-to-moderate functional tricuspid regurgitation in patients undergoing valve replacement for rheumatic mitral disease: the influence of tricuspid valve repair on clinical echocardiographic outcomes. Heart. 2012;98(1):24–30.
78. Kwon DA, Park JS, Chang HJ, et al. Prediction of outcome in patients undergoing surgery for severe tricuspid regurgitation following mitral valve surgery and role of tricuspid annular systolic velocity. Am J Cardiol. 2006;98:659–61.
79. Chikwe J, Itagaki S, Anyanwu A, Adams D. Impact of concomitant tricuspid annuloplasty on tricuspid regurgitation, right ventricular function, and pulmonary artery hypertension after repair of mitral valve prolapse. J Am Coll Cardiol. 2015;65(18):1931–8.
80. Vassileva CM, Shabosky J, Boley T, Markwell S, Hazelrigg S. Tricuspid valve surgery: the past 10 years from the Nationwide Inpatient Sample (NIS) database. J Thorac Cardiovasc Surg. 2012;143(5):1043–9.
81. Van Hare GF, Ackerman MJ, Evangelista JA, et al. Eligibility and disqualification recommendations for competitive athletes with cardiovascular abnormalities: Task Force 4: congenital heart disease: A scientific statement from the American Heart Association and American College of Cardiology. Circulation. 2015;132(22):e281–91.
82. Hayes CJ, Gersony WM, Driscoll DJ, et al. Second natural history study of congenital heart defects. Results of treatment of patients with pulmonary valvar stenosis. Circulation. 1993;87(2 Suppl):I28–37.
83. Oosterhof T, van Straten A, Vliegen HW, et al. Preoperative thresholds for pulmonary valve replacement in patients with corrected tetralogy of Fallot using cardiovascular magnetic resonance. Circulation. 2007;116(5):545–51.
84. Fathallah M, Krasuski RA. Pulmonic valve disease: review of pathology and current treatment options. Curr Cardiol Rep. 2017;19(11):108.

Index

B. A. Carabello (ed.), *Valvular Heart Disease*, Cardiovascular Medicine, https://doi.org/10.1007/978-1-4471-2840-3

D

E

Printed by Printforce, the Netherlands